AFTER-40
HEALTH
AND MEDICAL
GUIDE

Better Homes and Gardens®

AFTER-40 HEALTH AND MEDICAL GUIDE

Edited by
Donald G. Cooley

Illustrations by
Paul Zuckerman

BETTER HOMES AND GARDENS® BOOKS
Editor: Gerald M. Knox
Art Director: Ernest Shelton

Associate Art Directors:
  Neoma Alt West, Randall Yontz
Copy and Production Editors:
  David Kirchner, Lamont Olson,
  David A. Walsh
Assistant Art Director:
  Harijs Priekulis
Senior Graphic Designer:
  Faith Berven
Graphic Designers: Linda Ford,
  Sheryl Veenschoten, Tom Wegner

Editor-in-Chief: James A. Autry
Editorial Director: Neil Kuehnl
Executive Art Director:
  William J. Yates

After-40 Health and Medical Guide
Copy and Production Editor:
  David Kirchner

Additional medical illustrations by
  Marsha Dohrmann: color
  illustrations on pages 31, 34, 191,
  201, 212, 376, 385, 394, 405, and
  442; line and/or tinted
  illustrations on pages 14, 20, 26,
  32, 35, 39, 40, 63, 80, 91, 109, 113,
  170, 175, 183, 197, 204, 209, 215,
  218, 224, 226, 228, 231, 372, 377,
  378, 383, 386, 388, 389, 390, 393,
  394, 396, 397, 401, 417, 419, 424,
  427, 443, 444, 445, 448, 451, 452,
  454, 455, 457, and 460.

Special thanks to Chris Neubauer,
  Michael P. Scott, and Tom
  Wegner for their valuable
  assistance in producing this book.

FOREWORD

To everything there is a season. The purpose of this book is to help men and women to enjoy a healthful and happy season of maturity. To that end we invited specialists to share their knowledge and give friendly counsel about matters of mind and body that are especially pertinent to the middle and later years of life.

The likelihood that a fortyish reader of this book will live into his or her seventies and eighties, or even nineties, is very real. A generation ago this probability would have been less. The proportion of vigorous "over 65s" in our population continually increases. We are beneficiaries of remarkable advances in medicine, health care, sanitation, housing, nutrition, antibiotics, technology, immunization, surgery, and pharmacology — of innumerable interlinked benefits that were unknown a few decades ago but that are taken for granted today.

Many, probably most young adults have grown up in excellent health without suffering or encountering grave, life-threatening illnesses that were all too frequent in the families of our parents and grandparents, before modern medicine began. In today's world, everyone needs and profits from a little understanding of the structures and functions of body and mind and the processes of health and disease. The authors of this book were asked to share information that they believed a reasonably well-informed person should have.

Not every topic discussed in this book affects everybody — how very fortunate! An extensive index, together with cross-references within chapters, makes it easy to look up a subject of personal concern. Specially commissioned illustrations give visual clarity to the marvelous mechanisms of life. The text is easy to read, but medical words, always explained, are not avoided.

Many people are shy about asking questions of their doctor — questions that he would be happy to answer if he knew what was on his patient's mind. Conversations with one's physician are important to a patient's right to consent. What is the significance of symptoms, what treatment is proposed, what are the alternatives, what is a drug supposed to do, and what are its side effects, if any? Often, needless apprehensions are allayed if frank questions are asked and if the explanations are fully understood. The knowledge and reassurance one gains from reading these chapters can do much to foster this important patient-doctor communication.

Healthful attitudes, practices, and preventive measures are, of course, our own responsibility. The many things that the authors suggest we can do for ourselves yield continuing rewards as we mobilize the real assets of growing older from a rich store of experience.

We are confident that this book will contribute to a zestful design for living in the years ahead.

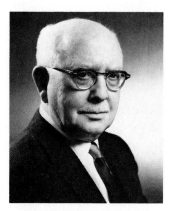

Donald G. Cooley, the editor of the Better Homes and Gardens *Family Medical Guide,* has had a distinguished career spanning over four decades as an editor and writer of medical subjects. Formerly science and medicine editor of *The Literary Digest,* he was the editor of *Your Health* and *Your Life* from 1938-60 and has written and edited more than twelve medical books.

ACKNOWLEDGMENTS

Owen Belmont, M.D. Associate Surgeon, E. Wills Eye Hospital; Associate Clinical Professor of Ophthalmology, Thomas Jefferson University. Philadelphia, Pennsylvania.

Lloyd E. Church, D.D.S., Ph.D. Oral Surgeon. Secretary, Academy of Medicine, Washington, D.C.; Associate Professorial Lecturer in Surgery, George Washington Medical Center, Washington, D.C.; Fellow, American College of Dentists. Bethesda, Maryland.

Donald G. Cooley. Fellow, American Association of Medical Writers; National Association of Science Writers. Aurora, Colorado.

David A. Culp, M.D. Professor and Head, Department of Urology, University Hospitals. Iowa City, Iowa.

Marsha J. Dohrmann, M.A. Medical Artist. Member, Association of Medical Illustrators. Mill Valley, California.

Bernard Fallon, M.D. Associate, Department of Urology, University Hospitals. Iowa City, Iowa.

Leon Goldman, M.D. Professor Emeritus of Dermatology, College of Medicine, University of Cincinnati; Director, Laser Laboratory, Medical Center, University of Cincinnati. Cincinnati, Ohio.

Robert P. Heaney, M.D. Professor of Medicine. Vice President for Health Sciences, Creighton University. Omaha, Nebraska.

Arno Karlen, writer, editor, teacher, and researcher. Author and editor of many books, articles, and scholarly papers on human behavior, human sexuality, and sex education. Formerly Associate Professor at Pennsylvania State University. Formerly Executive Editor of *Physicians' World.*

Leo P. Krall, M.D. Joslin Clinic and New England Deaconess Hospital; Director, Education Division, Joslin Diabetes Foundation; Lecturer in Medicine, Harvard Medical School; Editor in Chief, *Diabetes Forecast.* Boston, Massachusetts.

Robert J. Luby, M.D. Professor of Obstetrics and Gynecology; Assistant Dean for Graduate Medical Education, Creighton University. Omaha, Nebraska.

Clark H. Millikan, M.D. Professor of Neurology and head of stroke unit, University of Utah Medical Center. Formerly senior neurology consultant, Mayo Clinic. Salt Lake City, Utah.

Oglesby Paul, M.D. Professor of Medicine and Director of Admission, Harvard Medical School. Past president, American Heart Association. Boston, Massachusetts.

George E. Shambaugh, Jr., M.D. Professor Emeritus of Otolaryngology, Northwestern University; author, *Surgery of the Ear;* President, American Hearing Research Foundation. Introduced operating microscope to the United States. Chicago, Illinois.

Charley J. Smyth, M.D. Director, Arthritis Clinic, General Rose Memorial Hospital. Denver, Colorado.

Fredric J. Stare, M.D. Professor of Nutrition, Harvard School of Public Health. Boston, Massachusetts.

E. Clinton Texter, Jr., M.D. Professor of Medicine; Professor of Physiology and Biophysics; Head, Division of Gastroenterology, University of Arkansas for Medical Sciences; Fellow, American College of Physicians. Little Rock, Arkansas.

Jelia C. Witschi, M.S. Assistant Professor of Nutrition, Harvard School of Public Health, Boston, Massachusetts.

Paul Zuckerman, Medical Artist. President, Designs for Medicine, Inc., New York City and White Plains, New York.

TABLE OF CONTENTS

LIST OF ILLUSTRATIONS

INTRODUCTION   DONALD G. COOLEY

MIND
& BODY:
THE MIDDLE
YEARS
& BEYOND

Older people are simply young people who have lived longer.

With a little bit of luck, we too may live a long time. And with a little bit of wisdom, information, and effort, we may invigorate our years to come and brighten the lives of those around us, as well as our own.

Aging is a trait of the universe. The sun is aging—with only five billion good years left!—but its present shine sustains our lives. The specialists who have written chapters of this book give counsel that can help us make the most of our present brightness.

In our youth-oriented world, it is almost antisocial to say a good word for maturity. But is youth really the best time of life? Aren't you wiser now than you were at 21? At least you're beyond the disquiet of many young people who, as they tend to put it, are forever "trying to find out who I really am" and thereby risking the most humiliating discovery of their young lives.

By middle age, most of us have come to fairly reasonable terms with ourselves. We have surmounted enough to build a pretty sturdy self-image, perhaps as sturdy as that of Justice Oliver Wendell Holmes in his nineties. One day a law clerk asked Holmes, to whom one could talk about anything, how old he thought God was.

"About 70," Holmes replied. "Young enough to be vigorous and old enough to be wise."

There are comforting things to be said about reaching middle age and beyond. Thousands don't make it. We have built immunities to many diseases, have experienced much and learned something, may well be at the peak of our powers, and are nearing the time when we may reap what we have sown. By merely surviving, we have demonstrated a certain toughness.

Indeed, your life expectancy is greater than a newborn baby's.

Insurance companies, with a dollars-and-cents interest in the longevity of policyholders, have calculated the life expectancies of people at various ages. Their figures say quite a bit about the vitality of older people. Beginning with retirement age, arbitrarily taken to be 65 years, and rounding off the figures to tenths of a year, the years one has left come out like this:

REMAINING LIFE EXPECTANCY		
Age	**Men**	**Women**
65 years	15.9 years	19.1 years
66	15.2	18.3
67	14.6	17.5
68	13.9	16.7
69	13.3	15.9
70	12.7	15.2
71	12.0	14.4
72	11.5	13.7
73	10.9	13.0
74	10.3	12.3
75	9.8	11.6
76	9.3	11.0
77	8.7	10.4
78	8.3	9.8
79	7.8	9.2
80	7.3	8.6
81	6.9	8.0
82	6.5	7.6
83	6.1	7.0
84	5.7	6.6
85	5.4	6.0

A baby born in the United States in 1977 has a life expectancy of 73.2 years, according to a Congressional Committee on Population. Doesn't your present age plus remaining life expectancy add up to more than that? True, you have used up some of your allotment, but the odds are that you have a goodly number of happy and useful years ahead.

Averages say nothing about you personally. Still, insurance companies don't bet their money on long shots, and there is actuarial reason to feel that there's lots of good living ahead. Maybe you're not physically perfect. Were you ever? Was anybody? Virtually no newborn baby is physically perfect, except in the eyes of its parents. Aging begins before birth, and the newborn are several months into it.

Women outlive men, on the average. Women may feel that this indicates natural superiority; men, that males protect and shelter their women. Either opinion supports debate among chauvinists, but the biological reasons for female longevity are not known. One theory is that the paired sex chromosomes of women contain a little more genetic material than the matching chromosomes of men. One fact is relevant in looking toward the future: there are more widows than widowers.

Life is so chock-full of turning points that middle age can't be all-important. However, it is a time when the buildup processes of the body, which have been generally ascendant, come into a sort of plateau and begin to lose out ever so slightly to the processes of decline. It's not like a steep toboggan slide or a fall off a cliff, but more of a gradual change in the balance of forces that's entirely normal.

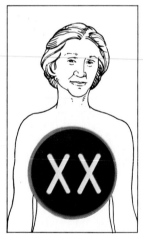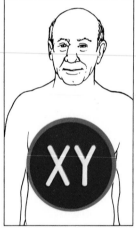

SEX CHROMOSOMES

Why do women live longer than men, on the average? A male cell contains paired X and Y sex chromosomes; a female cell contains two X chromosomes. The Y chromosome is smaller than the X and contains less genetic material, so men may lack a little of the life stuff that women get from a double complement of X chromosomes. Like other speculations on longevity, the theory is plausible but unproved.

Somewhere in mid-life, we may become aware of limitations, conscious of slight creaks and distempers we never had before, unhappy about a gray hair or well-earned wrinkle, sobered by some collisions of expectation with reality, or astonished that a bumptious young generation has grown up behind us. It is a time when myths and stereotypes about aging, of which there are many, may dishearten a feeble ego and leave no zest for adaptation to new and different challenges with compensating fulfillments.

But mostly, it is a good time to take stock and take steps, spelled out elsewhere in this book, to prevent or reduce the disabilities of advancing years, and have a lot of pleasure along the way.

Limits of Longevity

What is the natural span of human life? How long would people live if they were never affected by disease, accidents, or environment? No such persons exist, so the answer cannot be as definite as predicting the life-span of the May fly: one day.

Fascinating accounts of persons said to be 130, 140, 160, or more years old must be rejected as incredible. (A demised Russian tourist attraction, one Shirali Muslimov, claimed to be 168.) Alleged super-centenarians typically inhabit isolated, inaccessible, rather exotic regions where there are no city halls with birth records to discourage tall stories.

The most publicized people of astonishing longevity are the Hunzas, who live in a hard-to-reach mountain valley near Nepal; Russian peasants in parts of the Caucasus; and inhabitants of an Ecuadorian village, Vilcabamba, in the Andes. Word-of-mouth assertions of great age are suspect. The Hunzas do not have a written language. Documentation is lacking—except in the cases of many Caucasians whose carefully checked birth records proved to be bogus, forged during World War I to avoid service in the Russian army on grounds of over-age.

Undoubtedly there are many vigorous old people in these communities, just as there are in the United States. An age of 100 years is not at all incredible. There are 15,000 centenarians in this country alone.

Some evidence suggests that 100 years, plus a possible added decade, is the natural span of human life. Dr. Leonard Hayflick, research cell biologist at the Children's Hospital Medical Center at Oakland, California grew embryonic human cells in culture and found that the cells divided and replaced themselves about 50 times before dying out. In the living body, it would take 100 to 110 years to complete 50 cell divisions. This apparent maximum span of life has existed throughout history.

It is difficult to detect any master pattern of longevity in the life-styles of groups of aged people who have been studied, or in the whimsicalities of an occasional centenarian who, interviewed by his local paper, credits his long life to hush puppies or "corn likker." The diets of Hunzas, Russian peasants, and Vilcabambians vary in calories as well as composition. Some are teetotallers; others imbibe. Some smoke like chimneys; others abstain. But one factor is common to practically all the vigorous old people: they are physically active and are productive (and respected) members of their society.

Dr. Alexander Leaf, professor of clinical medicine at Harvard Medical School, visited, observed, and studied the people of the above-mentioned long-lived communities. His conclusions are interesting:

"A vigorous active life involving physical activity (sexual activity included) is possible for at least 100 years and in some instances for even longer."

Satisfactory?

Theories of Aging

A little is known about the "how" of aging. The "why" is for philosophers.

Rate of living. Forty years ago, the late Raymond Pearl observed that fruit flies kept in agitation died much sooner than inactive fruit flies. From this he speculated that organisms are endowed with a finite package of energy. When it is used up, they

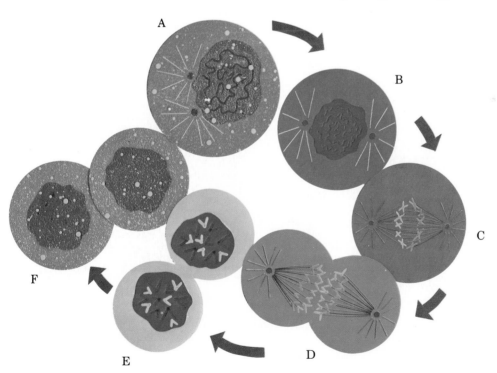

NEW CELLS FOR OLD

Most body cells divide and reproduce as long as we live. Phases of cell division are shown above. Chromosomes organize from nuclear materials (A, B), arrange in a single plane (C), move apart (D), reorganize (E), after which the cell divides into a new generation of daughter cells.

die. Like an unrefillable gas tank, the faster one drives, the sooner the tank runs dry. Or the slower one lives, the longer—a shabby appeal to the indolent.

Well known studies by Clive McKay of Cornell University in the 1930s give some indirect support to the rate-of-living hypothesis. McKay fed baby rats a nutritionally balanced diet sharply deficient in calories. This increased their life-spans as much as 40 percent. Starve a little, live slower, live longer.

More recent studies show that lowering body temperature a very few degrees slows the speed of living and increases life expectancy, at least in certain fishes. A more far-out idea is hibernation. Chill a person's body until he is unconscious, just barely alive, and he'll presumably grow older very slowly, if at all. Revive him years later to see how his great-grandchildren are doing. Unfortunately, this technology is not wholly impossible. Patients are deeply chilled in ice baths (hypothermia) to facilitate certain kinds of surgery. But any idea that the sudden appearance of a thawed great-grandfather would be greeted with unrestrained joy by his family is suspect.

Rate-of-living theories have little to offer to prolong life, other than suggesting that it may be prudent not to expend energies furiously and thus avoid becoming a burnt-out case too soon.

Heredity. All students of aging agree that heredity is an important factor. Long-lived parents ordinarily have long-lived offspring, though nothing is guaranteed.

Just what do we inherit, for good or ill? Inherited resistances and vulnerabilities make a mixed and murky bag. If fortunate, we may inherit a constitution with few "bad" genes that would make us susceptible to many big and little illnesses and stresses that, in the course of time, could erode life expectancy. Dr. Leaf's studies of the Hunzas suggested to him that these sturdy people originally had a good genetic background that, because of extreme isolation, remained uncontaminated by "foreign" genes from outsiders.

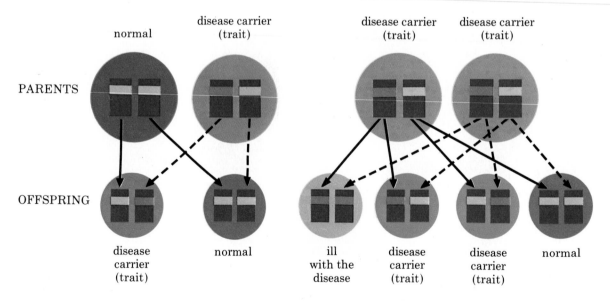

INHERITED TRAITS

Most inherited disease traits are recessive—that is, both parents must carry the trait to transmit frank disease to offspring. A carrier possesses the trait but is not harmed by it. At left, a normal and a trait-carrying parent can have offspring who do or do not carry the trait. Above, the chance that two trait-carrying parents will have a child with the disease is 1 in 4.

We can't choose our forebears or alter heredity. There are, however, clues in family histories that may be helpful in identifying ailments to which one may be more susceptible than the average person. What is inherited is not usually a specific disease, but increased likelihood that something that "runs in the family" may occur in blood relatives. Breast cancer, for instance, is more likely to occur in daughters of mothers who had breast cancer than in daughters of cancer-free mothers—which is far from saying that cancer is inevitable.

Physicians taking case histories usually ask about the health records of parents, brothers and sisters, and aunts and uncles. Not always, but often enough, a family history can give an early warning signal to be watchful in certain areas and to take prudent steps that a doctor advises.

Aging molecules. Scientists have tried to find mechanisms of aging in the marvelous chemical activities of human cells. Genes, the units of heredity, are strung along the structure of DNA (deoxyribonucleic acid), the "master molecule" of life. DNA in the nucleus of every cell contains the genetic code directing the production and assembly of myriads of molecules that, in far-flung interaction, make us what we uniquely are—blue-eyed or brown-eyed, or a human being instead of a rabbit.

One theory is that the genetic code has a built-in timetable for growing old: infancy, childhood, adolescence, maturity, and senescence. But genes do not exert all of their functions all of the time; "something" turns them on or off at appropriate times. Young adults stop growing taller, and puberty and menopause come uninvited. If a program for aging is built into the genetic code, it is like a phonograph record that can be played only once and comes to an end. The only way to make the music last longer is to play it more slowly.

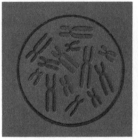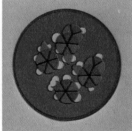

CHROMOSOMES AND GENES

DNA is contained in chromosomes, which are threadlike units in cell nuclei. We normally have 23 pairs of chromosomes, one in each pair from the mother, the other from the father. A gene is a tiny segment of DNA in which a sequential cluster of bases ("rungs" of the DNA ladder) specifies the synthesis of proteins that control life processes. We have about 50,000 genes; the locations of some 250 genes in chromosomes have been precisely mapped. Further mapping may pinpoint the genetic sites of life processes in health and disease.

GENETIC BLUEPRINTS

DNA (deoxyribonucleic acid) molecules contain the chemical codes that direct life functions and structures. Varying sequences of these units repeated thousands of times along the chain constitute the genetic code.

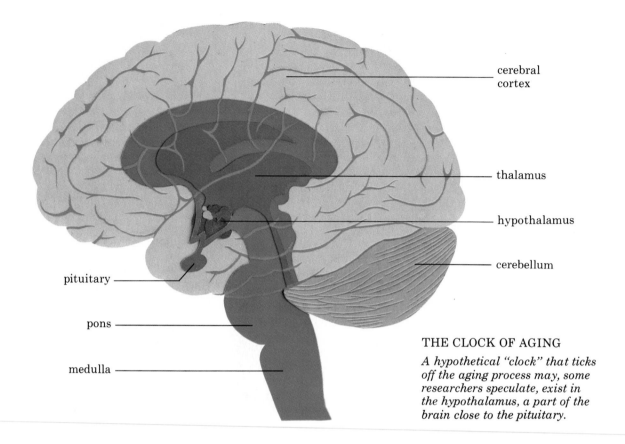

cerebral
cortex

thalamus

hypothalamus

cerebellum

pituitary

pons

medulla

THE CLOCK OF AGING

A hypothetical "clock" that ticks off the aging process may, some researchers speculate, exist in the hypothalamus, a part of the brain close to the pituitary.

On the other hand, the genetic code may be replayable indefinitely, but in the course of time, become more prone to error. The genes' machinery may be impaired, from exhaustion, wear and tear, mutations, insults of environment, or changes that accumulate as the machine gets older. The code, smudged by errors and full of misprints, sends defective directives to life processes. Aging, then, may be analogous to "background noise" that plays hob with harmony on a much-played phonograph record.

Not every investigator feels (none is sure) that a biological clock for aging is present in the nuclei of our cells. Some think that the hypothetical clock exists in a part of the brain, the hypothalamus.

Cell pollution. Erroneous information acted upon by cells may cause chemical mistakes, such as the synthesis of misshapen proteins and by-products that are not only useless, but probably harmful. There is evidence that aging cells do accumulate abnormal gene products, and this chemical sludge may depress vital processes such as self-repair and division.

Studies of the cell offer no present means of prolonging life, but studies of aging do shed light on the processes of growth. One aspect of growth is cancer. If every cell of your body divided 50 times, like those cultured by Dr. Hayflick, and all the cell generations accumulated, you would ultimately weigh 20 million tons and pose a serious housing problem. Fortunately, this doesn't happen.

Normal cells have growth restraints; cancer cells do not. How do normal cells "know" how to stop and go? If the answer is found, we may learn how to slow the aging process and lessen the risk of cancer.

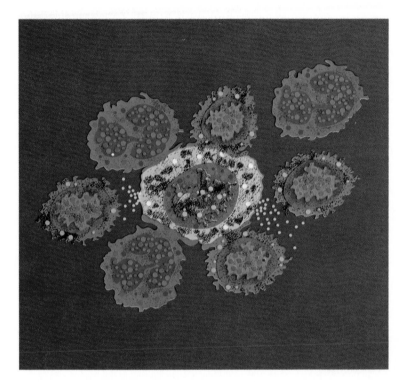

SYSTEMS THAT SEEK AND DESTROY

Powerful immune systems patrol the body and recognize, attack, and destroy cells and substances that are foreign to the "self." Cancer cells are abnormal, and doctors believe that a vigorous immune system destroys occasional malignant cells as they arise. Aging of the immune system may weaken it so that stray cancer cells escape detection and grow unrestrainedly. The drawing, based on an actual microphotograph, shows a cancer cell being attacked by normal cells (megakaryocytes and lymphocytes), which disrupt the wall of the cancer cell and spill its contents.

Cancer is an age-related phenomenon. Except for certain childhood malignancies, it is largely a problem of early middle age and later life.

Immune systems. A great protective system of the body recognizes materials that are foreign to it and rejects them. This immune system is powerful and complex. It has been suggested that the apparatus weakens or is thrown off kilter with age. One result could be that it then fails to deal properly with foreign invaders such as cancer cells. A current theory is that everybody produces a stray cancer cell now and then, but that a healthy immune system recognizes the malignant cell as abnormal and destroys it.

Another result could be that an aging immune system cannot distinguish between friend and foe and turns strangely against the body itself, inciting harmful reactions to perfectly normal body constituents. So-called "autoimmune" diseases of unknown cause are thought to be associated with a strange inability of the body to recognize parts of itself and establish specific sensitivity — with harmful reactions. It's not unlike an allergic reaction to ragweed pollen, except that the sensitizing substance is not foreign to the body, but is a part of it. Rheumatoid arthritis is apparently associated with autoimmune reactions, as are certain kidney and thyroid inflammations.

Ways of "normalizing" an old and possibly weakened immune system may be found. In fact, the system is regularly tampered with, to beneficial ends, by drugs that suppress its actions and increase the likelihood that an organ transplanted from a donor will not be rejected as foreign to the recipient.

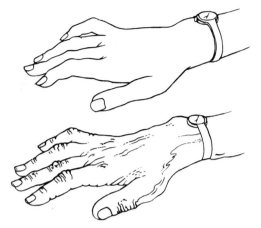

AGING HANDS

The skin of a young hand (top) is very flexible, and flattens quickly when pinched. The connective tissue of an old hand (bottom) is stiffened and inelastic from drying out and chemical changes in the interwoven fibers.

Connective tissue. Babies are wetter than grown-ups, in ways less obvious than those that every parent knows. Infants have a greater proportion of water in their tissues than adults, and children's tissues are more elastic and resilient. Some of this bounce disappears with age. Pinch and release the skin of the back of a young hand and it snaps back with alacrity; the skin of an old hand subsides slowly.

This reflects a drying-out that comes with age. Chemists have a name for the process: polymerization, a linking of molecules into long chains, with the elimination of water. It happens to rubber, paint, paper, and plastics, which become stiff and brittle with age, as well as to human beings. In people, stiffening changes occur in connective tissue (see page 234), of which the principal protein is collagen, which constitutes 30 percent of all body protein. The largest rate of increase of stiffening occurs from 30 to 50 years of age.

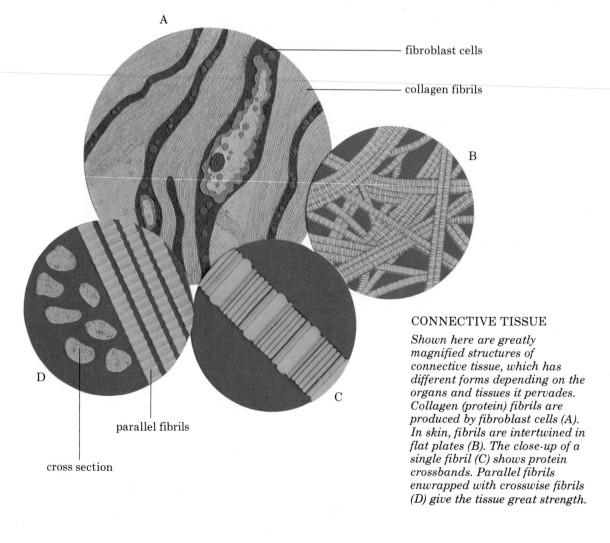

A

— fibroblast cells

— collagen fibrils

B

D

parallel fibrils

cross section

C

CONNECTIVE TISSUE

Shown here are greatly magnified structures of connective tissue, which has different forms depending on the organs and tissues it pervades. Collagen (protein) fibrils are produced by fibroblast cells (A). In skin, fibrils are intertwined in flat plates (B). The close-up of a single fibril (C) shows protein crossbands. Parallel fibrils enwrapped with crosswise fibrils (D) give the tissue great strength.

If one thinks of more or less rigid connective tissue clamping down on vessels, impeding blood flow, and cramping the processes of tissues and organs, it is understandable that lessened flexibility can underlie many conditions characteristic of the later years of life. Among these are high blood pressure, arthritis, hardening of the arteries, inadequate muscle contraction (the heart is a muscle), reduced lung elasticity (less breathing capacity), sluggish transport of blood and materials, and depression of cells and functions. Whether it is a cause or a result of aging, some loss of elasticity of connective tissue is an indubitable accompaniment.

THE MIND

There is splendid probability that you can keep your wits about you into advanced old age—provided you give them moderate exercise. In the absence of real physical impairment (and often, in its presence), a mind good enough to get one productively through turbulent youth into middle age generally is like a well broken-in engine: good for years of service if kept from rusting, and running, if not at maximum rpm, still at a very satisfactory rate for all the miles it's logged.

It is not possible to separate body and mind. Physical infirmities obviously can affect mental processes. A rare kind of atrophy of parts of the brain (Alzheimer's disease) is scarcely relevant to anyone who can read this book. Strokes, anything that decreases the oxygen supply to the brain, and bodily upsets consequent upon disease can all depress mental alertness. But a healthy mind will concentrate on leading an active and satisfying life rather than magnify the possible hazards of longevity.

A wise student of aging has remarked, "If a person can remember to get out of bed on time, wash, eat, and pay his bills when due, he's not mentally senile." Attitudes that help to keep the mind young and favor longevity, if several psychological studies are valid, are work satisfaction, happiness, and a *high level of self-esteem*. A robust ego is more appropriate to the old than the young, for the old have earned it. Ordinary sloppiness may be an early sign of aging. A physician who noticed the fast age deterioration of a friend long before fellow doctors saw any signs of it was asked how he knew. He answered, "Egg on his vest."

Skills. Our abilities are usually fully matured in the 50s, and if continuously exercised, do not decline to a significant degree at retirement age or later. One's capacity to maintain well-developed skills is quite remarkable, whether it's cabinet-making, dressmaking, fly-casting, typing, or whatever. It's not so easy, though certainly not impossible, to develop entirely new complex skills after retirement. Thus comes the wisdom of developing avocations, hobbies, and interests in younger years so that skills can be consolidated and extended after retirement.

Intelligence. Age does not universally bring a marked decline in intelligence. High intelligence is at least slightly associated with longevity, perhaps because intelligent people take care of themselves and likely have the means to do so. In general, the higher the original level of education and continued use of mental functions, the less the decline in sharp-wittedness with age. Thought processes may be a little slowed in some persons in their 60s; in others, scarcely at all.

Learning. An old dog can learn suitable new tricks if he takes his time. If slower, he tends to be more careful and accurate in performance, gaining quality at some cost in speed. Memory is the basis of learning, and short-term memory is usually excellent well into the 50s. Older people often fret about poor memory. They can't remember a name or fact that is on the tip of their tongues, or whether they turned off the gas. But young people have the same problems (and less to remember).

Memory is highly selective. We remember what is important to us. James Farley had a fabulous memory for names and faces, important to a politician; Einstein was an absentminded professor, but he remembered abstruse formulas. Short of brain damage or enfeebled circulation, memory in later years continues to serve well in matters that count, and our ability to learn is little impaired. What may slacken is the *drive* to learn, especially in

those who view education as something that happens in schools instead of as a lifetime process. The learning machine usually is quite adequate in later years—there are octogenarians in college—if it has a self-starter.

Work. By middle life, most people have established patterns of work (another term for careers) that earn a living and to some extent draw occupational boundaries for the future. Physical changes and modified views of one's role in life may require some adaptation, however. Power in later years shifts from what you can do (physical effort) to what you know. Professional and highly skilled workers often continue to rise in their careers until late in life, accustomed, as they are, to effort and challenge. Bureaucratic, supervisory, managerial, and similar workers may escape the sound and the fury by their willingness to delegate duties and share the perceptions and perspectives of maturity. The idea that re-

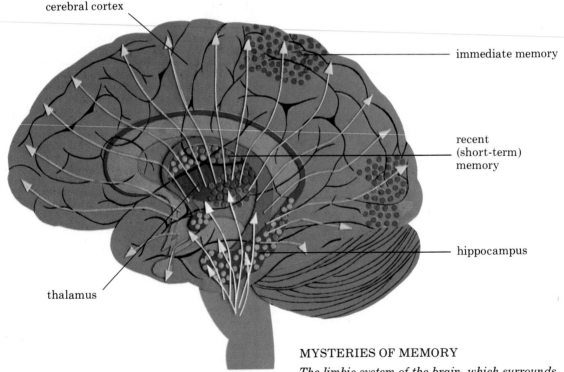

cerebral cortex

immediate memory

recent (short-term) memory

hippocampus

thalamus

MYSTERIES OF MEMORY

The limbic system of the brain, which surrounds the upper brain stem and includes the hippocampus, apparently is crucial to memory. Long-term memory is thought to spread diffusely through midbrain structures and cerebral cortex (white and yellow arrows). Colored dots suggest complex diffusion of memory processes.

tirement is the end of usefulness is, of course, nonsense. Innumerable men and women are fully capable of productive activity as contributing members of society well after retirement age.

What is one to make of these generalizations? Reasonable inferences may be: That the mental abilities of most older people are in good working order. That abilities may decline sadly if neither exercised nor challenged. That adaptation to changing circumstances is the trait of a matured personality. That learning, avocations, and interests nurtured in early years can be revived and returned to with great fulfillment in later life. And that drive, zest, participation, interest, and curiosity can transform the lives of motivated older people. Would you like to become a greater expert on a chosen subject than 99 percent of the population? Just spend a couple of days of research in a public library.

THE BODY

Do you feel much older today than yesterday? Not likely. One of the heartening facts about normal changes in maturing bodies is their generally slow progression. For instance, hearing begins to deteriorate at around ten years of age, but a ten-year-old knows nothing about it, and it may take another six or seven decades before any hearing impairment is a handicap to daily living, if it ever is.

A few natural changes of aging are briefly mentioned below. Until it is put to stress, the physiology of older people is not remarkably different from that of the young.

Circulation. We literally become less flexible with age from stiffening of connective tissue, as already mentioned. Loss of elasticity (there are other factors) ultimately burdens the great organs—heart, vessels, lungs, and kidneys—that transport oxygen and nutrients to all parts of the body and dispose of wastes.

The aorta, the great artery that arches from the heart and carries oxygen-rich blood through smaller and smaller pipelines to all parts of the body, begins to lose some elasticity as early as age 25; blood flow is just as great, but vessel flexibility is less. In time, stiffened sheaths around tiny capillaries make it harder for oxygen to diffuse into tissues, and increasingly rigid vessels resist blood flow and increase the work of the heart. The output of the heart is reduced to 70 percent after age 60.

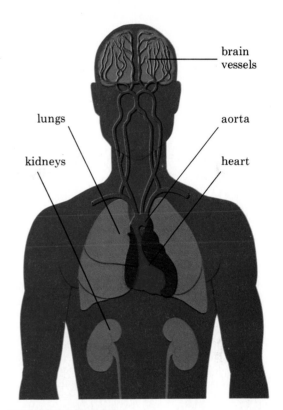

TARGET ORGANS

Great organs and vessels bear much of the brunt of living, but lose some efficiency and become more vulnerable to disease as we grow older. In themselves, changes with aging are natural and gradual, and generally do not preclude a satisfying, active life in later years.

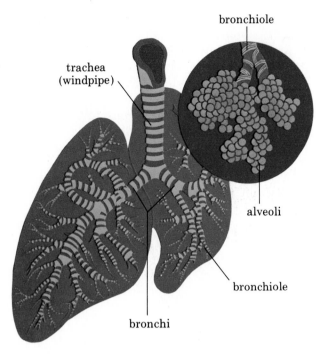

THE LUNGS

Alveoli are tiny air sacs (400 million of them) in the lungs, where gases are exchanged. (Blood is charged with oxygen and carbon dioxide is removed as a waste product.)

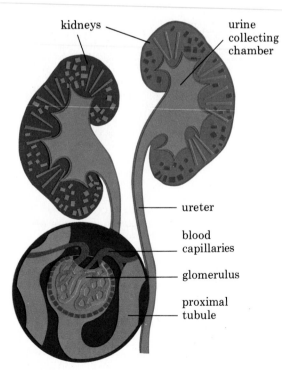

THE KIDNEYS

Blood from the cup-shaped glomeruli of the kidneys passes through tubules that reabsorb useful materials and filter out wastes, which are concentrated as urine.

Lungs gradually lose elasticity and their tiny air sacs (alveoli) thicken, impeding the passage of gases across membranes. The amount of oxygen the blood can carry is at its maximum at around age 50. Ultimately, more air has to be breathed through the lungs to oxygenate blood, even though breathing capacity is diminished some 40 percent in the 70s.

Blood pressure tends to increase slowly in healthy 30- and 40-year-olds. Sometimes blood pressure jumps rather sharply after menopause. Abnormally high blood pressure usually does not cause symptoms that alert the patient. Whether an increase in blood pressure is insignificant or dangerous is readily determined by one of the simplest procedures in a physical checkup.

Kidneys. These great filters work as hard as the heart; all the body's blood passes through them in a few minutes. Stiffening of circulatory pathways reduces the waste-filtering efficiency of the kidneys by about one-third by age 70. Worn-out kidney cells are never replaced, but fortunately, the paired kidneys have such ample reserves that a single healthy kidney is quite capable of doing all the work.

Strength. Sheer physical strength is well retained into the 60s, although back muscles may lose one-tenth of their power after 50. Diminished strength is not so much a matter of weak muscle fibers as loss of muscle cells (which are not replaced) together with reduced elasticity. The extent to which muscles can be strengthened begins to diminish in the late 30s.

Endurance. How long you can do hard physical work before stopping to rest is a measurement of endurance, a capacity that declines more significantly with age than does strength. A main factor is the reduced ability of the heart to circulate enough oxygen to keep effort going at full speed. Sedentary folk lose about one-third of their endurance by age 60. Usually they can work as hard as ever, but more intermittently, with longer rests between spurts. (The energy spent by muscular young workers in, say, digging ditches, is easily overestimated; there's quite a bit of leaning on the shovel.) If shortness of breath is a handicap to ordinary effort, a conditioning program is probably in order.

Digestion. Not much change attributable to age *per se* occurs in the digestive tract, except for slightly less secretion of hydrochloric acid. Cells of the digestive tract are prolific renewers of themselves. However, loss of taste buds may contribute to finicky or monotonous eating habits in older people. One meticulous bud-counter has calculated the rate of this loss: from 295 taste buds per given area in young adults to 88 in oldsters. Perhaps an old gourmet gets one-third of the savor from sauce Bearnaise. Some older people, not to mention some young ones, become almost obsessed with bowel function, and could profit from the terse remark of a gastroenterologist: "A healthy gut thrives on being ignored."

Basal metabolic rate (BMR). This is a measurement of the energy expended just to keep vital functions going, apart from energy spent in making beds, walking, talking, and so on. The BMR rate decreases about 20 percent by age 65. A natural result is diminishing desire to exert one's self prodigiously. If, however, one continues to eat as much as in the high-energy-output years of youth, obesity is in the offing.

Bones. Per decade, men lose 3 percent of bone substance after age 40; women, 8 percent. One result is that we get shorter after age 40; another, that bone and joint structures are vulnerable to thinning and forms of arthritis.

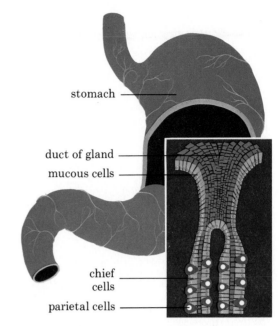

THE STOMACH

Secretory cells line the stomach and digestive tract. Parietal cells (red) produce hydrochloric acid, which is normal to the stomach and plays a role in peptic ulceration.

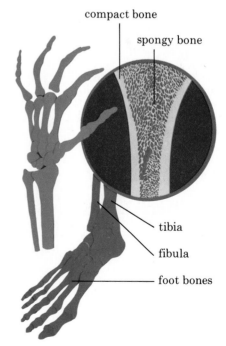

THE BONES

Some thinning of bone is to be expected after middle age, more so in women than in men. The quality of bone generally remains good, but there is a little less of it to withstand stresses.

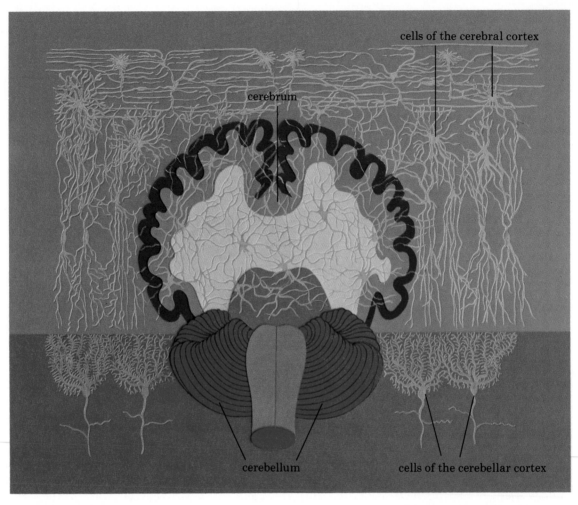

cells of the cerebral cortex

cerebrum

cerebellum

cells of the cerebellar cortex

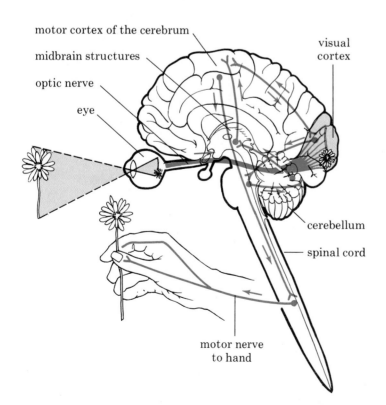

motor cortex of the cerebrum

midbrain structures

optic nerve

eye

visual cortex

cerebellum

spinal cord

motor nerve to hand

100 BILLION NEURONS

The brain contains billions of nerve cells (neurons) that convey impulses in response to chemical and electrical changes in and between them. Sensory messages that result in physical movement (dodge that car!) are mediated in the cerebellum, which controls muscle responses and coordination.

FROM SIGHT TO ACTION

To see and pick a flower is an incredibly complex act. Light waves from the flower reach the nerves of the retina and travel as impulses over the optic nerve to the visual cortex where they are "seen." Red arrows suggest the tortuous routes of information processing, resulting in a decision to pick the flower and appropriate orders to the muscles of the hand—all in a second or less.

Fertility. Many men remain fertile into old age, in the sense that they continue to produce sperm and may impregnate a suitable consort. A woman's fertility ends before she is really old, when, in fact, some of the most satisfying years of life are ahead of her. At puberty, the ovaries contain some 10,000 primitive egg cells; at age 50, none. Reduced functioning of the ovaries may begin as soon as five years before menopause, and ovulation—release of a fertilizable egg cell—may fail a year or two before menopause.

Brain and nervous system. The brain begins to lose weight in middle life. By age 60, its mass has shrunk about 5 percent. One estimate, that we lose 100,000 brain cells a day after the 20s, is frightening until we realize that the original quota of billions upon billions of brain cells hardly notices such a miniscule reduction. Depressed mental function is less associated with lost cells than with deficiency of oxygen, to which the brain is very sensitive.

Just as one cannot judge instantly where a tennis ball is heading the moment it leaves an opponent's racquet, it takes longer for nerve impulses to flash from the eyes to the brain and the spinal cord as we grow older. This slowing of split-second reactions—by as much as 15 percent—isn't a disaster, but can be a factor in accidents of the elderly, who usually learn to compensate by caution.

THE YEARS AHEAD

There is a certain risk involved in reading this book.

The chapters that follow give detailed information about a great number of ills and disabilities. Worse, hundreds of ailments that might befall anyone at any age are not mentioned; the authors limit their discussions to major conditions that become more common and important as time goes on. The risk is that an apprehensive reader might mistakenly feel that day-by-day living (the way everyone grows older) is an increasingly perilous and joyless venture, threatening that he or she will come apart at any instant.

Some bright perspective is in order.

For one thing, the health of the country can't be overwhelmingly bad, to judge by a 1977 death rate of 8.8 deaths per 1,000 population, the lowest ever recorded—and this in a population in which the number of people over 65 continually increases. Nor is there much substance in the fear that growing old inevitably means total helplessness in a wheelchair. Only 5 percent of people over 65 in this country are in nursing homes, many because there is simply nobody at home to lend a helping hand. And while poverty affects old as well as young people, the idea that all elderly people are victims of extreme deprivation is erasable by just looking around you.

One infirmity or another, some slowing down, some sensory or physical impairment, may, of course, lurk in the future. But most infirmities do not seriously interfere with satisfying life activities. Of those that do, many are correctable by measures, discussed in following chapters, that restore or improve function, ease distress, and slow or prevent the progress of some condition that could become serious.

Above all, never underestimate the wisdom of the body or its toughness. Far from being a fragile instrument, doomed to collapse if it isn't belabored by incessant efforts to prop it up, the body is astoundingly durable and its capacity to adapt to all sorts of insults is enormous. Count on it, along with your own wisdom, to sustain the quality of life in the long run.

Quite a tolerable prospect for tomorrow—and all of the tomorrows to come.

LOOK BETTER AS YOU GROW OLDER

By middle age, your skin doubtless shows some signs of growing older. You might be an exception if you have spent most of your life indoors out of the sun, but that would hardly be normal. And sometimes the facial skin of certain women who are overweight is surprisingly youthful as fatty layers tend to push out wrinkles from the inside.

But for most people, as the skin grows older, it loses some of its underlying layer of fat, becoming thinner and more transparent. Blue veins are then more noticeable, and spots and splotches may appear. The skin loses some of its elasticity or snap—a stiffening trait of older connective tissue (see page 234)—and doesn't instantly spring back into place when pinched. And it also loses moisture, becoming drier.

The consequences are most visible on exposed areas of skin—above the collar line, below the sleeves, and in women, on the V of the neck. Skin ordinarily covered by clothing can be quite supple in older people. It is clear that excessive exposure to sunlight speeds the normal aging process.

The skin includes such appendages as hair, nails, sweat glands, and tiny oil ducts that spread a thin lubricating film on the surface—in fact, all of your good looks that meet the eye, save the embellishments of tailors and dressmakers. If aging of the skin can't be completely stopped, a little informed and kindly care can do a lot to preserve its attractiveness, correct some defects, and revivify it.

Care of Dry Skin

To relieve dry skin, your cleansing routine should include the use of mild bland soaps, not-too-frequent bathing, and application of some of the creams we will suggest for dryness. In cold weather, when the heat goes on, house air becomes hot and dry and so does your skin. In the winter, then, a humidifier is a useful appliance for keeping room moisture at a desirable level that is pleasing to your skin.

If a "grease" or cream is applied to wet skin, it will penetrate more deeply, which is desirable. A common type of grease used by our grandparents' generation was heavy lanolin, or wool fat. Today, a more refined commercial product with a heavier feel is available; it can be thinned by beating a little water into it. Any edible oil or fat can penetrate the skin to some extent, though sometimes there's a risk of rancidity or olfactory offense.

You should keep a good grease handy in the bathroom and at sinks and basins so you can always apply a small amount after washing when the skin is wet. Pat dry with a towel. Also, apply some to dry skin before retiring at night.

A mild soap is one that your skin can tolerate. Sunbathers would do well to avoid soaps containing materials that can make the skin sensitive to sunlight. Certain substances (salicylanilides) are incorporated into soaps to increase their antiseptic quality, but they also can sensitize the skin to sun. The value of such agents is questionable since the soap is always rinsed off and this mechanical rinsing in itself helps to reduce the likelihood of skin infection.

The lower leg. Dry skin is not only a problem of the face and hands, but perhaps even more important, of the lower third of the leg. As the years roll on, circulation of the lower leg becomes less and less efficient. Blood tends to pool and vessels become weaker, leaving the skin more susceptible to irritation from dryness, cold, and the friction of rough clothes.

As a result, the lower part of the leg may begin to peel and scale, possibly leading to eczema and infection. If peeling is severe enough, ulcers may develop that, with poor circulation, can last a long time.

Also, you may notice little brown spots around your ankles that seem not to go away. These are often the result of slow-leaking blood vessels and some impairment of circulation—another important reason to keep the skin soft on the lower third of your legs. This can be done with steroid creams, but always have your doctor check the reasons for slow bleeding. Wear stockings, and if necessary, support hose if you are often on your feet.

"Rejuvenating" creams. Quite a variety of cosmetic creams containing estrogens (female hormones) or even more exotic ingredients are offered to women with claims that they soften the skin and keep it youthful. Sometimes such creams put moisture into the skin and make it a little bit softer (as does lanolin applied to wet skin). But unfortunately, very little else is accomplished.

The quantity of hormones in cosmetic creams is not great, but lavish use over large areas of the body can add up to a substantial dose. The Food and Drug Administration has warned that there is no evidence that estrogens can keep the skin soft or preserve youthfulness, and that long-term treatment carries a number of important risks.

Wrinkles

As children, we were told that if we worried and wrinkled our forehead, the wrinkles would become permanent. Brow furrowing, however, is hardly a cause of wrinkles. The common varieties of wrinkles reflect changes that aging brings about in connective tissues. Time, exposure, drying, and decreased flexibility allow the skin to fold in little pleats and crinkles.

Certain wrinkles that occur in association with hormone disturbances are not the wrinkles of aging. Another kind of facial wrinkling may sometimes be smoothed out by a dentist who corrects a "bad bite."

Prevention. Steps to prevent wrinkles should be taken early, even at a time when we are not concerned about them. Bathing with cream soaps and massaging the skin with hydrophilic salves that take up water are helpful measures. And as mentioned, there is no special magic in hormone creams, and their use may be hazardous.

Excessive exposure to the sun ages the skin prematurely. What's worse, the changes are irreversible. A coffee-brown suntan maintained season after season presages a leathery skin that is old beyond its years, so moderation is desirable. The legendary beautiful complexions of women of the British Isles are in part attributable to a cloudy, drizzly, moist climate that is kind to their skins.

The only worthwhile treatment of established wrinkles is surgery.

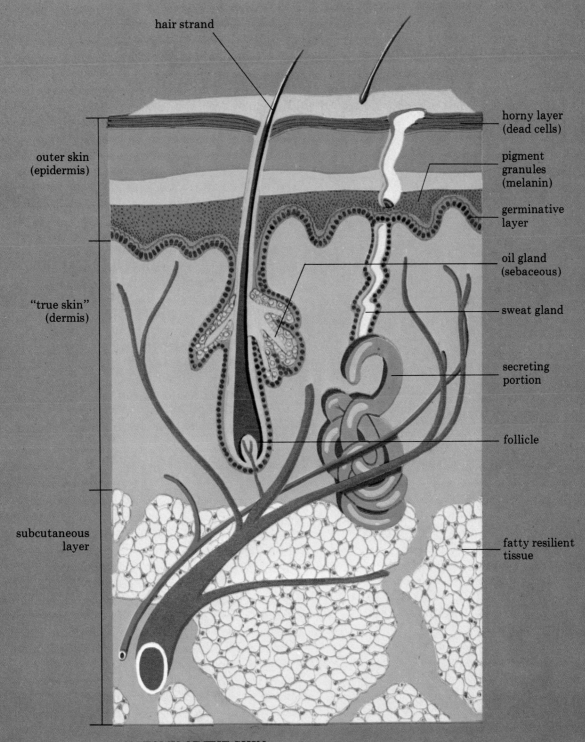

hair strand

horny layer
(dead cells)

outer skin
(epidermis)

pigment
granules
(melanin)

germinative
layer

"true skin"
(dermis)

oil gland
(sebaceous)

sweat gland

secreting
portion

follicle

subcutaneous
layer

fatty resilient
tissue

ANATOMY OF THE SKIN

*Surface layers of the skin
(epidermis) continuously shed
dead cells that are replaced from
the germinative layer below.
Sebaceous glands produce an
invisible moving film of skin oil.
Salty water from sweat glands
cools the body by evaporation.
Pigment granules exposed to
sunlight produce a tan or
freckles. Older exposed skin
becomes drier and stiffer. Loss of
cushioning fat may cause
shrinkage enfolded by wrinkles.*

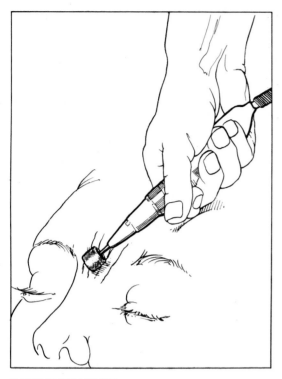

DERMABRASION

A rotating cutting instrument removes superficial skin layers, somewhat like sandpapering. Enough skin is removed to obliterate fine wrinkles but not deep pits or scars. Dermabrasion leaves a raw skin surface that requires proper postoperative care and bandaging for a few days.

Dermabrasion

In principle, dermabrasion is like sand-papering a rough piece of wood to smooth its surface. The procedure is best suited for removal of fine wrinkles around the mouth, eyes, and brow. Coarse scars of acne or accidents may be too deep for perfect smoothing.

The instrument used resembles a dentist's drill with a rapidly rotating button at its end. The button *(diamond fraise)* has a convex surface with a cutting edge. The patient's skin is superficially frozen with a Freon spray and the surgeon moves the skin-planing instrument over the surface, sanding off a layer of skin that, ideally, contains the wrinkles. The operation takes about half an hour and leaves a raw surface that regenerates baby-pink new skin, hopefully free of blemishes.

A possible drawback to dermabrasion is the development of small cysts in the treated area that leave spots of too much or too little pigmentation. And the patient may want to keep out of society for a couple of weeks or more while healing proceeds and discoloration decreases.

Skin Peeling

Peeling off the skin with chemicals is somewhat more hazardous than the mechanical peeling of dermabrasion, but successful results are similar—new skin for old. The usual chemical agent is a form of carbolic acid, a highly corrosive substance that requires the skills of a trained expert to prevent deep burns or systemic absorption. Careful application of the chemical will burn off a layer of skin—not very comfortably—and form a scab. In about ten days the scab drops off to reveal regenerated skin that is usually rather dark and red, but if all has gone well, devoid of fine wrinkles. It may take some weeks or months for the new skin to fade to its normal color, during which time the patient should avoid prolonged exposure to the sun and use a sunscreen ointment to avert discoloration.

Silicone Injections

Injection of liquid silicones to enlarge the breasts fell into disrepute with evidence of certain distressing long-term effects—nodules, thickening, and shifts of materials. As much as a half pint of liquid was injected into some breasts. However, the much more modest use of tiny amounts of the substance to fill out deep lines, wrinkles, and sunken scars of the face is another matter. Some practitioners report that a small amount of liquid silicone, properly injected into a deep wrinkle, smooths the defect and does not shift.

The technique would be most applicable to heavy, deep creases of an aging face that are too deep to be helped much by dermabrasion. However, liquid silicones of medical grade are not readily available to all qualified doctors, and the technique is considered experimental by the government.

Face Lift

This operation is pretty much what its name implies: a pulling-up of loose facial skin and tightening or removal of fatty tissues in the face and neck that tend to sag, creating wrinkles and, at worst, a jowled and wattled look. Most candidates are between 40 and 65 years of age—men as well as women—who don't want to look older than they really are.

The operation, performed by plastic surgeons and some dermatologists, is not a trifling one. Incisions must be made, but any remaining scars usually are well concealed under the hairline and around the ears. The operation takes three or more hours, with the patient under general anesthesia. He or she awakens with bandages around the entire face except for holes for the nose, mouth, and eyes.

When bandages are removed in three or four days, the first glimpse of the swollen, black, blue, red, and purple countenance is likely to be shocking. The hospital stay ranges from four days to a week, but the patient may desire seclusion at home or elsewhere until the improved visage is ready for public display.

What results can be expected? These vary with the skill and experience of the surgeon, the patient's health, age, bone structure, skin texture, and other factors. Over-tightening of the skin can give a mask-like look, and the operation itself may not be appropriate for some persons. But generally, the outcome is quite acceptable to most patients, who are pleased with their smoother skins and lost sag of the lower face and neck.

It should be understood, however, that a face lift is not permanent. Processes of skin aging and sagging continue, and good results lasting more than five years are uncommon. Longer-lasting benefits are more likely if the face is not naturally heavy. Or if desired, a second face lift can be done when the first one wears off.

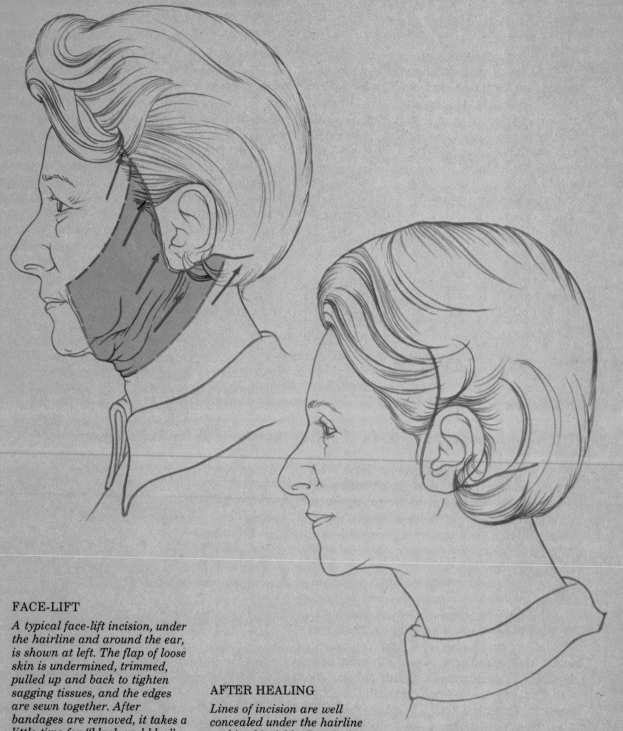

FACE-LIFT

A typical face-lift incision, under the hairline and around the ear, is shown at left. The flap of loose skin is undermined, trimmed, pulled up and back to tighten sagging tissues, and the edges are sewn together. After bandages are removed, it takes a little time for "black and blue" after effects to disappear. Care is taken not to over-tighten the skin, which would give a masklike look.

AFTER HEALING

Lines of incision are well concealed under the hairline and in skin folds. Results in the form of smooth unwrinkled skin are usually pleasing, but factors such as age, bone structure, type of skin, and others are considered in judging the desirability of surgery. In time, after a satisfactory face-lift, tissues tend to sag again as processes of skin aging continue, but the face-lift operation can be repeated.

Baggy Eyes

Excessive skin of the upper eyelids and bags below can give a hooded look of dissipation, obviously quite unwarranted. "Eye-lift" surgery, relatively simple as cosmetic surgery goes, can restore the wide-eyed view of the world associated with youth. A tendency toward excessive eyelid flesh may be hereditary or a consequence of sagging and reduced muscle tone associated with aging. The corrective operation, called *blepharoplasty,* is performed by ophthalmologists as well as by plastic surgeons.

An incision is made in a natural fold of the upper eyelid, where it will later be invisible. The surgeon removes redundant tissue, brings edges of the lid together, and sutures them. If the lower eyelid is involved, the incision is made just under the eyelashes. Immediately afterward, the sutured incisions have quite a red and battered appearance, but discoloration fades in about ten days, and sutures are removed in about four days.

No longer than a day's stay in a hospital is required. In fact, eye-lift surgery, which takes just over an hour to complete, is often performed on an outpatient basis. The patient returns home immediately after surgery with the doctor's directions, and there is no interference with vision.

A Word About Cosmetic Surgery

Be prepared to pay in advance for purely cosmetic surgery. Not all doctors request prepayment, but many do. The doctor's fee for elective surgery to improve appearance (unrelated to function, disease, or accident) is often not covered by insurance.

Doctors are usually concerned about the expectations of candidates for cosmetic surgery and the reasons why they seek it. An excellent technical result may be bitterly disappointing to a patient who expects too much. Improved appearance is a reasonable expectation, but not perfection. Nor can cosmetic improvement be expected to miraculously change the course of a life in which lack of success has been blamed on personal appearance. Some patients may be rejected for surgery because they expect unattainable benefits.

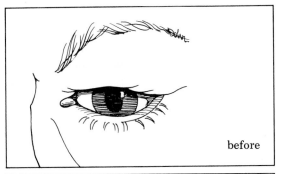

before

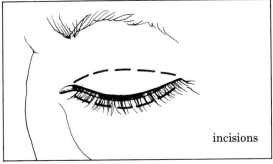

incisions

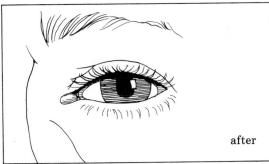

after

EYE-LIFT

Surgery to correct droopy, baggy eyelids is relatively simple and is often done on an outpatient basis. The middle drawing shows incision lines, either in a natural fold of the upper eyelid, under the eyelash line of the lower lid, or both. Excess skin is trimmed away and edges are drawn together and sutured. Below, incision lines in natural skin folds are entirely invisible after healing. Discoloration disappears in a few days. The eye itself is not touched nor is vision affected.

BROWN SPOTS

Most middle-aged people and nearly all older ones have at least a few "brown spots" on the skin—small, flat, brownish areas. The most common variety is freckles, which pop out on sensitive skin exposed to the sun and then fade away when protected from sunlight. There is nothing alarming about ordinary freckles, unless they are construed as beauty hazards. Light-skinned blondes and redheads and persons whose skin does not tan well are especially susceptible. However, the freckle-prone can reduce the crop by wearing long sleeves and broad-brimmed hats if they think it worth the trouble.

Another common type of brown spot has various popular names. These blotches, which appear early in some families but are more characteristic of middle age and later, are often called "old lady spots," "senile freckles," "beauty spots," and even "liver spots," although the liver has nothing to do with them. Typically, the spots appear on exposed parts of the body—the face, neck, backs of the hands, and arms.

Perhaps you can see some brown spots on the backs of your hands, but none on the fingers. This shows the effects of exposure in development of the spots. Brown spotting associated with seborrheic warty growth can expand into large black areas of roughness and scaling of the skin. In spite of their appearance, these are not at all dangerous or potentially cancerous, though cancer of the skin might possibly be a neighbor, detectable by a dermatologist.

Several things can be done if the spots are considered too cosmetically offensive. The simplest measure is to cover them with cosmetic creams or sticks. There also are various methods of removal: chemical peeling, burning with liquid nitrogen, use of electric needles, or removal by cutting. If spots are not removed deeply enough, however, they may recur. But to insure against spot recurrence, it is sometimes necessary to remove them so deeply that they leave little white spots.

Moles and warts. Practically everybody has a few moles scattered around the body; often they arise in youth and persist for years. Moles come in innumerable varieties—flat, soft and pulpy, light or dark colored, and with or without hairs. Seborrheic warts, or as some call them, senile warts, occur in older skin. Such "beauty spots" can be removed, as described, or they can be retained, like Abraham Lincoln's, for an honest portrait.

The great majority of moles and warts are harmless, doing principal damage to vanity, but there are exceptions. One should be watchful for changes in size or color, crusting, and bleeding, all of which call for examination by a dermatologist.

Prominent veins. Sometimes the little veins in the nose and cheeks become conspicuous. Certain hormone influences may initiate this, and heredity may play a part, as well as reactions to sun exposure. If prominent veins are a cause of concern, an effort should be made to block them out by fairly superficial techniques early in their development.

In general, it may be said that middle and later life is a time when protection of the skin becomes increasingly important.

Actinic Keratosis

Keratosis is a condition of overgrowth of the horny layer of the skin. A simple innocuous form is the callus that develops on a laborer's hands. But of more importance is actinic or solar keratosis, terms that imply a reaction of the skin to sunlight.

Such lesions—most apparent after middle age—are rough, brownish, scaly spots on the skin, often with a pinkish border, that take a long time to develop. They represent interference with cell growth at a very early stage, and are definitely precancerous—a frightening word that does not at all mean that cancer is inevitable, just that the possibility is there.

White-skinned persons who don't take a tan well are most prone to develop keratoses as they grow older, particularly if they live in sunny parts of the country or are sportively or occupationally exposed to lots of sun. The rough brownish spots appear on the neck, cheeks, brow, and scalp (especially a nude one). Persons who have driven a car for many years often have a preponderance of lesions on the left side of the face—the driver's side where the sun streams through.

If such spots develop, one will probably have to deal with them indefinitely. Removal of scattered spots by application of liquid nitrogen, which leaves no scar, is relatively easy and painless. Or an electric needle may be used. Spots with hardened skin around and beneath them will be removed more deeply, with the healed area appearing lighter in color than surrounding skin. The removed tissue will then be stained and examined under a microscope to check for any malignant changes.

Chemical treatment. An ointment containing fluorouracil (5-FU) is quite dramatic in its action. It is rubbed onto the affected skin for several days as the doctor directs, usually when rather large areas are involved. Gradually the spotted skin becomes lobster red, not only where spots are obvious, but also in seemingly normal areas where invisible spots are developing (fluorouracil does not inflame normal skin). At times, a corticosteroid is mixed with the 5-FU to reduce redness. After the redness fades, a more healthy skin surface is established. However, 5-FU is not reliably effective enough to penetrate deep spots where cancer may be developing, and during the inflamed stage, exposure to the sun must be avoided.

Protection. Sun-damaged skin needs more protection than "ordinary" skin. Of the innumerable sunscreen or suntan-sunscreen products now on the market, some are nearly useless for blocking out damaging rays. Studies indicate that aminobenzoic acid (PABA) is highly efficient protection against skin-reddening wavelengths of sunlight. And cream soaps and hydrophilic (water-absorbing) salves are helpful in keeping the skin soft. Generally, if skin protection is critical, it is better to have the advice of a dermatologist than a cosmetician.

THE REACTIVE SKIN

Your skin may react hypersensitively to an enormous variety of substances, both internal and external. As a result, you may experience itching, burning, pain, or blistering. And you probably won't look so good, either.

Contact dermatitis is skin irritation resulting from coming into contact with something in the environment. Poison ivy or poison oak is a familiar contactant. Generally there is no mystery as to the cause of the burning and weeping blisters typical of ivy poisoning. A mild attack can be eased with calamine lotion or aluminum acetate solution. But severely inflamed skin that becomes infected, with pus-filled blisters, needs medicines prescribed by a doctor.

Matters are worsened if highly reactive skin is subject to repeated attacks of ivy dermatitis season after season. Then one should consider measures of prevention, the most effective of which are preparations of poison ivy extracts taken by mouth for three or four months before the season.

Other hypersensitive skin reactions are more mysterious and take some detective work to track down. Such flare-ups occur from substances encountered in running a home, working, or pursuing a hobby. It is important to identify these offending substances to avoid a lingering chronic skin irritation that can cause loss of time from work and is a handicap to normal activity.

Skin tests can often detect irritating contact materials. In the patch test, for instance, suspected materials are applied to the skin and reactions are noted. Another test under controlled conditions is the usage test, in which the patient is instructed to use the suspected irritant, such as soaps and detergents found in the home. To test for suspected shoe dermatitis, one shoe should have the suspected material and the other should not. The search is then narrowed if only one foot breaks out. In dermatitis of the feet, many factors besides allergy can play a role, such as the environment, heat, and friction.

If rashes are caused by internal conditions, the problem is compounded. These conditions include drug allergies and may involve medicines often used for headaches or as laxatives or tranquilizers. All of them can cause rashes. Your physician can help you find the specific agent at fault.

Eczemas. Another type of skin reaction is often called eczema, a general term that means nothing but red, scaling skin. These are usually allergic or hypersensitive reactions to substances that are generally harmless, and may show up in childhood as repeated attacks of hives, hay fever, or asthma. One learns from experience that certain things cause reactions, and tries to avoid them. You can help your skin to defend itself by controlling excessive sweating in the elbows, armpits, behind the knees, and between the legs, and by not getting the skin too dry with strong soaps, detergents, and chemicals. Common sensitizers such as aspirin and penicillin should also be used very carefully and only when needed.

The commonest places to look for sensitivity reactions are on the hands, the elbows, behind the knees, the back of the neck, and around the lips. If you have a history of reactive skin, every little spot is a cause for concern and should be treated early. Don't wait until lesions are extensive, thickened, or very itchy. Your doctor and dermatologist can help you in intensive treatment of early lesions, usually with steroid creams to avoid protracted inflammation and skin infection. If there is not too much scarring or thickening, the skin can return to normal. But as long as there are brown or white spots in areas where trouble recurs, the skin is not completely cleared and treatment should be continued as long as necessary.

YOUR HAIR

On the sides of your forehead are graceful triangular areas called the "professor's corners" where early signs of hair loss can be seen. If you notice fine downy hairs in these areas, it may still be possible to arrest continued hair loss. Such hairs can be made more visible by holding a flashlight parallel to the surface. The back or crown of the head is harder to inspect, but sometimes can be done with mirrors or the help of a family member.

Male Pattern Baldness

After age 40, a man's hair loss is usually the type called male pattern baldness. Young boys don't have it. The process usually begins in the early 20s and by middle age is pretty well established. Typically, a persistent and reasonably thick fringe of hair remains around the sides of the head and above the neck in a pattern nobly known to medicine as the "Hippocratic tonsure."

Speculation and some evidence suggest that the cause is a tricky combination of heredity, hormones, and sufficient age, none of which is reversible. One should accept male pattern baldness as usually inevitable and progressive, and thereby save a great deal of aggravation and money that might otherwise be spent on hair-growing nostrums.

Certain types of nervous hair loss with spotty bald areas are known as *alopecia areata*. At times, a dermatologist can help to accelerate the regrowth of hair. But in mild cases, the hair eventually returns no matter what is done. Credit for magic hair-restoring properties may be wrongly given to goose grease, safflower oil, Abyssinian herbs, or whatever was applied just before the hair returned to life on its own. This type of hair loss is not at all the same as male pattern baldness.

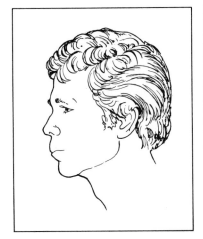 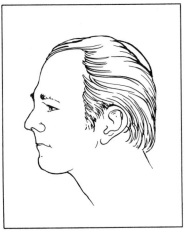 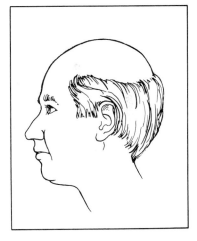

MALE PATTERN BALDNESS

A young head of hair, full at forehead, temples, and crown, usually shows no signs of male pattern baldness until the late teens or early 20s.

In encroaching male pattern baldness, hair gradually recedes from the forehead, temples, and the crown of the head (bald spot in back).

In full-blown male pattern baldness, hair is gone except for a fringe that stubbornly persists around the sides and back of the head.

Management. Scalp infections may co-exist with male pattern baldness. If so, mild medicated shampoos prescribed by a doctor will ease the infection and possibly slow the rate of hair loss. Excessive non-red scaling of the scalp—dandruff—can be suppressed with medicated shampoos and daily scalp medications recommended by your doctor.

Otherwise, if your scalp is absolutely clear and free of dandruff, just use a simple shampoo and rinse it out well. No proteins or other ingredients can feed a lifeless hair shaft that is dead when it is pushed out from its root, and no surface applications can significantly affect the growth of hair. At best, some substances may just coat hair shafts fairly agreeably, only to be washed away at the next shampoo. Vigorous scalp massage or rough toweling of wet hair can do more harm than good.

Instant hair. The safest and least painful way to flaunt an immediate head of hair is to have a hairpiece fitted by sympathetic hair people. Today's hairpieces are much improved over old-time "rugs," and when well chosen as to style, color, shape, and materials, they can be quite satisfactory. They do, of course, require special care, and a spare is advisable.

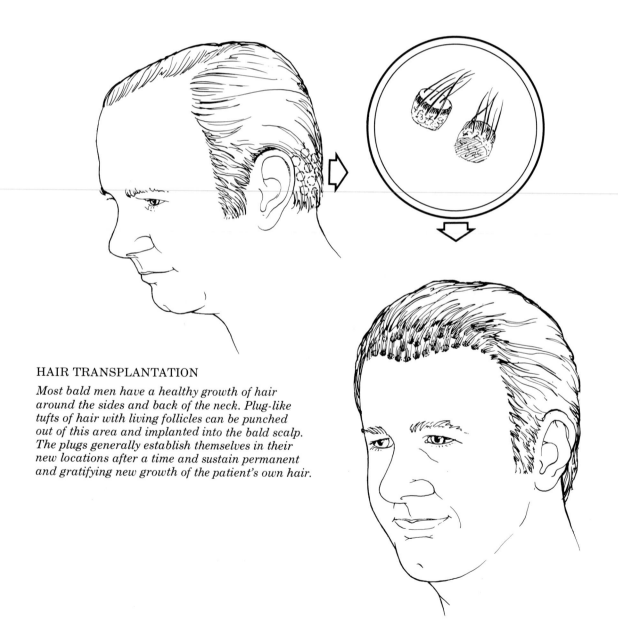

HAIR TRANSPLANTATION

Most bald men have a healthy growth of hair around the sides and back of the neck. Plug-like tufts of hair with living follicles can be punched out of this area and implanted into the bald scalp. The plugs generally establish themselves in their new locations after a time and sustain permanent and gratifying new growth of the patient's own hair.

Some unusual kinds of hairpieces offer permanent anchorage. One kind is tied to your scalp with your own existing hairs. Another is sewn around the scalp edge with heavy wires, or into the center of your scalp with heavy nylon. There are even ideas of tying hair to small gold wires inserted into the scalp, which would surely give an interesting X-ray picture.

But the potential for infection, especially with wire pieces sewn around the scalp, is painfully real. Deep scalp infections are no fun. They travel in devious pus-laden pathways down into the scalp, and treatment may leave considerable scarring and deformity.

Hair transplantation. Hair from the back of the neck will continue to grow if moved to the scalp. That's the principle of hair transplantation, a surgical procedure that has become available in recent years. Plugs of hair, not unlike plugs of grass, are cut from healthy hair on the sides and back of the head and implanted in bald spots. The hair usually falls out after the transplant but regrows in a few months, filling out the ragged look as growth continues. The ultimate head of hair is unlikely to be as luxuriant as in youth, but can still be gratifying.

Quite a few transplants containing hair follicles are necessary, depending on the size of the bald area, and the cost, around $10 per plug, is not trifling. Up to 50 plugs can be implanted at a sitting, and several sessions are usually necessary to cover bald areas satisfactorily. The transplanted hair, once established, is generally permanent.

Fiber implantation is a surgical procedure of implanting colored synthetic fibers into a bald scalp. Practically all of the artificial fibers fall out in a few weeks, and the risk of scalp infection and scarring is considerable. It should not be confused with hair transplantation, described above.

Research. Methods to stimulate hair growth continue to be investigated but are still experimental. Current studies involve materials antagonistic to male hormones for topical application, and progesterone (a female hormone) for injection into the scalp. Some men, however, are reluctant to have their male hormone production tampered with merely for the sake of hair.

Common Female Baldness

Common thinning of the hair in older women has some relationship to hair loss patterns in men, and is often called an androgenic (masculine) type of hair loss. Choosing one's ancestors to eliminate hereditary factors is clearly impossible.

The best defense is to avoid irritations that certainly aggravate hair loss. Repeated assaults on the hair are inflicted by rollers, especially brush rollers, and the practices of teasing, back-combing, and frosting. Permanents given by inept operators also can do much harm to silvered locks of hair.

Certainly, women who wish to avoid acceleration of hair loss as they grow older should treat their hair gently with bland shampoos and rinses. Care should also be taken to avoid rollers and heavy bristle brushes that may break hairs and pull forcefully at the roots.

Wigs and transformations can be worn without harm to the hair, unless they contain some adhesive to which the wearer is sensitive. Natural or synthetic hair is used in wigs, and neither does damage to natural hair. Their objective is to create a natural, unfaked look that does not proclaim "I'm wearing a wig."

Another type of hair loss, now vaguely called patterned hair loss, can occur in young women and even teen-agers. Although little is known about the mechanisms of patterned hair loss, it seems unrelated to hair damage caused by rollers, traction, or other cosmetic abuse.

Too Much Hair

Excessive or superfluous hair is primarily a concern of women, since men are more alarmed by paucity than abundance.

Superfluous hair of the face can be most distressing. Fine downy hairs in mustache areas may scarcely be noticed if they are light-colored, but are conspicuous if dark. If you notice a gradual increase of downy hairs as you get older, the chances are that the change is natural to your constitution, and little if anything can be done to stop the growth.

If excessive hairiness has come on recently and is associated with menstrual disturbances or related symptoms, the possibility of hormone imbalance should be investigated. Unfortunately, it is not common to find a definite cause.

The practical solution is to remove unwanted hairs, or cover them with heavy makeup. Besides the face, legs and armpits are other common sites for removal of unwanted hair.

Pulling out an individual hair—"plucking"—is one hair-removal technique. Another is to apply wax that hardens and pulls hairs out with it. Neither method is permanent, however.

Shaving. Probably the oldest method of removing surface hair is shaving, about which there are many myths. Shaving does not make the hair grow faster, nor does it make the hair more wiry, darker, or thicker in size. An ordinary safety razor is quite satisfactory for most skins if one does not try to cut too deeply. Avoid after-shave lotions, which often dry the skin severely.

Some women prefer creams such as barium sulphide that break off hair in the follicle; the deeper the break, the smoother the result. However, preparations of this type can irritate the skin and should be used with some caution. And as with shaving, the hair returns.

Electrolysis. This technique of hair removal employs an electrical current that travels down a needle adjacent to the hair shaft. A follicle hit by the current is put out of business and its hair will not regrow. But even though the operator uses multiple needles, hardly more than one-fourth of the hairs are effectively removed, since the needle is inserted blindly and burns the skin around it. There are also electrolysis needles that a woman can use herself. Generally, electrolysis is less suited to large hairy areas than local clusters of bristly hairs in public view.

New technologies may yield better methods of permanent hair removal. Ultrasonic devices have been tried with little benefit, but current studies of an epilating probe employing a laser beam look promising.

Coloring the Hair

Many kinds of hair-coloring products are available, ranging from temporary rinses to permanent dyes. The latter are permanent enough, except that the roots of the hair, as it grows, stubbornly retain their native color. Most of the products on the market are carefully tested and are not harmful, and occasional reactions that occur, as with some of the dark dyes, are allergic in nature.

For permanent hair coloring, a skin test should be done before any dye is used. A proper test is not simply dabbing some dye on the ear 15 to 20 minutes before hair coloring, as is the usual practice. A more reliable test is the patch test, in which the dye is put on a spot behind the ear or on the arm, covered, and left for 48 hours. If there is redness, puffiness, or itching when the covering is removed, the tested substance should under no circumstances be used. If you become sensitive to some types of black dyes used in hair washings, you may also react to a number of different colored materials, and—because of a fascinating crossover of materials—even to local anesthetics.

Watch for irritation, burning, itching, redness, and soreness, and advise your cosmetician about this as quickly as possible. If you get allergic reactions, your doctor will have to treat you and warn you what to stay away from in the future.

Trouble from Cosmetics

Cosmetics have been used for centuries and no doubt will be used for centuries to come. Even their use by men is not exactly new—dandies of the past used to powder their wigs and apply pleasing scents.

As a rule, cosmetics sold in the United States are not irritating, sensitizing, or toxic, assuming they're used according to directions on the label or package enclosure (read all cosmetics labels carefully before use).

But everyone's skin is different. Cosmetics may irritate the skin by causing dryness, or more importantly, some safe and commonly used ingredients may produce sensitive or allergic reactions. If so, the likely manifestation would be irritation of the skin, or incitement or aggravation of a rash. A simple test is to stop using a particular cosmetic for a while to see if the rash goes away. Still, however, cosmetics are compounded of dozens of ingredients and you won't know for sure which one you are sensitive to. To determine that, dermatological tests are necessary.

Unless your doctor so advises, cosmetics should never be applied directly to infected or irritated skin, or on top of medications.

Nails

Nails are medically described as flat, translucent, horny plates covering the ends of fingers and toes—hardly a definition of beauty. Nonetheless, in everyday life and especially for women, they are attractive and frequently embellished appendages that cause cosmetic concern if they become brittle, split, or broken at the tips.

Nails are much the same as hair, except that hair grows outward from a point while nails grow outward in a more or less flat horizontal line. Nails, like skin and connective tissue (see page 234), tend to become drier with age (compare your fingernails with a baby's). Many things can dry the nails, such as nail polish or, especially, the solvents in polish removers. Artificial nails applied with plastics of various types also are usually harmful.

The most common nail difficulties—brittleness, vertical or crosswise ridges, white spots, and the like—are usually related to internal conditions, poor circulation, and various deficiencies that can dry the skin and nails. For this reason, the cause should be sought. During such investigation, it is better for women to forgo nail polish. A little calamine lotion can be brushed on the nails to give a bit of glow and polish, or softening creams and medications may be prescribed.

White spots or ridges may persist for some time. You can determine for yourself whether or not a nail is getting better by watching the half-moon, the whitish crescent *(lunula)* at its base. If the portion around the moon gets smoother, it is growing toward the tip of the finger and will gradually get better. It takes about six months for a nail to grow full length, so if spots persist, the chances are that they are permanent markings in the nailbed.

It may seem strange, but it is sometimes very difficult to tell the difference between infection of the nail and dryness. This is true because the nail, like the skin, can react only in limited ways to many different kinds of injury or disease.

Infections are usually red with a blister-like swelling around the nail that is painful and exudes pus. Infection often spreads to other nails. These are problems of people whose hands are much in water and who work with strong chemicals. If fungus infection (ringworm) is suspected, medical care is required, and pieces of the nail and the skin around it are taken for testing.

Psoriasis

Psoriasis affects all ages, but when it first appears after 40, it is especially disturbing. It is a common chronic disease, very mild or quite severe, in which the "turnover" of skin cells is abnormally rapid and profuse. The primary lesion is a reddish flat-topped spot on the skin that becomes covered with an abundance of silvery scales. Affected areas enlarge as patches merge, and underlying skin gets thicker.

The cause of psoriasis is unknown. About one-fourth of all psoriasis patients have a family history of the disease, which suggests some inherited defect in the body's regulation of skin growth. Psoriasis is not dangerous or contagious, and indeed, most patients appear to be vigorously healthy. But profuse shedding of silvery scales is annoying and embarrassing, and patches on exposed skin detract from personal appearance.

Symptoms. An early sign of psoriasis may be stubborn dandruff that will not respond to conventional treatment. Although scalp psoriasis is common, it does not cause hair loss. Other signs may be a lingering rash around the nose and eyebrows, and scaling of the elbows, lower back, and lower leg. Persistence of scaling is characteristic; if scales are scraped off, small bleeding points often appear.

It is important to see a physician if psoriasis is suspected. If the diagnosis is confirmed, susceptibility remains for a lifetime. At times, the scaly patches may virtually disappear, only to return soon or after a very long time. The skin may clear up, stay the same, or become thicker.

Treatment. No miracle cure for psoriasis exists, but relatively new treatments have been developed. Medicines called *psoralens* are taken by mouth, and the whole body is then exposed to ultraviolet (UV-A) light. This is done in centers of dermatology with special equipment, and great care is taken to protect the eyes and the rest of the body. Medicines such as tar and salves may also be used in an effort to reduce the skin's too-rapid turnover time, but much basic research remains to be done in this field.

Persons with psoriasis tend to do better in sunny climates. Often the scaly patches diminish or disappear in summer, but return in winter. Clearly, sunlight has some beneficial effect, and a doctor may recommend judicious sun or sun lamp exposure to particular patients.

Prevention. A definite program to prevent recurrences should begin when the psoriasis is fully cleared. Heavy dandruff can be controlled with a bland oil used in the scalp after shampooing, and a bland cream will prevent dryness around the elbows and knees. When the skin is clear, use hydrophilic salves and creams that can be bought at drugstores. Apply these sparingly while the skin is still wet after washing, then dry. Such preventive treatment must be continued indefinitely to keep the skin clear; otherwise, psoriasis can flare up.

Seborrheic Dermatitis

A common disease about which little is known is seborrheic dermatitis. In a barber shop or beauty salon, one hears innumerable theories about scaling of the scalp. Everyone has a few white scalings. But if greasy scalings are thicker, or if the scalp is red, sore, and crusted, the condition is something more than ordinary dryness, and an infectious process is present.

If you notice a lot of scaling, you should watch around your nose, eyebrows, ears, chest, armpits, and groin because an active infection like seborrheic dermatitis can spread. Effective treatment includes shampoos, as well as daily medication prescribed by a physician that must stay a part of daily hygiene for months after the skin clears.

Intertrigo

Buildup of body fat, not uncommon as we grow older, has an obvious affect on appearance. Body fat can also, by its distribution, contribute to a condition known as *intertrigo*—redness of the skin, rawness, maceration, itching, and plain misery. Fat accumulates in the lower abdomen, between the legs, around the armpits, and in women, under the breasts. These are all areas where opposing skin surfaces rub together.

They are also areas that need ventilation. Obesity produces changes in heat regulation and sweat flow in fat-accumulating areas that easily become hot and sweaty, especially in humid heat waves. As a result of the stagnation of sweat and the friction of rubbing surfaces, normal skin flora, especially the yeasts, make the area "moldy." The skin gets raw and odorous, yeast cells proliferate, and certain types of fungus infections flourish.

Prevention is up to the individual. Diabetics are especially prone to intertrigo, and should try to keep skin-rubbing areas dry and cool. In the early phase, before there is redness and soreness, the skin can be washed with strong soaps, then patted dry and powdered with plain baby talcum powder.

However, if the skin becomes red and sore, simple measures are not effective and may even be uncomfortable. Your dermatologist can prescribe medications that tend to dry the skin. He may recommend the use of cool packs with the legs spread apart, or thin bands of washed linen placed underneath the breasts to keep the area dry. Some of the newer anti-yeast medications also may be prescribed. In general, reduction of weight in the obese helps to prevent recurrent episodes.

"Middle-Age Acne"

By 40, one has outgrown the common acne of adolescence, only to be susceptible to a quite different form that occurs in later years called acne *rosacea*. This takes the form of florid, pus-filled red spots (called "grog blossoms" in colonial America) that develop on the nose and face. Crops of such pustules somewhat resemble acne pimples, but there are no blackheads and usually no past history of acne.

Rosacea develops because of poor circulation and secondary infection, along with another development—a nose that gets redder, larger, coarsened, congested, and lumpy. This conspicuous condition is called *rhinophyma*.

Treatment. The most important aspect of rosacea is the relationship to internal conditions—possible liver disorder, poor digestion, nervousness, and anxiety. Treatment is essentially aimed at control of any factors that may be discovered, and medication to combat infection. The patient is advised to cut down on excessive consumption of strong coffees, teas, and alcohol, which increase flushing of the face. The relationship of bibulosity to rosacea is exemplified by W. C. Fields.

Clues in the Skin Mirror

Without being an expert, you can learn quite a bit from looking at your skin. If a skin eruption is symmetrical—that is, if it occurs on the same place on both legs, arms, or cheeks—the chances are that it originates internally. But if the eruption is in a line, with blisters, it is usually of external origin.

It is best not to irritate a rash until your doctor sees it because the early so-called primary spots often help in the diagnosis. If a rash is just red, it may be merely uncomfortable. But if the rash turns into blisters or bleeding spots, your doctor should examine this more severe reaction.

You can get some immediate relief without using powerful medicines. Do not suspect that every rash you have is ringworm or scabies or something serious. For temporary relief, apply ice cold witch hazel or aluminum acetate, a teaspoonful dissolved in a glass of water.

Drug eruptions can be caused by sensitivity to many common substances: aspirin; phenacetin and many headache medicines; antibiotics; or materials worked with in industry. Eruptions disappear when the offending substances are identified and contact discontinued.

"Sun" rashes. A prevalent kind of skin trouble called *photodermatitis* is caused by the reaction of sunlight with materials you have either applied to the skin, swallowed, or come into contact with. If you have a rash limited to the V of your neck, the cheeks, or outside surfaces of the arms—areas of sun exposure—you may have a photodermatitis.

Things that make your skin sensitive to light may not only come from pills, but also from soaps and perfumes used on the skin. People who work in gardens may know that certain plants, such as spoiled (pink) celery, make their skins sensitive to the sun. Berlock dermatitis is an interesting kind of light reaction that can be seen at lawn parties where lime drinks are prepared. Sprinkles of lime juice on the skin turn first into blisters and then brown spots when exposed to light.

It is important to discover the cause of photodermatitis so you can continue to enjoy the outdoors. Numerous brands of sun protectants are available at drugstores, but any that promises to be completely effective is usually also rather messy. Ingredients that are generally effective are para-aminobenzoic acid, benxophenoes, and methyl anthanilate; look for them on product labels. Sometimes, though, the best treatment for limiting sun exposure is to sit under an elm tree.

Other diseases are made worse by exposure to the sun. One is rosacea, previously described. Another is *lupus erythematosus,* related to rheumatoid arthritis (see page 242). It is sometimes called "butterfly disease" because the rash on the cheeks on either side of the nose resembles a butterfly's wings. Lupus is not a skin disease, but an internal condition with skin manifestations.

A peculiar type of allergy to drugs is the "fixed eruption." One or two brown spots appear anywhere on the body. Then, every time the offending drug is taken, the spots get redder and may even blister and burn, but quiet down again when the drug is stopped. The more frequently the reaction is produced, the darker the skin becomes. Phenacetin, aspirin, and phenolphthalein are often involved in fixed eruptions, and it is the doctor's job to find the exact cause.

Itching

Big itches from small irritations grow. For example, the skin may become a bit dry, mildly uncomfortable, or slightly irritated, causing the temptation to scratch. But the more itching, the more scratching, resulting in a vicious cycle that results in a purely secondary phenomenon known as "nerve itch." Soon scratching is continuous due to central fixation of the symptoms through repeated memory and imprint on the brain. This central fixation process is also evident in "phantom limb," a condition in which amputees feel pain in a limb that has been lost. Scratching without substantial cause can be similarly reinforced, so it is important to relieve itching as much as possible.

After age 40, itching can result from dry skin aggravated by frequent overzealous bathing with strong soaps and hot water, especially in the fall and winter. Unfortunately, this itching often affects the lower leg where poor circulation lowers body tolerance. So, with the onset of cool weather and heated houses, bathing should be reduced. Add oil to bath water and grease the skin frequently, paying special attention to red, rough, or scaly spots. If these are taken care of early, before they itch continuously, they should disappear.

Sometimes a person wakes from a deep sleep to find himself or herself scratching without having been aware of it. This is so-called "habit scratching," which demands detailed attention from patient and doctor to avert a habit that could become intractable.

The Foot: Corns and Warts

Anyone who walks may be distressed and even disabled by painful warts in the soles of the feet. A particularly trouble-some type is the plantar wart, so called because of its location in the forefoot where it is walked on every time one takes a step.

Ordinarily, warts display a small circle or circles in their center. Since warts are virus infections and are contagious, they should be covered. For want of anything else, a wart can be covered with adhesive plaster, plain adhesive, or medicated sali-cylic adhesive.

If there is pressure in the area, as with a plantar wart, it must be relieved if the wart is to heal. However, it's not always easy to eliminate pressure from an area where body weight keeps squeezing a wart, and sometimes an orthopedist must be con-sulted. No wonder some dermatologists would rather treat skin cancer than a pesky wart!

To get rid of the wart itself, there is need for a chemical that kills the virus in the wart without disturbing nearby skin and normal cells, and so far no such chemical exists. Most treatments today involve cau-terizing—removing and burning out the wart. But the wart may recur if infectious particles remain, and the area should be watched for signs of regrowth.

Corns are caused by pressure, usually from shoes. The top of the corn is generally smooth, but if pressure is continued and severe, a small clear spot called a "hen's eye" forms in the center. This area is very tender. Paring the corn gives temporary relief, but there is always recurrence if pressure is not relieved or if poor circulation complicates the healing process.

Painful foot troubles can distort the walk and sitting posture and give rise to pain in the ankles, back, and legs. A doctor should be consulted before such late com-plications appear.

SKIN CANCER
AND PRECANCER

Middle and later life is a time when many people become concerned about skin cancer and its prevention. Skin cancer may develop in the skin or may spread through the skin from the inside. Some types asso-ciated with exposure to the sun are more frequent in the South and Southwest.

As a practical matter, the area to watch for early signs of cancer is the skin above the collar line and below the sleeves. Most people have moles, warty spots, and brown markings without ever developing skin cancer. The suspicious spots are little hard bumps that you never had before but that seem to get larger; also, rough and irritated bits of skin that do not heal. Fortunately, common greasy and brown spots usually mean nothing at all.

The important precancerous spots are the actinic keratoses, previously discussed (see page 36). To repeat, if you have nu-merous keratoses on the face, scalp, or arms, your doctor will prescribe 5-Fluo-rouracil, which peels the skin selectively and improves the spots. If a precancerous spot develops into an invasive cancer of the squamous-cell type, 5-Fluorouracil will not help. Deeper removal is accomplished by surgery, electrosurgery with scraping, or other techniques that the doctor has used with good results. After treatment, a protective program is outlined to minimize solar insult and keep the skin soft.

Leukoplakia. Precancerous lesions occur not only in the skin, but also in mucous membranes of the mouth and genital area. A dentist may be the first to discover patches of white thickened scarring, known as *leukoplakia,* in a patient's mouth. If the white patches are sore, irritated, or bleeding, cancer may be developing. White patches may be secondary to local irritation, as from jagged teeth or ill-fitting dentures, or they may be directly related to smoking.

Tests must be done by the dentist and physician to determine the significance of leukoplakic patches, which may recede if irritations are corrected and smoking is given up.

Basal and squamous cancers. Basal and squamous skin cancers get their names from their respective cell types. Both are potentially invasive, meaning they can burrow and spread. But since their spread is not rapid, early treatment can almost always remove them completely. Although squamous-cell cancer may spread internally, about the only reason for disfigurement or more serious consequences is neglect.

Vital zones where early diagnosis of invasive skin cancer is important include the ears, the nose, eyelids, and around the lips.

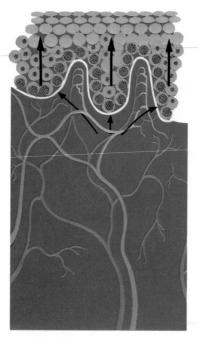
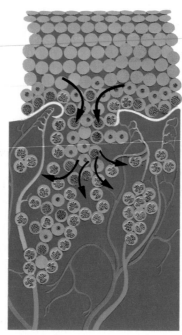

normal cells   cancer cells

INVASIVE CELLS

Normal cells occupy well-defined territories. Cells produced in the germinative layer of the skin (far left) migrate in orderly fashion toward the surface of the skin. Invasive cancer cells grow without restraint and break out of confinement, perhaps because of a defect in some mechanism that sets up territorial boundaries. Cancer cells escape and spread to other parts of the body (metastasis). The rate of growth and spread of different forms of cancer varies greatly. Most skin cancers develop slowly and can be removed completely if recognized early.

Tiny, scaling, thickened spots with a little rim, and spots with a pearly appearance are the important ones to recognize early. It may be necessary to remove a piece of tissue (biopsy) from a suspicious lesion to determine whether or not it is cancerous. This may leave a tiny scar, but one that is well tolerated if the diagnosis is negative. If a small lesion seems to be clearly cancerous to an experienced eye, it may be removed completely and studied later to confirm the diagnosis.

Melanoma. A serious form of cancer is *malignant melanoma,* sometimes called "black cancer," from its location in black or dark spots of the skin. It is not exclusively a skin cancer, since it can originate internally.

Most black areas on the skin mean nothing, being just warty spots or freckling. There is also a deep blue mark that looks like a piece of indelible pencil embedded in the skin. This is the "blue nevus," which only rarely becomes cancerous.

If a black spot develops a little redness, bleeding, or crusting, it should be investigated. See your doctor early if you are concerned or suspicious, and tell him of your anxieties.

Prevention. White skin that tans poorly, as in light-skinned blondes and redheads, is quite vulnerable to long-term damage by the sun. If excessively exposed, such skin tends in time to develop the actinic keratoses previously discussed. Many persons are aware that their skins can't take a bad sun-beating and either limit their exposure as a matter of comfort, or wear sleeves and broad-brimmed hats.

There is no reason to avoid outdoor pleasures. If you have sensitive skin, it's good practice to bathe with a cream soap and to use oils and sun protectants on exposed areas. If brown spots of keratosis begin to appear, keep the skin soft, well greased, and sun protected. This simple measure can often prevent progressive damage and possible subsequent cancerous changes.

A nice thing about skin cancer—if "nice" is a permissible word—is that it occurs where it is readily seen and inspected, leading, unless grossly neglected, to early treatment that affords a gratifyingly high rate of cure.

THE SKIN: TESTS & PROCEDURES

Biopsy. Removal under local anesthesia of a small piece of tissue to assist in diagnosis, especially of infections, precancer, and cancer. A tiny scar may be left.

Patch test. Suspected materials to which a patient may be sensitive are placed on the skin and covered, and then are examined for reactions after 48 hours. Sometimes it is necessary to wear or use the material; this is a *usage test.*

Allergy test. A test performed by an allergist to determine sensitivities, usually to internal materials.

Tests for bacterial, viral, or fungal infections. Small skin scrapings are fixed on slides and stained to determine if there is actual infection. It may be necessary to culture the skin scrapings to identify infectious organisms.

YOUR
HEART
& ITS
PIPELINES

A 40-year-old heart has beat 1½ billion times, give or take a few hundred million beats, and has pushed some 5 million barrels of blood through the body. Although the heart has worked hard, it has rested a lot between beats, too.

All of this is done by an ordinary normal heart with little or no complaint. Still, the heart grows older like the rest of the body, even if the development of abnormalities is usually a slow process.

Many subtle changes cause no apparent symptoms for a long time. Most people at age 50, if not earlier, have some degree of atherosclerosis (accumulation of plaques that narrow the bore of blood vessels) but don't "feel" it. Abnormally high blood pressure causes no symptoms while it is doing damage. Many persons with threateningly high blood pressure don't know they have it or what can be done about it. The uncomplaining heart adapts, enlarges, and works harder until signs of faltering appear.

The heart has great reserves of strength and can rebound from adversities with a little aid. It also takes kindly to improvements in its owner's living habits that can ease its stresses. And in crises, medical and surgical procedures now available very often sustain gratifying recoveries. A good heart at 40 may be good for another 40 . . . 50 . . . 60 years.

Courage is literally a word for the heart.

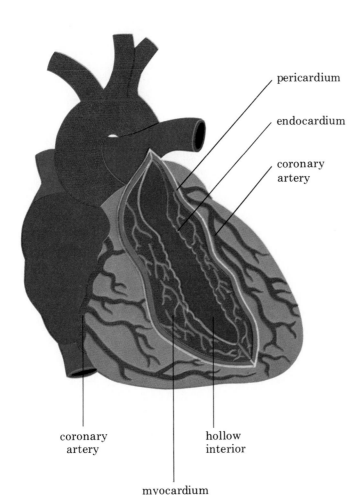

pericardium

endocardium

coronary artery

coronary artery

hollow interior

myocardium

PRIMARY HEART LAYERS

The cutaway view shows the three primary layers of the heart. The pericardium is a thin sac enveloping the heart. The myocardium is the thick specialized muscle of the heart. The endocardium is a membrane lining the interior of the heart. Coronary arteries supply blood to these tissues.

STRUCTURES OF THE HEART

The human heart is a sturdy organ and a rather simple one, compared to the chemical factories of the liver or the unfathomed complexities of the brain. Essentially, it's a pump with valves, a power plant, and an ignition system. Disturbances of the heart are best understood by some knowledge of the parts that are variously affected.

Anatomy. The heart is a hollow organ shaped somewhat like a large pear and situated mainly in the middle of the chest cavity but extending slightly to the left. Immediately below it is the diaphragm, the "breathing muscle," a large sheet that separates the chest and the abdominal cavities.

The heart is always full of blood that continually passes through it. Its outer wall is composed of specialized thick muscle called *myocardium,* as is a central partition or *septum,* which divides the heart into a right and a left side and prevents blood of the two sides from mixing.

Each side of the heart has two hollow chambers, one above the other. The upper chambers are called *atria* (another term is *auricles*). The atria receive blood that enters the heart and pump it into the lower chambers, called *ventricles.* The latter have thick muscular walls, since they do much of the hard work of pumping, particularly the left ventricle which pushes oxygen enriched blood to all parts of the body through the *aorta,* the great vessel that arches from the top of the heart.

Movement of blood between chambers is controlled by valves that snap open and shut at precise intervals to keep blood flowing in one direction and to prevent backflow. Valves of the left side are named *mitral* and *aortic*; of the right side, *tricuspid* and *pulmonary*.

The *pericardium* is a delicate, thin envelope surrounding the heart. The *endocardium* is a smooth layer of cells lining the inside of the heart and valve tissue.

Coronary arteries are small vessels that lie on the surface of the heart somewhat like a crown (hence the name). The coronaries deliver blood to the heart muscle, which cannot make use of blood inside the heart. Connecting with the arteries are still smaller vessels, the capillaries that actually nourish the heart muscle cells. Veins receive "used" blood from the capillaries and return it to circulation.

Rhythms of the heart. In the upper chamber of the right side of the heart, there is a tiny structure called the *sinus node* that controls the rate and rhythm of the heart. It sends out timed electrical impulses, not unlike the distributor of a car, at a rate of about once a second at rest but more rapidly during exercise or excitement. This signal spreads through the muscle of the atria, is picked up by a relay station called the *atrio-ventricular node* situated in the bottom of the right atrium, and then reaches the lower chambers or ventricles via threadlike tissues called conducting *bundles* in the septum, which act like very fine telephone wires.

These are the main structures that, in one way or another, may be involved in heart diseases. If the plumbing and circuits of the heart seem too complicated to understand, one need not feel chagrined. Circulation of the blood was a complete mystery until William Harvey, a British physician, described it fully in 1628. The drawings on the following pages should give some insight.

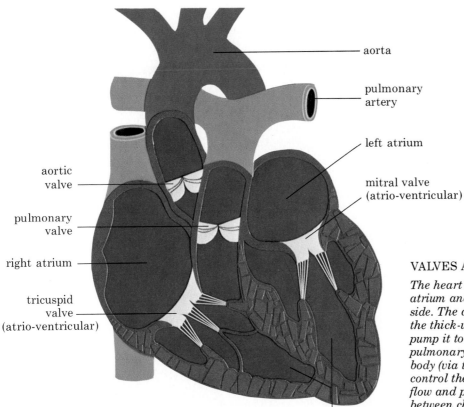

aorta

pulmonary artery

left atrium

mitral valve (atrio-ventricular)

aortic valve

pulmonary valve

right atrium

tricuspid valve (atrio-ventricular)

ventricles

VALVES AND CHAMBERS

The heart has four chambers—an atrium and a ventricle on each side. The atria push blood into the thick-walled ventricles that pump it to the lungs (via the pulmonary artery) and to the body (via the aorta). Valves control the direction of blood flow and prevent leakage between chambers.

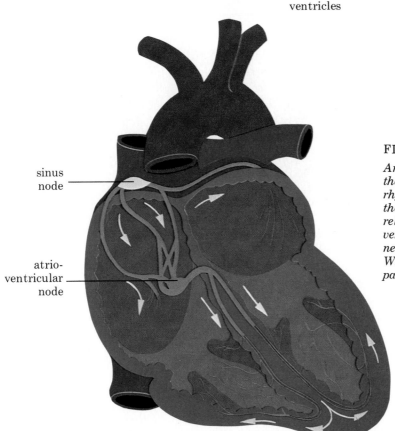

sinus node

atrio-ventricular node

FIRING THE HEART

An "ignition system" stimulates the heart to beat in regular rhythms. Timed impulses from the tiny sinus node spread to a relay station, the atrio-ventricular node, and over finer nerve fibers to the heart muscle. White arrows indicate the pathways of conduction.

Physiology and Function

The purpose of the heart is purely to push blood through the arteries and capillaries and back to the heart. Its complicated-looking plumbing is best understood if we remember that the heart is a two-sided organ. Its right side is solely designed to receive "used," bluish, venous blood, which has picked up waste products in its journey through the tissues, and to pump it to the lungs. There it unloads its wastes and takes on a load of oxygen, becoming bright crimson blood ready for delivery to the left side of the heart and a vitalizing round trip through the body.

In the right side, incoming blood from the veins is received in the right atrium, passed into the right ventricle through the tricuspid valve, and is pumped into blood vessels of the lungs via the pulmonic valve. Exchanges of carbon dioxide and oxygen occur in air sacs of the lungs called alveoli.

Blood that has picked up a new supply of oxygen in the lungs passes to the left side of the heart, is received in the left atrium,

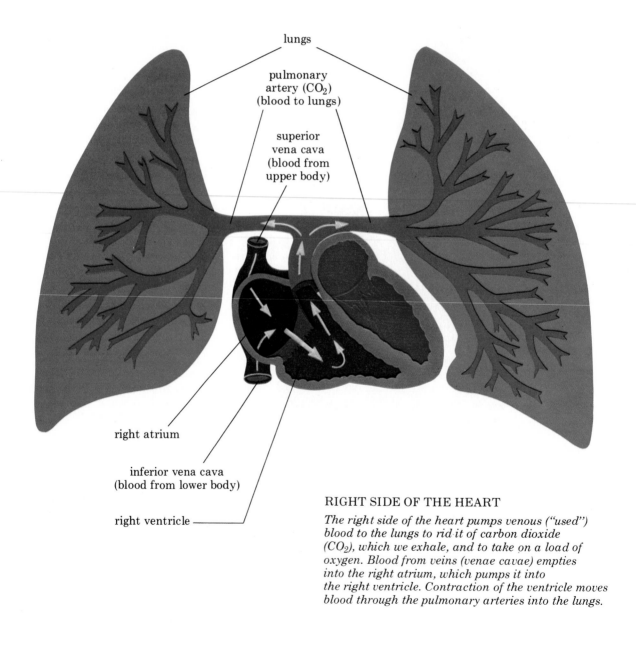

lungs

pulmonary
artery (CO_2)
(blood to lungs)

superior
vena cava
(blood from
upper body)

right atrium

inferior vena cava
(blood from lower body)

right ventricle

RIGHT SIDE OF THE HEART

The right side of the heart pumps venous ("used") blood to the lungs to rid it of carbon dioxide (CO_2), which we exhale, and to take on a load of oxygen. Blood from veins (venae cavae) empties into the right atrium, which pumps it into the right ventricle. Contraction of the ventricle moves blood through the pulmonary arteries into the lungs.

then passes through the mitral valve into the left ventricle and finally is pumped through the aortic valve into the aorta, the great artery that arches from the top of the heart. Thence it travels through progressively smaller and smaller conduits to all parts of the body.

The two atria are mainly receiving chambers, but their muscular walls contract to push blood into the ventricles. The two ventricles have much thicker muscular walls and provide the main pumping force for blood transport.

Fuel delivery. Blood inside the heart cannot nourish the heart muscle, which needs fuel to function. This is provided by an ingenious arrangement. A small portion of arterial blood propelled from the left ventricle via the aortic valve immediately enters two small coronary arteries which divide into several branches that spread over the surface of the heart muscle, delivering oxygen and nutrients to the heart. These vital coronary arteries are comparable to fuel lines delivering gasoline to an engine.

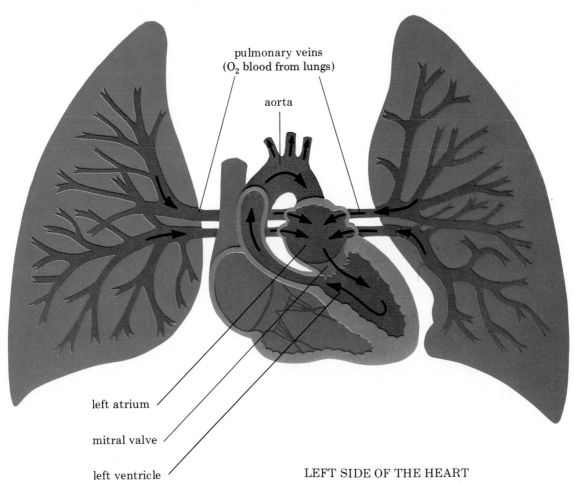

pulmonary veins
(O_2 blood from lungs)

aorta

left atrium

mitral valve

left ventricle

LEFT SIDE OF THE HEART

The left side of the heart is the half-side that pumps fresh arterial blood through the body. Pulmonary veins deliver oxygenated blood (O_2) from the lungs into the left atrium. Blood is pumped through the mitral valve into the left ventricle, which contracts powerfully to propel blood through the aorta to all parts of the body. Black arrows show the directions of flow.

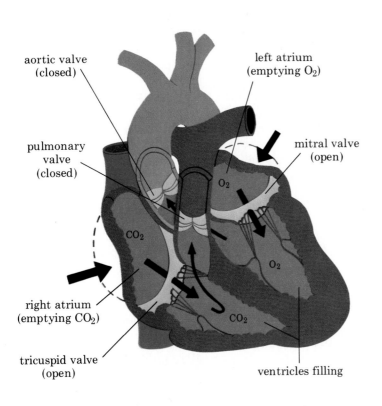

aortic valve
(closed)

left atrium
(emptying O₂)

pulmonary
valve
(closed)

mitral valve
(open)

O₂

CO₂

O₂

right atrium
(emptying CO₂)

CO₂

tricuspid valve
(open)

ventricles filling

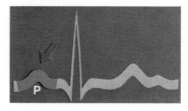

BEGINNING HEARTBEAT

*The first stage of a heartbeat.
Both atria (heavy black arrows)
contract simultaneously,
pumping blood through valves
into their respective ventricles
(CO₂ identifies blood that will go
to lungs; O₂, oxygenated blood
that will go to the body). An
electrocardiogram (ECG)
records the electrical activity of
the heart. Above, atrial
contraction is represented by the
P wave (red arrow).*

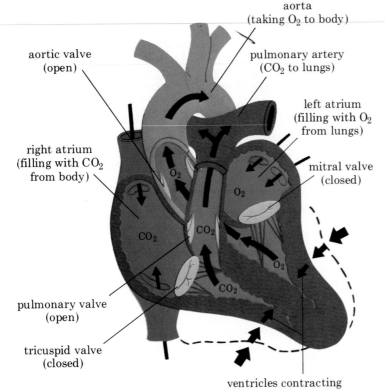

aorta
(taking O₂ to body)

aortic valve
(open)

pulmonary artery
(CO₂ to lungs)

left atrium
(filling with O₂
from lungs)

right atrium
(filling with CO₂
from body)

mitral valve
(closed)

O₂

O₂

CO₂

CO₂

O₂

CO₂

pulmonary valve
(open)

tricuspid valve
(closed)

ventricles contracting

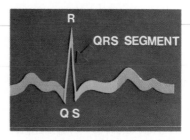

COMPLETED HEARTBEAT

*Following atrial contraction,
both ventricles contract
simultaneously, pumping
oxygenated blood (O₂) to the
body, and venous blood (CO₂) to
the lungs. Valves open and close
to control the direction of flow
and to prevent backflow
(compare with drawing above).
The "big squeeze" of ventricular
contraction registers as a spike
(QRS segment) on the
electrocardiogram pattern
shown above.*

Statistics of the heart are impressive. The adult heart, about the size of your fist, weighs 10 to 12 ounces; the left side is slightly heavier. Pressure inside the left ventricle is about 130 millimeters of mercury when the heart contracts, compared to about 24 millimeters of mercury inside the right ventricle—a fivefold difference. About 4 percent of the blood ejected by the left ventricle empties into the coronary arteries to feed the heart muscle, 30 percent is delivered to muscles of the body, 25 percent goes to assist digestion, and 20 percent travels to the brain.

The amount of blood ejected at rest by the left ventricle is about six quarts a minute for a six-foot 170-pound man. A trained athlete may pump as much as 25 quarts a minute. Finally, the heart may beat as fast as 200 times a minute with very vigorous exercise by a physically fit adult.

How a Doctor Rates Your Heart

When a doctor wants to know how a heart is performing, he asks wide-ranging questions of the patient. A complete history of current and past symptoms and illnesses is of the utmost importance. Indeed, more useful information is provided by a properly taken history than by any other measure. The interview should include matters of diet, habit, exercise, use of alcohol, smoking, psychological factors, and consideration of diseases or causes of death of family members.

A complete physical examination is a second and essential approach to the study of heart problems. "Complete" means just that, for both the history and physical examination. Evidences of thyroid disease, lung difficulties, diseases of the leg veins, and other conditions may be very significant in relation to heart trouble. The doctor will observe how you breathe, what your color is like, and will take your pulse and blood pressure.

Particular attention will be paid to any distention of the neck veins, and the doctor will listen to sounds over your lungs with a stethoscope, an instrument that transmits sounds from the chest to the ears via tubing. He will also "percuss" you, by tapping with the middle or index finger upon the fingers of the other hand that rest upon the chest wall, and he will feel the chest for heart impulses. These maneuvers give an estimate of the size of your heart.

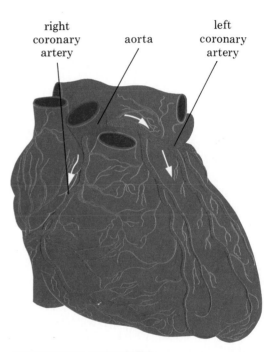

right coronary artery   aorta   left coronary artery

CORONARY ARTERIES

Coronary arteries, which encircle the heart like a crown, nourish the heart muscle (blood inside the heart is not available to the muscle). Two major arteries, the left and right coronaries, emerge from either side of the aorta and branch into progressively smaller vessels that spread over and into the entire heart muscle.

Sounds of your heart. Every heart makes "noises" while it works. These can be heard and differentiated through the stethoscope. A normal heart gives rise to two distinct short sounds—something like *lubb-dubb,* if you can spell a sound—when its valves open and close. If something is abnormal, the sounds may be altered or sounds that shouldn't be there are heard.

Murmurs are a series of long sounds occurring between the normal short heart sounds, often having a musical quality. Murmurs may at times occur in normal hearts, but they often indicate a disturbance of one or more heart valves.

There are many other tests and procedures in studying the heart; the most common are described on page 90.

VARIETIES OF DISORDER

What can go wrong with the heart? Some troubles arise from physical changes of heart structures. Others are functional—that is, structures are intact, but they misbehave or don't work together harmoniously. Specific disorders will be discussed later, but it may be helpful to review briefly some common categories of ills of the heart.

Abnormal heartbeat. The heartbeat rate is either too slow or too fast, making the heart less efficient. Examples: very slow rates of 20 to 40 beats a minute, or sustained very rapid rates, especially if over 150 beats per minute or even over 200 for short periods.

Rhythm upsets. Harmonious rhythms of the heart are disturbed so that pumping efficiency is decreased. Examples: *atrial fibrillation,* in which the upper chambers of the heart beat very rapidly but ineffectively; and complete *atrioventricular block,* in which contraction of the upper chambers is "out of sync" with contraction of the lower chambers.

Fuel line problems. Circulation of blood to the heart muscle is reduced so it cannot easily pump more blood when demanded by exercise or emotion. Example: coronary artery disease, in which vessels nourishing the heart muscle are narrowed or obstructed, slowing the flow of blood.

Muscle damage. Output of the heart is less than normal because of heart muscle disease. Examples: inflammation of the heart muscle (myocarditis) in rheumatic fever; loss of heart muscle and its replacement by scar tissue, as with a heart attack; damage to the heart muscle produced by a toxic substance such as alcohol.

Faulty valves. The heart is inefficient because of faulty opening and/or closing of its valves. Examples: rheumatic heart disease in which the valves may be damaged; syphilitic heart disease; heart trouble due to birth defects.

Defects. The heart may be inefficient because of "holes" in its central wall or septum. Example: birth defects in the septum between the upper or lower chambers.

Overwork. The heart has to work unduly hard to pump out blood because of increased resistance in arteries into which the blood is being ejected. Example: high blood pressure *(hypertension)* in which the heart muscle may become weakened from overwork.

Nevertheless, the heart muscle has great strength and large reserves of power, and can tolerate unfavorable circumstances for long periods of time without complaining.

HEART FAILURE

The terms *heart failure, decompensation,* and *congestive heart failure* are frequently used to describe the inability of the heart to do its work properly as a result of any of the above conditions. What do these terms mean? Essentially, that the great pump works hard but ultimately cannot propel enough blood to satisfy the body's needs. It begins to show fatigue.

Symptoms

Some symptoms of a failing heart are recognized by a doctor; others by the patient. Usually the heart is enlarged by its efforts to keep up with a heavy work load. At times, an abnormal sound, called a third sound, may be heard through a stethoscope. And, veins in the neck may be prominent because blood returning to the heart is not pushed forward efficiently.

The patient may complain of shortness of breath because the lungs are congested—again, because blood is not propelled forward normally. It backs up under increased pressure in the lungs. The abdomen, the liver within it, and the legs may swell due to the same factors.

Treatment

Heart failure does not mean that the organ is never going to recover. On the contrary, the condition is serious, but there are many measures to relieve it.

Simple rest programs are often greatly beneficial. Restriction of salt in the diet (specifically, the sodium component of table salt) may be advised. Sodium is an element that tends to hold water in the

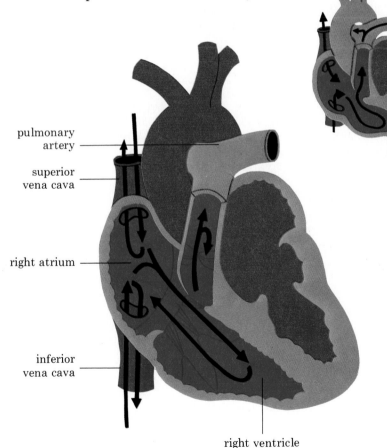

normal
circulation

pulmonary
artery

superior
vena cava

right atrium

inferior
vena cava

right ventricle

CONGESTIVE FAILURE

Congestive heart failure results from weakening of the heart as a pump, so it cannot propel enough blood to satisfy body needs. Either the left or right pumping chambers (ventricles) may be predominantly affected. The large drawing shows a congestive backup of venous blood in the right side of the heart, which may engorge organs to cause swelling of the abdomen, liver, or legs ("dropsy"). Compare this with the small drawing of normal right-sided circulation. Failure of the left side is likely to cause shortness of breath.

tissues. Moderate restriction can be attained by omitting salt in the preparation of foods or at the table, and by recognizing foods that have a high or low sodium content (see page 87).

Medicines. Extremely rigid low-sodium diets, difficult to follow, are prescribed less frequently since the advent of modern diuretic drugs. These are medicines that increase the loss of water from the body, lessen the burden on the heart, and diminish such signs as swollen legs and ankles.

Another often-prescribed drug is *digitalis.* Digoxin and digitoxin are forms of digitalis. The major effect of digitalis is to increase the strength and velocity of contractions of the heart muscle. Pumping power is thus enhanced.

A doctor's supervision is necessary in administering such drugs, which are not wholly innocuous. For instance, the toxic dose of digitalis is quite close to the effective dose. The dose must be individualized and, after initial determination, must be adjusted to maintenance levels. Digitalis may cause loss of appetite, nausea, and diarrhea. Another disconcerting effect of digitalis occasionally seen in male patients is enlargement of the breasts, which the patient may feel is cancer. It is not; the molecules of digitalis and sex hormones simply have some chemical similarities.

Long-term use of powerful diuretics may sometimes cause excessive loss of potassium, an electrolyte essential to many body processes, such as interaction with sodium in the transmission of nerve impulses. Heart patients are quite sensitive to potassium deficiency. Common foods, especially meat and fruits (see page 153), ordinarily furnish ample potassium to a healthy person, but drug-induced losses may be so severe as to require a potassium supplement. Excessively high levels of potassium in the blood can also be hazardous, and your doctor will be watchful of these possibilities.

Treatment of high blood pressure (see page 65) may take a big load off the heart and also help to relieve symptoms of heart weakness. Congenital defects and valve disease are often greatly improved with surgery, thus relieving heart failure. The heart indeed has an extraordinary ability to recover its pumping power with help.

It should be emphasized that symptoms of shortness of breath and swelling of the lower legs, ankles, and feet are by no means always due to heart failure. "Breathlessness" is often attributable to overweight, lung disease, and poor physical condition. Puffy legs and ankles are common consequences of prolonged standing, of sitting with the legs dependent, as in a bus or car, or of disorders of veins in the legs.

DISORDERS OF RHYTHM

What should your rate of heartbeat be? There is no single ideal rate. As a healthy adult, your heart may beat 50 times a minute while you sleep, 55 times while you awaken sluggishly, 60 times after eating breakfast, and 70 or 80 times during examination by a physician. Exercise, eating, and emotion all increase the heart rate, as do many illnesses such as infections, anemia, and overactivity of the thyroid gland. Long distance runners may have as few as 40 beats a minute. All of these are within the normal range.

We have already described the natural pacemaker that sparks the rhythms of the heart (see page 52). This remarkable electrical conductivity system can get out of kilter in several ways. Some symptoms may be scary but harmless; others are of more serious portent.

Too Fast

The word *tachycardia* is used to describe rapid beating of the heart, 100 or more beats per minute. You have doubtless experienced the kind called *sinus tachycardia* many times. Those big medical words merely mean that your heart responds to an increased number of electrical impulses arising from the sinus node—a healthy response to the normal rate-controlling mechanism speeded by exercise. You run fast, your heart beats fast.

Another kind of rapid beating—called *atrial tachycardia*—usually 150 to 200 regular beats per minute—can be quite frightening. Here the rapid beating comes from electrical impulses arising in the upper chambers of the heart, outside of the normally controlling sinus node. Attacks may come on suddenly and stop suddenly after minutes or hours. This kind of fast beating is common and rarely serious.

Atrial *flutter* and atrial *fibrillation* are also quite common. Here the upper chambers of the heart beat with great rapidity, 200 to 600 times a minute. Only a portion of these beats passes to the lower chambers so that these main pumps beat more slowly than the atria. The heart rate is usually rapid and the rhythm is often irregular. The medical terms may cause great anxiety in a patient who misconstrues them to mean that his heart is flapping wildly and may stop at any minute. The condition could be more comfortingly described as variations in heart rhythm, which may often occur without known cause but also may be present in various types of heart disease and with overactivity of the thyroid gland.

Management of the above conditions is accomplished by drugs such as digitalis, quinidine, and procainamide, and with electric devices that shock the heart back into a normal rhythm.

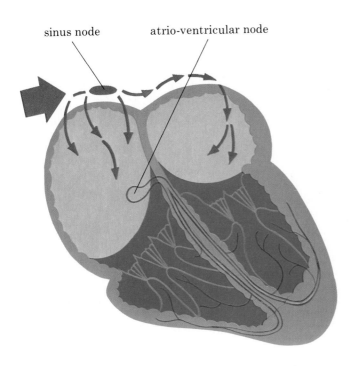

sinus node   atrio-ventricular node

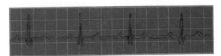

Normal EKG (60 beats per minute).

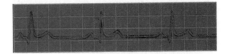

Sinus bradycardia (too slow). Less than 60 beats per minute.

Sinus tachycardia (too fast). More than 100 beats per minute.

HEART RHYTHM

The sinus node normally regulates the rate of heartbeat—for example, your heart beats faster when you jog or are excited. However, various disturbances of the sinus node (red arrow) may cause irregularities of rhythm.

"Skipped Beats"

The most common irregularity of the heart is that of premature beats or extra-systoles, often described by a patient as "skipped beats" because a beat seems to have been missed. What happens is that a beat comes earlier than expected in the heart cycle. At a rate of 60 beats per minute, there should be one second between beats. However, a premature beat may come one-half second after the preceding beat. This delays the next expected beat and is felt as an abnormally long pause.

The sensation described by patients is that the heart seems to "skip" or "jump," and after the skip, seems to stop momentarily. In words of the song, "my heart stood still." This premature beat may arise anywhere in the heart and is usually a single occurrence, but at times there may be several in succession.

Premature beats are exceedingly common events that often give rise to anxiety and alarm, usually needlessly. The vast majority are benign occurrences, not associated with organic disease, not in any way life-threatening, and requiring no treatment. In some persons they seem more frequent with fatigue or tension. If very frequent or if associated with significant heart muscle disease, they may require drug treatment.

Too Slow

A very slow heart rate *(bradycardia)* is not at all uncommon in older people. It may be associated with a disease (of unknown cause) of the bundle of pacemaker cells in the upper right chamber of the heart that trigger the heartbeat, or may be caused by "heart block"—interference with

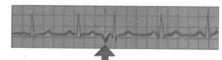

NORMAL HEARTBEAT

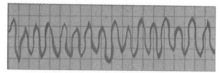

SKIPPED (PREMATURE) BEAT
A beat occurs before it normally would (green arrow) and the delay before the next beat is felt as if a beat were skipped or obliterated.

VENTRICULAR FIBRILLATION
Wild, rapid powerless quivering of the ventricle cannot effectively pump blood to the body.

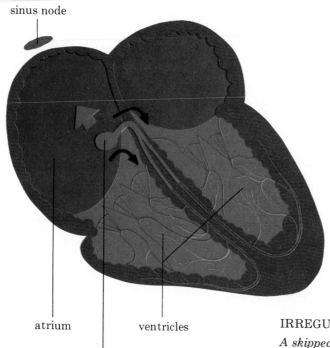

sinus node

atrium   ventricles

atrio-ventricular node

IRREGULAR HEARTBEATS

A skipped beat, usually harmless, is thought by some physicians to be caused by feedback from the AV node (green arrow). Ventricular fibrillation is a serious emergency, most often occurring in heart attacks or during surgery. Timely application of a defibrillating machine can usually shock the heart out of its standstill.

the downward passage of electrical impulses to the pumping chambers. The rate may be as slow as 20 to 30 beats per minute so that circulation of the blood is well below normal.

Not surprisingly, there are symptoms: weakness, light-headedness, dizziness, undue fatigue, exhaustion, lassitude, and even fainting or blackout spells. It is in this situation that artificial pacemakers are remarkably helpful.

Implanted Pacemakers

An artificial pacemaker is a battery-powered device about the size of a woman's compact. Besides batteries, it contains timing and responding elements. Its task is to deliver a properly timed electric charge that stimulates the heart to contract and push out an invigorating surge of blood.

Some pacemakers run steadily at a preset rate, but these are rarely used today. Much more common are the "demand" types. These go into action only when the heart's own rate of beating is inadequate.

How is a pacemaker connected with a beating heart? The necessary surgery takes about an hour and is done under local anesthesia. The unit is implanted under the skin of the upper chest (or it can be implanted in the abdomen). A fine wire from the unit is passed into and down a vein and thence through the right atrium into the right ventricle of the heart. The tip of the wire rests in contact with the wall of the right ventricle. The electrical impulse from the battery travels down the wire to the point of contact with the right ventricle. The impulse then leaks from the tip of the wire and stimulates the entire heart muscle to contract forcefully.

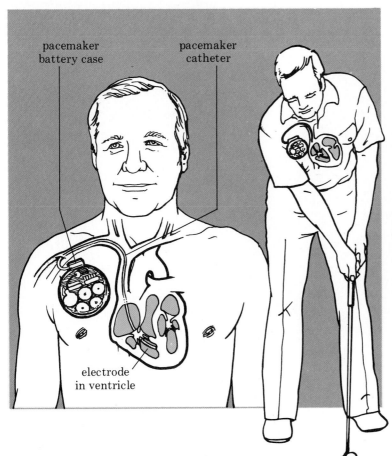

pacemaker
battery case

pacemaker
catheter

electrode
in ventricle

IMPLANTED PACEMAKER

The thin wire electrode of an implanted pacemaker is usually passed down the jugular vein just above the collarbone and thence into the right atrium and right ventricle, where its tip is in contact with the ventricle wall. The battery pack is usually implanted under the skin of the chest, and is not an impediment to a physically active life.

If the heart beats too slowly—below a predetermined rate of 65 times a minute, perhaps—the sensing mechanism of the pacemaker is activated and the battery discharges 65 times per minute. When the patient's own heart recovers and equals or exceeds the 65-beat threshold, the battery pacemaker shuts off until it is needed again. This very ingenious automatic device not only protects persons who have an intermittent slow heart, but becomes a permanent means of maintaining a more normal heart rate in those who constantly have very slow rates.

Types of pacemakers. Models differ in their power plants and refinements. Different types of batteries are available, all of which may be tested to see if they are "running down," and even a few nuclear-powered pacemakers have been implanted in patients.

Modern pacemakers are well shielded against outside electrical interference that might disturb their operation. There need be no apprehension whatever about interference from ordinary household appliances, radios, television sets, cars or airplanes. Possible leakage from a microwave oven is a matter to be discussed with your physician. In general, pacemakers have proved to be remarkably effective and safe.

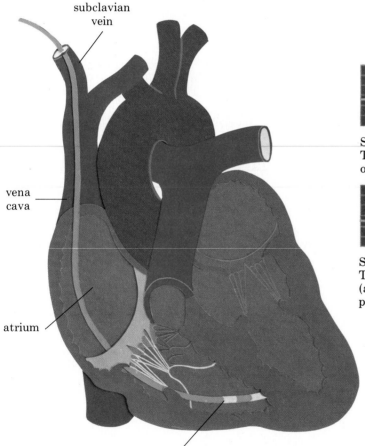

subclavian vein

vena cava

atrium

pacemaker electrode seated in ventricle

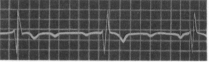

SLOW HEARTBEAT
The electrocardiogram shows a rate of 28 beats per minute.

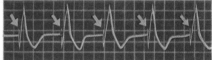

STIMULATED BEAT
Timed stimuli from the pacemaker (arrows) increase the rate to 60 beats per minute.

ELECTRODE PLACEMENT

This cutaway view shows the electrode of an artificial pacemaker in contact with the wall of the right ventricle. Most pacemakers are of the demand type, which go into action only when their sensors detect that the heart's own rate of beating is inadequate. Replacement of the battery pack is an operation that does not invade the heart.

An artificial pacemaker costs anywhere from $1,500 to $5,000 for exotic nuclear types that are not generally available but may become so as technology progresses. Their cost can be spread over the term of the manufacturer's warranty, commonly three or more years.

Living with a Pacemaker

Should you ever need an artificial pacemaker you will, if you are like most patients, be up and walking around the hospital the day after implantation. There will be a small flat bulge under the skin of your chest, undetectable under ordinary clothing, and the discolored suture lines will soon disappear. In a few weeks, you won't be as conscious of the device as you are of the watch on your wrist—less so, in fact, for the pacemaker is safe from fiddling and attention.

It's only natural to feel strange about a device that keeps your heart turned on properly, but this feeling disappears in a few weeks as continuously normal heartbeats sustain faith in technology. Probably the worst worry is over sudden battery failure. Will the heart stop dead? No. But the resulting symptoms of fatigue, dizziness, and slow pulse indicate that prompt checkup by your doctor is in order.

Batteries do run down and require periodic replacement every two to six years, a matter of a few days' stay in a hospital. The heart is not entered. The battery pack is replaced, wires thoroughly checked, and the skin covering is sewn back in place. To anticipate the need to replace batteries, the heart rate and rhythm and function of the pacemaker unit are checked periodically by the physician, through special pacemaker clinics, or even by regular telephone service.

Is a pacemaker a handicap to living the good life? The general condition of the heart and the patient's drives and interests have something to do with it. But the usual effects are a return of energies for preferred activities, and especially, freedom from spells of weakness or fainting. There are almost no limitations to an active life unless the heart is otherwise impaired or other disease is present.

HIGH BLOOD PRESSURE

(Hypertension)

Your blood pressure at 40 or 50 is almost surely a little higher than it was at 20. Blood pressure increases naturally with age. This does not mean that excessively high blood pressure, which doctors call hypertension, is normal or inevitable. But it is all too common, to some degree afflicting perhaps 20 percent of adults, at least half of whom don't know they have it.

Hypertension can seriously affect young people, but it's more common with advancing age. Although about 75 percent of hypertensives are over 40, many aren't recognized until their 50s and 60s. Hypertension is associated with obesity, with diabetes to some extent, and is more common among blacks than whites. And, it is more frequent in men than in women before the age of 50; after 50, women tend to have more hypertension.

Silent threats. High blood pressure is rarely listed as a cause of death. Its threat lies in the complications it may cause. It has been called the "silent disease" because it usually causes no distress while, over periods of time, it inflicts hidden damage on vital organs, notably the brain, heart, and kidneys.

Hypertension is a potent factor in promoting hardening of the arteries and often is an underlying condition in heart attacks. It is also associated with types of strokes (see page 115)—damage to and clotting in an artery of the brain, or actual rupture of an artery with bleeding in the brain.

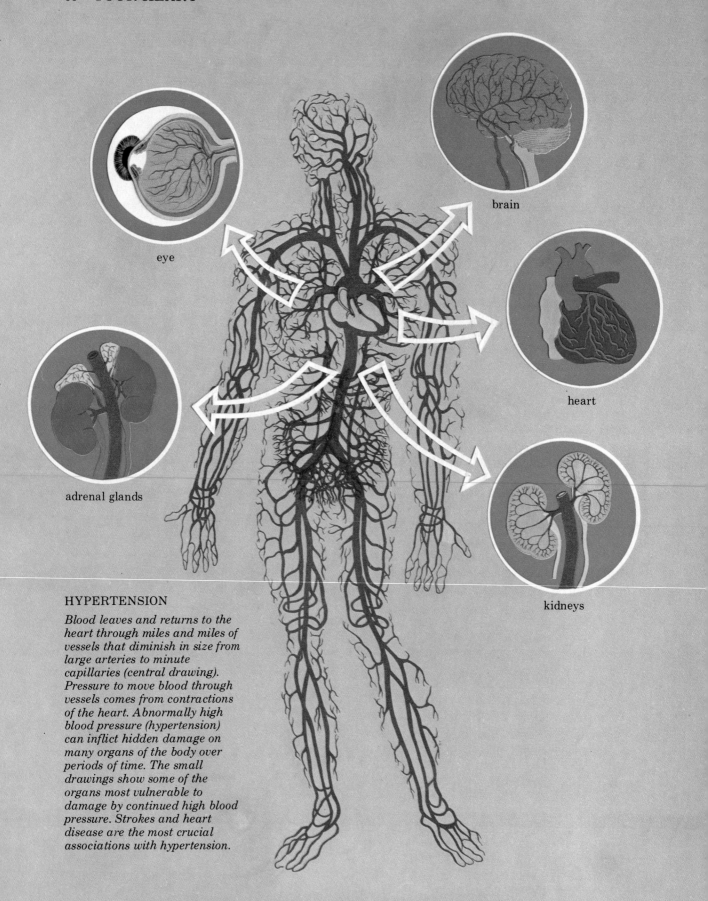

eye

brain

heart

adrenal glands

kidneys

HYPERTENSION

Blood leaves and returns to the heart through miles and miles of vessels that diminish in size from large arteries to minute capillaries (central drawing). Pressure to move blood through vessels comes from contractions of the heart. Abnormally high blood pressure (hypertension) can inflict hidden damage on many organs of the body over periods of time. The small drawings show some of the organs most vulnerable to damage by continued high blood pressure. Strokes and heart disease are the most crucial associations with hypertension.

High blood pressure may put severe strain on the heart muscle and damage the blood vessels of the eyes and kidneys, but the crucially important associations are with strokes and heart attacks.

A small percentage of cases of high blood pressure are attributable to physical conditions: inflammation and scarring of the kidneys, reduced blood supply to one or both kidneys, disease of the adrenal glands, and congenital blockage of the main artery leaving the heart. Some of these are correctable by surgery. But the great majority of cases are classed as essential hypertension, which doesn't mean that it is a necessary condition, just that the cause is presently unknown.

Symptoms. There are no symptoms at all in the vast majority of patients with hypertension. One cannot recognize the condition by a red face or obesity or fatigue or headaches or dizziness. It is recognized by the blood pressure reading, which indicates whether or not there is a need for studies or treatment.

When is pressure too high? There is no absolute division between normal and abnormally high blood pressure, no reading that is normal for everyone. Blood pressure rises with activity—even a simple one like standing up—and falls with rest. It also rises with anger, fright, and emotions.

In a blood pressure value expressed, let us say, as 140/90, the larger figure always represents systolic pressure, or the peak of pressure in the arteries when the heart contracts to pump blood. The smaller figure is the diastolic pressure, measured when the heart relaxes to fill with blood and rest between beats. Diastolic pressure is the measure of constant minimal pressure in the arteries.

In general and at any age, the systolic reading (the peak of pressure in the artery when the heart contracts) is desirably below 140 millimeters of mercury, and the diastolic pressure is desirably below 90. There is evidence that even lower values are favorable to longevity. Generally, the higher the blood pressure, the greater the possibility that hypertension may in time do harm to vital organs.

Predictions should not be made on the basis of a single blood pressure value. Several readings should be taken on different occasions to evaluate the outlook and possible need for treatment. Apprehension may push blood pressure to a higher than usual level when one is examined by a physician. Nevertheless, it is clear that an isolated high reading has important implications. Pressure may be 180/110 in a doctor's office and 140/90 when a patient has been lying in bed for some hours. This does not mean that the only value of significance is 140/90. On the contrary, the reading of 180/110 is in the long run most significant as to the likelihood of damage to health from hypertension.

Treatment. There is no cure for essential hypertension, the common variety of unknown cause. But in almost all cases, treatment is very effective in controlling the condition permanently, preventing complications, and generally making high blood pressure quite compatible with an active life.

There is one caveat: if treatment is needed, it must almost always be continued indefinitely for the rest of one's life. This is not necessarily an intolerable burden. Often it's simply a matter of remembering to take a pill a day.

If a patient is distinctly obese, a first approach is weight reduction. Excess fat means extra miles of vessels for blood to press through. Reducing weight may reduce blood pressure as well.

The role of dietary salt in hypertension has been investigated and debated for years. Extremely rigid low-salt diets are almost a thing of the past, largely because diuretic drugs do the job better and certainly more comfortably. But high salt intake is still quite undesirable. At present, it doesn't appear that a low salt intake will by itself lower elevated blood pressure adequately, or ensure against developing hypertension. However, most physicians advise against generous use of salt at the table and in food preparation. There are fairly satisfying salt substitutes, such as potassium chloride, that are available without a prescription.

Anti-hypertensive drugs. In addition to weight loss, the mainstay of therapy is medicines. There are a large number of useful drugs with different actions upon the diverse mechanisms of hypertension, and it is indeed rare when a physician cannot reduce a patient's blood pressure with well-chosen drugs.

Often the first drug to be prescribed is a diuretic that promotes the loss of water, sodium, and potassium. Since potassium loss is undesirable, diuretics are frequently combined with agents to reduce potassium loss, with potassium supplements, or with a diet high in potassium (see page 153). At times, diuretics may be sufficient to bring moderate hypertension under control.

Other drugs, singly or in combination, are highly effective in reducing blood pressure, and there is persuasive evidence that continued control prevents premature complications and death. No single drug is ideal; all have potential side effects. Frequently a single drug is ineffective, but in combination with one or two others, blood pressure may be reduced. It may take a period of trial and observation to determine what drug or combination is best for a patient, but it is practically certain that an effective choice can be made.

Life-style. Treatment of high blood pressure imposes few restrictions in the pursuit of work and pleasure, within the limits of one's physical condition. You can continue to play tennis if you're used to it, or golf or bowl if milder exercise is advised. Some specific diet suggestions may be made, and if you smoke cigarettes, you will be admonished to stop, since smoking and high blood pressure make an exceptionally bad combination. Frequent visits to the doctor will be necessary during the initial period of adjustment to treatment, and during this period you may not feel your best. Thereafter, as far as pressure is concerned, checkups three or four times a year are usually sufficient.

Probably the greatest threat to patients is the temptation to stop necessary treatment altogether. Daily pill-taking can be a bore. The patients feel good, and treatment may give an illusion of cure. But crippling or lethal complications may be ten or 20 years in the future.

For whatever reason, surprising numbers of patients drop out of treatment while hidden damage to organs goes on relentlessly. What is needed is better understanding of the seriousness of hypertension, its nature, and the effectiveness of treatment when it is followed faithfully by the patient.

Surgery is little employed today to control high blood pressure. It's limited to special circumstances, such as disease of one kidney, tumor of an adrenal gland, or a congenital block of the aorta.

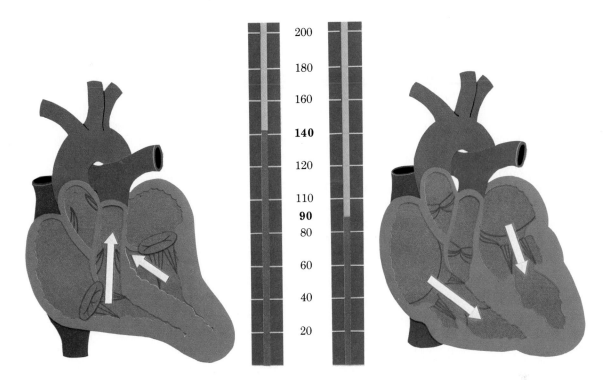

SYSTOLIC PRESSURE

Systolic pressure is the peak of pressure when the heart contracts to force blood into its pipelines. Pressure is measured by the rise, in millimeters, of a column of mercury (in the drawing, 140 mm).

DIASTOLIC PRESSURE

Diastolic pressure is the constant minimum pressure when the heart relaxes and fills its chambers. The column of mercury reads 90 mm; the combined reading, 140/90.

HOW A DOCTOR
READS BLOOD PRESSURE

Blood pressure is measured by pumping air into and out of an inflatable rubber cuff wrapped around the patient's upper arm. Pressures conducted through a tube register in millimeters of mercury on a manometer, which is somewhat like a tire pressure gauge.

A physician reads blood pressure by pumping air into the cuff while listening with a stethoscope placed below the bag. He inflates the cuff until pressure stops blood flow in an underlying artery and pulse sounds cannot be heard. Then he re-

leases air until the beat can again be heard. At this point, the gauge registers the peak of blood pressure (systolic pressure). He then releases more air until the artery is fully dilated and the sounds disappear. The gauge then registers the lower (diastolic) pressure. Blood pressure varies in normal healthy people and in the same person at different times, as when sleeping or exercising. Pressures vary from time to time, and repeated readings are usually taken if a diagnosis of hypertension is under consideration.

VALVE TROUBLE

Valves inside the heart (four of them) are floodgates that open to permit blood to flow in one direction and close to confine blood briefly in the appropriate heart chamber. The principle is something like that of a canal lock. A heart valve opens and closes 35 to 40 million times a year. Abnormalities of one or more valves may be of little consequence or may create serious problems. A valve may become narrowed or scarred so it cannot open wide enough to let blood through at a normal rate. Or it can become so flabby and stretched that its flaps cannot close tightly. It is then said to "leak," which doesn't mean that blood leaks from the heart into the chest cavity, but that there is slippage or regurgitation where there should be a tight valve lock. The faulty valve produces sounds that can be detected with a stethoscope.

Rheumatic Fever

Rheumatic fever is a disease of children and young people, rarely occurring after 30. Its significance to older persons is that long-term damage to the heart may not be seriously evident until years after the acute attack.

Acute rheumatic fever—which typically causes fever, fatigue, and hot, red, swollen, very painful joints at an elbow, wrist, knee, or ankle—is now uncommon in the United States. The disease is associated with infection by a common form of bacteria (beta hemolytic streptococcus), but is not directly caused by such infection. Rather, in susceptible persons, infection is followed in two or three weeks by a sensitivity reaction in the tissues. It is this altered sensitivity or allergic reaction that provokes rheumatic fever.

If a young person has a "strep throat" infection, and a culture identifies the beta hemolytic streptococcus bacteria, prompt treatment with an antibiotic, usually penicillin, will prevent rheumatic fever from developing. Prevention of recurrences after an attack of rheumatic fever is very important, as each recurrence may further damage the heart. This is accomplished by a regular program of medication, such as a daily dose of an antibiotic or a monthly injection of a long-lasting form of penicillin.

Target: the heart. Probably half of all rheumatic fever cases involve the heart. Joint complaints and other symptoms are transient and leave no permanent damage, but the heart is critically important. Its muscle mass, its inner lining, and its outer covering may be moderately or severely involved. Today, acute rheumatic heart disease is fortunately rare.

More important are long-term or chronic effects on the heart. When the acute process quiets down, it may leave a low-grade type of active inflammation as well as permanent scarring of the heart muscle and valves.

Most liable to damage are the two valves of the left side of the heart, the mitral and aortic valves. The tricuspid valve in the right side of the heart is not often involved, and there is no significant change in the pulmonic valve. Especially vulnerable is the mitral valve through which freshened blood from the lungs enters the left ventricle where it is pumped through the aortic valve to the body. Chronic effects tend to be leakage (regurgitation) of the mitral and aortic valves, and over the years, progressive valve deformity with scarring and gradual narrowing (stenosis).

There can be other forms of acquired valvular disease of obscure origin, and today a leakage of the mitral valve due to a type of degeneration making it "floppy" is often seen, which is not the result of rheumatic fever. An older patient may have no memory or apparent history of rheumatic fever, but an attack may not have been properly recognized at the time of its occurrence years before.

HOW HEART VALVES FUNCTION

*Four valves inside the heart control filling,
emptying, and the direction of blood flow. The
tricuspid valve in the right side of the heart and
the mitral valve in the left side control the flow
from atria to ventricles. The pulmonary valve
controls the flow of venous blood to the lungs; the
aortic valve, the flow of arterial (oxygen-laden)
blood to all parts of the body.*

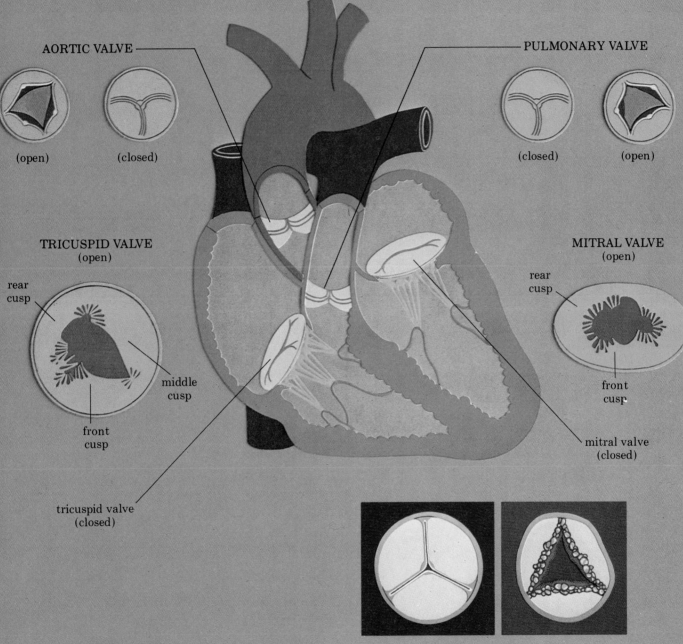

AORTIC VALVE

(open)   (closed)

PULMONARY VALVE

(closed)   (open)

TRICUSPID VALVE
(open)

rear
cusp

middle
cusp

front
cusp

tricuspid valve
(closed)

MITRAL VALVE
(open)

rear
cusp

front
cusp

mitral valve
(closed)

TRICUSPID VALVE

At left, a healthy tricuspid valve is shown in its
closed position. Its three leaflets open to permit
full flow of blood and close to seal tightly against
backflow. At right is a scarred, deformed tricuspid
valve that can neither open fully nor close tightly
enough to prevent leakage.

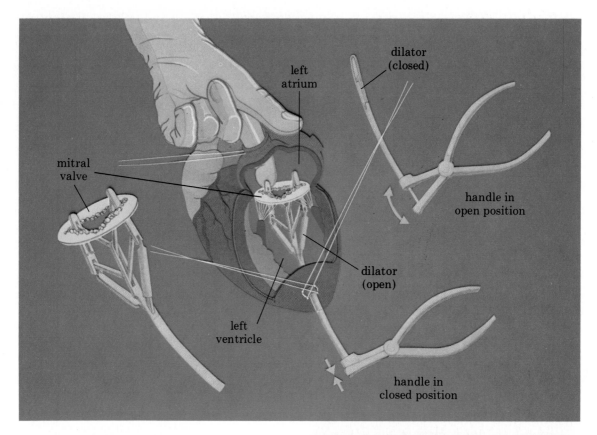

REAMING A MITRAL VALVE

A "sticky" mitral valve may be freed with the aid of a dilating instrument inserted into the heart chamber below the valve. The closed tip of the dilator, guided by the surgeon's finger, is pushed through the valve opening. Parts that resemble umbrella ribs cause the tip of the instrument to open and spread apart for effective reaming. If results are unsatisfactory, replacement with an artificial valve may be necessary.

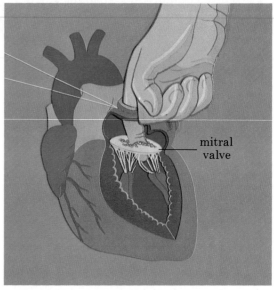

OPENING A MITRAL VALVE

The leaflets of a mitral valve that have become adherent and cannot open efficiently may sometimes be freed by a relatively simple operation called a commissurotomy. The surgeon inserts a finger into the chamber above the valve and attempts to free the "stuck-together" valve and restore satisfactory function.

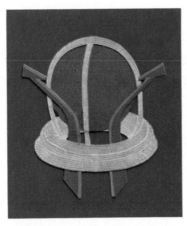 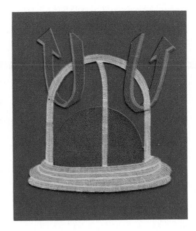 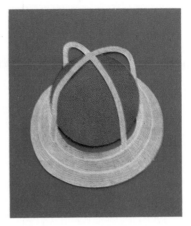

ARTIFICIAL HEART VALVES

A cage-ball valve moves up and down from a hole in its base to control the direction of blood flow. When the valve is open, above, blood flows in the direction of the arrows.

In the closed position, above, the ball is pushed down by blood pressure to block the opening below. The power to move the ball up and down comes from the heart's own contractions.

There are many refinements in the design of artificial heart valves. Above, the top view of a cage-ball valve shows the metal parts covered by fabric to retard blood-clotting.

In chronic cases, the valve deformities and muscle damage are often slight and require no specific changes in life-style or medicines for the heart. But a minority of patients with major valve damage may suffer severe limitation of activity. Abnormalities may eventually lead to signs of heart failure (see page 59); the patient may become short of breath, develop a cough, or have swelling of the abdomen and legs. At times blood may be coughed up, and quite often the normal heart rhythm is eventually replaced by irregular beating called atrial fibrillation (see page 58).

It is such patients with signs of heart failure and near-invalidism who are greatly benefited by valve surgery. One relatively simple operation consists merely of opening the leaflets of a mitral valve that have become adherent. This procedure, called a *commissurotomy,* is done only on the mitral valve. Usually, it is not in itself sufficient to restore good function, and in most cases one or more heart valves require replacement with prosthetic valves—artificial substitutes.

Valve Replacement

Valve replacement operations have been performed since about 1960 and have been remarkably successful, especially with improvements in techniques and in the design and materials of prosthetic valves.

Artificial valves are of several types. Some are metal, sometimes with synthetic cloth covering; some are animal tissues, including valves from a pig heart; and some are made of extremely smooth and chemically inert materials.

In principle, a valve has a moving part, a ball or disk called an occluder, which is a little gate that lets the blood through. The occluder is housed in a rigid cage to which a sewing ring is attached for implanting the valve in the heart.

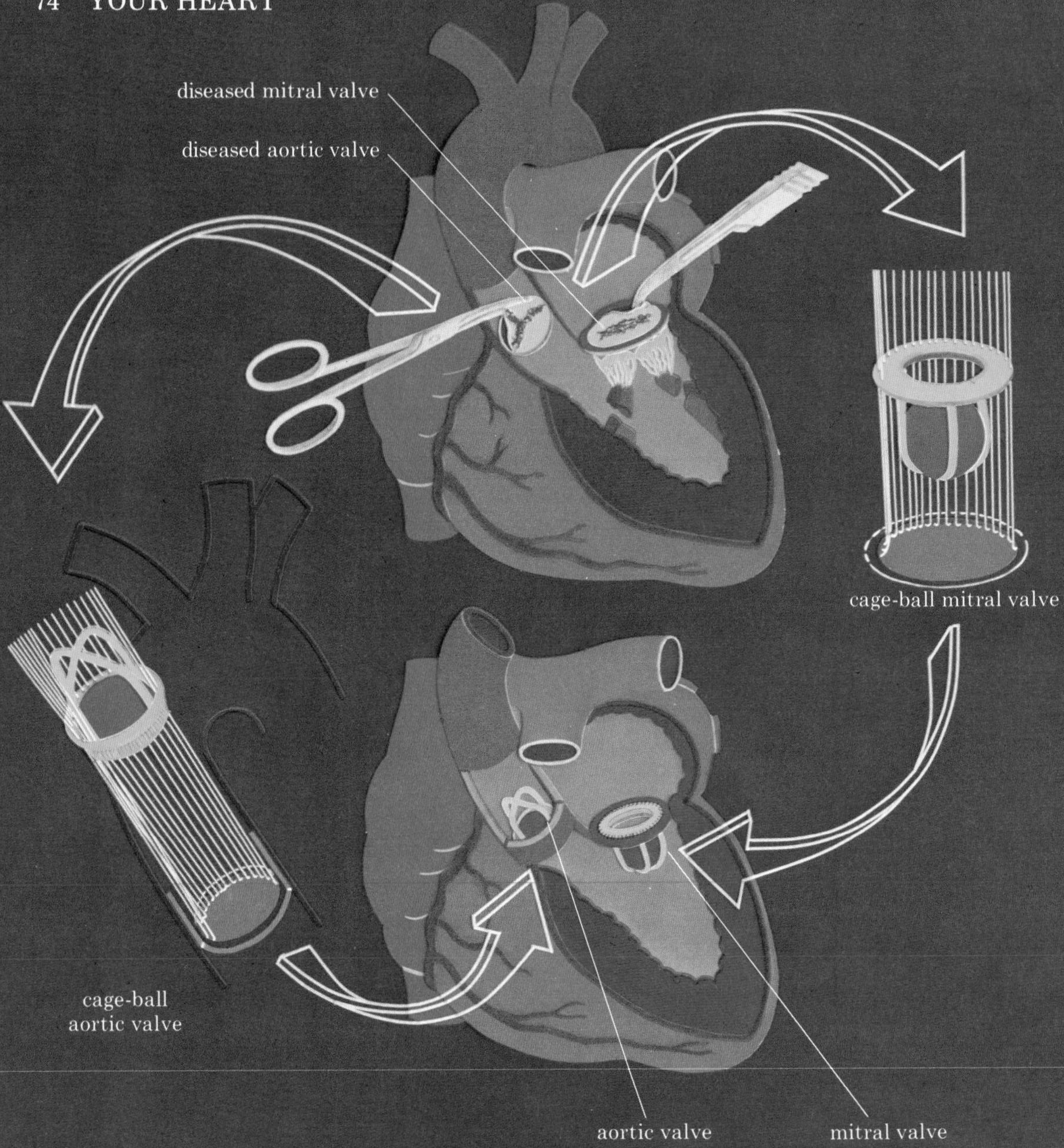

diseased mitral valve

diseased aortic valve

cage-ball mitral valve

cage-ball
aortic valve

aortic valve

mitral valve

REPLACING A HEART VALVE

*The top drawing shows the removal of diseased
mitral and aortic valves and the shaping of
adjacent healthy tissues for firm attachment of the
artificial valves. Either or both valves may be
diseased; more commonly, just the mitral valve.
The bottom drawing shows the cage-ball artificial
valves sewn into position inside the heart
(open-heart surgery). Complex suturing techniques
(small drawings) seal the valves securely to the
tissues where the diseased valves were removed.
The tops of the cages are oriented to stop-and-go
changes in the direction of blood flow, shown in
detail on the opposite page.*

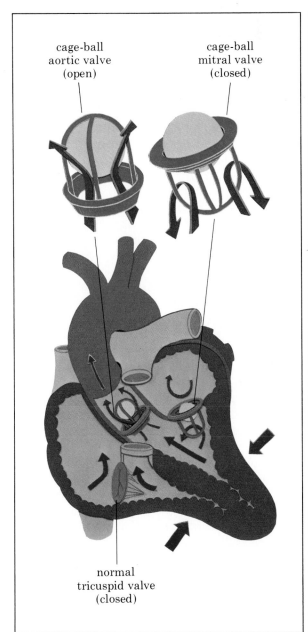

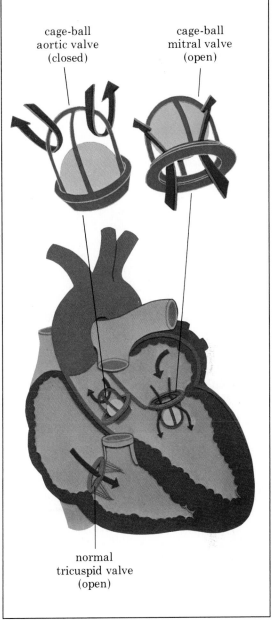

VALVE FUNCTION DURING HEARTBEAT

When the heart beats (systole), contraction of the left ventricle pushes the ball to the top of the aortic valve cage, opening the valve to admit blood to the aorta. Simultaneously, ventricular pressure pushes the ball into the opening of the mitral valve cage, closing it. The normal valves of the right side of the heart open and close in the same rhythm. Arrows show direction of flow.

VALVE FUNCTION DURING RELAXATION

When the heart relaxes (diastole), blood filling the atrium pushes down the ball of the artificial mitral valve so blood can fill the ventricle. At the same time, downward pressure of blood in the aorta drops the ball in its cage, closing it to prevent leakage into the relaxed ventricle.

The operation. Valve replacement is open heart surgery. A heart-lung machine temporarily provides oxygen to the blood and maintains circulation. The surgeon cuts into the heart, opens it, and works on it from the inside. He removes the diseased valve or valves, sews the replacement into position, and closes the heart—all of which is a good deal more delicate and exacting than this brief description suggests.

The breastbone must be split to expose the heart, and firm suturing and rejoining of structures is time-consuming. The entire procedure, performed by a skilled surgical team with extensive monitoring and life-support equipment, takes about four hours. The patient awakens in an intensive care unit, and in ten days to two weeks is ready to go home with the new valve working smoothly.

Power to run the artificial valve comes from the heart muscle, just as with a natural valve. Sometimes a heart may be so badly diseased that valve replacement would be unduly hazardous and unlikely to do much good. But in the more usual case, a doctor's knowledge of a patient's condition may indicate that an artificial valve is desirable or is likely to become so at some time in the future.

Valve implants greatly improve the mechanical efficiency of the heart and allow the patient to lead a more normal active life. They do not, of course, replace damaged heart muscle and thus do not restore the patient to perfectly normal health; there may be some limitation of activity and continuation of heart medicines. Infrequently, an implanted valve may be a site of infection and there is some tendency to clot formation, although the latter is less likely with valves that employ ultra-smooth inert materials. Patients may have to take anticoagulant drugs to reduce the blood clotting process.

CORONARY HEART DISEASE

Probably most people in general good health arrive at middle age without having been excessively preoccupied about the condition of their hearts. The organ has served them prodigiously and uncomplainingly, and there is every prospect that it will continue to do so for years and years.

Still, a certain informed awareness tends to come as one moves into and out of the 40s. A man reads of the death from heart attacks of friends, acquaintances, and strangers, no older than he is—premature by any definition. He may become concerned about heart thumpings, a fleeting chest pain, overweight, diet, smoking, the fact that long hours of work or play tire him as they never used to. A woman may know that the protection against heart attacks that her sex affords her dwindles after the menopause until in time she is just as susceptible as a man.

Heart attacks can be sudden, but in almost all cases the underlying factors have been building up for years and are present in large or small degree in most persons at age 50. Cardiovascular disease accounts for more than half of all deaths in the United States. A majority of these deaths is attributable to coronary artery disease, of which there are several types with varied manifestations.

The Heart's Fuel Lines

Coronary arteries are special supply lines that furnish blood, with its oxygen and nutrients, to the heart muscle. There are two sets of coronary arteries: one primarily feeds the left side of the heart; the other, chiefly the right side. The vessels branch into finer and finer subdivisions and connect with a vast number of tiny capillaries, through the walls of which the blood-fuel actually passes into groups of muscle fibers. The coronaries keep the heart muscle alive and functioning; any significant interruption of their services is a direct threat to the heart and to life.

The coronary arteries are quite small and prone to narrowing and obstruction. A common disease of the coronary arteries is *atherosclerosis,* of which more is mentioned later. This is a process in which the wall of an artery develops local degeneration (a plaque). The smooth inner lining of the artery becomes roughened and irregular as a substance called cholesterol is deposited in the walls, and as scar tissue is formed. Clots may form on the plaques, of which an artery may have several. The result is that the artery is less flexible and its channel is narrower in areas of plaque formation. A coronary artery may become completely blocked, chiefly when a clot forms on a plaque, plugging the channel and completely depriving a section of the heart muscle of blood.

Only rarely will a clot plug the coronary arteries in the absence of plaque formation. This has been noted in a few young women who were taking oral contraceptives. To a degree, a coronary artery can also narrow due to spasm, a reversible, temporary condition not dependent on plaque formation.

Manifestations of Coronary Disease

A sudden fatal heart attack may occur even when heart muscle is in good condition. This is possible when the heart may abruptly develop a very rapid, ineffective beating of the main pumping chambers

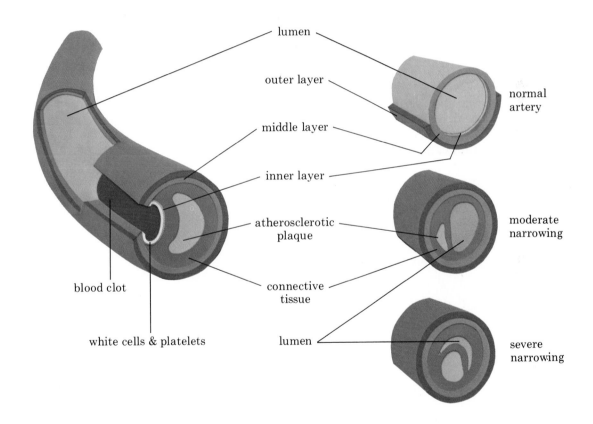

DEVELOPING ATHEROSCLEROSIS

Atherosclerosis precedes many heart attacks. Roughened deposits and scar tissue in the wall of the artery (plaques) can narrow its channel (lumen) and cause clots to form, sometimes large enough to plug the channel completely.

Progressive buildup of deposits takes place over a period of years, occurring earlier in some persons than in others, and affecting some vessels while sparing others. Coronary arteries are more vulnerable to obstruction than larger arteries.

called *ventricular fibrillation.* The fast fluttering of the muscle is incapable of giving a forceful push to the blood. Circulation ceases, and death may come in a few seconds or minutes, before any local damage can be inflicted on the heart muscle.

Sudden death may occur in persons who have no known history of heart disease, as well as in persons who have had prior heart attacks. Approximately half of all fatal heart attacks are sudden.

Chest Pain

(Angina Pectoris)

Angina pectoris literally means "constricting pain in the chest." It is a common but often misdiagnosed affliction that indicates the presence of an obstruction in the coronary arteries.

An artery that is 75 percent obstructed can transport enough blood to the heart muscle when one is at rest or inactive. But anything that increases the heart's work—exercise, emotion, stress—increases its need for blood. If obstructed coronaries cannot satisfy the heightened demand, the heart's protest is felt as angina.

Symptoms. Angina is not usually an extremely painful sensation. Typically, it is felt for one to several minutes as a tightness or vise-like sensation in the middle of the chest or across the whole front of the chest. The sensation may radiate to the neck and lower jaw, the shoulders, and one or both arms.

Some patients describe the sensation as pain, others as "burning," "pressing," "squeezing," or "heaviness." Sometimes the sensation is felt only in the left chest or one arm, and at times it may radiate to the back. There may be other occasional variations of these symptoms as well.

Angina is absent most of the time and an episode is characteristically brief. It is generally terminated by stopping to rest, and is notably provoked by emotion or effort such as walking—especially if walking briskly, carrying bundles, climbing stairs, walking in the cold or wind, or after eating. When angina occurs, the patient is ordinarily more comfortable when sitting or standing, and more uncomfortable when lying down.

Diagnosis. Angina is usually evident from the patient's history. Diagnosis may be supported by an electrocardiogram that may show abnormalities at rest, indicating insufficient blood supply to the heart muscle. A treadmill, two-step, or other exercise test may be given to demonstrate abnormalities more clearly. More rigorous tests will be given if surgical intervention is considered (see page 90).

Treatment. Anginal discomfort can be terminated very quickly by drugs that dilate the coronary vessels and enhance the blood supply. Tablets of nitroglycerin or isosorbide dinitrate, placed under the tongue, end an attack in a minute or two. The drugs may also be used preventively, as before some vigorous effort that might be expected to provoke an attack.

Another drug, propranolol, may be taken several times a day (usually four) to lessen the frequency and intensity of attacks. Regular exercise prescribed by one's physician also seems to be very helpful in permitting more vigorous effort and promoting physical fitness.

Living with angina. Although angina is a symptom to be taken seriously, it does not inevitably or usually lead to a life of invalidism. Innumerable patients lead entirely normal lives, working every day, pursuing favored activities, and only occasionally experiencing a twinge of anginal discomfort.

They should know that they are not alone. The majority of men over 40, and not a few women then and in later life, have some degree of obstructive process in their coronary arteries. Moreover, nature does its best to overcome the difficulty by opening competent new arterial branches (collateral circulation) to enhance the flow of blood.

There is another more drastic method of improving coronary circulation: surgery.

Coronary Bypass

The principle of coronary bypass surgery is easy to grasp. Blood is simply detoured around an obstruction. A segment of one of the patient's blood vessels is sewn to the base of the aorta (which supplies blood to the coronaries) and the other end is sewn to the coronary artery below the point of narrowing or obstruction. Blood is thus diverted to feed the heart muscle.

Older attempts to revascularize the heart by sprinkling irritating powder on its surface to stimulate new vessel formation, by reaming out obstructions, or by cutting out obstructions and making a patch graft have been abandoned as unsatisfactory. Coronary bypass surgery has become the accepted procedure for suitable patients. Skills have been perfected, operative risk is relatively low, and the quality of the patient's life is usually improved.

Who is suited? A person with "ordinary" angina usually does well with proper medical care. Some with severe, disabling angina—or possibly impending heart attack or signs of extensive coronary disease recognized by a doctor—may be candidates for coronary bypass surgery.

Great care is taken in selecting patients. An indispensable preliminary test, which to a great degree makes bypass surgery feasible, is the *coronary arteriogram*. This procedure gives X-ray visualization of the coronary circulation, and the location and extent of narrowings or obstructions. A coronary arteriogram is expensive and involves a small risk. It's done only in a hospital by a team with equipment that takes serial X-ray films and motion pictures of the heart's action.

Under local anesthesia, a catheter—a long, thin tube—is inserted into an artery of the groin or arm and gently worked into the aorta where the coronary arteries originate. The tip of the catheter is moved successively to the "mouths" or openings of the right and left coronary arteries and a dye is injected. The dye, which is opaque to X-rays, clearly delineates the size and location of plaques, narrowings, and obstructions of the coronaries. The dye is also injected into the left ventricle to give information about the condition of the main pumping chamber of the heart.

With precise knowledge of just where the coronary arteries are blocked, together with the patient's history, a decision can be made as to whether or not bypass surgery should be performed.

The bypass operation. To perform the bypass, the breastbone is split, the heart is exposed, and connections are made to a heart-lung machine. One of the surgeons removes a section of the saphenous vein in the leg (no problem because a deep vein takes over for it), and this vein is then used for the graft.

There are alternative vessels for grafting, particularly the right and left mammary arteries that descend down the chest under the breastbone. One advantage of a mammary artery is that it is already connected to a source of blood so that only its lower end needs to be attached below the point where coronary obstruction exists.

More than one area of the coronary system may be diseased. Two, three, even four or more grafts are often necessary to shunt blood around blocked parts of pipelines. Sewing leakproof ends of small vessels together requires delicacy and skill.

The entire operation, from the opening to the closing of the chest, takes about four hours. The patient, with various tubes attached to him, awakens in an intensive care unit where any emergency, such as disturbed heart rhythm, can be controlled. Ordinarily, the patient is out of the hospital and testing his new freedom for activity in a couple of weeks.

Upward of 50,000 bypass operations are performed yearly in the United States. No doubt the number will increase. The outlook for an individual patient varies with his general physical condition, his age, the presence of other disease, and other factors that are weighed in considering bypass surgery. But great improvements in skills and experience since 1974 have reduced operative mortality to an average of about 5 percent.

The operation, performed by specialized surgical teams, is expensive. The cost for surgeons and hospital is in the neighborhood of $8,000 to $12,000.

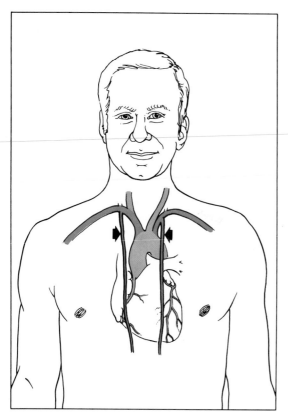

MAMMARY ARTERIES

Internal mammary arteries that run down inside the rib cage can be attached to a coronary vessel to carry blood around an obstructed area. The mammary operation is performed less frequently today than in the past.

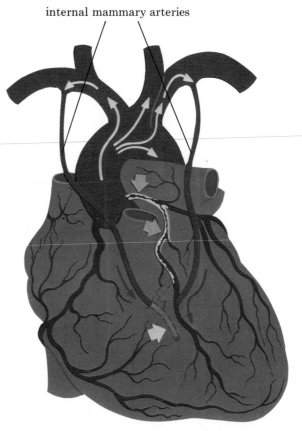

internal mammary arteries

BYPASS HEART SURGERY (MAMMARY)

A diseased portion of the left coronary artery (yellow arrows) is bypassed by internal mammary arteries attached to the heart (green and white arrows) below the obstruction. The left branch (green arrow) is attached to the vessel; the right branch (white arrow) is inserted in the heart.

Who will benefit? The consensus is that bypass surgery greatly improves the quality of a patient's life. In the great majority of suitable patients, angina tends to disappear to the extent that it is no longer a painful impediment to satisfying activity. In some patients, relief is partial but still highly gratifying. Quality of life can be measured by renewed ability to carry a work load, travel, dance, do housework, walk, or bowl, without fear of being stopped by crushing chest pain. Whether or not bypass surgery prolongs life is not known, but common sense suggests that it should. We also do not know for sure if bypass surgery prevents further heart attacks in a person who may already have experienced one.

Coronary heart disease is progressive; surgery does not cure the process. We know that bypass grafts themselves may become obstructed in time, and a person who has had successful bypass surgery should, of course, take prudent measures to lessen the risks of heart attacks—weight control, cessation of smoking, and proper diet (see page 137). Indeed, he may be more motivated than most because his renewed quality of life gives him a measure of what is at risk.

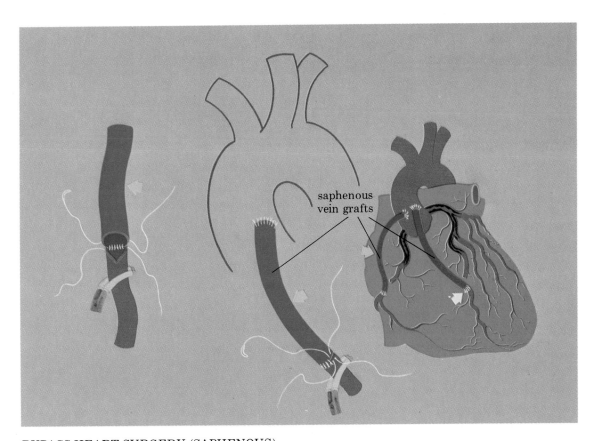

BYPASS HEART SURGERY (SAPHENOUS)

Segments of the saphenous vein from the patient's leg are now often preferred for bypass grafts. The segments have about the same caliber as the coronary arteries. Two, three, or more bypasses may be necessary. The drawing of the heart shows the connections from the aorta to the coronary arteries below the level of obstruction. Other drawings show fine details of the end-to-end joining of arteries and veins (anastomosis).

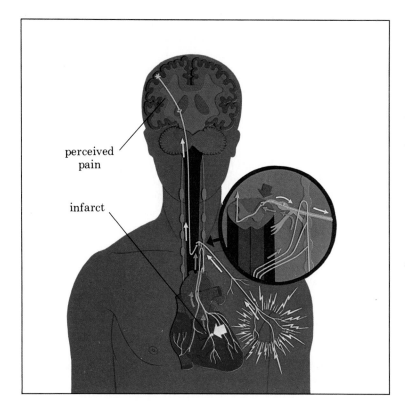

perceived
pain

infarct

REFERRED PAIN

Pain from a coronary infarct (white arrow) may seem to come from the left chest or armpit area. Nerves from the injured heart (pink arrows) and nerves serving the axillary area (small white arrows) merge in a "neuron pool" in the spinal cord (purple arrow in circle). Sensations of pain arriving from merged nerve pathways are perceived at higher brain centers as referred pain. Some heart attacks are "silent"; that is, without significant pain.

Heart Attack

(Myocardial infarction)

A man or woman suddenly feels severe, vise-like pain in the middle of the chest. The pain extends to the neck, lower jaw, one or both shoulders, and arms. There may be profuse sweating, shortness of breath, nausea or vomiting, faintness, or actual fainting.

Those are classic symptoms of a heart attack.

Not all attacks follow the classic pattern. Some are "silent," not recognized at the time for what they are. Discomfort may be mild, not interpreted as pain, and may go away without any treatment. Distress may be self-diagnosed as "indigestion," with a feeling that a big burp would give relief.

A heart attack may be triggered by unaccustomed strenuous exercise, such as shoveling snow or pushing a car out of a rut. But more often there is no association with effort or emotion. An attack may occur in the middle of the night and even wake the patient.

Heart attacks are most frequent in older age groups, but they by no means spare the relatively young and the middle-aged—persons in the prime of life. Statistically, a number of risk factors have been shown to be associated with liability to heart attack. A middle-aged man who is overweight, sedentary, diabetic, who is a heavy smoker, has high blood pressure, a high cholesterol level, and a family history of heart trouble is a prime candidate.

Some of these risk factors are controllable; others are not. The controllable factors, which we shall describe later on, give a reasonable chance that a heart attack may be forestalled for many years.

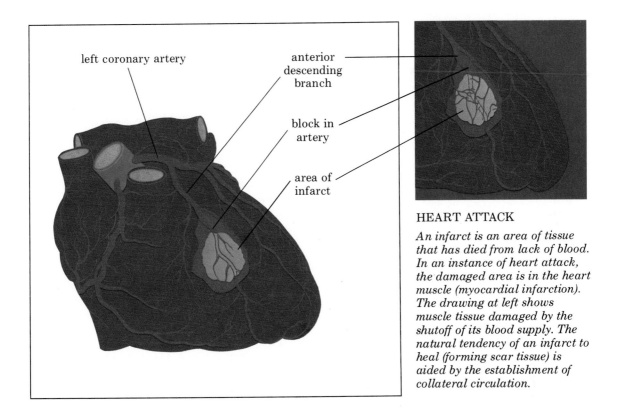

left coronary artery

anterior descending branch

block in artery

area of infarct

HEART ATTACK

An infarct is an area of tissue that has died from lack of blood. In an instance of heart attack, the damaged area is in the heart muscle (myocardial infarction). The drawing at left shows muscle tissue damaged by the shutoff of its blood supply. The natural tendency of an infarct to heal (forming scar tissue) is aided by the establishment of collateral circulation.

What is a heart attack? The medical term for a heart attack is *myocardial infarction.* A portion of the heart muscle (myocardium) dies from lack of blood; the dead tissue is an infarct. The damaged area is eventually replaced by a scar, which heals the tissue but cannot contract to help the work of the heart. Each scar weakens the action of the heart.

Coronary occlusion is a term for heart attack that was used in the past because a coronary artery was often found to be obstructed. *Coronary thrombosis* is another term, descriptive of a clot or thrombus as the cause of occlusion. However, it appears that some heart attacks are not initiated by a sudden blockage of a coronary artery; rather, the occlusion may follow the onset of the attack.

A myocardial infarction may be small and never be suspected by the patient. But most heart attacks that do significant damage are recognizable by the symptoms described. The fundamental disease is coronary atherosclerosis, as in angina pectoris, and symptoms of heart attack are similar to those of angina except that anginal twinges are brief, whereas symptoms of heart attack tend to persist for many minutes or hours.

Diagnosis of myocardial infarction, if not immediately obvious to a doctor, is made from the patient's history, a physical examination, an electrocardiogram that may show irregularities, and measurement of the amount of certain enzymes in the blood. These enzymes are released by damaged heart muscle cells, and their quantity gives an estimate of the amount of muscle that has died.

What To Do in Case of Heart Attack

The most important thing to do if a heart attack occurs or warning symptoms appear is to get medical help at once. Members of the family should know this as well as the patient. Life-threatening irregularity of the heartbeat is most likely to develop in the first few minutes or hours of a myocardial infarction. Immediate action is vital.

If symptoms are questionable, it is usually desirable to call one's doctor, but if he cannot be reached and symptoms are severe, the patient should go at once to a hospital emergency room. Call or have someone call an emergency ambulance service, if available. Most communities have trained ambulance, fire department, police, and other rescue teams. A trained ambulance crew can give oxygen and other supports while rushing a patient to a hospital. If an ambulance is not available or will be delayed, someone should drive the patient to the nearest hospital by car. Time is of the essence.

Most large hospitals have coronary care units. Know something about your local hospitals. Keep the phone numbers of your doctor, hospital, and emergency services in your purse or wallet and near your telephone.

The heartening fact is that about 85 percent of patients admitted to a hospital for treatment of a heart attack will survive, and the great majority return to active, satisfying lives.

Treatment. Hospital treatment of a heart attack includes bed rest and limited activity for ten days to a month, depending upon the severity of the attack. The critical first few days are typically spent in a coronary care unit with varieties of sophisticated monitoring equipment hooked to the patient. Complications, if any, are most likely to develop in the first 24 hours. Should serious irregularity of the heart occur, immediate electric shock treatment may be lifesaving.

A number of drugs—lidocaine, procainamide, or quinidine—may be used to control and prevent irregularities. Other medicines may be given to treat heart weakness and maintain adequate blood pressure.

The chief factor in recovery is time. In time, the body heals the damaged heart muscle and develops collateral channels to improve coronary circulation—in effect, performing its own bypass procedures.

A certain amount of anxiety is normal if you should find yourself in a coronary care unit with intravenous tubing, a picture tube on which your "heartbeat" jumps up and down, a respirator, an oxygen tank, a closed-circuit TV camera, and other mysterious technology. Some understanding of what the equipment does and what is happening helps to relieve apprehensions. And there's no harm in asking.

Recovery From Heart Attack

When a recovered heart attack patient is discharged from the hospital, six weeks or more of recuperation at home usually lie ahead. The patient may not understand why he feels as he does, may become depressed, irritable, worried about the future, or fearful of another attack and sudden death. There is little need for apprehension, but brooding about it can create a needless cardiac invalid.

Some physical weakness—dog-tiredness—is to be expected. This does not mean that the heart is getting worse. Ups and downs are normal and tolerable if the doctor makes it clear that he expects the patient to be back in harness in due time.

Restrictions may be resented and taken to mean that all the good things of life are forever in the past. But restrictions are temporary; most of them are modified or abolished as strength returns. It is important to know that one is not an invalid and that his life-style need not be bound in shallows and in miseries.

Four out of five recovered patients return to work, usually in a couple of months. A patient restored to substantially full activity may need little if any further treatment, aside from prudent medical checkups as a doctor recommends. Some patients, however, receive some form of digitalis, and most carry nitroglycerin tablets for use in the event of anginal pain. If present, other diseases or disabilities also are considered in planning reconditioning programs.

Can you have a cocktail if you are so inclined, enjoy good food, drive a car, try to improve your golf score, exert yourself on household chores or hobbies? Short of genuine invalidism, recovered patients can resume pleasurable activities within sensible limits, and not a few return to pretty strenuous athletics, such as tennis or handball, if that is their "bag."

In fact, many patients are urged to be more active physically than they were before their attacks. One thing that a doctor will almost surely recommend and give guidance to is a regular schedule of exercise. This may start with a daily walk of a mile or so and work up to jogging, bowling, or whatever is pleasing within one's increasing capacities. Exercise helps the heart muscle to gain strength and improve its collateral circulation.

Sometimes, and sometimes not, a man or woman who has recovered from a heart attack may ask his or her physician about sexual intercourse. Whether or not the question is asked, it is surely on the minds of marital partners who may have fantasies about sudden death during the act, inability to satisfy their partner, excessive demands, and apprehensions of doing or receiving harm.

It is realistic, if unromantic, to think of sexual intercourse as a form of work or exercise, not prolonged enough to have the rehabilitative value of a brisk long walk. The energy expended is about equal to climbing two flights of stairs, usually well within the patient's capacity. Should the act be followed by a twinge of angina, the patient learns to take a nitroglycerin tablet a few minutes before.

Can Heart Attacks Be Prevented?

The background of almost all heart attacks, and of other cardiovascular disease, is atherosclerosis, which we have alluded to (see page 76). If atherosclerosis could be prevented, perhaps so could heart attacks; and if the process could be slowed, heart attacks and circulatory diseases might be postponed until advanced old age.

A tremendous amount of research has been and continues to be exerted in the search for answers to cardiovascular disease. A number of "risk factors" have been shown to be statistically associated with a high incidence of heart attacks. Association is not absolute proof of cause and effect, but, in gambling terms, personal efforts to reduce risk factors should increase the odds in favor of the player instead of the house.

Coronary atherosclerosis is related to age. It is rare before 30, although there is evidence that the process may begin early in some young children, and that prevention of heart attacks in later years may fall within the domain of pediatricians. Any person of middle age can be rather sure that he or she has some degree of atherosclerosis, usually more extensive in men up to age 50 and thereafter increasing in frequency in women. This does not at all mean that a fatal heart attack is imminent. Autopsies have shown that a surprising amount of coronary atherosclerosis is compatible with a long and active life.

Risk factors. The usual form of coronary atherosclerosis is related to a number of factors, of which at least one, and often two or three, is present in most but not all patients with coronary heart disease. These factors are: heredity; diabetes; high levels of fatty substances (cholesterol and triglycerides) in the blood; high blood pressure; and cigarette smoking.

Heredity cannot be changed, but awareness can lead to medical examination that may confirm susceptibility and disclose risk factors that can be lessened. Heredity may be especially important if one or both parents or a brother or sister have died prematurely from coronary heart problems.

A person who has had diabetes for many years is more prone to coronary heart trouble than a non-diabetic. There is only limited evidence that treatment of diabetes reduces the mortality from coronary atherosclerosis.

Controllable Risks

High blood pressure (see page 65) is high on the list of risk factors. It is eminently controllable by a variety of medications; the patient merely takes pills as prescribed. The greatest threat is that a patient may stop taking medicines because symptoms disappear, pills are a bore, or the seriousness of high blood pressure is not understood. Dropouts from medication revert to their previous high-risk status.

Cigarette smoking is linked with lung cancer and chronic lung disease in the public mind. Less well known is the impressive accumulation of recent data that clearly indicates an association between coronary heart disease and cigarette smoking. The association is intensified in the presence of other risk factors, notably hypertension and high cholesterol levels. The risk seems directly related to the number of cigarettes smoked per day and the number of years of smoking. Pipes and cigars have less effect, but there is no clear evidence that low-tar and filter cigarettes are safer.

It is not easy to stop smoking, but awareness of risk should stimulate motivation. In limited groups who have given up the habit, there is definite evidence of a reduction in future risk of heart disease. Young people should be urged not to start the habit, and established smokers need to know the serious hazards of continuing.

Cholesterol and Fats

Blood taken from your arm during a medical examination goes to a laboratory where one of the things it discloses is the level of cholesterol in the serum. The finding is expressed as milligrams of cholesterol in 100 milliliters of blood. Many people are quite aware of their cholesterol values because of the association of high levels with atherosclerosis and heart attacks.

The most favorable reading of blood cholesterol is under 200. Most adults in the United States have readings of about 225; over 250 is in the unfavorable zone. Blood levels of triglycerides (neutral fats) have also been implicated in coronary atherosclerosis although they do not appear to be as potent a factor; a level above 150 is usually considered excessive.

So much for measurements. What is one to make of them?

Cholesterol is a normal and necessary fatlike substance that circulates in our blood. It is a constituent of nerve sheaths, a precursor of hormones, and is essential for many physiological processes.

The body manufactures cholesterol, mainly in the liver, but small amounts are furnished by certain foods. In some people who have too much cholesterol or can't handle it properly, the substance may settle down in plaques inside blood vessels and lead to premature hardening of arteries.

Cholesterol levels can be reduced somewhat by dietary modifications and even drugs. Absolute proof that reducing high cholesterol levels prevents heart attacks or slows the progress of atherosclerosis is lacking. Most people have no reason to radically change their diet. But cholesterol levels are to some degree controllable, and many physicians feel that persons with excessively high levels, in conjunction with other risk factors, would do well to make the effort.

Dietary measures tend to put emphasis both on avoiding cholesterol-containing foods and on increasing the proportion of unsaturated fatty acids of vegetable origin over saturated fatty acids. You will see that highly palatable menus can be put together, or low-fat diets of the type available from the American Heart Association or its affiliates can be followed.

Obesity. An additional virtue of low-fat diets is that they ordinarily produce desirable weight loss in obese persons. Excess weight makes the heart work harder, and if the heart is already damaged, the added burden is more serious. Grossly overweight persons have been found to have increased heart work rate, blood volume, and size.

Obesity is commonly associated with high blood pressure, a significant risk factor. A person with angina pectoris frequently finds that eating a large meal aggravates his symptoms. Regardless of the ultimate cause of death, the life expectancy of greatly overweight people is less than average, according to actuarial figures. It is not possible to say that obesity results in this or that specific disease, but there are overall good reasons to avoid excess weight and its cause, overeating.

Exercise. The role of physical exercise in the prevention and management of heart disease is one of wide discussion and opinion. It is possible that a life of regular activity may help to prevent coronary heart trouble, but there is no conclusive scientific proof that exercise conditioning delays the progress of atherosclerosis or prevents the recurrence of heart attack in persons who have already had one.

Unquestionably, many people in this automobile age are rather flabby and out of condition. What can they accomplish if they exercise more regularly? Certain benefits can be expected. There is no doubt that a sense of physical and mental well-being is imparted by an appropriate and regular exercise program, which also helps in weight control and improvement of circulation in the legs. Many persons with coronary heart disease and angina pectoris find that an exercise program seems to lessen the frequency of chest pain.

The special matter of exercise after a heart attack involves the condition of the individual patient and the counsel of his or her doctor. To be of value, an exercise program must be safe and suitable. Walking is often recommended—not into an icy wind, however, and always stopping short of excessive fatigue. All too often, vigorous exercise is undertaken by persons with serious heart trouble who are out of condition—with disastrous results.

Jogging or running is *not* for everyone. Some patients with severe heart disease need rest, not exercise. Before initiating an exercise program, it is important that anyone with heart disease, or for that matter any middle-aged or older person without heart disease, seek the advice of a physician as to the type, frequency, intensity, and duration of physical activity. For some, formal supervised group exercise programs may be available in the vicinity. For others, individual programs may be undertaken on a graduated basis.

Salt. Table salt, which is sodium chloride, also has a role in heart disease. A person with a weakened heart may tend to retain both water and sodium in his tissues, giving rise to swelling of the abdomen and legs, congestion of the lungs, or shortness of breath. Restriction of *sodium* intake may be very helpful in preventing or controlling such congestion.

The usual American diet provides about four grams of sodium daily. It's often wise to reduce this intake to two grams, one gram, or even one-half gram. Extremely rigid restriction is often less necessary if a patient is on diuretic drugs.

A strict low-sodium diet requires that no salt be added to foods, and that naturally salt-containing foods be avoided. It is not easy to follow, but is perfectly feasible and practicable with planning and a little knowledge of foods, as from labels (see page 149). Non-salty flavorings such as lemon juice, onions, herbs, and wine enhance palatability to a highly satisfying level. Some restriction of fluid intake may at times be needed for persons with very advanced heart disease.

Alcohol and the Heart

Alcohol is well known for its assaults upon the liver, but in the past little notice was paid to its effects on the heart. Now we recognize that, for some persons, alcoholic beverages have the potential for creating true heart problems. Alcoholic deterioration of the heart may be manifested as irregularities of rhythm, weakness of the heart muscle, and even death.

Exactly how alcohol works such injury in certain susceptible persons is not clear. Some heavy drinkers are poorly nourished, not getting enough vitamins and other nutrients, but this does not explain abnormal heart function in most cases. Possibly more important is the direct toxic effect of alcohol on the heart muscle.

Whatever the underlying cause, it is apparent that certain heavy drinkers develop serious, and at times, fatal heart disease that can only be blamed on excessive alcohol intake. Once this is recognized, the treatment is complete abstinence. If detected early, alcoholic heart disease appears to be reversible.

Mysterious Myocardopathy

A quite obscure and not uncommon group of heart problems is grouped under the general name of *myocardopathy,* also called cardiomyopathy. The terms apply to a disease of the heart muscle of unknown origin. The patient may have a family history of heart disease of indeterminable cause.

Typically, the heart muscle may thicken or dilate, or the mitral valve may leak. The heart gradually becomes inefficient and death may occur after a few or many years. The disease may be seen at all ages, and ranges in seriousness from a minor disturbance tolerated for a long time, to a grave disorder that greatly shortens the life-span.

The diagnosis is readily made by use of the echocardiogram. No medicines are clearly effective, although the drug propranolol has been employed in some cases. Surgery may be performed when there is a major malfunction of the mitral valve, or when the heart muscle is so thickened that it actually obstructs the internal flow of blood.

This group of entities comprises a mystery area of heart disease that requires much further study.

Stress and Personality

The concept that stresses and personal temperaments have a lot to do with liability to heart disease is attractive and quite controversial.

It has been suggested that tensions of modern life in a troubled world are responsible for "our epidemic of coronary disease." And that the way we behave—that is, our personality type—is associated, for better or worse, with proneness to heart trouble. The "heart attack personality" is said to be ridden by deadlines, impatient, ambitious, and aggressive. The opposite behavior type, presumably with a quiet heart, is said to be relaxed and passive.

The personality theory does not have enough serious support to justify constant worry about your heart if you are a deadline fighter, or to feel that you are immune if you like to take it easy. For one thing, it is admittedly very difficult to measure personality variants with any precision. Most physicians don't feel that any one personality type is associated with high blood pressure.

It is also believed by some that tremendous personal stresses—the death of a spouse or child, divorce, or the loss of a job—may precipitate a heart attack in a susceptible individual. It is not clear how one scientifically quantitates stress, although certain measures have been used.

These concepts have merit and may have some validity. But their true importance and precipitative influence in high blood pressure, coronary artery disease, and heart attacks is difficult to define. It is true that an attack of angina pectoris may be brought on by emotion. Is the same true for a heart attack? It would not appear so. Blood pressure rises with anger and excitement, yet there is little evidence that permanent high blood pressure results from such influences.

One may agree that equanimity and freedom from constant tensions, frustrations, and embattled deadlines are desirable objectives. But success in a job, and even with one's family, generally demands hard work with inescapable tensions, competitiveness, and intense effort to resolve problems. A torpid, tension-free life is usually incompatible with economic survival and the satisfying exercise of innate abilities. Body and mind are at their best when functioning actively.

Some compromises are needed. Perhaps a useful and practical standard is that your heart and blood vessels may be best protected by a way of life that yields personal satisfaction and accomplishment without inordinate physical and mental fatigue, but by the same token without excesses of stimulation or tranquillity.

It is heartening to know that nationwide deaths from heart disease and strokes reversed a continuing upward trend and began to decline in 1975. The decline was substantial enough to persuade some hardheaded life insurance companies to revise their mortality tables and increase dividends to policyholders. It's tempting to credit at least part of this decline to improved care of cardiac and hypertensive patients and to the efforts of many thousands of people to modify their risk factors.

Somebody must be doing something right.

THE HEART: TESTS & PROCEDURES

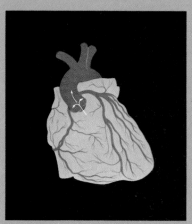

HEART X RAY

The black-and-white drawing shows the front of the heart as it would appear in an X-ray picture (angiogram) of coronary circulation. The location, size, and nature of obstructions and abnormalities of vessels can be recognized in this way.

X rays of the chest give information about the size and shape of the heart, as well as circulation to the lungs.

The electrocardiogram (ECG or EKG) is a record of the electrical activity of the heart, and is imprinted on a tape strip as a series of peaks and valleys. Electrical impulses are picked up through electrodes placed on the surface of the body, arms, legs, and chest. The ECG gives information about heart rate and rhythm, enlargement of or damage to heart muscle, and abnormalities in conduction of electrical impulses within the heart.

An echocardiogram, a relatively new technique, utilizes the properties of ultrasound—very high-frequency sound waves that enter the body and return as echoes. These can be analyzed to give data on heart muscle size and movement, on valve motion, and on the pericardium surrounding the heart.

A phonocardiogram is a recording of heart sounds and murmurs, especially useful in studying disease of the heart valves.

A treadmill, or other exercise test such as the two-step test, provides a record of changes in the electrocardiogram that may occur during the stress of exercise. It gives information about heart rate, rhythm, and blood pressure responses to physical effort—information that may be important in assessing physical fitness, as well as in disclosing signs of disorders that may not show up at rest (such as significant disease of the coronary arteries).

Catheterization is a sophisticated procedure performed only in a hospital. Small long tubes called catheters are passed under X-ray visualization through veins and arteries into the heart. Direct measurements of oxygen levels and pressures are taken within chambers of the heart and within the large blood vessels entering and leaving the heart. With X-ray pictures taken at the same time, it is possible to get valuable data about the competence of the heart and specific abnormalities of the valves and heart muscle.

An angiogram is a special X-ray picture of an artery or vein taken by injecting into the blood vessel a liquid that is opaque to X rays to delineate vessel structure.

An arteriogram is an angiogram of an artery; a *venogram,* of a vein. Arteriograms of the coronary arteries are frequently done as part of catheterization of the heart, to disclose narrowing or obstruction of these arteries.

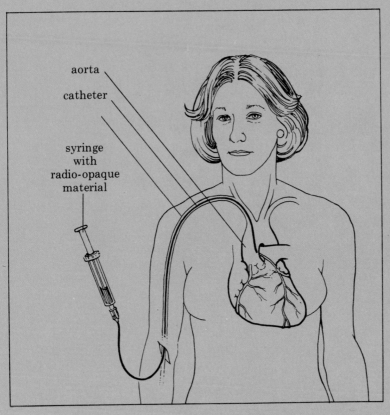

aorta

catheter

syringe with radio-opaque material

ANGIOGRAPHY

As the heart beats, X-ray stills and motion pictures of its circulation are taken by angiographic techniques. A catheter is inserted into an artery of the arm and threaded through the vessel to the aorta at the top of the heart, and thence to the small openings of coronary arteries where they join the aorta. A dye opaque to X rays, injected through the catheter, gives a clear picture of the living events.

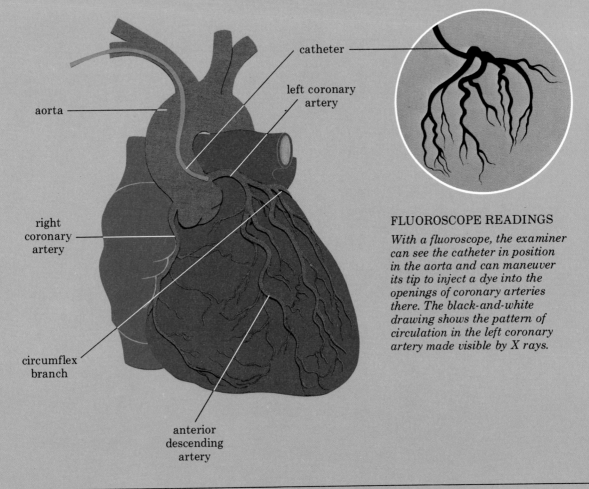

catheter

left coronary artery

aorta

right coronary artery

circumflex branch

anterior descending artery

FLUOROSCOPE READINGS

With a fluoroscope, the examiner can see the catheter in position in the aorta and can maneuver its tip to inject a dye into the openings of coronary arteries there. The black-and-white drawing shows the pattern of circulation in the left coronary artery made visible by X rays.

EXERCISE AND FITNESS

Physical fitness is more than just avoiding disease; it is a state of body and mind, a positive way of life involving one from head to foot and from inside out. It means good appearance—no unattractive fat or skinniness, clear skin, and good posture—as well as grace, agility, endurance, lack of tension, sound sleep, zestful days, and unfatigued evenings. But most important, it means healthy heart, lungs, and blood vessels, improved resistance to disease and better recuperative power. All these add up to a longer and more enjoyable life. As researcher J. P. Hracovec has said, "Exercise is the closest thing to an anti-aging pill now available. It acts like a miracle drug, and it's free for the doing."

To some people, the words fitness and exercise mean dutiful hours, boredom, sacrificed pleasure, and a history of failed resolves. They are wrong. Nature would be stupid to make something so vital a joyless chore. To reach and maintain it, one should have a variety of exercises, games, and sports that fit one's own physical endowment, personality, and life-style. And since these change through life, the program should be periodically retailored. Fitness can thus be a venture in self-discovery as well as a source of health and daily satisfaction. People who say they hate exercise have forgotten how good fitness feels—or perhaps have never known.

No one is too old to pursue fitness. Tolstoi learned to ride a bicycle at 67. President Harry Truman used to leave a wake of winded young reporters during his brisk morning walks. Other recent presidents have been avid golfers and swimmers. They knew that fitness means vigor and pleasure, not grudging effort and discomfort. But it must be regular, not a weekend or summer outing or a fad. And it must start not tomorrow but today.

Before we look at specific exercises, let's see what needs they must fill and the great variety of choices available, so that you can better tailor a program to fit your individual needs and interests.

Judge Your Fitness

A look in the mirror and at your daily life tells much about your fitness.

• Does your abdomen bulge or sag? A "spare tire" may be part fat and part weakened muscle. The abdominal muscles are a natural girdle supporting the internal organs and helping many body movements. A weak abdomen may lead to a hernia, lower-back strain, and other disorders.

• Do you stand straight? Slumping and letting a bulging belly exaggerate the spine's S-curve may show weak muscles in both abdomen and back.

• Are there deposits of excess fat on your thighs, hips, or upper arms?

• Are parts of your body undesirably thin and slack? This shows loss of muscular development and tone.

• Can you reach and stretch freely without strains, aches, and puffing? Or has disuse robbed your body of suppleness, efficiency, and grace? At 40 or 60, one naturally lacks the elasticity of youngsters, but still one needn't wince, redden, and pant.

• Does your body feel or look tense? If so, it is vulnerable to back spasms, muscle and joint disorders, insomnia, and the many ills that may reflect stress, from ulcers to colitis.

• Is your weight twenty pounds above or below that suggested by your doctor? Has it changed 10 percent or more since you turned 40? If so, both your appearance and health are probably suffering.

• Does exertion leave you stiff and aching?

• Are you easily winded?

• Do you sleep poorly, drag through the day, and often feel fatigued and apathetic?

• Is it an effort getting in and out of chairs and cars, dancing, walking up stairs, bending and lifting, or doing other things that demand flexibility and muscle tone?

• Have you become more susceptible to minor aches and ills?

There is much evidence about your fitness in the annual or semiannual medical examination that everyone over 40 should seek. If you haven't had an exam recently, arrange for one now. It should include an electrocardiogram and tests for blood pressure, cholesterol, and other factors affecting circulation. Since you are estimating your fitness and training aims, the exam probably should include a vital capacity (lung capacity) test and, if possible, a treadmill electrocardiogram or some equivalent (for instance, a step-walking test). Learn to take your own pulse; this is easy and a good precaution as you proceed with a conditioning program.

If you're already fit, you must remain so. But if your muscles, heart, lungs, and blood vessels aren't fit, you need conditioning. Failing to keep them healthy leaves you prey to injury and illness, especially high blood pressure, angina, coronary artery disease, and stroke. There is everything to gain, and even people with special physical problems can create interesting fitness programs to preserve and probably improve their health (see page 98).

Why Fitness Fades

Eons of evolution have shaped us to function best when active—walking, running, hunting, swimming, crafting, or carrying. A few decades of laborsaving devices, quick-food industries, and turning from participants into spectators haven't undone that inheritance. We've become a society of smokers, drinkers, and lazy overeaters. We snack on sugar and carbohydrates, ride when we could walk, watch sports instead of play them, work at sedentary jobs, and live in tension-producing environments.

Journalistic myth says that we are a nation faddishly seeking fitness, yet half of our adult population is out of shape. As much as our society emphasizes good looks and physical prowess, it does little to teach us how to stay fit. Therefore we are left to educate ourselves, especially in the middle and later years, when we burn fewer calories and have reduced physical capacities.

In youth, many people live and eat as they please without overweight or physical problems; in middle age, this is no longer possible. They tend to eat as much as before, but to use their bodies less. Confusing tension with tiredness, they fail to see that their sense of fatigue is too rarely caused by healthful exertion. While they may use certain muscles at a job or hobby, they gain no muscle and heart-lung conditioning.

Some people want to seek fitness but don't feel they have the time, facilities, or money. Others just don't know how to start. And all too many imagine fitness as a punishing grind. For them, the greatest problem is inertia.

Overcoming Inertia

However comfortable a lazy, unfit life may seem, it is finally no comfort to let the body deteriorate. How much more fun it is to wake up fresh, able to fully enjoy activities from chores to vacations, and still have energy left at the end of a day—in short, to feel good, look good, and be charged with vitality.

Lose the idea that fitness requires expensive equipment and lots of money and time. If you want and can afford any of these, that's fine but not essential. If you're stymied by the lack of a pleasant route to jog or a convenient swimming pool, gymnasium, or tennis court, either you haven't looked hard enough or haven't used enough imagination in creating an individual fitness program.

Some people's inertia grows from imagined problems and irrational fears. The very words physical fitness rouse their reluctance, guilt, and even dread. Some imagine boring calisthenics and see no alternatives; perhaps they tried jogging or working out at a commercial gym (or "spa") only to quit after a few weeks or months. If so, they may feel a guilt akin to that of people who often try and fail to lose weight or to give up smoking. Such people may never have felt confident about their appearance, strength, grace, or athletic ability, and may secretly fear to be seen jiggling when they jog or falling when they skate.

Such feelings may be rooted in youthful uncertainty about appearance and effectiveness. However, these ghosts of adolescent fears and broken promises to oneself should not be allowed to tyrannize the present. Old inhibitions and doubts tend to wither as one feels increased vigor and flexibility and sees the results in a mirror. If stress or mild depression adds to inertia, learn to recognize it and be aware of its self-perpetuating quality. Exercise is an excellent mental tonic, too.

Starting today, set aside a specific time for exercise and continue it for a while with regularity. Don't let stress or mild depression dampen your energy. If you're very competitive and perfectionistic, don't give up in frustration if you're not a star after a few weeks. After all, it may have taken twenty years to get out of shape, so allow a while to make a comeback. And if you are one of those who actually fear the attractive and vigorous self that lies dormant within you, take your chances. Keeping one foot in fantasies of the past (or future) will keep fitness a dream instead of a reality. So set realistic short-term goals and meet them. Don't wait until a disturbing image in the mirror, inability to wear your clothes, or even failure to walk or keep your heart beating tells you you're unfit.

The Elements of Fitness

Fitness, of course, consists of many elements—weight control, muscle tone, strength, muscular endurance, agility, balance, coordination, flexibility, lack of tension, and healthy organs. In the past, many fitness programs overemphasized strength, through calisthenics, isotonics, and weight lifting. There may now be an overcorrection in the direction of heart-lung health and endurance through jogging and aerobic exercise. Recently an interest in flexibility and relaxation has appeared, through yoga, meditation, and other techniques.

Each of these elements is necessary, but none is enough by itself. Jogging promotes strong legs and a healthy cardiovascular system, but it doesn't increase flexibility and upper-body strength. Yoga gives flexibility and relaxation, but does not provide peak exertion to build endurance. And few calisthenics programs promote balance and coordination.

Most people can't spend great amounts of time at physical conditioning, but with a little thought, anyone can create a program that fits his special needs for most or all of the elements of fitness. In planning such a program, the following points should be kept in mind:

Weight control. One cannot be fit and underweight or overweight at the same time. The chapter on diet and nutrition (see page 135) discusses this in detail, emphasizing that a fitness program *must* include adequate nutrition and weight control, but must *not* depend on crash or fad diets. A sensible diet and adequate exercise will automatically bring most people to the right weight after a while, and one needn't gain or lose more than a pound a week. You may see discouraging figures about how many miles you must run to lose an ounce, but don't be bothered. Regular exercise decreases overeating; it is boredom and inactivity that overstimulate appetite.

If you are at or below your best body weight, exercise will bring you bonuses in health and appearance. Muscle is denser (heavier) than fat; it takes up less space and creates trim lines instead of sags and bulges. Therefore exercise builds up undesirably thin arms and legs and may increase weight. Even though it cannot make the breasts larger or smaller, it can improve their contours by giving firmer muscular support.

Strength. Many fitness programs used to advertise photos of hulking former "weaklings" with necks bigger than most men's thighs. These inspired some men, discouraged others, and made women feel that corseted flab was a better alternative than this brand of fitness. We now seek not body building but necessary basic strength.

There are more than 600 muscles in the body, constituting half its weight, and their good condition is vital for health and attractiveness. Dr. Kenneth Cooper writes:

"When you see a woman of 50 looking like 30, or a woman of 60 looking—and acting—like 40, chances are that she is one of the growing number of middle-aged women who prolong their youthfulness by preventive health care, including regular exercise. Their outward signs of age-defying youthfulness—the straight back, taut, smooth skin on face, neck, arms and legs, and supple muscle contours—are evidence that these women don't spend all their spare time sitting before a TV set, moping over their lost youth."

As previously mentioned, muscle forms nature's girdle, holding in the abdomen and keeping the back straight and free of pain. Muscle strength means the ability to work and play without strain, discomfort, or fatigue. And strength in the limbs and trunk helps give suppleness for moving easily and gracefully. Some women fear that developing muscular strength and endurance will give them an unfeminine appearance. Nothing could be less true; men seldom avert their eyes from the legs of swimmers and dancers. The few women who do start developing unwanted muscle definition need only revise their programs away from isotonic and isometric exercise (see page 101) and more toward exercises for flexibility and endurance.

As you build greater strength, you will see that few job or housework patterns use more than a small fraction of the body's muscles. Much of the day-end fatigue people feel rises not from exhaustion, but from boredom, mental strain, and lack of zest and overall conditioning. For these people, the best cure is not rest, but exercise to build strength and vitality.

The mind and emotions. An unused body produces both tension and apathy. Inactivity and stress finally have the same symptoms as chronic mild depression. As exercise improves attractiveness and physical capability, one feels greater enjoyment of life. A recent study at Purdue University dramatically showed how fitness refreshes the mind as well as the body. The subjects of the experiment (by Drs. A. H. Ismail and Robert Young) were 60 middle-aged men, most of them professors and administrators, and all sedentary and unfit. Most couldn't run more than a quarter mile. But after working out for an hour and a half a day several times a week for four months, they were averaging runs of two and three miles. At that point they reported that they felt more independent and in control of their lives, and that their imaginations and creative energies had greatly increased.

Cardiovascular health. The body can function only if the heart, blood vessels, and lungs supply it with oxygen and energy. Therefore endurance depends chiefly on heart-lung health, the absence of artery and blood-pressure problems, and not forcing the heart to labor moving extra pounds of fat. Cardiovascular ills—heart attack, hypertension, stroke, etc.—kill a million Americans each year, and women are quickly catching up to men in susceptibility. Therefore building endurance has become a major or even the chief aim of fitness programs.

Endurance is usually measured by ability to walk, jog, or swim. In the past, people with cardiovascular problems were told to take it easy. But now it seems that deterioration, not exertion, is the worse threat, and that medically supervised exercise is usually part of the route to recovery. Exercise not only strengthens the heart and improves vessels, it also increases vital capacity and actually helps reduce blood cholesterol. Moderate exercise can take ten or fifteen years off one's cardiovascular age—and perhaps add them to one's lifespan. Endurance can be increased as late in life as the sixties, and by people with almost any medical history.

Tailoring Your Own Program

Obviously, different fitness programs are needed by different people: the housebound but active woman; someone who spends the day at a desk; the once-athletic man of 40, now sedentary and wheezy; the underweight woman who never trusted her coordination and grace; the 60-year-old woman who walks a great deal and occasionally swims; someone with the legs of a postman or waitress who rarely uses the torso or arm muscles; the impatient perfectionist; and the slow starter. Some points to consider are:

Men and women. Men have a higher muscle-to-fat ratio than women, and over their lifetimes use their large muscle masses harder and oftener. Well conditioned men can also extend peak efforts harder and longer. On the other hand, most women have greater flexibility and grace. Therefore men's exercises and sports demand greater strength and endurance, while women's require more suppleness. This doesn't mean that both sexes should stick to what comes easiest. Women as well as men need muscle tone, and shouldn't feel it is unfeminine to exert themselves and work up a sweat. And men shouldn't lose their balance and agility or feel that flexibility and grace are unmanly.

Some women are uncomfortable exercising just before or during their menstrual periods. Whether to do so is a matter of individual choice.

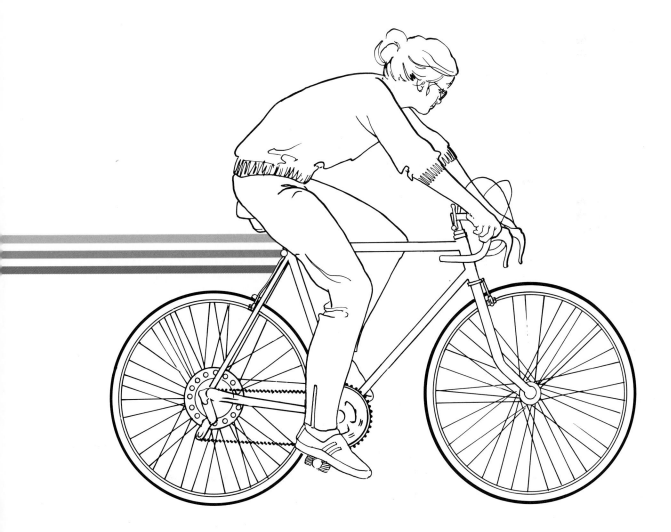

Age. No one is ever too old to become fit or stay fit. We all age differently, and even the various parts of our bodies age differently. Within approved medical limits, one should follow the sports and exercises that are most comfortable and enjoyable—at any age.

A fit person of forty to fifty can begin or continue almost any sport. This is also true through the fifties, though the fine edge of endurance and coordination may be gone. Even a vigorous sexagenarian can enjoy all but the most violent competitive sports, though it is wise for some people of this age group to limit themselves to walking, hiking, cycling, and swimming.

Someone who is out of shape should begin slowly and with medical approval, avoiding demanding sports until a fair level of fitness is reached. After fifty, it is best to begin with walking, swimming, golf, and similar activities.

Most exercise programs suggest age-graded walking, jogging, swimming, or calisthenics. However, comfort and medical supervision are the best guides, regardless of charts. Endurance capacities and appropriate exercise will change with advancing age; accepting these limits keeps activity safe and enjoyable and should not be resented.

Past and present fitness. People who were athletic in youth may overestimate their present abilities and underestimate the effects of sedentary years and normal aging. Part of us remains youthful and cannot believe that reflexes are a bit slower and that endurance is no longer a bottomless well. As a result, there is a chance of severely overtaxing the cardiovascular system, joints, and tendons.

Those who have not been athletic should not drag past insecurities with them. Most of us will never be superb athletes, just as we will not be musical virtuosos or mathematical wizards. But that shouldn't deny us the pleasures of feeling our bodies become stronger, sounder, and quicker.

Special health conditions. Some special health conditions may limit or modify fitness programs, but few make exercise impossible, and many will benefit from it. Various kinds and degrees of arthritis, rheumatism, diabetes, and kidney, lung, and cardiovascular disease require medical approval and monitoring of one's exercise program.

One should not exercise during or soon after any acute illness or infection. People who are grossly overweight may have to knock off some pounds even before going beyond walking. All such decisions must be made by you and your doctor during the consultation preceding your fitness program. For many people, and especially those with special health conditions, this exam should include an ECG taken during exercise.

Personality. Many people have dropped out of fitness programs for the simple, sensible reason that they just didn't enjoy them. Fitness should not be grimly swallowed medicine, but should rise naturally from your personality. With the wide variety of sports and exercises available, not to mention all the different ways of enjoying them, there's something for everyone.

Some people enjoy disciplined solitary effort and a regular routine; they do well with jogging, calisthenics, and charted programs, checking off each daily stint and competing with their own records. Others enjoy solitary workouts but with a sense of play—exercising to music, skating or walking alone—creating a private island of time that is more relaxation than measured discipline. Some find fun only in competitive games, such as tennis, squash, handball, and golf. People who are bored by solitary exercise and who want conviviality can obviously find it in sports for two or more, but really there's almost nothing you can't do in a group. You and your family, a few friends or neighbors, or the members of a health club or other community group can join in anything from yoga to jogging to dancing. Almost all sports can be done in a variety of ways, and one can easily change if a particular style becomes boring.

Aims: balance and variety. Few people's daily activities use all the major muscle groups, develop all the elements of fitness, or sustain effort long enough to have a conditioning effect. Housework, a job, hobbies, and even most sports cannot bring total fitness. One must plan a balanced variety of activities.

> ## "EXERCISE IS THE CLOSEST THING TO AN ANTI-AGING PILL NOW AVAILABLE."

First, you and your doctor can set priorities. After you have maintained some degree of fitness, you may choose to emphasize increasing flexibility, building up the legs, or reducing tension. With time, your aims and needs will change, and so should your sports and exercises. Perhaps at first you will need better endurance, lower blood pressure, and firmer abdominal muscles. After they are achieved, you may want to strengthen your upper torso and arms.

If an injury or change of schedule or environment makes some sport or exercise difficult, switch to another. For instance, if walking or jogging becomes difficult, switch to stationary running, swimming, or golf.

Keep up your enthusiasm by taking every opportunity for variety. Whenever you can, walk a new street or route; even take a brief auto or public-transit ride to reach another area to explore. Play sports with new partners, exercise at different times of the day, or use the "hidden calisthenics" described on page 102. From all the sports and exercises available, there may be a half dozen to help you reach your fitness goals.

How much, where, and when. The old Spartan fitness program called for leaping out of bed, throwing open the window, and plunging into exercise. For some people that's fine, but for others it's appalling. It doesn't really matter when one exercises—on waking, before lunch, in the afternoon or evening, or before bed. Some people recommend late morning or late afternoon, since exercise tends to reduce the appetite and thus keep down the size of the next meal. Others suggest evening, to dissipate the day's accumulated tensions. When you exercise is less important than maintaining a regular schedule.

Where to exercise is partly dictated by one's daily routine. A housebound woman may enjoy working out at home, to music or TV; or she may look forward to visiting a health club or pool or just taking a long walk to break her domestic routine. If she works away from home, she may find lunchtime a welcome exercise period to break up the day and avoid tension and monotony.

Various programs call for 45 minutes of exercise three times a week, 11 minutes every day, or intermediate amounts. Some people thrive on regularity and habit, others on variety. Don't fit yourself into a rigid program, but select a time and place that suit you. We do suggest a minimum of three days a week; more, of course, is better, but less will produce little or no conditioning. The weekend athlete and sporadic exerciser cannot achieve proper conditioning, and in over-exercising, may take their lives in their hands. Your doctor should advise a schedule of frequency and duration suited to your particular condition, and it should be regularly adhered to. If inconvenience or boredom is making you skip workouts, try to figure out why and shift your activities, time, or place until you have the program you enjoy and can keep.

Remember that exercise needn't hurt to be effective, but it must be strenuous and sustained enough to have a conditioning effect, which happens only when one uses one's capacities beyond their present level.

Exercise and Sports

There are three basic types of exercise: warm-up, strength-building, and endurance or heart-lung conditioning. Many exercise programs divide each workout about evenly among warm-up, muscle and endurance work, and a cooling-off period. As one's fitness improves, more time can be given to the second part.

Warming up and cooling off. One should not eat, smoke, or drink alcohol for an hour or two before exercise, because of their effects on the arteries.

It is uncomfortable and even risky to omit the warm-up before peak exertion and the cooling off afterward. Even young professional athletes begin a workout with a gradual warm-up to stretch the muscles and tendons. This avoids painful injuries, especially to the Achilles and hamstring tendons, to such major joints as the ankle, knee, and shoulder, and to the neck and back. As the warm-up progresses, the small blood vessels of the heart and limbs begin to dilate, helping the body meet its higher oxygen demand. The warm-up is especially important after age 40, when abrupt stress or strain to any part of the body is less easily tolerated.

The first warming-up exercises should loosen the body gradually; the movements shouldn't be forced. After a few stretches, the body reaches farther and more comfortably, and after a few more stretches it extends farther still. These exercises should move all parts of the body through their full range without such muscular efforts as push-ups and weight lifting. Never strain; let the body unwind naturally. Some days this will happen more quickly and fully than others. Some good warm-up exercises are:

• Stride briskly with long, rhythmic steps, swinging the arms high.
• Rotate the head, turning it gently from side to side.
• Side bends. With arms above head, bend from side to side at the hips.
• Stretch the head back and the abdomen forward, to loosen the lower back and calves.
• Toe touching. Bend at the waist and reach for the toes, bending at the knees at first if necessary.
• Knee hug. While sitting, standing, or lying on the back, raise the knees alternately and hug them to the chest.
• Arm lifts. Lift the arms sideward to shoulder level or above the head; also forward to those levels.
• Jog in place lightly, flat-footed at first, to slowly stretch the foot and ankle tendons.

These warm-up exercises should be done for at least five minutes before mild exercise, and certainly for ten minutes before strenuous efforts such as tennis, handball, skiing, and jogging. For some sports, extra leg-stretching is a good idea; for instance, walk first on the toes and then on the heels, then lie on the back and lift the legs alternately. Other stretching exercises can be added as desired. Be especially careful to limber up adequately in cold weather and when feeling tense (see page 106).

Cooling off is also a matter of both comfort and health. After peak exertion, an athlete always "walks it off" for a while; the nonathlete must do the same, with a slow jog, a walk, or light exercise (perhaps tapering off with light warm-up exercises). This allows the body to return comfortably to normal temperature and heart rate. Cooling off should continue until heavy perspiring has stopped and the pulse is down to about 100 to 110.

Failing to cool off can cause dizziness, fainting, cardiac stress, and even a heart attack. If one stops exercise abruptly, the heart and arteries are still pumping blood hard and fast, but the veins have ceased returning it quickly; therefore blood pools in the small vessels of the legs. Tapering off with light exercise slows the arterial flow and keeps the veins at work until normal circulation is restored.

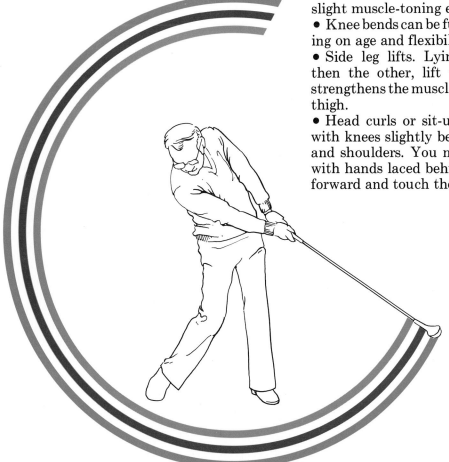

Strength. After warming up, proceed to sports and exercises that build muscular strength and endurance. Isometric exercises (also called dynamic tension) enjoyed an almost faddish popularity not many years ago. These exercises tone and strengthen muscles by exerting them against a stationary object or against other muscles—for instance, pushing with one hand against a wall or against the resistance of the other hand. While they do build strength, they may raise blood pressure enough to cause faintness or even a heart attack in susceptible people. Perform them only with a doctor's approval and without holding the breath.

More common are isotonic exercises, such as most calisthenics and weight lifting, in which the muscles push through their full range of motion. The following isotonics give a strengthening workout to most major muscle groups.
• Toe-touching, side bends, knee hugging, and some other warm-up exercises have slight muscle-toning effects.
• Knee bends can be full or partial, depending on age and flexibility.
• Side leg lifts. Lying on one side and then the other, lift the upper leg. This strengthens the muscles on the inside of the thigh.
• Head curls or sit-ups. Lie on the back with knees slightly bent and lift the head and shoulders. You may also sit up fully with hands laced behind the head or lean forward and touch the toes.

• Body twists. Turn the body from side to side at the waist, with feet apart and arms extended overhead.

• Prone arch. Lie on the stomach and raise both head and legs from the floor. This can be extended to raising the chest and thighs and adding a flutter kick.

• Leg lifts. Lie on the back and lift the legs to a 90-degree angle with the floor, alternately or together.

• Push-ups range from easy (knees fixed on the ground) to difficult (entire body straight, only the chest touching floor).

Working one's way up from ten to twenty of each of these exercises (again, with a doctor's approval) will be quite adequate for building overall muscle tone and strength. As your strength grows, you can move from mild to more demanding forms of any exercise. For instance, if your abdominal muscles are out of shape, begin with head curls. Lying supine with arms at your sides, lift the head and shoulders just enough to see your toes. Then progress until you can rise halfway and then fully to a sitting position, with hands behind the head. Finally, sit up, reach forward, and touch the ankles; then touch the toes. You should feel perfectly comfortable at each level of difficulty before moving to another.

Other exercises can be substituted for variety or added to build certain muscles:

• Shoulder squeeze is a mild isotonic for strengthening the shoulders: hug your arms about yourself and squeeze the shoulders.

• Pull-ups. With hands facing toward the body, hang from a bar and lift the body till the chin reaches the bar. Be sure the bar is secure and cannot fall. This strengthens the arms and shoulders.

• Arm circles. Extend the arms sideward or frontward and turn them in large circles, first forward and then in the reverse direction. If this seems easy, try it with a magazine or light book in each hand. This builds up the shoulder muscles and helps release tension.

• Side arm lifts build up the pectoral muscles that support the breasts. Lie on the back, arms extended at the sides, and raise them till they meet overhead. Once this seems easy, hold a light book in each hand.

There are other isometric and isotonic exercises that specifically develop the chest muscles, prepare the wrists for tennis and golf, the legs for jogging, and the ankles for skiing.

Hidden calisthenics. You can enjoy brief relaxing, stretching, and strengthening exercises during the course of any day. This is especially good when events interfere with your usual exercise and when you are tense or tired.

To relax at home or office, take five long, deep breaths and release them fully. Roll the head loosely to the left and right. Stand and do a few easy toe-touches and side-bends. Cover the eyes with the palms of the hands for a half minute; then exercise tired eye muscles by gently rolling the eyes to left and right, top and bottom.

You can do some exercises sitting in a chair. Lift the legs alternately or together for a count of three or six. Tighten the abdominal muscles for a count of six. Do a few knee hugs with each leg. If your doctor says you can do mild isometrics, clasp your hands behind your head and push the head back while resisting the movement with your hands. Put your hands on top of a desk or table, bend the elbows, and press down as if trying to lift your body from the chair; do this for a count of three. Place your palms against the underside of a heavy desk and push up as if trying to lift it.

While standing, tense the abdominal muscles for a count of six; do the same with the muscles of the buttocks. Stand with your back to a wall and try to flatten the small of the back against it for a count of six. Rise on your toes for a count of six, then on your heels. If your doctor advises isometrics, put your hands against opposite sides of a door jamb or file cabinet and press inward for a count of three.

These little exercise sessions performed while dressing, waiting in a line, working, and performing routine tasks, are enough to help keep muscle tone, reduce tension, and leave you more refreshed.

Endurance: the lifelong conditioners. Walking, jogging, and swimming are inexpensive or free, and they can be done all life long to build heart-lung health and muscular endurance.

> ## "No one is ever too old to become fit or stay fit."

Walking is a fine way for an out-of-condition person to start back to fitness. You can begin with short strolls and gradually go on to a comfortable but brisk pace, timing your distance. Once the legs are in good condition, you can jog outdoors or run in place indoors. Many people find walking and jogging boring, can't find congenial routes, or hesitate to brave hot or cold weather. Although jogging is enjoyed more by some people than others, walking certainly should be given a chance. For variety, try it in new and interesting places—down different streets, beside a river, or in a park. Even drive a few miles from home to explore a new route on foot. Alternate jogging and walking every block or every hundred steps. Or if you are in good enough condition, run backward or hike or run cross-country. Like all other exercise, walking and jogging should be a pleasure and an adventure, not a grind.

When you walk or jog, always wear snug but comfortable socks and well cushioned athletic shoes. Go with a natural heel-to-toe step, breathing as normally as possible, in through the nose and out through the mouth, until inhaling through the mouth becomes necessary.

Those who find that walking and jogging just don't hold their interest should consider bicycling and swimming. The latter is especially good, for it improves overall muscle strength and vital capacity as well as endurance. Even people who have never been comfortable in the water can learn a few basic strokes in the shallow end of a pool, and many facilities offer inexpensive or free lessons. Like walking, swimming can be enjoyed at almost any level, from a slow easy paddle to a strenuous workout to build endurance and strength. It also produces flexibility and muscular endurance, especially if one learns a few different strokes, such as the breaststroke, crawl, and backstroke. All are excellent for the muscles of the legs, arms, shoulders, back, and abdomen. Under medical supervision, swimming and walking are fine therapy for many health conditions that often discourage people from exercise.

How far and how long to walk, jog, swim, or cycle is easy to determine. Your physician, as part of your physical exam, will give you guidelines based on your vital capacity and cardiovascular condition. He will probably suggest a short distance and comfortable rate at the beginning and then have you gradually increase distance and shorten time. Almost all systematic programs—aerobics, the Royal Canadian Air Force exercises, and YMCA programs—give time and distance charts adapted for age, sex, and condition. The YMCA, for instance, sets up a fifty-mile swim that can be done over a few months or a few years, depending on age and fitness.

Similar effects can be reached through rope jumping, rowing machines, bicycling exercisers, and other methods, but don't buy expensive equipment unless you are quite sure of using it long and regularly. Besides, a walk, jog, or swim offers more variety, change of scene, and human contact.

Sports. Many sports offer a combination of muscular and endurance conditioning, and they add to calisthenics and aerobics the elements of agility, balance, flexibility, and grace—to say nothing of fun. They can supplement, accompany, or even partly replace calisthenics and endurance training.

• Games to leave behind. In the forties, certain sports should be discontinued or modified. Among these are football, basketball, hockey, soccer, and strenuous gymnastics. Middle-aged bones are a bit more brittle, and tendons and ligaments are less elastic. There is also greater risk of injury and cardiac strain, and injuries heal more slowly.

• Strenuous sports build endurance, agility, and strength, especially in the legs and lower torso. They include handball, tennis singles, and skiing, which should be played after young adulthood only by those who have remained fit or have reconditioned themselves first. People in good condition can enjoy these sports well into their fifties and even beyond. But they should bear in mind that in exhilarating, competitive sports, one tends to play in hard spurts, increasing vulnerability to falls, injuries, and cardiovascular stress.

• The lifetime sports. Many other sports, however, can be enjoyed throughout life, at a level suitable to one's age and fitness. Swimming, walking, running, skating, golf, cycling, and modified tennis and skiing all offer opportunities for sociability and change of scene.

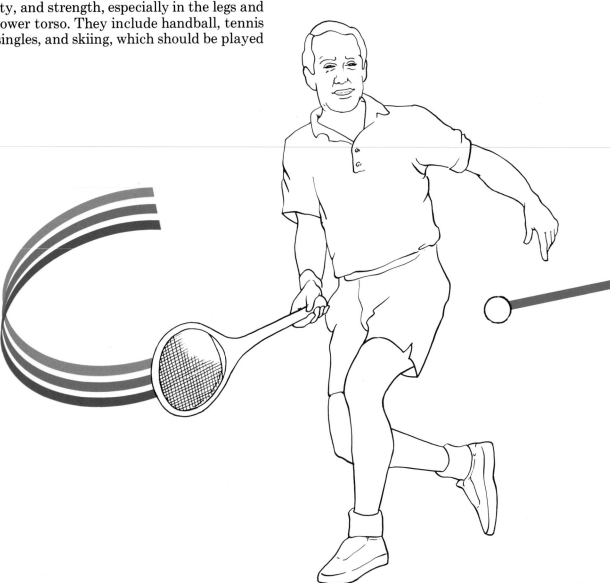

Tennis is becoming one of our most popular sports. Municipal, school, and other free or inexpensive courts now exist in many communities. Singles can be intense and grueling, but can also be played moderately through most of life. The late King Gustav of Sweden played tennis into his nineties. Many people switch in middle age to the less strenuous doubles, which can be enjoyed by couples, parents and children, and friends.

Although tennis carries some risk of injury, especially to the shoulder, elbow, knee, and ankle, it is a fine conditioner for endurance and the muscles of the lower body. It stretches the entire body and increases agility, coordination, and grace. Squash, paddle tennis, and other variations share the advantages of tennis and can be played indoors or out.

We should add a point that applies also to many other games of skill. Each year many new players try tennis, play sporadically, and give up. The first few months may frustrate beginners, especially if they play only once a week—too little to improve skill but enough to endanger the heart. Hitting a tennis or golf ball or gliding down a gentle ski slope looks relatively easy, but many skills must be mastered and coordinated. It takes persistence to get beyond lobbing the ball around the court wildly, but it's worth it. Games of skill are far more satisfying when played well rather than in slapdash sallies. So if you take up tennis or other sports requiring acquired skill, obtain a few lessons. These often are available free or inexpensively, and they get one off to a more promising start.

Skiing has many of tennis's advantages in conditioning, change of scene, and choice of individual, family, or social participation. And because of the effort required in poling, it also develops the upper body.

Many people are rightly intimidated by downhill skiing. Those who have already mastered downhill skiing can continue on gentle slopes into their middle or even later years. Ski lifts and artificially maintained slopes have made it safe for fit people of ordinary athletic ability. There is still some risk of injury, but less if one skis sensibly.

At any age, however, one can enjoy cross-country skiing, which doesn't call for slopes and their attendant risk of injury. Wherever there is snow, people can simply put on their skis and glide as small or great a distance as they like across any terrain, even a golf course or neighborhood park. It is an excellent family and group activity, noncompetitive and safe.

As with tennis, one should have a doctor's approval, buy proper equipment, and seek some initial instruction. Cross-country skiing requires a rather high level of fitness, and special exercises may be needed to strengthen certain muscles and tendons, such as the hamstrings, calves, and ankles.

Golf is a thoroughly involving game to those who know it. Some who have never played it may think it boring, but that's hardly true for those who've learned the many subtle skills involved. This is an excellent game for the middle and later years as it promotes coordination, aids flexibility, and offers miles of pleasant walking. So don't ride in a golf cart, and don't begin with eighteen holes.

• Hidden exercise. You don't need a gymnasium to use your body well throughout the day. Dozens of daily opportunities exist for stretching and strengthening the body.

The best basic exercise is a brisk walk. Don't drive to the store, office, or mailbox if you can walk. If you use a car or public transportation, park or debark a few blocks from where you're heading. Climb stairs instead of using elevators; if possible, take them two at a time.

Lose the habit of avoiding effort. You will come to enjoy using your body and feeling its vigor. Laborsaving devices are fine for eliminating pointless drudgery, but they become a curse when they make laziness a way of life. In fact, you can remove some of the boredom from tasks by thinking of them as useful exercise. Keep yourself fit, not delivery boys and your children. Bend to tie your shoes instead of sitting down to do so. Don't push things when you can lift them (remember to bend the knees, not the back, and lift with the legs). Dr. Robert Butler writes:

"Emptying the trash, mowing the lawn and walking upstairs instead of taking the elevator should follow a redefinition of what is called drudgery and what is exercise. . . . Gardening is a fine hobby that gives pleasure to oneself and others. It saves money to garden, cut the grass, pull weeds, do household chores. Purchase of a handyman's guide for work around the house can lead to exercise and save repair costs too." He adds that dancing and hiking are fine exercise at any age.

Such a life lifts one from passive habits that take a great toll in our society, bringing one back into the world of the active, the confident, and the rewarded.

• Tension and relaxation are barometers of fitness. Try to notice whether feeling tired or tense results from too little sleep, physical fatigue, worry, mild depression, or tuning out with exasperation from unwanted, boring tasks. Sometimes the best cure for apathy, depression, or tension is vigorous exercise, but one must first undo the feeling of being tied in a knot. Such distinctions are important because exercising while tense can cause stiff, sore muscles, especially in the lower back and joints.

Experiment and discover what works for you. Meditation or yoga may be useful. Although some people think yoga demands slithering into reverse pretzel position and living on rice husks, basic Hatha yoga is actually an easily learned relaxer and muscle-toner. Gentle or deep-muscle massage relieves tension for some; others find that sexual activity helps them relax, mildly stimulates their circulation, and leaves them refreshed.

Coping with Heat and Cold

In the middle and later years, one adapts less quickly and easily to severe heat and cold. Dealing with them inadequately can have serious results.

When the body works, it generates heat, which is dissipated when perspiration evaporates. Obviously heat and humidity slow the process. Profuse sweating also causes dehydration and salt loss, which may produce heat cramps in the abdominal and leg muscles, weakness, nausea, and fainting. Without causing such symptoms, heat exhaustion can build over days or weeks. Sunstroke must be avoided by those unused to outdoor exposure. Most important, dehydration is dangerous to people with cardiovascular problems.

• Condition yourself slowly to sun exposure and exertion in the heat. Always stop if nausea, extreme fatigue, or other signs of heat exhaustion appear. Then, over weeks and months, your heat tolerance will increase.

• Don't try to sweat away weight. Before day's end, normal eating and drinking will restore the fluid weight loss, and dehydration is dangerous. Avoid rubber "reducing" belts; they only increase perspiration.

• Wear loose, comfortable clothes to prevent chafing, heat rash, and extra sweating.

• Avoid sauna and steam baths and very long hot showers after a heavy workout. Again, increased dehydration may raise your blood pressure.

• If you sweat heavily, take one or two salt tablets with a meal or medium-size glass of water. During prolonged exercise, pause for occasional sips of water (slightly salted if necessary), orange juice, or a medically approved commercial product containing salt, minerals, and sugar.

Once accustomed to outdoor exercise, be guided by the temperature-humidity index (THI), which is given in many summer weather reports. When the THI goes above 70, reduce exercise to swimming and light calisthenics; above 80, engage in swimming only. At 90 degree temperature and 80 per cent humidity, even with a light breeze to aid cooling, you run the risk of heat cramps and cardiovascular strain. In such periods of great heat, try to exercise in the cool of the morning or evening.

Exercising in the cold also requires precautions. Do a thorough warm-up routine before all exertion on cool days, when muscles and tendons stretch less easily. Even young athletes suffer snapped tendons, torn ligaments, and joint injuries if they skip warming up on cool days.

Cold air sometimes causes rapid pulse, flushing, faintness, and a drop in blood pressure. This is increasingly likely as the temperature goes well below freezing. Inhaling a lot of very cold air, as when jogging or working strenuously into a freezing wind, can trigger a heart attack. When exercising in below-freezing weather, avoid heading into strong winds, working till you pant for breath, and holding your breath (as in some moments of shoveling snow). You may increase comfort and health by covering the mouth loosely with a scarf.

After exercise, always cool off slowly without becoming chilled.

Sticking With It

When unused muscles are put to use, there will be some minor aches, but exercise shouldn't be severely uncomfortable. Never force stretching, muscular effort, and endurance. If you feel exhaustion or strain halfway through an exercise, stop and rest, then pick up where you left off. If pain, fatigue, or breathlessness is persistent, see your physician at once. You may have merely tried too much too soon; if so, exercise at a less demanding level and work your way back up. When work, illness, or vacation breaks your routine, drop back and return to your old level at a comfortable rate. Never exercise when suffering any chronic or acute illness or during convalescence.

If you have been out of condition for some time, the first month of exercise will be the hardest. You will be breaking years-long patterns with unaccustomed effort and discipline. To avoid flagging, try to vary the kinds of exercise and time of day, or switch to exercising alone or with family or friends—whatever adds to your interest and enjoyment. Do remember that any new sport or exercise stresses a new set of muscles and must be adapted to slowly.

Having achieved basic conditioning, you'll come to miss working out when you skip it. Even three or four weeks of exercise will bring you a new measure of strength, vigor, and bounce—probably a better appearance, too.

The second difficult point comes after three to six months of fitness training. Now you feel and look better, and like the dieter who has lost half the weight he should, you may become overconfident and backslide. Maintain fun and involvement in workouts and sports so that fitness is not a routine or duty, but a way of life. At every stage, design and redesign your program so that it keeps offering motivation and rewards. Aim for a slightly better walking time or distance, a better tennis stroke, or another inch on or off some part of the body.

One advantage of some popular exercise programs (for instance, aerobics and the RCAF system) is their specific, progressive goals. Every week one can say, "I've just done better than I could last week." But for this very reason, they can also become monotonous. That's why we suggest eventually combining their goals and methods with sports, games, and creative personal efforts to achieve a fit life that is fun.

CHAPTER 4   CLARK H. MILLIKAN, M.D.

PIPELINES TO THE BRAIN: STROKES

The Greeks had a word for it—*apoplexy,* meaning "struck down." The word was an apt description of an occasional dramatic event: a man or woman suddenly falling to the ground, as if poleaxed or clubbed down, lying there paralyzed, unconscious, and perhaps dead. Today we commonly call such an event a *stroke.* Some doctors use the term *cerebrovascular accident.*

Not all or most strokes are immediately fatal. They range from transient "little strokes" that may not even be recognized, to massive strokes that are quickly lethal. In between are hundreds of variations. Probably as many as two million Americans have some trouble from stroke each year. Many patients recover and return to their usual work or to modified activity, but for others, disability may make it impossible to hold a job and may require the constant care of others.

We are more vulnerable to strokes as we get older. Although the peak incidence is at about 60 years of age, the groundwork is usually laid much earlier, and strokes are not uncommon in fortyish and younger persons. Great emphasis is currently directed toward prevention of strokes by identifying people at high risk—those with a "stroke-prone profile"—and instituting protective measures.

In most respects, protective and preventive measures against strokes are the same as those against heart attacks. Most of the risk factors are similar if not identical. The main difference is that heart attacks affect vessels that serve the heart, while strokes result from damage to vessels that supply blood to the brain.

BRAIN CIRCULATION

The heart pumps oxygenated blood upward through the neck to finely branched arteries that serve the brain and head. Any impairment of the brain's blood supply can cause minor or major symptoms of stroke.

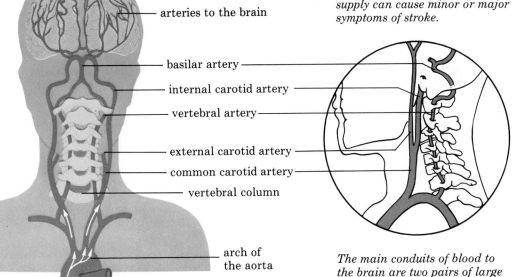

arteries to the brain

basilar artery

internal carotid artery

vertebral artery

external carotid artery

common carotid artery

vertebral column

arch of the aorta

heart

The main conduits of blood to the brain are two pairs of large arteries (right- and left-sided) that emerge from the arch of the aorta. The vertebral arteries travel upward through openings in the neck vertebrae. The common carotid artery on each side of the neck divides into the external carotid and the internal carotid, which branches inward and upward.

BLOOD SUPPLY TO THE BRAIN

The brain is extremely sensitive to its blood supply. Shutting off its oxygen-enriched blood for a very few minutes results in irreparable damage. Arteries that supply the brain arise from the arch of the aorta, the great output vessel of the heart through which oxygenated blood is pumped, and branch in complicated ways in their upward course.

Pipelines to the Brain

You can think of your brain as getting its blood through two pairs of large arteries. One pair—the *carotid arteries*—is at the sides of the neck. The *external* carotid is near the surface where, at a Y-shaped junction, the *internal* carotid branches inward and upward. "Carotid" derives from a Greek word meaning "to put to sleep," corroborative of the legend that pressure of a hand on the artery produces unconsciousness. Manual pressure impedes blood flow in a way similar to obstruction of the artery in some forms of stroke.

The *vertebral arteries,* the other major system, travel upward to the base of the skull through a series of holes in the sides of the neck vertebrae. The arrangement gives bony protection to the arteries and keeps them from being compressed or kinked whenever we twist or turn the head. Inside the head, the two vertebral arteries join to form the basilar artery. The combination is called the *vertebro-basilar* system, a term so technical and hard to remember that we shall simply call it "vertebral" or "VB." The arteries are strung through our neck bones somewhat like thread through the eyes of needles.

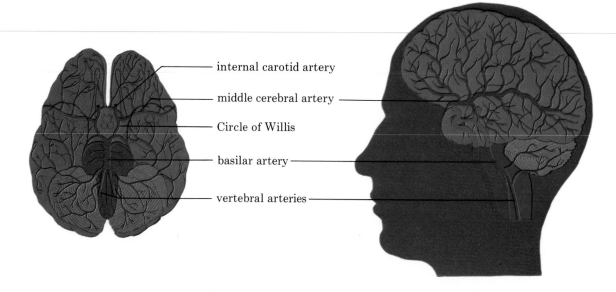

internal carotid artery

middle cerebral artery

Circle of Willis

basilar artery

vertebral arteries

BLOOD FLOW TO THE BRAIN

This bottom view of the brain (above left) shows the Circle of Willis, where four major arteries join to create a rotary traffic circle of blood flow. Here, blood is channeled to both sides of the brain, even though an artery farther down is obstructed. The paired vertebral arteries emerge from the vertebrae of the neck and join to form a basilar artery (VB system). The carotid and VB systems supply blood to different parts of the brain; hence, the area affected by stroke may be suggested by characteristic symptoms.

On the underside of the brain, the four major arteries join a structure shaped like a rotary traffic circle and appropriately called the Circle of Willis. This is a protective system that supplies blood to both sides of the brain even when something plugs an artery farther down so its blood cannot reach the "rotary."

The structures described are the principal ones affected by stroke in all of its many variations.

Marvels of Brain Function

A stroke is a condition in which an acute local disruption of blood supply produces local damage to the brain.

Someone has described the brain as "that miraculous black box between our ears." Miraculous indeed! To oversimplify, the brain is a receiver and interpreter of stimuli from our senses, and an instigator of whatever action it deems appropriate.

To trigger an action, the brain sends out messages to selected muscles to produce the movement. The action may be a simple reflex, such as jerking the hand from a hot object, or one as complex as mobilizing all the speech-producing muscles to deliver a lecture (an action presumably involved with the thought process as well). Symptoms of stroke give some clues as to the part of the brain that is damaged.

Locations of damage. The abnormalities of function that are produced by an injury to a part of the brain depend on the part involved. In general, the left side of the brain controls the right side of the body, and vice versa.

In right-handed people, faculties for understanding and formulating speech are located in the left side of the brain. Speech defects resulting from stroke depend on the extent and severity of brain damage. A very little bit of damage in the dominant (usually left) side of the brain may cause a minor defect in speech, such as inability to name objects. The person may, for instance, recognize a pencil but be unable to name it. More extensive damage may cause loss of all understanding and production of speech *(global aphasia)*.

Motor impairments—paralysis, weakness, and numbness—likewise vary with the extent and location of brain damage. A small bit of damage to the motor system in one side of the brain may cause only slight weakness or numbness of the opposite hand. More devastating damage may produce more profound weakness or paralysis of the opposite side of the body. Vision to one side or the other also may be involved to varying degrees.

In a very bad stroke—a relatively large area of severe brain damage—speech, movement, vision, and sensation all may be gravely impaired. The extraordinary complexity of brain function provides the matrix for thousands of different symptoms and neurological defects.

Local brain damage may vary from a brief change in brain function, completely reversible so that the patient returns to normal, to severe permanent damage, such as the inability to speak in a patient who has had one side of his body completely paralyzed. Brain cells do not reproduce or regenerate, and when brain tissue is deprived of blood for even a few minutes, there is risk of permanent change.

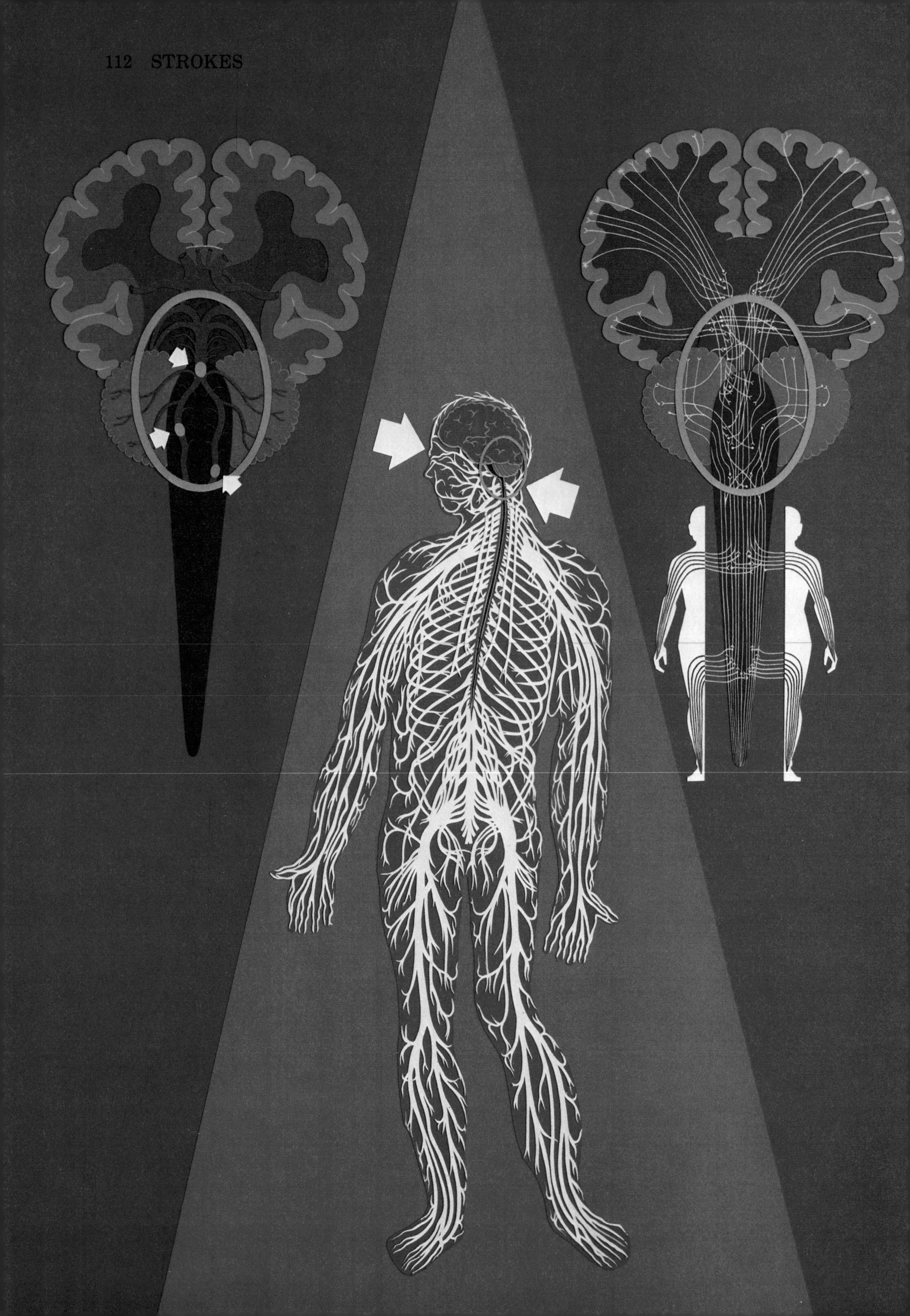

SWITCHING CENTERS OF THE BRAIN

The left drawing on the opposite page shows the blood supply to the brainstem from the vertebral-basilar arteries. Clots (white arrows) obstruct the blood supply and cause almost limitless combinations of symptoms. The nerve tracts of the entire brain and entire body (center figure) converge in the brainstem with cascades of incoming and outgoing messages that demand interpretation and action. The right drawing suggests the switchboard function of the brainstem (circle), where torrents of nerve impulses, coming and going, make connections, cross to the opposite side, receive sensations, and activate muscles. Nerve impulses from the brain to the muscles produce movement (motor function), and from the body to the brain convey feelings of pain, heat, touch, etc. (sensory function). A minor decrease of the blood supply to the switching station can cause major trouble.

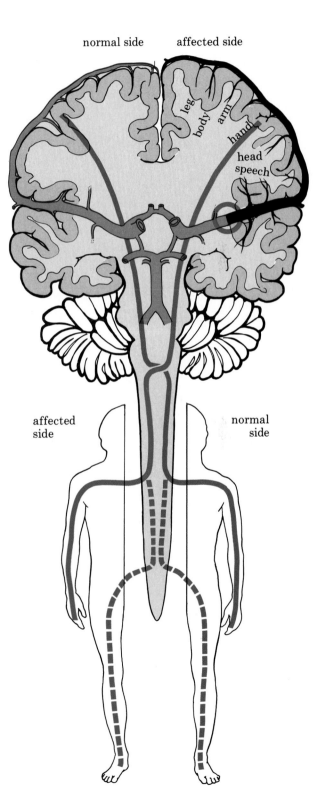

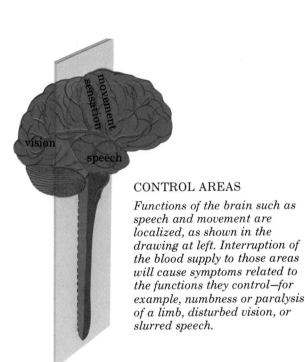

CONTROL AREAS

Functions of the brain such as speech and movement are localized, as shown in the drawing at left. Interruption of the blood supply to those areas will cause symptoms related to the functions they control—for example, numbness or paralysis of a limb, disturbed vision, or slurred speech.

CROSSOVER

At right, the left side of the brain (labeled "normal side") shows blood circulation and the transmission of nerve impulses (blue line) to muscles on the opposite side of the body. The right side of the brain (labeled "affected side") shows blood flow obstructed by a clot in the middle cerebral artery (encircled). This interrupts the blood flow to brain cells that control movements of limbs on the opposite side of the body, while functions controlled by the normal side of the brain are unimpaired.

NORMAL EYE FIELDS

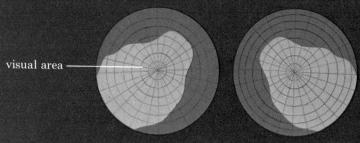

visual area

AFFECTED EYE FIELDS

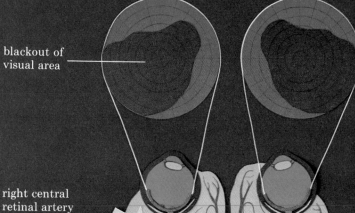

blackout of
visual area

STROKE-AFFECTED VISION

*Examination of the eye fields
(the area encompassed by vision)
following stroke, together with
the patient's recollection of
visual impairment, help the
physician to pinpoint the site of
blood-vessel obstruction. An
embolus (clot fragment) traveling
up the left internal carotid artery
may lodge in a bend of the vessel
(white arrow). The obstruction
interrupts blood flow to parts of
the brain and to the central
retinal artery, causing temporary
loss of vision in either eye.
Similarly, obstruction of the
right central retinal artery
(yellow arrow) by a smaller clot
will cause loss of vision in the
right eye.*

right central
retinal artery
(obstructed)

left internal
carotid artery
(obstructed)

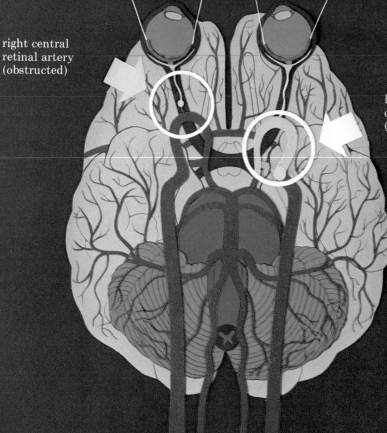

TYPES OF STROKE

By definition, the word "acute" in reference to stroke has to do with the span of time during which disturbance of blood supply to a local area of the brain comes on, commonly a few minutes to a few hours. Fundamentally, there are two types of strokes: occlusive strokes, in which an artery supplying a particular area of the brain is obstructed, and hemorrhagic strokes, in which an artery breaks and blood rushes out, causing damage to an area of the brain.

Mechanisms of Stroke

Occlusive stroke. By far, the most common type of stroke is the one in which there's obstruction of an artery supplying blood to a part of the brain. The blocking of an artery must ordinarily occur quite suddenly to produce local brain damage. This sudden blocking comes about in two ways: a clot *(thrombus)* occurs, or an *embolus* lodges, obstructing blood flow.

An embolus is a particle of material moving in the bloodstream. It may consist of a piece of clot that has broken off from the main thrombus—one carried in the blood through smaller and smaller arteries until it becomes stuck in a vessel too small to traverse. Or it may be another type that is made from cholesterol and occurs when there is ulceration of an atherosclerotic plaque inside an artery. Still another kind of embolus may form from particles—red blood cells, fibrin, and formed blood elements called platelets—that are just beginning to form a clot.

If a block occurs in an artery, additional disruption of blood flow may be produced by downstream formation of clots below the original obstruction—clots that can close off openings into other arterial branches. Because there is this definite relationship between clotting and embolus formation, the two processes are often referred to as "thrombosis-embolism."

Hemorrhagic stroke. The other major mechanism of stroke is rupture of an artery that spills blood into areas of the brain. Hemorrhage most often occurs inside the brain and is a devastating disorder. Occasionally the bleeding takes place on the surface of the brain, in which instance it is called a *subarachnoid hemorrhage.* This condition is often caused by the breaking of an *aneurysm,* which is a ballooned-out portion of an artery.

Even though blood pressure may be abnormally high, an artery must be defective to break. But if there is a defect in the arterial wall, high blood pressure greatly increases the risk of hemorrhage. In some instances, hemorrhage occurs from an abnormal connection between arteries and veins—an *arteriovenous malformation*—but this is not a common cause of stroke.

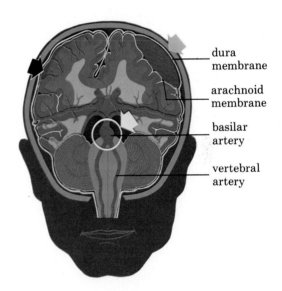

dura
membrane

arachnoid
membrane

basilar
artery

vertebral
artery

HEMORRHAGIC STROKE

Rupture of a vessel that spills blood onto the surface of the brain or deep inside it causes hemorrhagic stroke. The schematic drawing shows a subarachnoid hemorrhage (black arrow) and a subdural hemorrhage (yellow arrow). The arachnoid and dura membranes are coverings of the brain, also called meninges. The white arrow points to an aneurysm—a weakened, ballooned-out part of an artery that can burst and spill blood inside the brain.

Background of Strokes

Two primary factors figure prominently in the background of stroke patients: *atherosclerosis* and *hypertension* or high blood pressure. We shall be brief in our mention, since both factors are equally involved in heart attacks and are discussed in detail elsewhere in this book (see pages 65 and 76).

It is true that a great many people who have atherosclerosis will never experience a stroke or heart attack. But it is also true that strokes do not occur in people who are free of atherosclerosis unless there is an uncommon obstruction by an embolus arising in the heart or elsewhere. It is the atherosclerotic plaque that is commonly the site of clot formation, with or without development of an embolus.

It is easy to conceive how high blood pressure might produce a hemorrhage in an artery that's ripe for a blowout. But it is not so obvious how high blood pressure is a factor in the common type of stroke caused by obstruction in an artery. The statistical relationship between such strokes and high blood pressure, however, is quite clear. It appears that in many instances, hypertension increases the amount of atherosclerosis that is present.

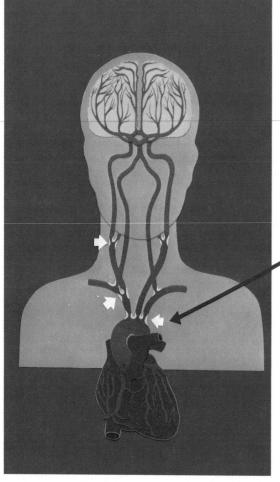

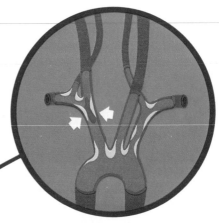

VESSEL BLOCKAGE

Atherosclerosis is the underlying condition of many strokes. Fatty plaques in artery walls may accumulate at critical junctions of the vessels carrying blood to the head, especially at bifurcations where vessels branch and become smaller (white arrows). The drawing above is a close-up view of blood vessels dividing into smaller and smaller branches. Atherosclerotic plaques (yellow) narrow the internal diameter of blood vessels and impede blood flow. A clot may form (white arrows) and obstruct blood flow, or part of a clot (embolus) may break off and travel in the bloodstream until it is trapped in a vessel too small for it to pass through.

The vital point is that current treatment to control high blood pressure, discussed elsewhere with respect to heart disease, is effective and available, and is a prudent precaution against strokes.

Diagnosing strokes. Early diagnosis of stroke is very important, because once brain softening has occurred, it is permanent. However, diagnosis is difficult: there's no definitive test for atherosclerosis in the arteries of hidden organs, and many people with atherosclerosis never suffer a stroke.

Clues to atherosclerotic involvement are derived by assessing changes in brain function, i.e., keeping a meticulous history of the patient's symptoms and administering careful physical and neurological examinations. It is now customary to group types of stroke into three categories:

Incipient or impending stroke. These patients, particularly those who have had transient ischemic attacks (see this page and page 118), seem most likely to have a stroke in the near future.

Advancing or progressing stroke. These patients have active progression of symptoms and physical disability, such as increasing weakness of one side of the body over a short period of observation, perhaps a few hours.

Completed stroke. These patients have suffered damage that is no longer progressing, and there is the possibility of improvement over ensuing days or months.

In taking the patient's history, inferences can be drawn from the "temporal profile" of the disorder: the length of time during which symptoms—from weakness to paralysis, for instance—have developed. Symptoms resulting from a stroke usually occur relatively quickly, in minutes or hours, whereas symptoms of a brain tumor ordinarily come on over many weeks or months. A brain tumor may mimic a stroke by suddenly obstructing an artery, but fortunately, this is uncommon.

INCIPIENT OR IMPENDING STROKE

The concept of predicting a stroke before permanent brain damage has been done has matured in the past two or three decades. Many persons vulnerable to stroke because of obstruction of an artery have important episodes, brief symptoms, or other "red flags" that give advance warning of possible catastrophic stroke.

Warning Episodes

(transient ischemic attacks)

Members of the family or a person himself may be aware of sudden brief changes of sensation or function that give fair warning of a possible serious stroke in the future. The person may suddenly feel dizzy, unsteady, numb, or have difficulty in speaking. Typically, the warning episode comes and goes rather quickly; afterward the person is perfectly normal but may be puzzled about what has happened.

What *has* happened? Blood supply to a local area of the brain has been impaired. This is also what happens in a major stroke, but the warning episode is too brief to cause permanent damage to the brain. We could call such attacks small strokes, miniature strokes, little blackouts, or something else, but the descriptive medical name—technical but not hard to understand—is *transient ischemic attacks (TIA)*. "Ischemia" means insufficient blood flow due to mechanical obstruction. The TIA concept is new to the layman, but very important in the symptomatology of strokes because of its "red flag" value.

Rarely does a physician see a patient during one of these episodes; symptoms soon disappear and the patient is back to normal. The patient himself is often the best observer, but family and friends may sometimes notice lapses and changes in behavior without understanding their significance. A family physician may be the first to recognize warning signs over a period of time.

Symptoms. Signs of little strokes may appear before age 40. These do not invariably end in a catastrophic stroke, but they may indicate incipient or impending stroke, and they give fair warning that preventive care is essential. Some of the warning signs are:

- Sudden temporary weakness or numbness of the face or an arm or leg
- Temporary loss of speech or trouble in speaking or understanding speech
- An episode of double vision
- Temporary dimness or loss of vision, particularly in one eye
- Unexplained dizziness or unsteadiness, or momentary blackout
- Confusion or personality changes: a previously stable and cheerful person may become irritable, sloppy, suspicious, or behave in ways inconsistent with his previous life pattern.

These symptoms depend on the parts of the brain affected by an insufficiency of blood—parts that can be identified by careful diagnosis.

Identifying the Source

There are two types of transient ischemic attacks, recognizable from the brain territories served by the carotid and vertebral arteries (shown in the drawing on page 110). Each type of attack is treated differently.

Each carotid artery supplies about three-fourths of the side of the brain that it serves. The vertebral (VB) system carries blood to the *brainstem* above the spinal cord, to the back portion of the brain, and to the *cerebellum,* a structure underlying the back of the brain that governs balance and coordination.

Carotid Warning Attacks

The symptoms arising from an attack in the carotid system depend on what portion of the brain suffers the temporary decrease in blood flow. If the entire carotid system is affected, there will be a sudden onset of weakness or paralysis. The patient may describe this as a "deadness" or a "numbness" of the face, arm, or leg, and be more impressed by this sensation than the fact that he cannot move those parts.

If he attempts to talk during the few minutes of the attack, he may have poor control of one side of his mouth, with slurring and mushiness of speech. In right-handed people (left-brain dominant), decrease of flow in the left carotid artery may cause difficulty in formulating speech—in putting syllables together, as distinguished from slurring—as well as in comprehending the speech of others.

Vision, too, may be affected. The artery that supplies blood to the eye is the first major branch of the carotid artery inside the head. Insufficient flow of blood in this artery may produce a sudden, painless loss of vision in one eye, ordinarily lasting only three to ten minutes. Frequently the patient describes the loss of vision as "a shade being pulled over the eye."

Occasionally vision may be affected in another fashion. Objects situated in the field of vision opposite to the involved carotid artery may not be seen at all. For example, if the right carotid is affected, the patient may not see objects to his left when he looks straight ahead. Each attack lasts less than half an hour, so the physician must get his understanding from a precise account furnished by the patient.

Transient ischemia commonly affects only a portion of the carotid system, and an attack may exhibit only a fraction of the picture described. For instance, there may be only mild clumsiness or weakness of a hand, foot, or one side of the face. There may be defective speech alone, or mild impairment of speaking and a weak right hand. There are dozens of variations, although an individual patient usually has episodes that are similar to one another if not commonly identical.

One person may have tens or dozens of transient episodes and never have a stroke, while another may have a single episode and then a permanent serious stroke. A high percentage of patients who have a serious stroke have a previous history of transient ischemic attacks. This means that the attacks are very significant and that great attention should promptly be paid to them.

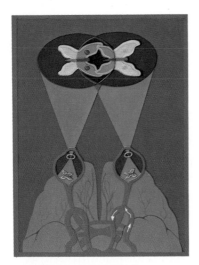

CAROTID WARNING ATTACKS

Normal full-color binocular vision and normal circulation of blood to the arteries of the eye are shown in the drawing above. At right, obstruction of the internal carotid artery is indicated by the yellow dot. This causes temporary loss of vision in only one eye, usually for a few minutes. Other symptoms, typically one-sided, have many variations: clumsiness of one side of the body, a weak hand or leg, or defective speech.

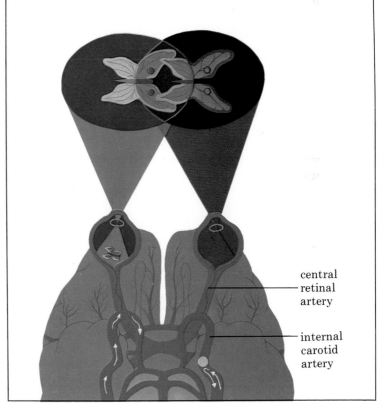

central retinal artery

internal carotid artery

Follow-up. If a person has had one or several attacks of transient ischemia in the carotid system, a thorough examination should be performed. There will be no neurological abnormalities—by definition, each attack abates and leaves the patient functioning normally.

The physician will probably feel for pulsation of the carotid artery on each side of the neck—very gently, since marked pressure may actually break off a piece of a clot, which can then act as an embolus capable of causing a stroke. Through a stethoscope, he may hear a noise over the diseased portion of the artery, a swishing sound called a *bruit,* produced by blood streaming over the rough inner surface of the vessel or through a narrowed place in the artery.

Probably the physician will test the blood pressure in each eyeball for an indication of which carotid artery is affected. Narrowing in one artery may cause a decrease of blood pressure in the eyeball on the side of the narrowing. He will look into the back of the eye with an ophthalmoscope to examine tiny arteries and veins in the retina. If cholesterol emboli are coming from a fatty deposit in the carotid artery, the emboli will lodge in retinal vessels (commonly with no change in vision) and may easily be seen. Detection of such emboli in the retina is of great importance, as their presence indicates ulceration of an atherosclerotic plaque in the carotid artery on that same side.

Other tests will be mentioned subsequently, but a *history* of these short attacks is paramount in establishing a diagnosis. The experienced physician will distinguish the confusions of speech and movement associated with transient ischemic attacks from the deceptively similar mumblings, clumsiness, and mental sluggishness of persons who have a high fever, who have taken too many sleeping pills, or who are simply inebriated.

Migraine mimic. Sufferers from migraine headache occasionally develop symptoms that might seem to presage a stroke. In these unusual instances, the migraine may begin with numbness and weakness in one side of the body, but the symptoms soon fade away and are followed by the sick headache. Such strange events are thought to be due to spasm or brief narrowing of one of the brain arteries.

A physician can generally recognize this condition on the basis of a history that informs him that relatives have had sick headaches, that the patient always has such headaches following the numbness and weakness symptoms mentioned, and that the patient is much younger than persons who commonly fall into the stroke category. It is rare for a stroke to develop in anyone who still experiences migraine episodes.

Vertebral Warning Attacks

Another cluster of warning signs of an impending stroke involves the vertebral-basilar (VB) system of blood supply to the brain, previously described. The VB system supplies different parts of the brain than the carotid system, and brief interruption of blood flow produces symptoms sufficiently different to distinguish the source.

The VB system serves the portion of the brain at the back of the head where nerve signals from the eyes are transmuted into vision. It also supplies the brainstem, an incredible switchboard that sends millions of nerve impulses from both sides of the brain to the spinal cord, and also transmits messages from all over the body to the brain—orders to move a muscle, or to take action on a message sent by an itchy nose. At its largest point, the brainstem is about the diameter of a 50-cent piece, which means that torrents of transactions incessantly take place in a very small volume of tissue. Therefore, a minor decrease in blood supply can cause major trouble.

Symptoms. As any infinitesimal part of this complex system can be involved during an episode of decreased blood flow, the possible combinations of symptoms are almost without limit. However, some symptoms or combinations are of particular importance.

A patient may suffer momentary impairment or complete loss of vision in both eyes, which he may describe as dimness, haziness, blurring, or blacking-out. This particular symptom is seldom the result of any other disease process. Double vision—the patient sees two objects clearly when there is only one—is another symptom of VB transient ischemia.

Nerve impulses that control voluntary muscles also pass through the brainstem. Thus, there may be weakness of a limb or limbs during an episode. When such weakness involves both sides of the body simultaneously, it indicates trouble in the brainstem, in contrast to impaired flow in a carotid artery where there is weakness on only one side. Difficulty on both sides of the body is peculiar to VB disease when there are concurrent sensory disturbances—sensations of numbness, prickling, tingling, burning, or coldness. Staggering or faulty control of a limb may be a part of such attacks. Another symptom is difficulty in swallowing; if moderately severe, it may be accompanied by drooling of saliva.

Dizziness is the most common of all symptoms of little strokes involving the VB system, but it is dizziness of a very distinctive form. The patient feels that objects are whirling around him, or he around them. He has irregular sensations of movement, as if walking in a speeding train or lurching on a ship at sea. The sensations are strong enough to make the patient grasp for support, sit down, sway, lurch, or otherwise adapt his behavior to the brief emergency. These uncomfortable and distressing sensations of movement are often accompanied by nausea that may progress to vomiting.

In some attacks, the person may have difficulty in talking, with severe mushiness and slurring of speech rather than an incapacity to think of words, form sentences, or understand others. However, it is unusual for deafness or unconsciousness to occur. As mentioned, the characteristic that most distinguishes involvement of the VB system from that of the carotid system is the involvement of both sides of the body. As with carotid-system episodes, symptoms differ greatly from one person to another, but there is often considerable similarity of symptoms in the same person.

Prognosis. Transient ischemic attacks are important warnings of impending stroke, but they are not inevitably followed by a "real" stroke, which implies damage to some part of the brain. Such transient episodes are too brief to inflict damage, unless they persist as long as 24 hours, which is rare. However, well over one-third of all persons who have such warning attacks will suffer a catastrophic stroke at some time in their future.

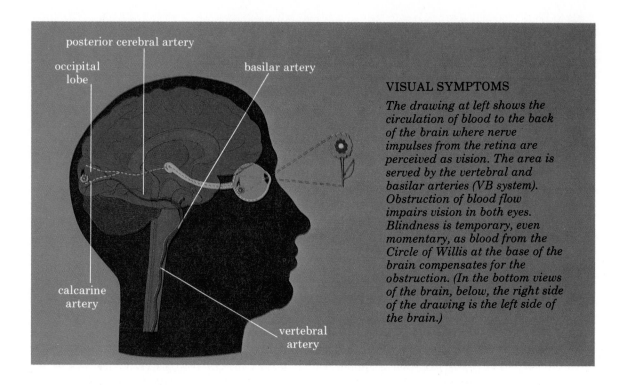

VISUAL SYMPTOMS

The drawing at left shows the circulation of blood to the back of the brain where nerve impulses from the retina are perceived as vision. The area is served by the vertebral and basilar arteries (VB system). Obstruction of blood flow impairs vision in both eyes. Blindness is temporary, even momentary, as blood from the Circle of Willis at the base of the brain compensates for the obstruction. (In the bottom views of the brain, below, the right side of the drawing is the left side of the brain.)

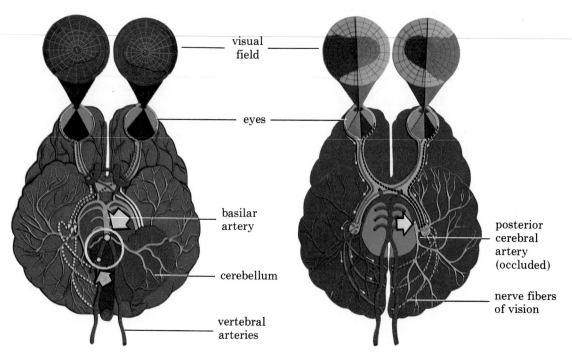

VISION IMPAIRMENT: BOTH EYES

This bottom view of the brain has the right half of the cerebellum removed to show the nerve fibers of vision. A clot in the basilar artery (white arrow) can cause a temporary loss of vision in both eyes. Obstruction of a vertebral artery (yellow arrow) will cause a less severe visual impairment.

VISION IMPAIRMENT: HALF OF EACH EYE

The drawing shows an obstruction of an artery on the left side of the brain, shutting off the blood supply to visual centers of the brain. But since nerve fibers from the affected area divide (dotted lines) and send impulses to each side of the eye, only half of the field of vision in each eye suffers.

ADVANCING OR PROGRESSING STROKE

Since nine out of ten strokes are due to thrombosis, embolism, or hemorrhage, a swift and accurate diagnosis of the type of stroke may permit treatment prompt enough to prevent it from worsening.

A progressing stroke due to clotting may occur in either the carotid or vertebral blood-supply systems. While the technical aspects of distinguishing the two are beyond the scope of this chapter, certain hallmarks can be mentioned.

Indications of thrombosis in the carotid system include weakness or paralysis limited to one side of the body, impaired sensation on only one side, typical difficulty in speaking and understanding speech if the dominant side of the brain is affected, impaired vision in only one eye, a decrease of blood pressure in one eye compared to the other, and an occasional swishing sound called a bruit. Thus, carotid thrombosis could be called a *one-sided stroke.*

Hallmarks of progressing stroke in the vertebral system are impairment of strength and sensation on both sides of the body, impairment of vision throughout the entire fields of both eyes, double vision, certain impairments of ability to move the eyes, trouble in swallowing, and occasionally, slurred or mushy speech. Vertebral thrombosis, then, may be thought of as a *two-sided stroke.*

Hemorrhagic Stroke

The speed with which a stroke develops when an artery breaks and spills blood into the brain varies with the size of the defect in the arterial wall. Hemorrhage *into* the brain, as distinguished from hemorrhage *around* the brain, is almost always associated with high blood pressure and is commonly very severe.

Usually there are no warning signs to herald the approaching event, and the hemorrhage almost always occurs while the patient is awake and active, rarely during sleep. There seems to be no relationship to intensity of activity.

Symptoms begin after blood starts to escape into or around the brain. Often there is severe headache that may be accompanied by nausea and vomiting. As the mass of blood collecting in brain tissue increases, the patient experiences weakness or shows other signs of disturbed nervous-system function.

If bleeding continues, pressure increases inside the head and the brain may actually be squeezed to the side opposite the bleeding. Overall brain function is disturbed, and the patient may fall into a coma. Blood then may break into one of the cavities of the brain, travel to its surface, and be found in the spinal fluid. Such is the case in about three-fourths of brain-hemorrhage cases, and a discovery of blood in the spinal fluid may be of great help in making the diagnosis.

Aneurysm. If bleeding is *around* the brain, it is called *subarachnoid hemorrhage* and commonly comes from a thin-walled balloon or blister-like formation—an *aneurysm*—usually located at the point where an artery divides into two other arteries.

Aneurysms seldom cause difficulty before they actually rupture, and ordinarily do not give warning of attacks. When an aneurysm breaks, a stream of blood spurts into the space between the covering of the brain and the brain itself, like water squirting from a hose. This sudden escape of blood produces an excruciating headache—often in the back of the head—that comes on almost instantaneously.

Some patients immediately become unconscious, but many remain lucid and complain of a stiff neck, nausea, and vomiting. Occasionally, lost consciousness is regained in a few minutes, with the patient again entirely lucid.

An aneurysm is a serious disorder, fatal in 30 to 40 percent of instances.

Stroke from the heart. Special mention should be made of a type of progressing stroke produced by a fragment of a clot—an embolus—that comes from the heart. This occurs so frequently that careful attention should always be devoted to heart examination. Because an embolus to the brain may be the very first sign of a heart attack, many physicians take an electrocardiogram in all stroke patients.

The importance of accurate diagnosis in this situation lies in the fact that administration of an anticoagulant drug, which decreases the clotting power of the blood, may prevent further emboli from coming from the heart.

COMPLETED STROKE

A completed stroke is one that has run its course and will inflict no further damage. It is not necessarily one that has left the patient dead or with total functions of vision, sensation, speech, or movement permanently destroyed. After a completed stroke, the reparative processes of the body come into play, and, with appropriate aid, progress is made in returning the patient to normal activity, whether partially or completely. To determine whether a stroke is progressing or completed, the physician may need to observe the patient over a period of several hours, as is also true in many types of heart attack.

Spontaneous improvement. An important characteristic of completed stroke is the beginning of improvement some hours or days after impairment has reached a maximum. This is evinced in innumerable ways, varying with the severity of damage and the functions affected—perhaps in movement restored to a limb, return of sensation, clearing of vision and speech, or regained coordination.

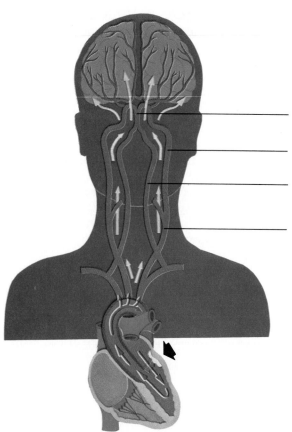

basilar artery

internal carotid artery

vertebral artery

common carotid artery

STROKE FROM THE HEART

Not infrequently, a stroke originates from a clot in one of the heart chambers (black arrow). A small piece of the clot may break off and travel upward to the head and brain, obstructing blood flow along the line. Studies of the heart are commonly a part of the examination of stroke patients.

It is highly encouraging that completed-stroke patients not only improve, but do so to the extent that they can resume their previous occupations and activities. Treatment and rehabilitative measures are important, but the body's own self-repair efforts are truly remarkable.

It is important to note that this common and spontaneous improvement often makes it difficult to assess the value of new methods of therapy. The unwary physician may assume that a new approach to therapy produced benefit, when it was really the result of spontaneous improvement—the natural course of the recovery process.

TREATMENT OF STROKES

In contrast to two decades ago, today there are a number of valuable treatments for different types of strokes. We will discuss these rather complex matters under the general categories of prevention, treatment of acute stroke, and rehabilitation from completed stroke.

Prevention

Specific measures of prevention involve the treatment of transient ischemic attacks that are warnings of possible stroke to come—incipient or impending strokes. We have previously discussed such attacks in detail; obviously, it is important that they be recognized for what they are. Since recovery is prompt and the person is soon back to normal, it is easy to brush off such attacks as having no significance. But if you experience typical symptoms (see page 118), it is prudent to seek treatment that might keep a stroke out of your future.

In a very general way, susceptibility to stroke—what is sometimes designated as the "stroke-prone personality"—is suggested by the following:
- advancing age
- a family history of strokes
- heavy cigarette smoking
- known ischemic heart disease (angina or heart attack)
- high blood pressure
- diabetes

Treatment

What can be done preventively if warning attacks occur? There are three general categories of treatment:
- Administration of oral anticoagulants that decrease the clotting power of the blood.
- Surgical reconstruction of the carotid artery (see page 128).
- Medicines that affect the clotting power of the blood in a different way than anticoagulants—by interfering with the aggregation of blood platelets that, in turn, affect clotting power.

Anticoagulants must be given with care—administering too much will cause dangerous bleeding, but too little will not sufficiently inhibit clotting to prevent a possible stroke. Anticoagulants should not be used if the patient will not meticulously follow directions for their use, or if a patient's laboratory reports cannot suggest a precise dosage. Periodic blood studies are necessary to measure the effects of anticoagulants in each particular patient.

Anticoagulants are most commonly used to treat transient ischemic attacks in the vertebral system. For such attacks in the carotid system, the treatment of choice is often surgery, which will be discussed later.

Hypertension—abnormally high blood pressure—should always receive treatment whenever it is observed. We have seen that high blood pressure is a potent risk factor in strokes as well as heart attacks. Treatment (see page 67) is highly effective and is a preventive measure of great value.

Medications. During the past decade, three medicines that affect blood platelets have been investigated for their possible benefit in preventing strokes and related conditions involving the formation of obstructive clots inside the arteries. The medicines are: aspirin; dipyridamole (Persantine); and sulfinpyrazone (Anturane).

Blood platelets are formed elements in the blood, as are red and white blood cells. They help to initiate the very intricate process of blood clotting. Under certain circumstances, platelets stick to each other in clumps (aggregate); but in other instances, they stick to the very smooth wall of blood vessels (adhesive capacity). The above-mentioned medicines affect the clumping and adhesive capacity of platelets, and are called *platelet antiaggregating agents.*

A positive relationship between these characteristics of platelets and the mechanism of warning attacks is not firmly established. However, it seems likely that the "stickiness" of platelets, to each other and to vessel walls, could result in clotted obstructions provocative of stroke. Plausibly, then, reduction of platelet stickiness might inhibit the clotting process.

Drugs to accomplish this are not routinely used in medical practice, but two collaborative studies of such agents are under way. Initial evidence from one group that worked with patients who received aspirin suggests that this familiar drug was of little value in patients who had single transient ischemic attacks, but of some value in those who had a series of such attacks. It appears unlikely that any of the three drugs, or others to be discovered, will give a full answer to the extremely complex matter of stroke prevention.

ACUTE PROGRESSING STROKE

Someone collapses on the street or is found unconscious on the floor at home. An acute stroke is under way, progressing and continuing to do damage to the nervous system. Good medical care is obviously important at this juncture, to slow the progress of stroke and to minimize its after-effects as much as possible.

General treatment of stroke has improved greatly in the past two decades. Better nursing care and detailed attention to supportive measures have virtually become standard in most hospitals.

Treatment should first keep the heart and blood pressure mechanisms normal, or as near normal as possible: the heart-pump supplies blood to the brain and, of course, sustains life. The patient's airway also must be attended to promptly. This simply means careful protection of his ability to inhale air with its oxygen through the mouth, windpipe, and other parts of the respiratory system—in short, to breathe effectively. If breathing muscles are impaired, oxygen may be provided, possibly through a tube in the windpipe, or by some form of artificial respiration. Possible infection in the urinary system, skin, or lungs must be guarded against through antibiotic therapy. And, bladder and bowel functions may need special care.

In patients who are very ill, great attention must be paid to fluid intake to assure the correct balance of nutrients, minerals, and calories. Periodic blood studies may be made to check the levels of certain chemicals, especially electrolytes (minerals such as potassium, sodium, calcium, and many others) that are essential to the normal composition of internal body fluids. Adjustments can then be made to provide these essentials in correct amounts.

Stiffening of muscles and joints often occurs quite soon, so it is important to provide early physical therapy. This may consist only of moving each leg and arm through its range of joint motion, which could prevent the contraction of tendons, ligaments, and muscles, and avert considerable pain.

Specific therapy. A number of specific forms of treatment depend upon an accurate diagnosis of the particular type of stroke. For instance, in unusual instances, blood pressure is elevated well above a level that was already abnormally high. This produces symptoms indicative of damage to a local area of the brain, among other things. Such a condition constitutes a medical emergency that demands immediate control of the high blood pressure. Fortunately, there are excellent medicines to treat this particular complication of stroke.

Although there is not absolute agreement, most authorities believe that many instances of progressing stroke (due to the closing off of a blood vessel) should be treated with an anticoagulant drug. The drugs may be injected into the muscle or skin, or be taken intravenously or orally. It is imperative that the diagnosis be absolutely correct, for if an anticoagulant is given to a person who has a bleeding problem, it can only make matters worse—even disastrous.

If the patient has a kind of "super-rich" blood, thickened by excessive numbers of red blood cells *(polycythemia),* it may be important to dilute this concentration of cells. Generally, however, this condition is quite rare in stroke patients.

Projections. Chemicals that dissolve fresh blood clots have been available for some years, and have been looked to with hope that they could help the patient with an acute stroke. So far, however, their use has created more problems than it has solved.

Blood vessels, especially arteries, expand and contract, and the idea of alleviating a stroke by expanding a closed vessel so that some blood can get through is an attractive one. A number of methods of increasing the size of a blood vessel *(vasodilatation)* are available, including the administration of carbon dioxide gas (which we exhale with every breath). But there is no convincing evidence that these methods significantly alter the progress of stroke, and none of them is widely used today.

Another attractive concept involves the use of some chemical or physical method to put the brain at rest—almost in hibernation—during the serious acute period following the onset of stroke. Theoretically, the resting brain would need less blood, and its recovery might be enhanced. Ways to rest the brain have included extreme cooling of the body *(hypothermia),* continued anesthesia (sedation), oxygen under increased atmospheric pressure *(hyperbaric oxygenation),* as well as the intensive administration of oxygen under normal pressure. None of these methods has been effective in preventing significant amounts of brain damage, however.

One of the great problems of serious stroke is swelling of the brain, which can compress adjacent areas and cause further damage. A number of drugs—mannitol, glycerol, and cortisone-like medicines—have been used in an attempt to prevent, alleviate, or reverse this swelling, but unfortunately, results are unconvincing. Once the swelling begins, no method is fully effective at combating it.

Rehabilitation

Variation in the outcome of strokes is enormous. Some patients leave the hospital, go back to work, and resume their usual life-styles. Some die. Between these extremes are hundreds of varieties of slight or severe residual damage, and hundreds of ways to cope with it.

During the past 40 years, rehabilitative measures of physical medicine have developed greatly and now are of tremendous assistance in restoring a satisfying quality of life to stroke patients. The goal is to help each patient develop the very best use of some function that has been impaired, and to return him to the highest possible level of activity, consonant with the damage that has taken place.

Physical medicine programs of rehabilitation are almost always centered in special hospitals or in portions of major general hospitals that are equipped with special apparatus and are staffed with specialists in rehabilitation to help the patient regain some function to the maximum degree possible.

Evaluation comes first, after which an appropriate program is built to develop the highest degree of skill possible with the brain function that remains. This complex assessment of capacities is made by a team headed by skilled physicians, often including a physical therapist, an occupational therapist, a speech therapist, a psychologist, a social worker, and a vocational counselor.

A word to the family. After weeks or months on a rehabilitation program, the greatest possible improvement has probably occurred. Brain cells do not regenerate; if a major area of cell death has occurred, there will be a residual defect that is permanent in spite of every effort at rehabilitation. There are limits to what can be done, and specialists may have to counsel against treatment they know cannot help matters.

However, a gratifying number of patients who do not need constant nursing care return to a home environment and do very well, particularly if family and friends are understanding and supportive. The family should know that the patient is often quite capable of carrying out certain activities such as dressing or feeding himself — provided he is given enough time and the task is not taken over by someone impatient to get it done. Perhaps the patient cannot speak well or at all, but can understand what he or she hears. Wants can be determined by questions answerable by simple "yes" or "no" signals, such as a hand or head movement.

A stroke patient's improvement is less a matter of dramatic increase in muscle strength or coordination than of finding new ways of adapting to the world around him. An atmosphere of encouragement and support is vital to fend off depression. The stroke patient needs a feeling of self-esteem and independence just as much as the next person—probably more.

SURGERY FOR STROKE

One type of threatened stroke, presaged by transient ischemic attacks, is accessible to surgery. The area involved is the carotid artery system, previously described, part of which lies close to the skin surface at the sides of the neck. Obstruction or narrowing of vessels by atherosclerotic plaque is particularly likely to occur at a junction where the arteries diverge in the shape of a Y. This area is *extracranial,* or outside of the head, and within easy range of surgery.

Diagnosis. Whether or not a patient is suitable for such surgery depends upon an accurate determination that the principal site of trouble lies in the carotid system, on one or both sides. We have mentioned tests and examinations that enable a physician to distinguish between carotid and vertebral types of stroke in 90 percent of cases. However, before surgery is undertaken, a procedure to visualize blood vessels is an absolute requirement.

Arteriography. In the 1920s, a technique was devised to display the pattern of blood vessels in the brain. Normally, these arteries and veins do not show up in a head X ray unless the vessel wall contains calcium, which casts a shadow on the film. Such shadows, however, are of little diagnostic help. The technique consists of injecting a dye, which is opaque to X rays, into one of the carotid or vertebral arteries in the neck and then taking a rapid series of X-ray pictures *(angiogram* or *arteriogram).* The course of the dye displays the pattern of the blood vessels as the dye is carried by the bloodstream into the head.

The question of whether arteriography should be performed on all stroke patients is not firmly answered. The test is not without risk for the patient. Strokes—and in rare instances, death—have been associated with the procedure. In the great majority of cases, an experienced physician can diagnose the type of stroke without doing an arteriogram. However, prior to carotid surgery, the test is essential to accurately define the extent and location of lesions in the arteries and to evaluate probable surgical benefit. If the test indicates that a patient is suitable for surgery, a favorable outcome is likely.

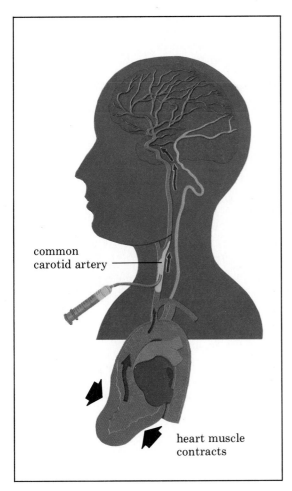

ARTERIOGRAPHY

Arteriography is the procedure of taking X rays after injecting into the bloodstream a dye that is opaque to the rays. Contraction of the heart (black arrows) forces the dye in the bloodstream into higher vessels.

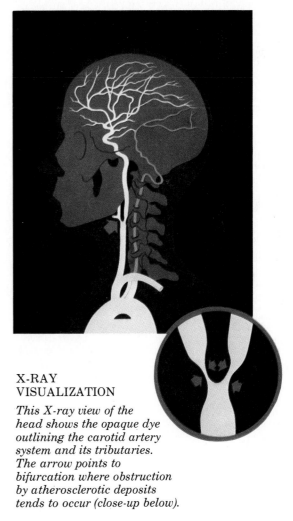

X-RAY
VISUALIZATION

This X-ray view of the head shows the opaque dye outlining the carotid artery system and its tributaries. The arrow points to bifurcation where obstruction by atherosclerotic deposits tends to occur (close-up below).

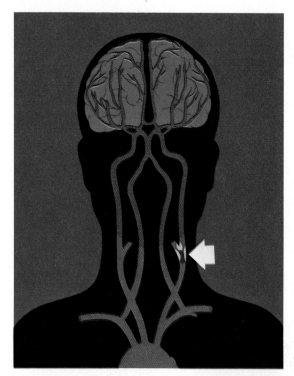

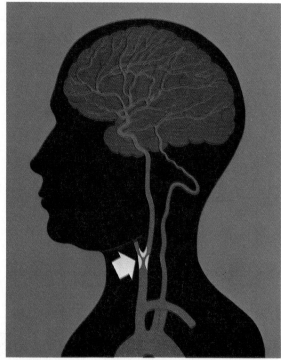

CAROTID OBSTRUCTION

Arteriography and other studies—taking physical condition, age, acuteness, and other factors into consideration—may indicate that a patient is a good candidate for surgery on an obstruction that is close to the surface of the neck (white arrow). Compare the side view of an obstructed carotid artery (top right) with the front view at top left to visualize the depth and location of an area that is readily accessible to surgical treatment.

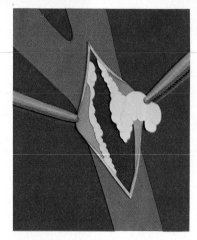

CLOT REMOVAL

Endarterectomy is accomplished by making an incision in the wall of the affected artery and cutting out the obstruction to restore adequate blood flow through the vessel. Patients most likely to benefit from the operation are thought to be those who have had transient warning attacks and are at risk of a major stroke.

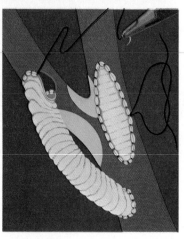

RESTORED BLOOD FLOW

The cleaned-out artery may be enlarged and strengthened by a patch graft. Or, the blocked segment may be bypassed with a vein graft or a prosthetic tube.

Less irritating dyes and improved X-ray techniques have substantially lessened the risk of the test. And, it is not given if the patient has had a recent heart attack, is allergic to the dyes, or has other complications. Since arteriography is used primarily to gain precise information leading to successful carotid surgery, there is no point in doing such a test if the patient's age, general health, or seriousness of existing brain damage makes surgical treatment unwise. Impending stroke is the category for which arteriography provides the most useful information.

Arteriography is the best test for determining the nature of the defect in the carotid arteries, and of judging whether it is possible to restore normal blood flow by a surgical procedure. It also gives information about other major arteries that must supply blood to the head during the minutes when the surgeon shuts off the affected vessel for operative repair.

Procedures. If a patient is a good prospect for carotid-artery surgery, just what is done? The surgeon may open up the artery and clean out the obstructing clot or plaque *(thrombo-endarterectomy),* with the patient out of the hospital in a week or so and back to work in a month. Complications are rare. If the lesion is extensive, an artificial blood vessel made of Dacron or a similar inert material may be implanted to bypass the area.

What benefits may be hoped for from carotid-artery surgery? The objective is to prevent a major stroke in a patient who is likely to have one, as indicated by a history of transient attacks. Although thousands of such operations have been performed since the first was reported from England in 1954, predictive knowledge of long-term effects in patients of greatly varied physical status is still limited. One factor that makes prognosis uncertain is that atherosclerosis, the usual underlying condition, is a progressive disorder.

In a collaborative study conducted by a number of institutions a few years ago, the investigators reported a four-year follow-up of two groups of patients who were treated either by surgical or medical means. During the period, 15 percent of the surgically treated patients and 14 percent of those medically treated had a stroke. Unfortunately, no long-term follow-up of precisely studied groups is available, but it seems likely that results have improved since the investigation mentioned.

It is apparent from reports in the literature that many physicians who are active in the stroke field are moderately to greatly enthusiastic about surgical treatment for carotid-system transient ischemic attacks. Recently, at a meeting of the American College of Surgeons, it was reported that a small group of ten elderly patients who had carotid endarterectomies showed a marked increase in mental alertness, with an average jump of 18 points in their IQs after six weeks!

THE STROKE-PRONE PROFILE

A number of phenomena that suggest proneness to stroke have been mentioned earlier in this chapter. Transient ischemic attacks rank so high as a risk factor that the cause of these episodes should be searched for immediately so that steps to prevent a big stroke can be taken. Increasing age is another risk factor, but since nothing can be done about it, the only healthy attitude to take is acknowledgment that it will continue to increase. For the most part, risk factors are related to occlusive or vessel-obstructive stroke and not to cerebral hemorrhage (except high blood pressure).

Obesity *per se* is not linked directly to increased risk of stroke. However, because obesity usually leads to decreased physical activity and is often accompanied by an increase in blood pressure, heart work load, and risk of angina pectoris, it is prudent for an obese person to go on an appropriate weight-reduction program.

Blood pressure. The interrelationship of high blood pressure and stroke is not completely understood, but it is generally agreed that sustained hypertension is an important risk factor. Fortunately, hypertension is readily recognized, and almost always responds well to medical treatment. However, it should be carefully studied in each patient to ascertain the cause and the appropriate management (see page 65).

Various forms of heart disease and certain abnormalities of the electrocardiogram are statistically associated with stroke-proneness. Here, the stroke-preventive aspect is an added plus with the treatment of whatever abnormality may be discovered on medical examination.

Cholesterol is incriminated as a factor in atherosclerotic plaque formation, thrombosis, and embolism, and is discussed elsewhere in this book (see page 153). Elevated blood cholesterol in relation to stroke is another factor about which there is no unanimity of opinion. Data from one study indicate that elevated blood cholesterol in patients under 50 years of age is strongly associated with increased risk of stroke, but after 50, very little relationship could be demonstrated. The combination of elevated blood cholesterol and high blood pressure was judged to be substantially more serious than either condition alone.

Diabetes. Complications of vascular disease, affecting blood vessels of many different organs and tissues, occur eventually in many diabetics (see Chapter 12). It appears that the risk of stroke is increased by diabetes even with only slight elevation of the blood sugar after fasting. Persons with both diabetes and high blood pressure have about a 600 percent greater risk of stroke than the general population. Medical management of both conditions is very important, but it is uncertain whether precise control of diabetes also will reduce the risk of stroke. The mechanisms of interaction are not known.

"Thick blood"—an excessive number of red blood cells with increased tendency for clots to form—is a risk factor for strokes. There are various types of this disorder *(polycythemia)* that should be precisely ascertained and appropriate treatment instituted.

Cigarette smoking is significantly implicated in a number of disorders. Many now believe that it is also a risk factor for stroke. The habit clearly is not conducive to health, and advice not to smoke is well based, if not always well taken.

Oral contraceptives. Studies of oral contraceptives in relation to strokes suggest that they should not be used by women who have had emboli or clot formation in blood vessels of any part of the body, any suggestion of a temporary brain or vision attack, high blood pressure, or migraine headaches.

PIPELINES TO THE BRAIN:
TESTS & PROCEDURES

In addition to the examinations described under the various categories of stroke, a number of laboratory tests and special procedures are of value in diagnosing and managing the disease.

Urine tests should be conducted to check for sugar, protein, and microscopic sediment. It is important to know whether the patient has active diabetes, abnormal kidney function, or the presence of certain kinds of cells that may indicate inflammation of small arteries.

Blood tests include the usual red and white cell counts, and tests for syphilis and hemoglobin concentration. Too much hemoglobin indicates blood that is too thick and tends to form clots. The *sedimentation rate* (precipitation time of red blood cells) is checked to rule out active inflammation of small arteries. Blood sugar and levels of cholesterol and triglycerides (fat-like substances) also should be tested.

Prothrombin time measures the intricate process of blood clotting. If an anticoagulant drug that decreases the clotting power of the blood is administered, it is essential that the dose of the drug be very precise, so it will not provoke excessive bleeding. Prothrombin tests give information for proper dosage calculations.

An electrocardiogram should be obtained in virtually all patients suspected of having any category of stroke, due to the active interrelationship between various forms of heart trouble and stroke. If the heart is of normal size with normal sounds, rhythm, and blood pressure, active heart disease is unlikely. But in rare instances, a "silent" heart attack may have occurred and there may be some change in the rhythm system that cannot be detected by physical examination. That is the reason for routinely taking the electrocardiogram.

Angiography (arteriography) refers to an X-ray technique that employs a radio-opaque dye for visualizing the patterns of blood vessels in the brain. It is mainly used in evaluating candidates for carotid-artery surgery (see page 129).

Computerized tomography. This remarkable and entirely new X-ray device became available in the summer of 1973 and is truly revolutionizing the differential diagnosis of various kinds of trouble inside the head. The technique is often called "CAT-scanning" (for computer-assisted tomography) or CT (for computerized tomography).

The equipment employs a narrow beam of X rays to scan a patient's head in a series of flat sections, much like slices. Thousands of tiny X-ray readings are passed into a computer that calculates the absorption values—different densities—of tissues the X rays have passed through. From these calculations, a three-dimensional picture matrix is built that displays and differentiates the X-ray "densities" of tissues inside the head in a way never before possible.

The system is a hundred times more sensitive than conventional X-ray systems, and it enables small changes in tissue densities to be recognized and localized. Cavities in the brain are accurately displayed, as is blood outside of a blood vessel, which has a greater density than the brain. As yet, circulating blood is not displayed, and it is still necessary to use arteriography to discern blisters on blood vessels (aneurysms) within the head.

CHAPTER **5** FREDRICK J. STARE, M.D.
JELIA C. WITSCHI, M.S.

EATING FOR YEARS & YEARS

By the time you are 40 years old, you have eaten about 45,000 meals and uncountable snacks. This massive repetitious experience no doubt exceeds the time and effort devoted to any other activity, and it is natural to feel that one has become quite expert in food selection. We know what we like, we avoid what doesn't "set well" on the stomach, and our eating habits, including eccentricities, are usually pleasing.

To a young appetite, almost anything that is edible is enjoyable. Relatively few persons give serious thought to the nutritional quality of diet in younger years. But this happy indifference begins to change for many persons around middle age and later. It is a time when intimations of maturity encroach, when the metabolism slows a bit, and when vague discomforts get preoccupied attention. Some people actually get into a panic over their eating habits and grasp for some wonder diet, "health" food, magic nutrient, or exotic supplement that will increase vigor, promote longevity, and mitigate the decline into old age. No such miraculous products exist, but countless dollars are invested uselessly in their pursuit nonetheless.

Good nutrition is not so unfathomably complex or bound in rituals or promoters' promises as it sometimes may appear. The purpose of this chapter is to discuss food habits, simple ways of evaluating and obtaining adequate nutrition, and some current theories that may be helpful in developing and enjoying a sound and satisfying personal diet.

How's Your Diet

Many people believe that "diet" means a rigidly prescribed program of eating, distressingly different from accustomed habits and designed to correct some physical problem—commonly, overweight. Actually, everybody has a diet: a set of habits and customs around which daily food choices are made. Your own diet, if not quite so unique as your thumbprint, is nevertheless highly individual. It may or may not be a very good one.

Innumerable factors affect our food preferences, not the least of which is availability. We in the United States are fortunate to have a wondrously wide array of available foods. People now living can remember when an orange was a once-a-year treat found in a Christmas stocking. Taste affects food choices very powerfully, both in preferences and aversions. Most of us know of a food or two that we wouldn't eat short of starvation.

Cost is of course important, but the most expensive foods are not necessarily the best nutritionally, or even necessary. A serving of lean beef or chicken breast is about equal in nutrients to a $10 lobster tail. Lobster with melted butter is considered to be a gourmet item, but we can thrive wonderfully without it.

Cultural, family, ethnic, and social backgrounds determine our food preferences unconsciously. We learn to like what family and friends serve and like. So-called ethnic foods or unusual ones—maybe eel or squid, or local specialties such as gumbo or buffalo steak—are as good as any in a mixed diet. The body doesn't care whether its carbohydrates come from johnnycake or a hush puppy. Only our taste buds care.

Conscious choices about nutrition are likely to be the least powerful force in shaping food habits for most people until, as mentioned, we come of a certain age and begin to wonder whether attention to diet may work an amazing transformation in our lives. What about the quality of your own diet? A survey of diets of middle-aged and older men and women, done by the United States Department of Agriculture in 1965-66, is interesting. Men fared better than women, perhaps because a lot of them eat more of everything. Women in the older age group tended to get less than optimal amounts of calcium, iron, and vitamin A. And the poorest diets were found among persons with the lowest incomes and the least education.

Age-Related Changes

Since the environment and functioning of every body cell is dependent upon nutrition, what we eat affects the aging process. The biological processes of aging are not completely understood; theories and speculations are discussed in the opening chapter of this book. The effects of nutrition on these processes may be direct or indirect.

Some decreases in physiologic function accompany the aging process, but their timing does not correlate exactly with chronological age. Thus, a person may be biologically younger or older than others of the same age. The rate and extent of physiologic decrements vary with individuals, as do the incessant chemical activities of a body of which we are the unique possessor.

With the years, there comes some loss of functioning cells with concomitant changes in the size and capabilities of organs. Muscle and nerve cells gradually deteriorate; the amount of collagen (see page 234) gradually increases and becomes less elastic; and connective tissues of tendons, ligaments, skin, and blood vessels become stiffened.

Blood glucose levels also tend to rise and to be sustained as we grow older. This does not necessarily portend diabetes, but about 80 percent of diabetes is the maturity-onset type that occurs around middle age, commonly in obese persons (see page 407).

Greasy foods may not be well tolerated if the biliary system is sluggish. The body's handling of fats is less efficient with age, commonly reflected in a rise of blood levels of *cholesterol* and *triglycerides*. The latter are fatty elements, less-familiar to the public than cholesterol, but of helpful significance in a doctor's assessment of possible need of control by dietary modification or medication.

In addition, decreases in the acuity of taste and smell may lessen appetite. Missing teeth or difficulties with dentures may lead to a preponderance of soft and watery foods in the diet, over those of greater nutrient density. Gastric juices are reduced in volume, acidity, and pepsin content, so that digestion of foods and hence absorption of nutrients may be impaired. And reduced muscle tone of the gastrointestinal tract conduces to distention and constipation.

Energy needs diminish with aging as both physical activity and thyroid activity lessen. The body fires are less fiery! Measurable decreases in the rate of metabolism indicate a reduction of about 20 percent in caloric needs over a 60-year span from age 30 to 90. Body fat increases in proportion to lean tissue, and physical activity usually slackens. We don't run so fast for a bus, or we wait philosophically for the next one.

The message is clear. After 40, or not long after, most people require less energy and hence need less food (calories) than when they "hit the ball harder" in younger years. For healthy persons, reduced caloric intake should be gradual, comfortable, and conscious. The most reliable indicator is the bathroom scales. If a man or woman continues to eat as much as he or she did in youth and does not compensate by adequate physical effort—generally beyond the dedication of the average person—the result is overweight.

What if one does reduce food intake little by little over the years so that weight remains normal? Requirements for many nutrients remain pretty much the same, but they must be provided by lesser amounts of food. There isn't as much tolerance for foods low in nutrient content as there was when calorie intake was more generous. The inference is that *quality* of diet is very important as we grow older.

Never too late. Anyone who has reached middle age with a lifetime of poor eating habits behind him or her is less likely to enjoy good health than someone who has consistently eaten wisely and well. A good diet in later years cannot completely make up for years of nutritional inadequacy. Middle life and later is a time when many people seek a dietary fountain of youth, hoping to discover foods that impart boundless vigor, cure arthritis or colds, and turn back the clock. Unfortunately, diet is not capable of such miracles.

Nevertheless, it is never too late to benefit from an improved day-to-day quality of diet. Especially, older persons with poor food habits who are not in too-robust health may well benefit from improved diet. Special diets, under medical supervision, are important parts of the treatment of many conditions, mentioned elsewhere in this book. The following comments, directed to the average person in reasonably good health, concern the everyday eating of everyday foods that are the foundations of good nutrition. A little attention to nutritional quality can do nothing but good for anyone.

A Simple Plan for Diet Quality

The quest for food has always been, and still is, a basic drive of human beings. Primitive man recognized the root, the berry, the leaf, and the meat that he chewed and swallowed. But he could not identify the "thing" contained in these very different, unrelated foods that supported life and strength. Belief in food magic perhaps began then, and has not totally vanished from civilized man. Even when food studies began to become scientific, early theorists promoted the concept of "nutriment" as the intangible, unknown, unmeasurable element of food.

Today there are more than 50 identified nutrients in foods. Many of their functions and complex interactions are quite well understood. All the nutrients may be grouped into six major categories: *proteins* (amino acids), *carbohydrates* (sugars and starches), *fats* (fatty acids), *vitamins, minerals,* and *water.* Health and proper functioning of the body depend upon adequate amounts of these known nutrients, and probably a few others that have not yet been discovered but are no doubt present in a varied diet.

No single nutrient or group of nutrients can nourish the body adequately. All of them are necessary, not at every meal or even every day, but certainly over a period of days or weeks. These nutrients are widely distributed in foods, but no single food contains all of them or all of them in proper amounts.

Because few of us have the time, knowledge, or motivation to calculate each nutrient in our daily food, the simplest and most practical way to assure excellent nutrient content is to make our choices from a wide *variety* of foods—what nutritionists call a mixed diet, not unbalanced by over-dependence on a few favorite foods. Thus, reliable guides have been developed for selecting foods according to their average nutrient content.

The Basic Four Food Groups is such a guide, developed about 25 years ago by Harvard's Department of Nutrition. It provides a baseline diet that will meet all the nutrient needs of the average healthy person. Foods are categorized, according to origin, into four groups:

- Meat, fish, poultry and other high-protein foods
- Dairy foods
- Breads and cereals
- Fruits and vegetables

The Basic Four guide is sometimes criticized on grounds that prepackaged meals and take-out and convenience foods can't be fitted into single categories. But of course they can. A cheeseburger on a bun provides meat, cereal, and dairy groups. A frozen beef pie provides meat, vegetable, and cereal groups. Anyone who makes a sandwich knows what goes into it.

A 1,200-Calorie diet*. A basic diet of approximately 1,200 Calories, balanced in nutrients, is supplied by the following selections from the Basic Four groups:

Bread and cereals, 4 servings
Dairy foods, 2 servings
Meats or meat substitutes, 2 servings
Fruits and vegetables, 4 servings

---

*Calorie with a capital C is the kilocalorie or large calorie, the unit of heat measurement that refers to a specific number of Calories in studies of food, metabolism, and nutrition. It is one thousand times larger than the small calorie, which is the amount of heat needed to raise the temperature of one gram of water one degree Centigrade. The small calorie is often used as a general term to mean "calorific" or heat-yielding.

A 1,200-Calorie diet is a reducing diet for practically anybody who is overweight due to excess calories. The Basic Four listings just given can be used as a framework for a reducing diet of high nutrient quality and considerable flexibility, since any preferred or available foods that fit the categories will serve. Note, however, that *fats* and *sugars* are not part of the Basic Four groups. Nor are the Basic Four intended to restrict food selection; rather, the groups serve as a checklist or planning guide to ensure that *basic* supplies of major nutrients will be provided by the day's meals. Fats are obtained from meats and many dairy products, and sugars from fruits. In addition, extra fat from margarine or butter and extra sugar are usually added to foods of the Basic Four for palatability.

Most people of normal weight need more than 1,200 Calories a day to replenish their energy expenditures. Thus, as mentioned, additional calories are usually obtained from extra fats and sugars, by increasing the size of servings, or both. A closer examination of the Basic Four groups and their characteristic nutrients may be helpful.

Bread and cereals. A combination of any four servings of bread and cereals provides approximately 300 Calories and valuable carbohydrates, protein, iron, and vitamins of the B-complex group. In fact, it is difficult to obtain sufficient thiamine and iron if this group is excluded from the diet.

Bread and cereals are often maligned as overprocessed, full of air, and fattening to boot—quite a paradox! Three ounces of "average" beef (a small serving) provide about 300 Calories, while two slices of bread might average only half that number. On a daily basis, the extra 150 Calories saved by such a substitution would result in the loss of a pound of body fat every 23 days or about 16 pounds in a year. The body is not a "nitpicker" about calories. Extra calories are extra calories.

Whole grain breads are increasing in popularity, but enriched white bread is still the best seller. Enrichment laws enacted in about half of the states, and practiced voluntarily in many others, require that major nutrients that are partially removed in flour milling—iron and the vitamins thiamine, riboflavin, and niacin—be replaced at a level equivalent to whole wheat flour. Proposals are pending to include other nutrients in the enrichment program, to increase the amount of iron, and to extend enrichment to other bakery products such as rolls, crackers, doughnuts, and pastries, some of which are now enriched.

Whole grain cereals and bran-containing products are generous and convenient sources of dietary fiber, which has gained renewed interest as a desirable non-nutrient constituent of foods. Adequate fiber intake is thought to be associated with less disease of the lower bowel, such as cancer of the colon, diverticulosis, and constipation.

Fruits and vegetables. Four servings of fruit and/or vegetables provide an average of 160 Calories, 90 percent or more of the vitamin C, and at least 60 percent of the vitamin A in the daily diet. There should be one serving of a vitamin C-rich food every day or so. Many people prefer citrus juices, but other fruit and vegetable juices also are valuable sources of vitamin C; some juices and foods are fortified with the vitamin. Useful amounts are provided by green leafy vegetables, and even potatoes when cooked in their skins.

One serving of a vitamin A-rich food at least every other day is sufficient for almost everyone. Dark green or deep yellow vegetables—for instance, carrots, broccoli, squash, or spinach—contribute substances *(carotenes)* that the body converts into vitamin A. A daily or alternate-day serving of one of these is desirable. Two or three additional daily servings of fruits or vegetables, or both, provide crunchiness, color, texture, taste appeal, and variety in the diet.

In addition to vitamins A and C, the fruit-vegetable group furnishes important minerals, folic acid, and carbohydrates, which are the principal fuel for energy. Peas and beans *(legumes)* contribute significant amounts of protein *(amino acids)* in a mixed diet. Many vegetables are good—indeed superior—sources of dietary fiber.

Contrary to popular belief, the kind and amount of fertilizer or pest control employed in growing fruits and vegetables has little or no effect on their nutritive value. This is the one food group that consumers can produce pleasurably on their own while enjoying the exercise, sunshine, and fresh air bestowed by labor in a small garden plot. It's a rare home gardener who doesn't believe that his vegetables are bigger, better, more flavorful, more nutritious, and incomparably superior to those produced by his neighbor or bought at a produce counter.

Dairy foods. Milk and milk products are the principal sources of calcium in American diets, and it's difficult to get enough calcium if this food group is avoided or underutilized. The group includes fluid milk and products such as cheese, yogurt, and ice cream, of varying caloric value, that can be substituted for part of the milk.

Two servings (8-ounce glasses) of whole milk provide about 320 Calories. Skim milk contains about half the calories, but still furnishes practically all of the major nutrients except vitamin A (unless it is fortified). Vitamin A is fat-soluble, and is contained in the butterfat part of the milk that is removed by skimming.

All of the foods in this group are excellent sources of protein, of many of the B vitamins (especially riboflavin), of vitamin A (in whole milk or fortified low-fat milk), and of vitamin D if that has been added as it should be.

Some of the dairy substitutes such as "creamers," coffee whiteners, and whipped toppings are not dairy products at all. They are convenient to use but do not have the nutritional advantages that might be hoped for. In addition, they do not offer fewer calories or reduced cholesterol levels, since their principal ingredient is a highly saturated fat—coconut oil. Some of the newer creamers, frozen products made from soy or safflower oils, do offer a good source of polyunsaturated fat and, when used to replace real cream, may help in lowering blood levels of cholesterol.

THE BASIC 4 FOOD GROUPS

MEAT GROUP

Provides complete protein, iron, thiamine, riboflavin, niacin, and several other nutrients.

Beef
Veal
Lamb
Pork
Organ meats (liver, heart, kidney)
Fish
Shellfish
Poultry

Meat substitutes:
Dry beans
Dry peas
Lentils
Peanut butter
Eggs

Serving units:
2 to 3 ounces (without bone) of
    cooked meat, poultry, or fish
2 eggs
1 cup cooked beans, dry peas, or
    lentils
4 tablespoons peanut butter

Recommended intake:
2 or more servings daily. Note that a serving of meat is only 2 to 3 ounces.

VEGETABLE/ FRUIT GROUP

Provides carbohydrates, minerals, and vitamins, particularly vitamins C and A.

All vegetables and fruits

Good sources of vitamin C:
Citrus fruits and juices
Melons
Fresh berries
Broccoli
Brussels sprouts
Leafy greens
Potatoes cooked in jackets
Cabbage
Cauliflower
Spinach
Peppers
Tomatoes or tomato juice

Good sources of vitamin A:
Apricots
Broccoli
Cantaloupe
Carrots
Pumpkin
Sweet potatoes
Winter squash
Dark green leaves

Serving units:
½ cup vegetables or fruit
Customary serving; e.g., a medium
    apple, banana, orange, potato,
    half grapefruit or cantaloupe

Recommended intake:
4 or more servings daily
Include 1 serving each of a good
    source of vitamin C and of
    vitamin A.

BREAD/CEREAL GROUP

Furnishes worthwhile protein, iron, several B vitamins, carbohydrate, calories, and fiber.

All whole grain, enriched, or restored
    breads and cereals
Ready-to-eat or cooked cereals
Cornmeal
Crackers
Flour
Macaroni
Spaghetti
Noodles
Rice
Rolled oats
Baked goods made with whole grain
    or enriched flour

Serving units:
1 slice of bread
1 ounce ready-to-eat-cereal
½ to ¾ cup cooked cereal, macaroni,
    noodles, rice, or spaghetti

Recommended intake:
4 or more servings daily

MILK GROUP

Provides complete protein, riboflavin, vitamin A, vitamin D (if fortified), and most importantly, calcium.

Milk
    Whole
    Skim
    Low-fat
    Evaporated
    Dry
    Buttermilk

Milk alternates of equivalent calcium content:
Cheddar-type cheese, 1-inch cube =
    ½ cup milk
Cream cheese, 2 tablespoons = 1
    tablespoon milk
Cottage cheese, ½ cup = ⅓ cup milk
Ice cream, ½ cup = ⅓ cup milk
Ice milk, ½ cup = ⅓ cup milk

Recommended intake:
2 or more cups of milk or equivalent
    every day

OTHER FOODS

Most people, unless reducing, will need more calories than the minimum specified servings of the Basic Four Food Groups provide and will round out their diets with judicious choices of foods not included in the groups—butter, margarine, salad and cooking oils, jams, jellies, and sweets in moderation.

Meat and meat substitutes. This food group is not all red meat, or exclusively meat, but it is the major source of biologically complete protein (that is, it furnishes all of the essential amino acids). It includes fish, eggs, and poultry, as well as common meats.

At an average of 90 to 100 Calories per ounce, meat contributes more calories to most diets than any of the other basic food groups. This is because of the fat that meat contains. Even lean meats may be 10 percent fat, and most meats contain 20 to 30 percent fat.

Five ounces of meat provide about 425 Calories. The same amount of fish or poultry has fewer calories because of its lesser fat content. This amount of fish, meat, or poultry is quite enough to satisfy the protein needs of almost everyone, assuming that foods from the other Basic Four groups are included as recommended.

Other nutrients of meat and meat substitutes include B vitamins such as thiamine, riboflavin, niacin, B_6, B_{12}, and iron. Meat is a main source of saturated fats and contains modest amounts of cholesterol, although egg yolk is the main source of dietary cholesterol; the whites are almost pure protein and are devoid of cholesterol.

Continuing research indicates the desirability of replacing some of the *saturated fat* in the diet with *unsaturated fat,* particularly *polyunsaturated fat.* Our body tissues make more cholesterol when saturated fats predominate in the diet, but less from unsaturated fats. Low blood cholesterol is thought to lessen the extent of fatty deposits in the arteries. A rough guide is that saturated fats are of animal origin, while unsaturated or polyunsaturated fats are of vegetable origin (except coconut and palm oils).

It is of course possible, and advisable, to trim visible fat from meats, but a well-marbled steak has streaks of fat that can't be cut out and that indeed help to make the meat tender and flavorful. Broiling and roasting remove some of the fat in the form of drippings, the base for gravies. A simple way to get most of the fat out of drippings is to pour the drippings into a container and set it in the freezer part of a refrigerator. Soon the fat will rise to the top and congeal so that it can readily be removed and discarded, leaving the taste-rich extractives that make fine gravy.

Most people enjoy the flavor and texture of meat and consume large quantities of it—more than good nutrition demands, and far more than the five ounces per day that we have suggested. As far as nutrition is concerned, two small servings of meat or one moderate serving daily will be quite enough. Beyond that, personal preferences and pocketbook considerations come into play.

Other foods. Seldom are meals or snacks eaten without a host of "complements" outside of the Basic Four Food Groups— fats, sweets, dressings, sauces, gravies, and spreads. Such extras are by no means prohibited—some supply essential fatty acids and other important nutrients—but they should be taken account of as additions to basic food group choices. On the average, extras may boost daily calorie intake by 25 percent or more. An obvious route to weight control with a well-balanced diet is to keep the basic diet intact, restrict the calories from extras, and keep meat portions small.

(The Basic Four Food Groups do not arbitrarily specify particular foods, but categories of foods that collectively assure the quality of the daily diet. Substitution of one food or combination for another that has virtually the same nutrient and calorie value can be made with the Exchange Systems shown on pages 143 to 148.)

FOOD EXCHANGE LISTS

Food Exchanges give you an accurate, easy-to-use method of meal planning. The Exchange System was designed for diabetics who, as their doctors determine, may need rather precisely calculated amounts of protein, fat, carbohydrate, and calories to maintain normal weight and blood sugar. The Exchanges include the great range of everyday foods, and the system is so flexible that it is very easy to use in planning normal, well-balanced family meals, as well as in special circumstances, such as reducing diets with restricted calories (see page 148).

In principle, Food Exchanges are measured servings of general classes of foods (meat, vegetables, fat, etc.). Every food within a single Exchange List provides substantially the same package of nutrients and calories; the values have been analyzed for you. Any food may be substituted for any other within the same Exchange List, according to choice or availability in the larder.

Because saturated fat may be associated with an increase in blood cholesterol (a possible risk factor in coronary heart disease), a physician may recommend decreased intake of saturated fat and relative replacement with polyunsaturated fats. The Exchange System was recently revised to incorporate less fat, fewer calories, and more carbohydrates into the diet. Foods listed in **boldface** type under each exchange are either **nonfat** or **low-fat** foods, or they contain **polyunsaturated fats.** To eat a diet low in saturated fats, simply select foods that appear in **boldface** in the Exchange Lists.

The diabetic Exchange Lists are reproduced with the permission of the American Diabetic Association.

Fruit Exchange

1 Exchange contains 40 Calories and 10 grams of carbohydrate.

The amount of each fruit listed below (no sugar added) counts as *1 Fruit Exchange.* Fruits are **nonfat.**

Apple	1 small
Apple Juice or Cider	⅓ cup
Applesauce (unsweetened)	½ cup
Apricots, fresh	2 medium
Apricots, dried	4 halves
Banana	½ small
Berries	
Strawberries	¾ cup
Other Berries	½ cup
Cherries	10 large
Dates	2
Figs, fresh or dried	1
Grapefruit	½
Grapefruit Juice	½ cup
Grapes	12
Grape Juice	¼ cup
Mango	½ small
Melon	
Cantaloupe	¼ small
Honeydew	⅛ medium
Watermelon	1 cup
Nectarine	1 small
Orange	1 small
Orange Juice	½ cup
Papaya	¾ cup
Peach	1 medium
Pear	1 small
Persimmon, native	1 medium
Pineapple	½ cup
Pineapple Juice	⅓ cup
Plums	2 medium
Prunes	2 medium
Prune Juice	¼ cup
Raisins	2 tablespoons
Tangerine	1 medium

Cranberries may be used as desired if no sugar is added.

Vegetable Exchange

1 Exchange contains 25 Calories, 5 grams of carbohydrate, and 2 grams of protein.

Each ½-cup serving of the vegetables listed below counts as *1 Vegetable Exchange*. Unless cooked with fat, all vegetables are **nonfat**.

Asparagus
Bean Sprouts
Beans, green or yellow
Beets
Broccoli
Brussels Sprouts
Cabbage
Carrots
Cauliflower
Celery
Chilies
Cucumbers
Eggplant
Mushrooms
Okra
Onions
Peppers
Rhubarb
Rutabaga
Sauerkraut
Spinach and other greens
Summer Squash
Tomatoes
Tomato Juice
Turnips
Vegetable Juice Cocktail
Zucchini

The following raw vegetables are all free exchanges and may be eaten in any amounts:
Chicory, Chinese Cabbage, Endive, Escarole, Lettuce, Parsley, Radishes, Watercress
Starchy Vegetables are found in the Bread Exchange List.

Milk Exchange

1 Exchange contains 80 Calories, 12 grams of carbohydrate, 8 grams of protein, and a trace of fat.

This list shows the kinds and amounts of milk or milk products to use for *1 Milk Exchange*. The items in **boldface** are **nonfat**.

Nonfat fortified milk:	
Skim or nonfat milk	1 cup
Powdered (nonfat dry, before adding liquid)	⅓ cup
Canned, evaporated— skim milk	½ cup
Buttermilk made from skim milk	1 cup
Yogurt made from skim milk (plain, unflavored)	1 cup
Lowfat fortified milk:	
1% fat fortified milk (omit ½ Fat Exchange)	1 cup
2% fat fortified milk (omit 1 Fat Exchange)	1 cup
Yogurt made from 2% fortified milk (plain, unflavored) (omit 1 Fat Exchange)	1 cup
Whole milk (omit 2 Fat Exchanges):	
Whole milk	1 cup
Canned, evaporated whole milk	½ cup
Buttermilk made from whole milk	1 cup
Yogurt made from whole milk (plain, unflavored)	1 cup

Bread Exchange

1 Exchange contains 70 Calories, 15 grams of carbohydrate, and 2 grams of protein.

A serving of the following breads, cereals, starchy vegetables, and prepared foods counts as *1 Bread Exchange*. **Boldface** items are **low-fat** foods.

Bread:

White, Whole Wheat, Rye, Pumpernickel, or Raisin	1 slice
Bagel, small	½
English Muffin, small	½
Plain Roll, Bread	1
Frankfurter Roll	½
Hamburger Bun	½
Dried Bread Crumbs	3 tablespoons
Taco Shell	1

Cereal:

Bran Flakes	½ cup
Other ready-to-eat unsweetened cereal	¾ cup
Puffed Cereal (unfrosted)	1 cup
Cereal (cooked)	½ cup
Grits (cooked)	½ cup
Rice or Barley (cooked)	½ cup
Pasta (cooked)	½ cup
Popcorn (popped, no fat added)	3 cups
Cornmeal (dry)	2 tablespoons
Flour	2½ tablespoons
Wheat Germ	¼ cup

Crackers:

Arrowroot	3
Graham, 2½-inch	2
Matzo, 6x4-inch	½
Oyster	20
Pretzels, 3⅛ inches long, ⅛-inch diameter	25
Rye Wafers, 3½x2	3
Saltines	6
Soda, 2½-inch square	4

Dried Beans, Peas, and Lentils:

Beans, Peas, Lentils (dried, cooked)	½ cup
Baked Beans, no pork (canned)	¼ cup

Starchy Vegetables:

Corn	⅓ cup
Corn on the Cob	1 small
Lima Beans	½ cup
Parsnips	⅔ cup
Peas, Green (canned or frozen)	½ cup
Potato, White	1 small
Potato (mashed)	½ cup
Pumpkin	¾ cup
Winter Squash	½ cup
Yam or Sweet Potato	¼ cup

Prepared Foods:

Biscuit, 2-inch diameter (omit 1 Fat Exchange)	1
Corn bread, 2x2x1-inch (omit 1 Fat Exchange)	1
Corn Muffin, 2-inch diameter (omit 1 Fat Exchange)	1
Crackers, round butter type (omit 1 Fat Exchange)	5
Muffin, plain small (omit 1 Fat Exchange)	1
Potatoes, French-fried (omit 1 Fat Exchange)	8
Potato or Corn Chips (omit 2 Fat Exchanges)	15
Pancake, 5x½-inch (omit 1 Fat Exchange)	1
Waffle, 5x½-inch (omit 1 Fat Exchange)	1

Lean Meat Exchange

1 Exchange contains 55 Calories, 7 grams of protein, and 3 grams of fat.

Each serving below is for *cooked meat* and counts as *1 Low-Fat Meat Exchange*. All lean meats are **low in saturated fat and cholesterol.**

Beef: Baby Beef (very lean), Chipped Beef, Flank Steak, Tenderloin, Steaks (Sirloin and T-Bone, trimmed), Plate Ribs, Plate Skirt Steak, Round (bottom, top), all cuts Rump, Tripe	1 ounce
Lamb: Leg, Rib, Sirloin, Loin, Shank, Shoulder	1 ounce
Pork: Leg (Whole Rump, Center Shank), Ham, Smoked (center slices)	1 ounce
Veal: Leg, Loin, Rib, Shank, Shoulder, Cutlets	1 ounce
Poultry: Meat without skin of Chicken, Turkey, Cornish Hen, Guinea Hen, Pheasant	1 ounce
Fish: Any fresh or frozen	1 ounce
Canned Salmon, Tuna, Mackerel, Crab, Lobster	¼ cup
Clams, Oysters, Scallops, Shrimp	5 or 1 ounce
Sardines, drained	3
Cheeses containing less than 5% butterfat	1 ounce
Cottage Cheese, Dry and 2% butterfat	¼ cup
Dried Beans and Peas (omit 1 Bread Exchange)	½ cup

Medium-Fat Meat Exchange

1 Exchange contains 75 Calories, 7 grams of protein, and 5.5 grams of fat.

Each serving below is for *cooked meat* and counts as *1 Medium-Fat Meat Exchange*. Because of additional fat in these items, charge yourself for both 1 Meat Exchange and ½ *Fat Exchange* for each medium-fat meat serving. The item in **boldface** is **low in saturated fat and cholesterol.**

Beef: Ground (15% fat), Corned Beef (canned), Rib Eye, Round (ground commercial)	1 ounce
Pork: Loin (all cuts Tenderloin), Shoulder Arm (picnic), Shoulder Blade, Boston Butt, Canadian Bacon, Boiled Ham	1 ounce
Variety Meat: Liver, Heart, Kidney, and Sweetbreads (high in cholesterol)	1 ounce
Cottage Cheese, creamed	¼ cup
Cheese: Mozzarella, Ricotta, Farmer's Cheese, Neufchâtel	1 ounce
Parmesan	3 tablespoons
Egg (high in cholesterol)	1
Peanut Butter (omit 2 additional Fat Exchanges)	2 tablespoons

High-Fat Meat Exchange

1 Exchange contains 100 Calories, 7 grams of protein, and 5.5 grams of fat.

Each serving below is for *cooked meat* and counts as *1 High-Fat Meat Exchange*. Because of added fat content, charge yourself for both 1 Meat Exchange and *1 Fat Exchange* for each high-fat meat serving.

Beef: Brisket, Corned Beef (Brisket), Ground Beef (more than 20% fat), Hamburger (commercial), Chuck (ground commercial), Roasts (Rib), Steaks (Club, Rib)	1 ounce
Lamb: Breast	1 ounce
Pork: Spareribs, Loin (Back Ribs), Pork (ground), Country-Style Ham, Deviled Ham	1 ounce
Veal: Breast	1 ounce
Poultry: Capon, Duck (domestic), Goose	1 ounce
Cheese: Cheddar types	1 ounce
Cold Cuts	4½x⅛-inch slice
Frankfurter	1 small

Fat Exchange

1 Exchange contains 45 Calories and 5 grams of fat.

Foods that appear in **boldface** are **polyunsaturated**.

Margarine, soft, tub, or stick*	1 teaspoon
Margarine, regular stick	1 teaspoon
Avocado (4-inch diameter)**	⅛
Butter	1 teaspoon
Bacon Fat	1 teaspoon
Bacon, crisp-cooked	1 strip
Cream, Light or Sour	2 tablespoons
Cream, Heavy	1 tablespoon
Cream Cheese	1 tablespoon
French or Italian Dressing***	1 tablespoon
Lard	1 teaspoon
Mayonnaise***	1 teaspoon
Nuts:	
Almonds**	10 whole
Pecans**	2 large whole
Peanuts**	
Spanish	20 whole
Virginia	10 whole
Walnuts	6 small
Other**	6 small
Oil: Corn, Cottonseed, Safflower, Soy, Sunflower, Olive**, **Peanut****	1 teaspoon
Olives**	5 small
Salad dressing, mayonnaise-type***	2 teaspoons
Salt pork	¾-inch cube

*Made with corn, cottonseed, safflower, soy, or sunflower oil only.
**Fat content is primarily monounsaturated.
***If made with corn, cottonseed, safflower, soy, or sunflower oil, can be used on fat-modified diet.

The following items do not provide any calories or nutrients. They may be used freely to add spice to your cooking and to enhance flavors.

Salt
Pepper
Herbs
Spices
Parsley
Lemon
Horseradish
Vinegar
Mustard
Celery salt
Onion salt or powder
Garlic
Bottled hot pepper sauce
Calorie-free beverages and foods include:
  Tea
  Coffee
  Nonfat bouillon
  Calorie-free soft drinks
Unsweetened gelatin
Unsweetened pickles

Foods to Avoid

Avoid any foods with concentrated sugar such as cookies, candy, cake, pie, jelly, jam, honey, syrup, soft drinks, chewing gum, cough medicine, and sweetened condensed milk.

Key

Fruit Exchange
Vegetable Exchange
Milk Exchange
Bread Exchange
Meat Exchange
Fat Exchange
Free Exchange

A Sample Day's Menu (1,500 Calories)

Breakfast

½ cup orange juice
½ cup cooked cereal
½ cup skim milk
1 slice toast
1 teaspoon butter
Coffee or tea

Lunch

1 turkey sandwich
  (2 slices bread,
  2 teaspoons butter,
  lettuce,
  2 tomato slices,
  2 ounces turkey)
2 peach halves
  (fresh or packed in water)
  filled with ½ cup cottage cheese
½ cup skim milk
1 cup beef bouillon
Coffee or tea

Dinner

3 ounces broiled fish
  with lemon wedge
1 medium boiled potato
  with chives
½ cup cooked carrots
1 biscuit
  with 2 teaspoons butter
Tossed salad
  with low-calorie dressing
Unsweetened pear slices
Coffee or tea

Evening Snack

½ cup milk
6 saltine crackers
1 teaspoon butter

Read the Labels

Most canned items have nutritional information printed on the label. If sugar is used as an ingredient, it will be listed in the ingredient listing on the can. Calories, carbohydrates, protein, and fats are given for a serving as well as other nutrients. If the label states that the product is a "dietetic" or "diabetic" food, read the fine print carefully. Dietetic green beans, for instance, may be the same as the ordinary canned product but at a higher cost. Ice milk contains about the same number of calories as ice cream—it simply uses increased sugar in place of decreased fat.

Nutrition Labeling

As of June 30, 1975, every company that labels or advertises special nutritional qualities or that adds vitamins or minerals to its food has to label its products according to a standard format. Any other food company also may voluntarily label its products, but the label must conform to a uniform format.

For one-serving amounts, the calories and the gram weights of protein, fat, and carbohydrates must be listed. The percentages in terms of the U.S. RDA of protein and seven vitamins and minerals must follow. The vitamins are A and C and the three B vitamins—thiamine, riboflavin, and niacin; minerals are calcium and iron. Any of 12 other nutrients must be listed on the label when added by the food manufacturer.

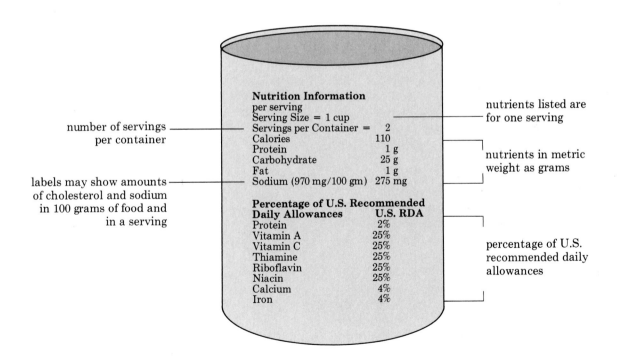

number of servings per container

labels may show amounts of cholesterol and sodium in 100 grams of food and in a serving

Nutrition Information
per serving
Serving Size = 1 cup
Servings per Container =   2
Calories   110
Protein   1 g
Carbohydrate   25 g
Fat   1 g
Sodium (970 mg/100 gm)   275 mg

Percentage of U.S. Recommended Daily Allowances   U.S. RDA
Protein   2%
Vitamin A   25%
Vitamin C   25%
Thiamine   25%
Riboflavin   25%
Niacin   25%
Calcium   4%
Iron   4%

nutrients listed are for one serving

nutrients in metric weight as grams

percentage of U.S. recommended daily allowances

The label may include the amounts of polyunsaturated fat and saturated fat and also the cholesterol content. The following statement must then be included. "Information on fat (and/or cholesterol) content is provided for individuals who, on the advice of a physician, are modifying their total dietary intake of fat (and/or cholesterol)." Sodium content may be given both per serving and per 100 grams of food.

Remaining on all the labels except those on standard foods is a listing of ingredients in descending order of amounts. Thus a listing for spaghetti with meat sauce may read: Ingredients: Water, tomatoes, spaghetti, beef, food starch—modified (from corn), carrots, celery, cheese, non-fat dry milk, onion flavoring, and salt. This means there is more water than tomatoes, more spaghetti than beef, more carrots than cheese, etc.

With the percentages of nutrients listed on the packages, you can calculate the amounts in each category and with proper menu planning, serve all the nutrients you need in one day. However, don't be alarmed if you don't have 100 percent of each nutrient. Different people have different requirements, and the U.S. RDA doesn't discriminate according to sex, age, or size. It takes the highest value in most categories and sets that figure as the standard U.S. RDA. So while women need more iron than men, men need slightly more protein and vitamin C than women, and teen-age boys require more thiamine than both, the standard for each nutrient takes into consideration the highest amount that is recommended for most population groups.

Since no one food is nutritionally complete, you need a wide variety of foods daily. Maybe today you will select orange juice for the vitamin C, but tomorrow choose broccoli and tomatoes. With nutrition labeling, comparing food values and counting calories should be easier.

REDUCING OR
CALORIE-RESTRICTED DIETS

A reducing diet is any diet that restricts calories sufficiently to produce weight loss. A very bad diet can do that just as effectively (but dangerously) as a very good diet. Dozens of allegedly miraculous slimming diets come and go in bewildering succession. It is neither necessary nor desirable to follow a diet that extols a singularly virtuous food or two, requires exotic and expensive supplements or ingredients, or espouses some gimmick or asserted scientific discovery that makes reducing effortless.

A sensible reducing diet, besides being well balanced, should allow wide and changing choices of foods one likes, and should be simple to follow. The Food Exchange System described in preceding pages helps you to choose (and stay on!) just such a diet.

The 1,200-Calorie diet on the facing page is, for most people, a moderately fast reducing diet. At first glance, it looks like an ordinary menu plan for breakfast, lunch, and dinner. But it's really a framework within which you can freely substitute foods that are equal to each other. This allows an almost endless variety of choices and may even produce some surprises—would you think that three sardines are equal to one-fourth cup of cottage cheese? Nice to know if you have sardines but no cottage cheese, and if you like sardines.

This is how it works:

Each item in the diet plan is identified by its color-coded Exchange category, and the number of Exchange units allowed is given. Any food in the same Exchange can be substituted for another (see the Exchange Lists on pages 143 to 148).

Thus, one day's meals can be entirely different from the next day's, but the calorie and nutrient values will be the same. Include foods from the Basic Four Food Groups (see page 140) to maintain balanced nutrition.

Total calories for the day can be figured by simple addition of calories per Exchange Unit, which have been calculated for you. If desired, you also can add up the given nutrient values to figure your day's intake of fat, protein, and carbohydrate.

In a reducing diet, there's no reason to limit yourself to three squares a day—as long as the calories stay the same. Divide up the foods you had planned for the three large meals into four, five, or even six sittings.

Take your time when eating, and savor every morsel. Be watchful for the "I'm full" signal, and stop eating when you're aware of it. You can save any food from your allotted meal for a snack when you're again hungry.

Keep a supply of "as desired" vegetables on hand and at easy access for nibbling or to fill out a meal. These vegetables include asparagus, bean sprouts, green or wax beans, broccoli, Brussels sprouts, cabbage, cauliflower, celery, chicory, cucumber, eggplant, endive, escarole, greens, lettuce, mushrooms, okra, parsley, green pepper, pimiento, radish, romaine, and sauerkraut.

Check the Free Exchange List of the Exchange System for seasonings to spark up foods. Also included are calorie-free beverages and foods.

A Sample Day's Menu (1,200 Calories)

Breakfast

½ cup orange juice
½ cup cooked cereal
½ cup skim milk
1 poached egg
1 slice toast
1 teaspoon butter
Coffee or tea

Lunch

1 turkey sandwich
    (2 ounces turkey,
    lettuce,
    2 tomato slices,
    2 slices bread,
    2 teaspoons butter)
Fresh peach half
    (or other fresh fruit in season)
    topped with ½ cup cottage cheese
½ cup skim milk
1 cup hot beef bouillon

Dinner

3 ounces broiled fish
    with lemon wedge
1 medium boiled potato
    with snipped chives
½ cup cooked carrots
Tossed salad
    with low-calorie salad dressing
½ cup skim milk
Coffee or tea

Evening Snack

½ grapefruit

Key

Fruit Exchange
Vegetable Exchange
Milk Exchange
Bread Exchange
Meat Exchange
Fat Exchange
Free Exchange

WAYS TO HELP YOURSELF

Don't Follow the Fads

A fad can be defined as a "silly custom" followed for a time with exaggerated zeal. Of the making of food fads, there is no end. To watch food fads as they come and go is like oscillating the head at a tennis match. A great deal of excellent counsel about diets, meal planning, and cookery is available to the public through books, magazines, newspapers, and government pamphlets but so is a lot of nutritional nonsense. How can one tell the sound from the unsound?

A faddist food plan or diet program, most often a reducing diet, generally has a distinctive "gimmick" to which wondrous virtues are ascribed. Most fad diets extol the value of special products, preferably exotic and expensive ones, that assertedly have health-giving or restorative properties confirmed by testimonials (but by no documentation of lasting benefit). The gimmick may be some ritual of drinking or eating, limitation to one or two foods, exclusion of carbohydrate or protein or fat, fasting, allowance of alcohol, and oddities beyond the scope of a nutritionist's imagination. Promoters of such diets may be sincere but uninformed. Some earnest faddists are convinced that foods bought in the ordinary marketplace are devastating the nation's health and that the only recourse is to eat "natural" or "health foods" or "organically grown" food. Someone has said perceptively that more organically grown food is sold than is grown!

Food fads, as the Surgeon General might say, can be dangerous to your health—not because they furnish anything toxic (although some herbal concoctions have been found to contain "natural" mind-altering drugs), but because they encourage self-experimentation while postponing proper medical attention to a condition that may not be responsive to diet, even a good one. Too, a faddist diet that restricts foods to a limited variety or overemphasizes others may itself cause nutritional deficiencies.

The birth rate of fad diets is about the same as the death rate—easy come, easy go. Meanwhile, reducing or "regular" diets, nutritionally well-balanced but gimmickless, go on and on without raising any fanfare.

Food fads are usually expensive. Money spent for products that are useless (unless psychologically) leaves less for the purchase of good nourishing foods. It is estimated that 10 million people spend large sums every year for nostrums that are worthless or unnecessary. Vitamin and mineral supplements, adjusted to variable dosage needs of individual patients, are important in medical practice. However, self-chosen supplements may fall wide of the mark, may be used by persons whose diets are perfectly adequate, may be inappropriate to dietary needs, and may provide too little of a needed vitamin or too much of one that is already adequate.

No food, nutrient, elixir, drug, or medication will reverse or halt the process of aging. The best formula known is far too simple to be hailed as a miracle: over a lifetime, it calls for a well-balanced diet, moderate exercise, adequate rest and relaxation, and prompt medical attention to conditions that may occur.

Weight Control

Legend has it that delicious foods are fattening and nutritious ones are a chore to eat. Nonsense! A calorie is a calorie, whether it comes from something appetizing or repellent. Extra weight comes when we consume more calories than we expend in energy, although there is a natural tendency to put on weight after the 20s merge into the 30s. It is easier and much more healthful to keep weight at a desirable level than to reduce repeatedly—gaining weight, dieting, regaining weight, and dieting again.

Calories that we consume from any source will be used for energy to do body work, and will disappear. Or, they will be stored as fat if they are not needed for energy. Excess fat can be regarded as spilled-over calories that had no other place to go.

We do a good deal of unconscious, internal body work without thinking about it. We burn energy to breathe, to maintain the heartbeat, circulation, body temperature, and other subtle body activities over which we have little or no control. The sum of such energies burned just to stay alive is called the basal metabolism, which is all involuntary work.

Exercise is external or voluntary work done outside of the body. Exercise burns calories, and is something we can control, sometimes by exercising will power. A person who stays at normal weight exhibits a fine balance between physical exertion and food intake. A fat person can reduce by decreasing calorie intake (from food and drink) or by increasing exercise, with a physician's approval. Theoretically, exercise could do it all, but as a practical matter, the great majority of obese persons will need to reduce their calorie intake as well as increase physical activity.

Reducing doesn't require an unusual or bizzare diet, as will be seen from the examples on pages 148 to 151. The most long-lasting weight loss results from adjustments to foods the dieter likes, is accustomed to, and that fit familiar patterns. This usually means smaller food portions and a reduction of extras, treats, snacks, and "reward" foods. Foods from the Basic Four Food Groups, necessary for nutrient quality and balance, should not be omitted, although servings should be smaller.

Fats and Cholesterol

Various fats and oils in the diet contribute a few essentials, greatly enhance the flavor and "richness" of foods, and carry a big load of calories, more than twice as many as carbohydrates and protein, gram for gram. There are many different food sources of fats and oils, as well as technical differences in their composition and action.

The association of some dietary fats with blood cholesterol levels, atherosclerosis, heart attacks, and strokes is an area under intense medical investigation. The hope is that dietary modifications might reduce the risk of heart attacks and strokes. It seems prudent to reduce total calories, dietary cholesterol, and saturated fat, but final answers are not yet in. Studies are currently under way to test the hypothesis that lessening the various risk factors, of which elevated blood cholesterol is only one, will reduce the risk of heart attack. A large scale coordinated study involving some twenty medical centers is under way, financed by the National Heart and Lung Institute of the United States Public Health Service. Some definitive answers may come from the conclusion of this study, which is still some years away.

Potassium in Foods

Diuretic drugs known as thiazides are often prescribed for patients with waterlogged tissues, hypertension, and heart ailments to remove excess water from the body. Sodium, an element of common salt, has water-binding properties that hold fluids in tissues. The diuretic drugs wash some sodium from the body and thereby promote the excretion of water.

At the same time, the drugs wash out some potassium, the major electrolyte of fluids inside body cells. Potassium is absolutely essential to life and health. It participates in transmission of nerve impulses, muscle contraction, and other vital functions. Depletion of bodily potassium can result in weakness, fatigue, faintness, slow reflexes, and irregularities of the heart's rhythm.

For this reason, physicians monitor the blood potassium levels of patients on thiazide diuretics. If tests show a deficit, the doctor may prescribe a potassium supplement in tablet form and will probably recommend a diet high in potassium-rich foods to offset losses. Frequently, such a diet is all that is necessary to maintain normal potassium levels, but this should be confirmed by tests and the doctor's knowledge of the condition for which diuretics are taken. An inexpensive non-prescription supplement that furnishes generous amounts of potassium is the most common type of salt substitute, which contains potassium chloride; this ingredient will be listed on the label.

In general, foods high in potassium are meats, nuts, whole grain cereals, and certain fruits and vegetables. Listed at right are representative everyday foods that provide liberal amounts of potassium. Avoid obviously salty foods and canned vegetables that usually contain salt added in the canning process.

Change the chewability. A primary reason for inferior diets of some elderly people is difficulty in chewing, because of missing teeth, ill-fitting dentures, or reluctance or inability to obtain reconstructive dental care (see page 167). The tendency is to avoid foods that take effort to chew—crunchy vegetables, crisp fruits, seeds, meat, and things that must be "bitten off" like corn on the cob—and to make very soft, easily chewed foods the principal if not exclusive components of the diet. These soft foods are usually high in carbohydrate and, while they are perfectly good foods, excessive intake with avoidance of other foods prevents a sufficiently varied diet that provides necessary nutrients.

It is not at all necessary to exclude good foods because they are hard to chew. Use a tenderizer or blender to grind hard-to-eat meats or vegetables to any consistency, from small pieces to liquids. The texture is different, but the flavor and the nutrient value are intact. If you don't have a blender or grinder, commercially strained, chopped, or pureed foods may be used.

Strained or liquefied foods also can give nutritional support when used temporarily during periods of acute oral problems, or permanently if problems remain. Persons using such foods should not feel that they have reverted to "baby foods." Other foods of excellent nutrient value for people with chewing or swallowing problems include stews, rich soups, casseroles, puddings, custards, soft desserts, fruit juices, and a wide variety of dairy foods.

Food	Amount	Potassium (mg)
All-bran cereals	½ cup	336
Avocado	½	600
Bread, whole grain	1 slice	128
Apricots, dried	4 halves	196
Bananas	1 small, ½ cup	370
Apples, raw	1 medium, ½ cup	110
Peaches, raw	1 medium	202
Cantaloupe, raw	¼, 6-inch diameter	376
Orange juice	½ cup	200
Watermelon	1 slice, 6-inch diameter x 1½ inches	600
Spinach, cooked	½ cup	291
Squash, winter, baked	½ cup	461
Potatoes, white, baked in skin	1, 2½-inch diameter	407
Beans, dry, cooked	½ cup	416
Peanuts, roasted, with skin, unsalted	3½ ounces	740
Salmon, baked, broiled	3½ ounces	443
Halibut, cooked	3½ ounces	525
Hamburger, medium	1 patty, 3-inch diameter x 1 inch	382
Beef, sirloin, broiled	1 slice, 3 x 2½ inches	545
Ham, fresh, cooked	3½ ounces	434
Chicken	4 ounces	430

Buy smartly. Nutrition problems rarely exist in isolation. They are complicated by such prosaic matters as transportation to markets, housing, storage, money, and physical handicaps. Any of these can affect the purchase or preparation of food. Individual circumstances differ, but some general guidelines may be helpful:

- Shop by list; check supplies and plan menus before going to the store. Planned menus are usually more nutritious and varied than those made on impulse.
- Buy only what you can use quickly or store properly. Most spoilage and nutritional deterioration occur in our own kitchens.
- Get the most for your money—shop comparatively if you have the time and energy. Unit prices disclose differences in costs, brands, and content weights. It is a good habit to read labels that list ingredients and thus encourage interest in nutrition.
- Buy the food form best suited to you. Many people, especially in households of one or two persons, enjoy the convenience of frozen meals or entrées that can be prepared with very little effort, time, or equipment. They cost slightly more than the raw materials of unprepared meals, but the saving in time and labor may well be worth the difference. Also, convenience foods can mean little or no waste. Hundreds of choices can be made to suit any taste or nutritional need.
- Shop at off-peak times, if time permits. It is more pleasurable to shop in unhurried, uncongested surroundings than when the store is overcrowded and noisy, and sometimes there are more bargains then, too.
- In cooking, consider preparing enough for more than one meal. "Leftovers" are not to be sneered at, and in fact can be delicious if they are not pushed to the back of a refrigerator and forgotten for days. If storage permits, freeze your own convenience meals for quick and easy use at a later time.

How others may help you. Practical ways of helping older people satisfy their nutritional needs are being expanded widely. *Group meals* are one way of providing not only food but companionship, new interests, and a place to go. Many group meal programs are conducted in the readily available facilities of schools in early or mid-afternoon after the school children have been fed lunch.

Home-delivered meals for shut-ins are available in many communities. Government agencies are developing a project for shipping freeze-dried foods to consumers by mail. Freeze-dried foods do not require refrigeration until they have been reconstituted with water in the home kitchen. A variety of such foods, enough to last a week or more, can be shipped in a package of moderate size.

In all of these programs, a nominal fee is paid for meals and there are varying arrangements for requesting specific foods. The goal is to assist people in meeting their nutritional needs. Information about the programs can be obtained from local hospitals, health departments, or community service organizations.

In summary, good nutrition is the foundation of good health, and the improvement of a poor diet can do nothing but good—although it should not be expected of itself to cure conditions that need medical attention.

Good nutrition consists of eating a varied diet that furnishes all essential nutrients. High quality is attained by daily choices from the Basic Four Food Groups:

- Meats, poultry, fish, dried peas and beans
- Dairy products
- Fruits and vegetables
- Cereal foods

Vary the choices within food groups, and don't eat so much as to become obese. Control weight by adjusting the size of food portions and by moderate daily physical activity. Food supplements of various types are rarely necessary; if they should be, a physician should determine what is needed. A poor selection of foods cannot be made into a good one by supplements.

CHAPTER **6**   LLOYD E. CHURCH, D.D.S., Ph.D.

THE
TEETH
IN
MATURITY

If you are middle-aged and have all your natural teeth in prime condition, except, perhaps, for wisdom teeth, you are either an exceptional person who knows a lot about dental care or you're extraordinarily lucky. Unfortunately, the chances of your being such a person are very small. Dismal statistics from the Department of Health, Education, and Welfare tell us that 23 million people in the United States have lost all their teeth—are edentulous—and that four million of them do not have artificial dentures or false teeth, and have to "gum it."

Does this mean that loss of teeth is a natural result of growing older? No, aging itself does not destroy teeth. What happens is that year after year, there is more and more time for neglect, poor care, and even fear of dentists to mount up to dental disaster.

This is not to say that an older mouth is identical to a young one. Middle age is a time when new cavities are less of a threat to teeth than loss of support from gum and bone disease. No two mouths are alike. Very likely you have had some dental work, extractions, or conditions that at some time in the future will affect decisions about what should be done to keep your teeth in best condition. Also, the mouth, excluding the teeth, may show signs of chronic disease, which tends to be more frequent in older age groups.

Changes in an Older Mouth

Don't expect a 40-year-old mouth to be perfect, but do expect it to be healthy and efficient. Around middle age, a mouth in reasonably good condition will have several teeth with restorations—fillings, inlays, or crowns—and there may be a bridge or partial denture filling the space of an extracted tooth or teeth. Some persons may have full upper and lower dentures, which are no longer an indication of old age.

A physical change associated with age is some recession of the gums, which exposes more of the roots of the teeth and makes them look longer. Such recession will be less noticeable if the teeth are well cared for and the preventive measures discussed under *periodontal disease* are followed.

Recession of the gums means that bone around the teeth has also receded. This may occur in one or more small areas, or may involve all of the teeth. It is due to changes in the "bite,"—the way uppers and lowers mesh together—and to spaces left by extracted teeth, which allow adjoining teeth to drift, causing excessive stress and movement.

"In the pink." Everything you see when you open your mouth and look into a mirror should be a glistening pink color, except for your teeth. There should be no dark spots, ulcers, or sores on the lips, cheeks, or tongue. The top of the mouth (palate) is hard to see, but the back part is visible. Stick out your tongue, move it from side to side, and look underneath it. This occasional self-examination will reassure you that your mouth is in the pink, or if not, that a visit to your dentist is in order.

Cavities. Tooth decay *(dental caries)* tends to be somewhat different in older people. Cavities in young persons generally occur in the crown of the tooth, especially in pits and fissures of the chewing surface. These are the kind avoided by the toothpaste-conscious youngster who comes home from the dentist with the glowing report, "Look, Mom, no cavities!"

Caries in older persons typically occur in the *cementum* layer of the tooth, in the root area, at or near the gum line, or under it. The lower part of the crown may also decay near the gums. These cavities are often quite sensitive to temperature (hot or cold food or drink may cause pain) and should be filled.

Erosions and V-shaped etchings also occur at the gum line. Presumptive causes are faulty brushing, acids, and patterns of saliva flow. Technically, these are not decayed areas, but they should be filled to save the tooth. A preserved tooth may be priceless in years to come as an anchor for a bridge or a preventive of drift that could distort the bite.

An impression that tooth decay is not exactly rampant among older people may or may not have some validity. Some evidence suggests that older teeth are more caries-resistant, perhaps because of slow changes in mineralization or a shift in dietary habits, as from sugar-loaded soft drinks to more spirited forms. However, an older mouth is likely to have a substantial number of fillings, crowns, jackets, or spaces where teeth once were, so there is less left for decay processes to work on.

How to Find a Good Dentist

You will probably have to find a new dentist someday. You may move to a new town; an old dentist may die, retire, or get a bit out-of-date in his training; or maybe you just don't like him anymore.

If you don't know of a reputable dentist and need immediate attention, there are standard ways of locating one. Call your local dental or medical society. If there is a hospital in your area that provides dental service, call the dentist on the staff and ask for names of qualified dentists. Or if you live near a dental school, there will likely be several faculty members who practice general dentistry in your vicinity.

Better yet, anticipate your need of a dentist before a tooth hurts. Ask your physician what dentist he and his family use. Also neighbors and fellow members of a church or service club are usually pleased to be asked about a dentist. Obviously, word-of-mouth well applies to dentistry.

The first visit. Your first impression of a dentist's office should be one of orderliness, pleasant surroundings, and modern equipment, with waiting room reading matter not more than a few months out-of-date.

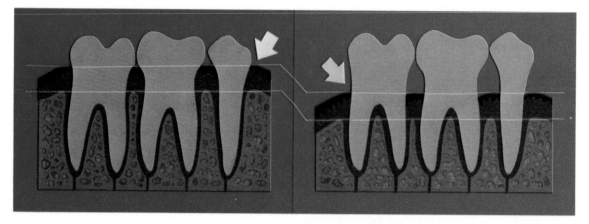

CHANGES WITH AGE

In a young mouth, the normal gum line (white arrow) meets the enamel at the base of the crowns of the teeth, and the surrounding bone support is intact. Gums tend to recede as we grow older, exposing more of the roots of the teeth (yellow arrow). The bone around the teeth also recedes.

The dentist's nurse or assistant should be neat and pleasant, as it is important that you be at ease with the staff. A good dentist is concerned about the welfare of every patient, and is well aware that many patients have fears and misapprehensions that are largely needless.

The initial examination will include a full-mouth set of X rays and special X rays if needed. The teeth will get a detailed examination, and the mouth will be checked for possible ulcers, sores, swellings, or lumps. You will probably be asked to answer questions and volunteer information about your dental and medical history. Don't hold anything back, as some middle-aged and older patients may have chronic diseases which require that dental treatment be planned in consultation with a physician. Be very skeptical of a dentist who is content just to treat symptoms and doesn't bother to do an initial work-up.

Prevention is very much to the forefront in dental care today. Your dental and dietary habits afford great opportunity for applying preventive measures that save the teeth. Regular self-care procedures will be explained (see pages 186 and 187), but a dentist can't do it all. The patient must do much of the preventive work at home.

What's to be done? When the X rays, laboratory work, medical history, and examination are completed, the dentist will review his findings with you in detail and tell you what he thinks should be done. Perhaps nothing, other than a recommendation to return in four to six months for prophylaxis and examination.

More likely, particularly if some tooth problem prompted your visit, he will recommend one or more courses of treatment. A good dentist takes plenty of time to explain a patient's condition, the treatment he proposes, the alternatives, and the basis for choices.

Be wary of a dentist who leans toward extracting teeth rather than saving them. Regard the loss of a salvageable tooth as a tragedy: you can't chew on a cavern or attach a bridge to it. It is often possible to save a damaged tooth by root-canal therapy (see page 163), or to rescue one that is threatened by gum disease. A general dentist may or may not perform some specialized procedures, but may refer you to a tooth-saving specialist.

Once a course of treatment is agreed upon, ask what it will cost, or at least get an estimate. This is absolutely essential for a good relationship between dentist and patient, and for a satisfying outcome.

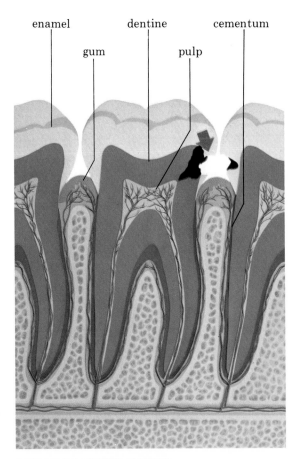

DECAY IN OLDER TEETH

Cavities (dental caries) in older persons occur more often at or under the gum line (red arrow) than on the chewing surfaces. They undermine the cementum, which is bone deposited on the roots of the teeth. Dentine, related to bone, forms the major part of a tooth.

PERIODONTAL DISEASE

(Pyorrhea)

Seventy-five percent of tooth loss after age 40 is caused by destruction of tissues that hold teeth in their sockets. Thousands of these lost teeth are cavity-free and absolutely beautiful. According to the National Institute of Dental Research, two out of three middle-aged Americans are affected by periodontal disease.

"Periodontal" means "around the teeth" and refers to the gums, bone, and surrounding tissues. Laymen simply call it gum disease, or *pyorrhea,* a condition in which pus flows from pockets under the gums.

There is good news and bad news concerning periodontal disease. The good news is that gum disease is preventable and controllable by a regular program of self-care and periodic professional attention. The bad news is that periodontal disease is insidious, that it worsens with age, that prevention requires personal effort, and that people generally are more worried about cavities than gum disease until their teeth begin to wobble.

A good general dentist is quite competent to recognize, treat, and give counsel about early gum disease. Or, he may prefer to limit his practice and to refer patients who need specialized care to a *periodontist,* a dentist with special training in treating diseases of the gums and surrounding tissues.

Anatomy. Teeth are not anchored solidly to the jawbone, but move slightly when you chew. A tooth rests in a bony socket a little larger than its roots, and between the root and the socket there is a tough muscular cushion, somewhat like a powerful sling, called the *periodontal membrane.* The protein fibers of this membrane give strong support, with the principal protein being collagen, a component of connective tissues that is involved in a great variety of disorders (see page 234).

Periodontal disease commonly begins with *gingivitis,* an inflammation of the gums. Then it progresses to create pockets between gums and teeth in which germs and food particles collect. As the pockets get wider and deeper, pus may form in them (pyorrhea). Finally, supporting fibers and bone are destroyed and the tooth falls out.

Causes. Most of the causes of gum disease are preventable and correctable if steps are taken in time.

The most common cause of gum irritation is *tartar* (calculus). Tartar is a hard, crust-like material formed from substances normally found in the mouth. It is deposited on the teeth and under the gums, hardens in a very short time, and cannot be removed by a toothbrush. *Plaque* is a thin film attached to the surfaces of teeth that is a breeding-ground for bacteria, linked with tooth decay and gum disease (see page 186). Tartar at the base of the teeth is an accumulation of plaque that has hardened and become mineralized.

Missing and improperly spaced teeth will cause adjacent teeth to drift toward the open space, rotating as they move. When this happens, upper and lower teeth do not meet properly and cause uneven pressure during chewing. This, too, damages the gums and bone surrounding the teeth.

Everyday wear and tear on fillings, crowns, bridgework, and dentures is considerable and can also cause irritation of gum tissue. Adjustments will be necessary to keep up with changes in the mouth that normally occur with age.

Likewise, harmful dental habits may be injurious to the gums and surrounding bone. Examples are: chewing on one side of the mouth, mouth breathing, lip biting, bottle opening, grinding of teeth, and biting on pencils.

Some systemic diseases — tuberculosis, diabetes, and blood diseases, to mention a few—also cause changes in the gums and adjacent bone, as may pregnancy and vitamin deficiencies.

In addition, improper diet is often associated with gum disease in older people. Inadequate chewing ability, too many soft foods, and imbalanced nutrition all contribute to gum and digestive disorders and lower the general state of health.

Prevention. Implicit in a discussion of causes are rational and effective measures for preventing periodontal disease. As mentioned previously, you can't do it all by yourself. Tartar must be removed by a dentist in periodic tooth-cleaning sessions. You must also count on him to correct a bad bite, to fill the space of a missing tooth as soon as possible, to recognize systemic disease and consult with your physician, and of course, to alert and advise you about incipient gum disorders before you are aware of any symptoms.

The rest is primarily your continuing responsibility. You should faithfully apply the routine procedures explained in detail on pages 186 and 187, which will promote general dental health as well as healthy gums. *Flossing* is particularly important, and water jets and power brushes also have their roles.

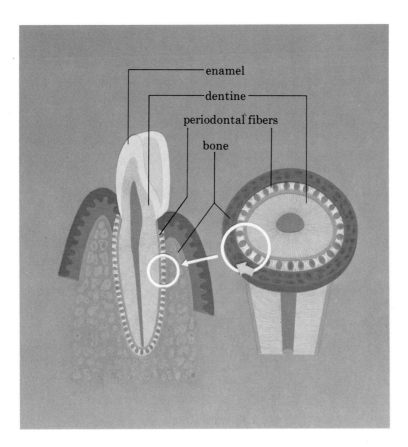

enamel
dentine
periodontal fibers
bone

TOOTH SUPPORTS

The far left drawing shows a front tooth with its root resting in a bone socket. The root and bone do not touch, but are separated by a strong sling-like cushion (periodontal membrane) that allows some movement. The closeup drawing shows a cross section of a root slung in a loose, strong network of tiny fibers (yellow arrow) between the root and bone.

A gentle *gum massage* and cleansing of pockets can be accomplished with a soft-bristle brush rocked slowly back and forth at the gum line. Devices with a soft rubber cone, sometimes attached to a toothbrush handle, are useful for gentle massage between the teeth and help to stimulate blood circulation in the area.

Symptoms. The very earliest stages of gum disease give no signal of pain or anything to warn that trouble is brewing. The simplest and most common early indicator is *gingivitis,* an inflammation of the gingiva (gums) that may have its onset as early as the mid-teens but which may not be noticed by the patient until the 30s or even later. Previously, the patient may only have been bothered by painless mild gum infections that "come and go."

Normally pink gums have smooth edges that cling to the teeth. Inflammation begins with a reddening and swelling along this gum margin, and gradually the gum tissue loosens from the tooth surface, leaving a slight crevice. The first and probably the only symptom that the patient notices is that the gums bleed easily when the teeth are brushed. At this stage, simple treatment effectively checks the disease.

If neglected, however, the gums become puffed up, bleed easily, and lose their normal pink color. Debris-collecting pockets between teeth and gums, often filled with pus, are a source of constant bad breath, and usually cause some pain. But the ultimate symptom of a deep-seated condition is a loosened tooth or teeth or the opening of spaces between teeth.

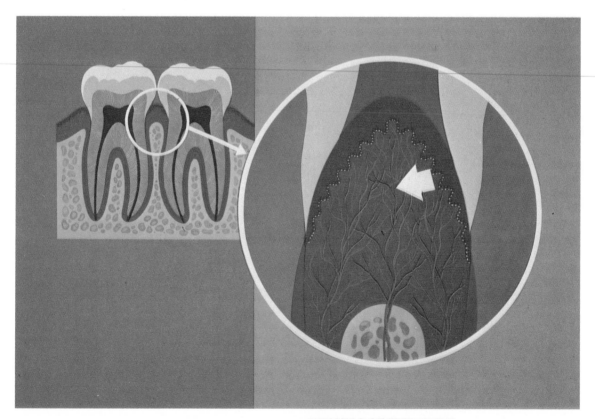

VESSELS OF THE GUMS

Normal gums have smooth edges that cling to the teeth, and a uniformly pink color given by a rich network of blood vessels (closeup in circle). Changes in color and easy bleeding of the gums are typical early signs of periodontal disease.

Treatment. Destroyed tissue cannot be restored, but usually a good deal can be done, depending on the condition of the patient's mouth. Severe gum conditions can be treated and restored to a healthy state by a surgical procedure done in the dentist's office. He cuts away the excessive gum tissue and deep pockets that have formed, and then cleans the tooth roots. This removes areas of inflammation and irritation. Although this procedure leaves a larger area of the tooth exposed, the surface is accessible to good care and treatment. The operation itself causes almost no pain, which is well-controlled with medication. And the chances that periodontal surgery will be successful in preserving the teeth indefinitely or for a long time are very good.

The dental procedures already described can help to keep a mouth in good chewing condition even though some teeth are moderately loose or threatened. In biting, certain teeth may "hit" each other too powerfully or at an angle that puts abnormal stress on their supports. A dentist may correct this by careful grinding of opposing surfaces. He may also splint a couple of teeth together for extended service, or put a bridge in the space of a missing tooth, to save adjacent teeth from the strains of tilting and drifting that can damage supporting tissues.

Some people have an unconscious habit of grinding their teeth together *(bruxism)*. The hard jaw-clenching, which often occurs during sleep, puts damaging strains on periodontal structures. It may be desirable to overcome the habit with the aid of a device, somewhat comparable to a boxer's mouthpiece, that is worn only at night.

Advanced periodontal disease, with some teeth lost and others ready to go, brings the patient and dentist to some hard decisions. Should the teeth be retained as long as possible, or should one give up and go to artificial dentures (false teeth)? The feeling of some people that dentures will solve their problems permanently is not always well-based, and alternatives should be discussed. It may be feasible to retain the superior performance of natural teeth if there are enough of them in reasonably good or repairable condition to serve as anchors for bridgework.

SAVE THAT "DEAD" TOOTH

It is a common belief that a tooth that has lost its nerve or pulp is dead and useless. This is not true. The life of a tooth does not depend upon the contents of its pulp chamber, which is tissue containing nerves, blood vessels, and lymphatics. A tooth is kept alive by its root covering, which keeps the tooth attached to bone, and it is through this covering that the tooth receives its nourishment. As long as a tooth has a living root covering, it will stay in the jaw as long as any healthy tooth, it will feel good, and it will be strong enough to chew with and to support bridgework.

These facts are the basis for *root-canal therapy,* a procedure that in its modern form saves thousands of teeth and gives valuable options for restoration of the mouth to its best capacity. Extracting teeth because of pulp problems is now considered old-fashioned dentistry. In the past, if a tooth was broken, abscessed, or had a deep cavity, it was simply extracted. Today these teeth are completely restored and serve a long useful life. An *endodontist* is a dentist who has had special training in the prevention, diagnosis, and treatment of diseases of the pulp and surrounding tissue.

Anatomy. The nerve or pulp of a tooth is located in the center of the crown and the roots, and is enclosed within the pulp chamber. This chamber narrows as it reaches the tip of the root, and this narrowed extension of the pulp chamber in the root or roots is the root canal. Each tooth root has its own canal, and possibly more than one.

The pulp of a tooth may be damaged by deep decay, trauma, or loss of circulation from many causes, and may become invaded by bacteria, leading to abscess formation and loss of the tooth. Root-canal therapy aims to save the tooth and avoid its extraction and replacement with a false tooth or denture.

Treatment. Root-canal work is usually not painful, but may require anesthesia. Local anesthesia is usually sufficient, but sometimes general anesthesia is required. The work is done in several visits, and after it is completed, any remaining work is usually done by the patient's own dentist.

Endodontia requires sterility of all instruments and of the area of operation. The dentist isolates the tooth by a rubber dam or cotton rolls, and then drills an opening directly into the pulp chamber. He uses fine delicate instruments such as broaches, reamers, and files to remove the entire pulp content, and enlarges the canal and smooths its walls to make it easy to fill.

Frequent X rays are taken to determine the right length for the canal-filling material and the position of instruments. The canal is irrigated several times, dried, and medicaments are sealed into it for interim protection between visits.

When the canal is ready for permanent filling, it is isolated, cleaned, and dried, and a filling material—commonly gutta percha or silver point—is inserted to completely fill the canal and pulp chamber. X rays are taken to ensure that the canal is totally filled, as incomplete filling may mean future pain and infection. Once the canals are filled and sealed, the opening in the crown through which the dentist worked is sealed with a permanent filling.

A one-root tooth, as found in the front of the mouth, may require fewer treatments than a multi-rooted tooth in the side or back of the mouth. Front teeth with single, straight, large root canals are easier to fill than back teeth with multiple, curved, and narrow canals. Also, front teeth are more accessible to instruments, making them easier to treat.

Root-canal therapy has the greatest chance of success in healthy patients whose roots are straight and not too narrow. Treatment will usually be difficult and not be advised for elderly, chronically ill, or extremely nervous persons, nor will it be suggested if root canals are extremely irregular, blocked, or curved. In these extreme cases, root resection or tooth extraction may be the only alternative.

Complications. Infrequently, despite good root-canal treatment, an infection will appear at the tip of the root or be of such magnitude that it must be surgically corrected by a minor office procedure called an *apioectomy*. The dentist removes the tip of the root and all infected tissue, after which the bone grows back normally with the infection gone.

It is not true that a tooth that has had root-canal work will eventually turn black. Sometimes a tooth will darken, but never to a black color. And any darkening can be corrected by bleaching, a simple procedure done through a tiny opening in the back of the tooth. The procedure may be repeated if necessary.

In the early days of root-canal treatment, before modern materials were developed, silver and mercury amalgams were used to fill the opening in the crown after the root-canal filling was completed. They discolored the tooth in some instances, usually to a shade of gray, but this type of filling is never used today. Now, when the opening is filled with newer plastic material, it can hardly be detected and does not stain or discolor the tooth.

ROOT-CANAL THERAPY: SAVING A TOOTH

Root-canal treatment often can save a "dead" or badly diseased tooth from extraction and restore it to comfortable service. Drawing A shows a tooth with a deep cavity, infection, and abscess. An opening is drilled into the pulp chamber, the contents are totally removed with delicate files and instruments (B) down through the root canal at the tip of the root, and a filling is placed in the entire chamber (C).

Subsequently, the crown of the tooth is drilled away and the pulp chamber is cleaned out about two-thirds of the way up (D). The completed restoration might be a crown and post, as shown in drawing E.

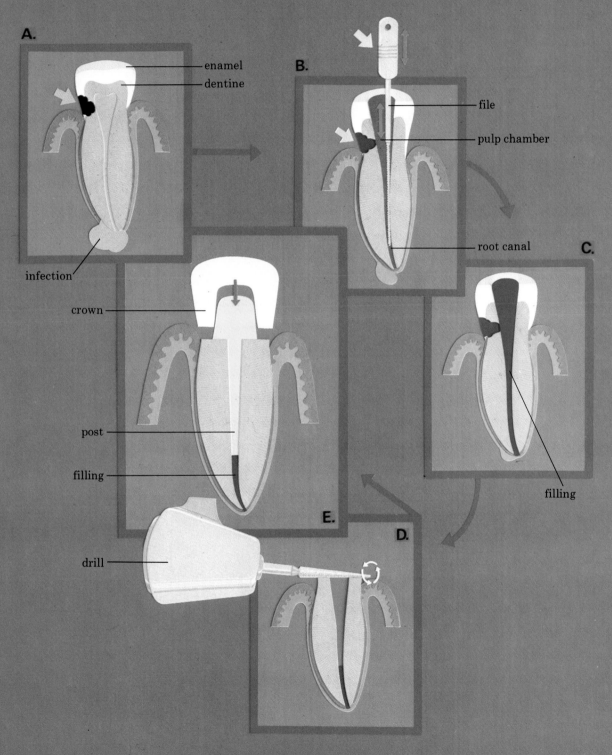

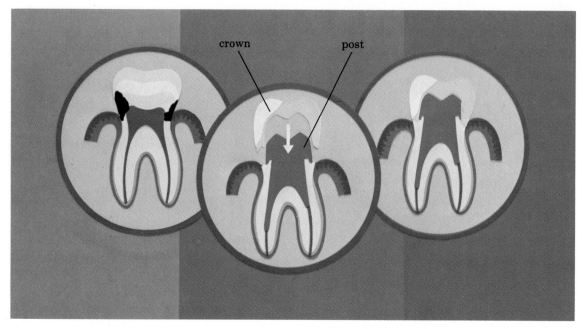

crown   post

DOUBLE ROOT CANAL WITH POST SUPPORT

A tooth with two or more roots usually requires more treatments to clean out and fill the pulp chamber and root canals than a single-rooted tooth. The drawing at left shows a decaying tooth with a double root. After root-canal preparation, center, a double-pronged post is sealed into the chamber (crown is above). At right is the completed restoration. The side of the tooth that shows when speaking or laughing is white; the chewing and inside surfaces are of gold. Extremely irregular, narrow, or curved canals may make root-canal therapy inadvisable.

Root-canal therapy is not cheap, and any subsequent work in the way of a crown, jacket, or other procedure must be added to the cost. But the cost of saving a tooth is usually less than the cost of replacing it. And although today's artificial teeth are skillfully made and fitted, they do not compare with natural teeth.

Knocked-out (avulsed) teeth. Root-canal treatment can even save a tooth that has been knocked completely out of the mouth, but quick action is necessary. Put the tooth into a glass of water to which a pinch of salt has been added. This simulates body fluids the teeth are accustomed to. Then rush the tooth in the fluid—and the patient—to the dentist.

The root of a tooth has a covering *(cementum)* that can aid in reattaching the root to the bone. The dentist will clean the socket and the tooth, and then put the tooth back in the socket the way it fit before the injury. Healing takes many weeks, and often the tooth will need support until it becomes firm and attaches itself to the bone. Support is given by wiring the tooth to adjacent teeth and applying a protective covering, usually a type of dental paste. The refitted tooth must then have the same absolute rest and quiet that a broken bone needs.

A dislodged or avulsed tooth will need root-canal treatment because of injury to the contents of the canal. The dentist will either wait until the tooth attaches itself, or do the root-canal treatment with the tooth in his hand, place it back in the socket, and wire it in place.

CAPS AND CROWNS

If you're over 40, fillings, caps and crowns, and perhaps some bridgework are probably a part of your life experience. We will therefore be brief in discussing the modern restoration of a chipped, discolored, worn-down, poorly shaped, badly decayed, or partially destroyed tooth to its natural appearance and function.

An artificial crown is commonly known as a cap or jacket. It is prepared and fitted over a defective tooth, but looks as lifelike, feels as comfortable, and functions as well as a healthy natural tooth.

Crowns are made of a variety of materials. *Porcelain-jacket crowns* are primarily used on the front teeth. They can hardly be distinguished from natural teeth. With today's dentistry, there is no reason for one to have unsightly or malformed front teeth. "Capping" gives the equivalent of a face-lift with renewed encouragement to smile. You can see the results of capping on almost any TV show that employs actors and actresses.

Crowns for the larger back teeth are made from cast gold, which has great strength, often combined with an acrylic veneer so that gold does not show on a visible part of the tooth. A *pivot or post crown* is used on a tooth that has had root-canal treatment.

Fitting a crown. To make a crown or cap requires two to four visits to a dentist. The tooth is prepared by shaping it so that the crown will fit over it flush. Then the patient bites down on plaster to produce an impression from which a model is made. Since it takes a little time to make the crown, a temporary crown is placed over the prepared tooth to protect it and keep it clean. When the completed crown is ready, it is adjusted for proper fit and cemented permanently in place. Food cannot get under it, and the patient cannot remove it.

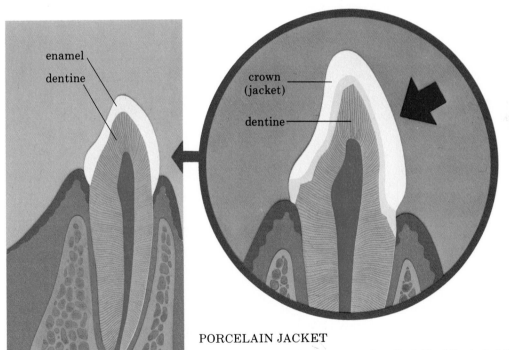

PORCELAIN JACKET

"Caps" (porcelain-jacket crowns) are used mainly on front teeth. Such a tooth may be normal (left drawing) but may have fillings and be misshapen, chipped, or discolored. A porcelain jacket can improve appearance and protect the tooth. At right, the tooth is ground down a bit for *flush fit of the jacket that is cemented over it (blue arrow). The capped tooth is sturdy and usually looks better than the original tooth in shape and alignment.*

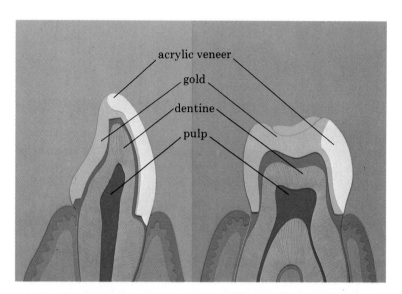

NATURAL APPEARANCE

The veneer side (outside surface) of a jacketed front tooth is white. The gold on the inside surfaces is soft enough to cushion stresses that could crack the veneer. At right, an artifical crown is fitted over a molar. Cast gold, used for strength and ductility, continues around the entire crown; veneer is fused to the outside surface for a natural appearance.

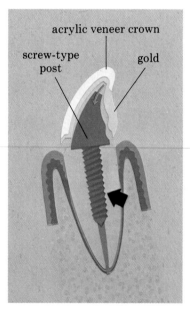

BROKEN-OFF TOOTH

Here is a restoration of a tooth broken off at the gum line. An artificial crown is cemented to a projecting screw-type post fitted into the prepared root-canal chamber. Or, several small screws may be used to secure the crown to an intact root.

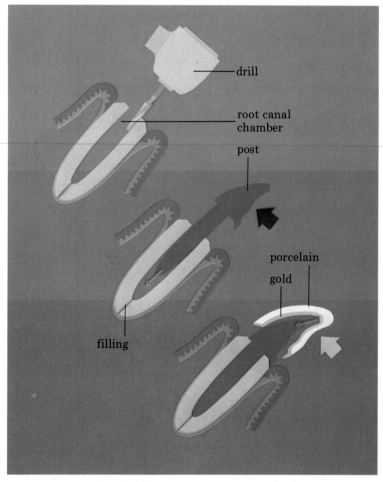

PIVOT OR POST CROWN

A pivot or post crown is fitted to a tooth that has had root-canal therapy. Burrs, files, and fine instruments are used to excavate, smooth, and enlarge the pulp chamber and canal after removal of the decayed top of the tooth (top drawing). A post is then fitted and sealed into the chamber (center). Below, a crown of gold with porcelain veneer is cemented over the post. Food debris cannot get under it and it can't work loose.

Old tales that caps and crowns harm the teeth are based on methods used more than 50 years ago. Today's dentistry is quite different. Caps are not placed on teeth unless they are clean and free of infection. Rather than harming teeth, they prolong their life. Crowns are strong enough to support bridgework, and once in place will give many years of service.

Considering the work involved, caps and crowns are not unreasonably expensive. However, the cost should be discussed before any work is started.

Broken-off teeth. A front tooth may be broken off even with the gum line as the result of an accident. Even if only the tooth root remains, a crown can be fitted to it. The root is prepared by the root-canal treatment previously described, and a metal post is then fitted into about half the length of the canal. The top of the post projects from the tooth above the gum line and a crown is prepared to fit over it. This is called a *dowel* or *pivot tooth.*

BRIDGES AND PARTIAL DENTURES

Nearly half of all adult dental patients need replacements for one or more missing teeth. A great many after-40 patients already have such replacements. Proper vanity spurs us to have a missing front tooth replaced immediately. But the gap of a missing back tooth is ordinarily not seen by others, and there is some inclination to temporize and put off doing anything about it. That, however, is a mistake.

With back teeth, replacement is more important to function than to appearance. Teeth may drift toward the space of a missing tooth and set the stage for future trouble. Chewing becomes distorted and inefficient when opposing surfaces meet empty space. And since digestion begins in the mouth, poorly masticated foods and excesses of soft and liquid foods can impair nutrition. To keep yourself and your mouth healthy, you must have 28 properly functioning teeth—all that nature originally provided, less wisdom teeth.

Sometimes a single tooth can be replaced by an implanted substitute, such as the pivot tooth described above. But by far the most common replacements are fixed bridges and partial dentures, which are artificial teeth inserted into the spaces from which natural teeth have been extracted. A removable bridge and a partial denture are the same thing.

Fixed bridge. Teeth on either side of the space must be reduced so that a crown will fit over them. Impressions are then taken, from which permanent supporting crowns of gold or stainless steel are made. The replacement teeth of a bridge are made of plastic or porcelain. The permanent crowns are soldered to the artificial teeth, and the completed bridge is cemented to the supporting teeth. It is immovable.

Advantages of fixed bridgework are: ease of cleaning, minimum adjustment and repair, immovability, strengthening of adjacent teeth, and natural feel and appearance. A disadvantage is that fixed bridgework, being precision work, is expensive. Also, a fixed bridge cannot span too large a space because there is a limit to the stress that can be placed on supporting teeth.

Partial denture. A removable bridge or partial denture is kept in place by support of the gums and attachment to sound adjacent teeth by means of metal clasps. The usual materials are metal—which may be gold, stainless steel, or a cobalt-chromium alloy—and plastic.

Clasps may be visible when a person talks, smiles, or laughs. However, they may be designed to hide most of their bulk. Precision attachments may reduce or eliminate the need for clasps or keep them out of sight, but such attachments require special preparation and are very expensive.

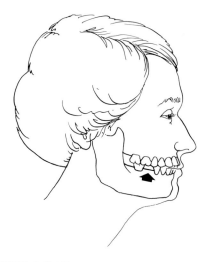

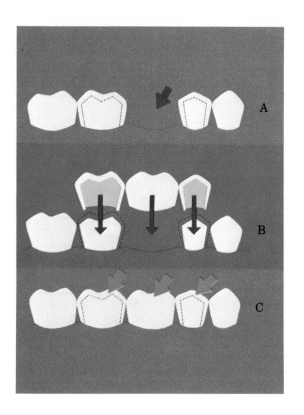

BRIDGING A GAP

A missing first molar leaves a gap at the gum line (arrow). Adjacent teeth will begin to drift, rotate, and tilt into the open space, and the upper molar above the gap will drift downward. Occlusion can be seriously distorted. At right, the purple arrow marks the gap of the missing tooth; the dotted lines indicate the surfaces of adjacent teeth to be cut away to accommodate a fixed bridge (A). At center, crowns with an artificial tooth between them (blue arrows) are ready for cementing to supporting teeth (B). The completed bridge in place is shown in drawing C.

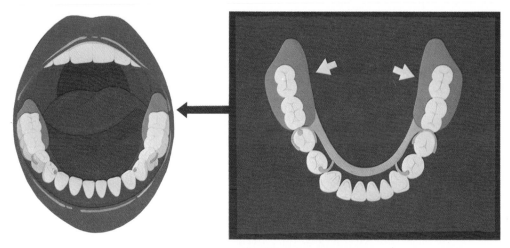

REMOVABLE BRIDGE

A partial denture, often called a removable bridge, is shown in place in a lower jaw. The denture is held in place by clasps that partially encircle sound teeth, and is supported by the gums. At right, artificial teeth attached to the denture replace missing first and second molars (white arrows). Dentures usually can be designed so that clasps are not conspicuously visible, depending on the position and condition of remaining natural teeth.

Adjacent teeth that support a partial denture need not be ground down; the clasps slip over healthy teeth. Other advantages are that the removable bridge is supported by gums as well as adjacent teeth, is less expensive, is easily cleaned, and can be repaired outside of the mouth. Additional teeth and clasps can be added if necessary.

Fixed and removable bridgework should receive careful cleaning. If it's not possible to do this after eating, at least rinse the mouth. Clasps tend to catch bits of food, and bridgework that is not taken out of the mouth for cleaning can give rise to offensive breath odor. Your dentist will advise periodic checkup for adjustment and repair. Bridges can be constructed so that they can be inserted immediately after tooth extraction.

Fixed or removable bridge? Should you be a candidate for bridgework, your dentist will help you consider factors that could affect the choice between a permanent and a removable type. Supporting teeth and gums must be healthy and clean. The number and size of spaces between teeth must be considered, along with the sturdiness of supporting teeth, because not every tooth can support a bridge. And supporting teeth may need fillings or other treatment that must be done before the bridgework is begun.

Your life-style may also affect the decision. Participation in contact sports or vigorous physical action suggests that a removable bridge is desirable since it can be taken out before contact. Repeated jarring and bodily contact will dislodge even the best fixed bridge, usually requiring extensive and expensive repair. However, musicians, singers, and public speakers may prefer fixed bridgework in the front of the mouth for good articulation or tongue-work on a reed instrument.

FULL DENTURES

It isn't age *per se* that brings a need for full-mouth artificial dentures, uppers and lowers. It's a mouth, and it can be a quite young mouth, that has reached such a state that there is no other alternative.

Psychic shock. Anyone who thinks that full dentures are a symbol of old age is mistaken. While most dentures are made for people over 40, thousands of younger persons wear them without the slightest feeling of senility.

Still, to be told that one needs dentures is to suffer a great psychological shock, especially if "middle-age crisis" has brought worries about one's work, prestige, future, or declining vigor, or if "menopause blues" have set a woman to brooding about waning attractiveness and advancing age. Dentures may seem like an affirmation that everything is going downhill.

Many people have a dread of dentures, based largely on things they have heard or observed. They may remember friends or relatives whose "plates" are kept mostly in a glass of water, whose facial and jaw lines have sagged and look old, whose speech is affected, or who complain of pain and an inability to chew foods they used to enjoy.

Poorly fitted dentures can indeed cause much trouble and dissatisfaction. But expertly fitted dentures made by a conscientious dentist (the specialist in this field is a *prosthodontist*) are quite another matter. They fit, function, and flatter, often looking better than the natural teeth. Once a patient adapts to dentures, they become a comfortable habit, like wearing glasses.

Do you really need dentures? Reasons why full dentures should be considered will be discussed by your dentist. Are there alternatives? Often there are. A key tooth or two may be saved by a crown or by root-canal therapy to support bridgework. Or periodontal treatment may give weak teeth better support. Bridges and partial dentures may support and restore function without the need to extract all of the teeth, so you should keep your natural teeth as long as you can.

It is cheaper, often very much cheaper, to extract all the teeth and replace them with dentures than to do extensive rehabilitative work. But be wary if extraction is the first and only recommendation. All dentures require an initial period of adaptation, and for physical or psychological reasons, some people cannot wear dentures at all. They have many sets in a drawer at home and have generally given up hope of wearing them comfortably. For such persons, there are newer techniques of implanting dentures in the bone with metallic screws and inserts.

Full dentures are necessary only when the natural teeth and gums are beyond rational treatment.

Materials. Dentures are as individual to you as your fingerprints. Modern materials allow a great variety of choices, and your dentist will respect your preferences, even for a false tooth with a crack or stain in it, if you confide in him.

The denture base is made from pink acrylic, virtually indistinguishable from natural healthy gum tissue, and the teeth are porcelain or plastic. Porcelain teeth tend to click if the denture is a little loose. Plastic teeth wear down a bit during chewing so that small defects are worked out, but they discolor more readily.

Perfectly regular, dazzlingly white teeth almost shout "dentures!", hence you can choose replacements from almost unlimited shades of color. Ordinarily, the colors will be those of the natural teeth that are being replaced. Natural teeth tend to become a bit yellow with age, and to acquire stains, cracks, chips, fissures, and other distinguishing marks. You can reproduce these in your dentures if you choose to and are willing to pay for it, so that when you start to wear them, hardly anybody will notice a difference. However, a "defective" artificial tooth is much more expensive than a perfect one.

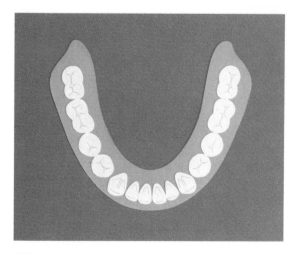

FULL DENTURE

This full artifical denture has a pink acrylic base that looks like healthy gum tissue. Selections of tooth color, size, and shape are harmonious with the structures of the mouth, and do not distort face or lip muscles.

Care is taken to assure that the color of your artificial teeth will harmonize with the color of your skin and hair. The size of your upper and lower jaws, the size of your lips, and the length of your teeth are also evaluated to ensure that the dentures will not distort facial and jaw lines. The shape of your face—square, oval, or tapered—is also considered, since it is generally related to the shape of your teeth.

It is essential that dentures give proper support to the face and lip muscles. Poorly fitted dentures do not give this support, and as a result, the face looks much older and its whole expression changes. The upper lip becomes thin and straight; the chin moves forward and seems to be trying to touch the nose; and age lines appear between the nose and upper lip. A badly fitted denture need not always be replaced, however; many times, only a relining of the base part of the denture is necessary.

Immediate dentures. In the past, patients had to go toothless for many weeks while their gums healed after extraction. Their speech was affected, and their diet was limited to baby foods, mush, and liquids. During the healing period, their facial muscles caved in and their faces aged.

This situation is a thing of the past. Today, with careful preoperative planning, you can wear new dentures as soon as the last tooth is extracted. Impressions are taken and dentures are made before the teeth are removed.

There are many advantages to immediate dentures. The gums heal more rapidly and more comfortably; adjustment is usually quicker and easier than if the patient went without teeth for a time; and appearance, of course, is better, as are speech and eating. However, immediate dentures need to be relined sooner than other dentures since gum tissues shrink after extractions.

Careful evaluations must be made before immediate dentures are recommended. Multiple extractions at one time may be too stressful for some people to stand. In that case, the back teeth will be extracted first and the gums allowed to heal before extracting the remaining teeth and inserting the immediate denture.

Adjustment to dentures. New dentures require a period of adjustment or "breaking in." At first they may rub or irritate the gums, but these sore spots will be corrected by the dentist in postoperative visits. Some persons have gums that are tender and bone that projects, making it difficult to wear dentures. This can be corrected by trimming the bone and smoothing out the ridges, a minor office procedure.

Psychological problems also may be disturbing—self-consciousness, feelings that the face is "different," that everybody is staring at your new teeth, or that dentures have not dramatically improved one's occupational and social life. It may help to discuss such feelings with your dentist.

When you first start to wear new dentures, there are certain steps you should take to attain comfort and satisfaction. This is true whether you have worn dentures before or are adjusting to a new set. The muscles of your lips, cheeks, and tongue must get used to the new shape and bulk of dentures. The tongue and teeth interact in speech, an extraordinarily complex achievement, and the strange feel of dentures may cause some slurring. The best way to learn to speak clearly and distinctly is to read aloud. Pronounce each word clearly and your speech should improve rapidly and present no problem.

Usually it is easier to adjust to an upper than a lower denture. The reason is that the upper denture covers the entire roof of the mouth and has a greater area to adhere to by suction. Lower dentures are smaller and have less surface area because they must leave room for the tongue. The tongue is in almost continuous motion, which tends to dislodge the "floating denture," as old-timers called it. While you may not get the same suction in both dentures, in time they can be well controlled, if necessary with the aid of the dentist to improve the "grip."

Eating is the most common difficulty for new denture wearers. This can be managed by beginning with soft foods and working up to a regular diet. During the first few days, select foods that need little chewing—cereals, soft-boiled eggs, soups, beverages, stewed fruits, custards, and most desserts. Chewing will be easier if you take small bites, dividing each bite of food.

One of the most effective tricks in eating with dentures is to divide each mouthful of food into two equal parts. Put one half on one side of the mouth, the other half on the other side, and chew. This equalizes pressure, makes eating easier, and helps to keep dentures from rocking or slipping.

As your gums harden and you become more accustomed to your dentures, you can increase the pressure of your biting, but be cautious. Biting too hard can cause sore gums and harm the tissues on which dentures rest. Chew slowly, without trying to keep up with the rest of the diners until you can match their speed comfortably.

Dentures do not change, but your mouth tissues do; the gums are subject to continuing normal change and shrinkage. If dentures seem to move and slip and do not fit as properly as they used to, see your dentist for minor corrections to restore their original comfort.

Many people believe that with full dentures their tooth problems are gone for good and they have no further need of a dentist. Good-fitting dentures will last for years, but the tissues of the mouth should be examined at least once a year. As you grow older, the gum tissues shrink and change shape so that the dentures may lose some or quite a bit of their original fit. Continued irritation by poor-fitting dentures may cause harmful growths to occur, and is one of the possible causes of cancer of the mouth.

In general, new full or partial dentures can be worn day and night for two or three weeks. Thereafter, they can be removed at night and submerged in a container of water to prevent drying out. Dentures should be cleaned after every meal with soap and water or one of many denture cleaners, using a stiff brush. In addition to your own cleaning, your dentist will do a thorough cleaning at each visit and will examine them to be sure they are in good condition. A clean denture has no odor; if yours has, it isn't clean.

DENTAL IMPLANTS

The concept of an artificial tooth firmly implanted in the jaw is an appealing alternative if, for some reason, dentures or bridges are ruled out. Dental implants are not routine or widespread procedures as yet, but at times they can be the answer to rehabilitating a mouth, and there is substantial progress in the search for better materials and techniques.

Currently, the most common metal used for implants is a cobalt-chromium alloy. It is employed in what is called the *subperiosteal denture*. The periosteum is a fibrous membrane covering the bone surface. A metal frame is designed to fit snugly between the membrane and the bone. This reduces the volume of pink acrylic material used in a conventional denture. The procedure is especially useful for patients who are missing all or almost all of the teeth in one jaw.

Single tooth implants are less satisfactory. *Endosseous* (in the bone) methods are used today. One of these is a "blade vent" method in which a metallic blade is inserted into a prepared slot in the bone, leaving a small part projecting above the gum to which the tooth is attached. Vents or openings in the submerged blade encourage the growth of tissue and increase the stability of the implant.

In a mechanical sense, tooth implantation is not very complicated. A plug-like unit of metal or other material is inserted into the jawbone. This unit holds a steel post that is a base for the attachment of an artificial cap or crown. The surgery is fairly complicated, requires hospitalization, and risks other drawbacks. Bone may shrink away and undermine the metal supports, and some materials are not stable in the aqueous environment of the mouth.

Many materials are being experimented with in the hope of finding one or more that will be inert and permanently stable in tooth implants. Porous ceramic is used on the premise that surrounding fibrous tissue may grow into it. Vitreous carbon, epoxy resins, and metals coated with various materials also are being tried. Synthetic fibers are being studied, as well as the mineral hydroxyapatite, which is the main inorganic constituent of bones and teeth. Even barnacle secretions, which resemble the components of teeth, are being investigated as possible solutions.

The prospect for successful permanent inplantation seems promising, and future tooth banks for implants are not wholly visionary. Transplants of a person's own teeth from one area to another, transplants of donated teeth from another person, and even transplants of animal teeth have been attempted. But much work lies ahead before such transplants become widely accepted procedures.

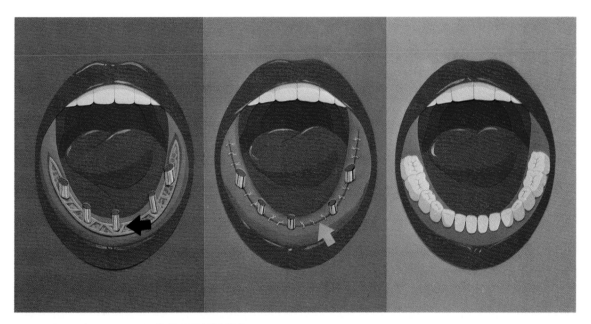

ONE TYPE OF IMPLANTED DENTURE

One method of anchoring a denture so that it won't wobble employs a metal frame fitted with protruding posts, implanted between the bone of the jaw (blue arrow) and a membrane that covers the bone. At center, gum flaps (yellow arrow) are sutured over the metal frame. At right, the denture is secured firmly by frame and posts. The procedure is not common, but in some instances where there is no other alternative, it can restore a mouth to comfort and efficiency.

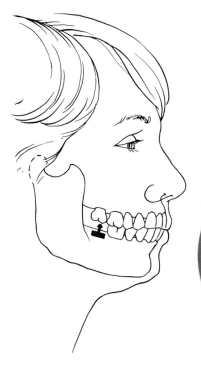

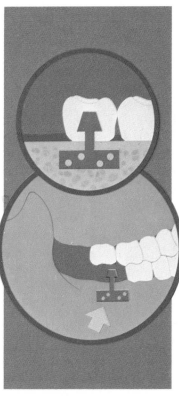

A SINGLE IMPLANT

Implantation of a single tooth is feasible, but should become more successful as researchers discover inert materials that are stable in the mouth and do not permit the surrounding bone to shrink. The drawings show the "blade vent" procedure, in which a metal blade with vents or openings in it is inserted in a slot in the bone (yellow arrows). The vents are intended to encourage fibrous tissue to grow around and anchor the blade. A metal part protrudes above the gum line for attachment of an artificial crown (top circle at left). This fairly complicated surgery is done in a hospital.

STRAIGHTENING
OLDER TEETH

Mention "orthodontia" and the picture that comes to mind is that of a school child or teen-ager with metal bands strung like railroad tracks along his or her teeth. Most orthodontia treatment is indeed done on young patients. But about 15 percent of patients are adults, and their numbers are increasing. Orthodontic treatment for adults is one of the most rapidly expanding areas of dental health services, although only a fraction of adults who have malocclusions severe enough to benefit from treatment have received care.

Malocclusion, a faulty or irregular arrangement of the teeth, develops gradually during childhood and is often made worse by adult dental disease. The result may be excessive space between teeth, protrusions ("buck teeth"), rotation of a tooth, or decay. Not all malocculsions are extreme. Slightly irregular teeth can be uniquely attractive and give a touch of distinction to a personality.

Many malocclusions, however, affect personality adversely. Men and women may suffer anxieties about personal attractiveness, job associations, and professional security; confidence and self-esteem may be badly shaken. Too frequently, adults feel that straightening crooked teeth in grownups is sheer vanity or "kid stuff," unworthy of professional attention. They do not seek treatment that could help them psychologically as well as medically.

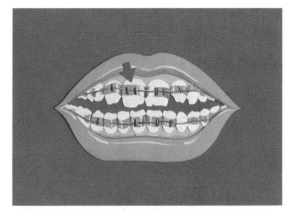

A RANGE OF DEVICES

The familiar "tooth braces" of school children are not always necessary in adult orthodontia. Brackets and fixed appliances may contain very little visible material. The devices exert gentle pressure that gradually nudges teeth into felicitous positions.

If you have a malocclusion that troubles you, the chances are that it can be corrected. Your dentist will tell you. The fact that you are no longer a child does not of itself rule out orthodontic treatment. Bones are pliable, and mouth structures allow the position of teeth to be changed, within reasonable limits, regardless of age.

Improved appearance is no doubt the greatest motivation for having orthodontic treatment. But there are other benefits. Treatment may very well help to prevent periodontal disease, which is characteristic of middle life.

How long, how much? Many family dentists have been trained to treat and diagnose orthodontic problems. Your dentist may refer you to a specialist, an *orthodontist.* In contrast to the past, an orthodontist is within easy traveling distance in most communities today, a factor to be considered since you will pay him many visits.

How long will it take to straighten your teeth? How much will it cost? It is important to clear up such matters in advance, since the answers are highly variable, depending on the condition of your mouth and the customary charges in your locality. Most health insurance does not cover the cost of orthodontia, and you will have to stand the expense yourself.

Initially, the dentist will take X rays and plastic casts of your upper and lower jaws as well as precise measurements of your head and jaws. The space a tooth occupies is changed by moving a tooth, and the new space has to be filled gradually by regeneration of tissue. Obviously it takes longer to change an entire bite than to move a tooth or two. The dentist will want to be sure that you have a positive attitude about what he proposes to do and that you will not be continually morbid and resentful of the procedures.

Many orthodontic problems of adults are relatively minor, such as closing a gap between teeth or straightening a crooked tooth. This takes up to six months and costs in the neighborhood of $500 to $750. Major problems that require the movement of many teeth in both jaws and the extraction of several teeth to eliminate overcrowding take two years or even more to complete and cost at least $1,500, usually on a pay-as-you-go basis. If standard orthodontic treatment is too slow and the patient is suitable, techniques of oral surgery may get results more quickly or serve if conventional treatment is impracticable.

One reason why orthodontic care seems expensive is that most adults who need it also require extensive gum treatment, tooth restoration, or replacement—expensive services in themselves. Because moving the teeth is the most dramatic aspect, many people attribute the entire cost to orthodontic treatment alone.

"BAD BITES"

Age, within reason, cannot wither the prospects of successful tooth-straightening in adults. In the large circle, normal occlusion (contact of chewing surfaces of upper and lower teeth) is shown. Common malocclusions are: overbite ("buck teeth," yellow arrow); crooked teeth; overlaps; excessive space between teeth; and misalignment. Timely orthodontia may help to prevent worsening of periodontal disease.

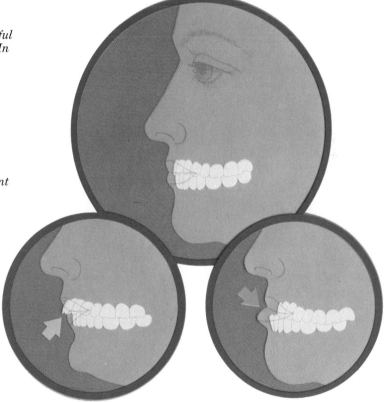

Many adults are deterred from orthodontic treatment by their unwillingness to wear conspicuous "bands" on their teeth. Bands and other devices exert gentle pressure on teeth to move them gradually to desired positions. Metal bands may sometimes be necessary, but often they are not. New materials and devices offer procedural choices. A removable retainer that is virtually invisible may serve the purpose. Brackets and fixed appliances are made of plastics that greatly reduce the amount of visible material. When tooth repositioning is completed, invisible *retainers* are worn to support the teeth while they become secure in their new position. After a while, the retainers are worn only at night, and eventually are dispensed with entirely.

ORAL SURGERY

You might someday be referred to an oral surgeon for treatment of a condition that could require hospitalization and is more complicated than the routine procedures of dentistry. An oral surgeon is trained to diagnose and treat all diseases, injuries, and defects of the oral cavity and related tissues. He is a graduate dentist with an additional three years of study with extensive hospital training, and is on the staff of one or more hospitals to serve patients who need treatment outside the office.

Most general dentists handle all routine dental procedures, including minor oral surgery. Lengthy and complex procedures are usually referred to an oral surgeon.

Extractions. Difficult extractions and impacted teeth are usually handled by an oral surgeon (a specialist in extraction is called an *exodontist)*.

The patient's medical history may require consultation with the family physician before an extraction is undertaken. Conditions such as pregnancy, excessive bleeding, high blood pressure, diabetes, kidney ailments, prior history of rheumatic fever, valvular heart disease, and others may affect the course and outcome of tooth extractions. Antibiotics and appropriate medications may be prescribed before extraction, or it may be desirable to delay the procedure until the patient's medical condition is under better control.

Before an oral surgeon removes a tooth, he takes X rays to establish the exact position of the tooth and its roots and the condition of the tooth and surrounding structures. This gives him a complete picture of the problem so he can accurately plan the procedure and know the kind and extent of any possible complications. He gives a general or local anesthetic. A general anesthetic—usually a "shot in the arm" into a vein—will put you into a pleasant sleep and you will feel nothing. If a local anesthetic is used, the area will be numb and you will not feel pain, only slight pressure when the tooth is removed. He may give a whiff of "laughing gas" (nitrous oxide), which puts you into a brief sleep from which you awaken with a giggly feeling that soon passes.

Teeth are removed by application of gentle pressure in definite directions, calculated according to the underlying positions of parts. The bone is not damaged, and the soft tissue is handled with great gentleness. An instrument called an *elevator* is used first to separate the gum attachment from the tooth and to loosen it. Elevators may be used to raise the tooth completely out of its socket if it is at all loose. Or if it is more firmly attached to the socket, forceps are used to grip the tooth firmly and lift it out.

Aftercare. Tiny blood vessels severed by the extraction cause some bleeding that lasts only a few minutes while a blood clot forms in the socket. The clot is nature's way of protecting the exposed socket by sealing it off from food, germs, and saliva.

If the clot does not form properly or is dislodged, a painful condition known as *dry socket* develops. The bare, unprotected socket is exposed to irritants and becomes inflamed. Not much can be done except to use pain-relieving medications and antibiotics, if prescribed, and to keep the area clean. Pain gradually disappears after several days as the area heals.

Proper aftercare helps to prevent disturbance of the blood clot. You will be advised not to chew in the area of extraction and to follow a soft diet—soft-boiled eggs, soups, custards, and ground meats—for a day or two. Over-vigorous rinsing of the mouth should be postponed to the day after extraction, and the socket with its clot should not be explored by the tongue.

Some swelling may occur after tooth extraction and is usually nothing to worry about. Ice packs or cloths soaked with cold water can be applied to the face over the affected region to help keep pain and swelling to a minimum.

Although most extractions are short minor surgical procedures, complications do occur. A root may fracture, a crown may break, or a nerve may be injured. These are quickly corrected so that no permanent damage is done.

Wisdom teeth. If you are over 40 and still have all or some of your wisdom teeth, the probability that they will cause some trouble in the future is quite high. Wisdom teeth (technically, third molars) get their name from the fact that they erupt between 17 and 21 years of age, a time when wisdom is supposed to descend upon us—a debatable assumption that nevertheless persists in popular terminology.

Wisdom teeth come in after all the others and usurp whatever space is left. It is likely to be crowded space. No doubt wisdom teeth were highly serviceable to our prognathous ancestors, but the jaws of modern man and woman—at least most of them—are too small to accommodate useful third molars. For the most part, wisdom teeth are potential troublemakers of little functional value.

If there is not enough space for a wisdom tooth that tries to erupt, it may come in out of alignment. It may be *impacted,* embedded so it cannot erupt in normal position. The tooth may erupt only partially, it may be embedded in the gum, or it may be completely embedded in bone.

Erupted wisdom teeth are difficult to reach for proper cleaning and thus are more likely to decay. An angulated wisdom tooth may press harmfully upon an adjacent tooth. And sometimes a wisdom tooth is so inaccessible that the dentist cannot reach it to insert a filling or to do root-canal therapy. Is such a tooth worth saving? Probably not.

If an impacted tooth gives no difficulty, it can simply be left alone. However it should be checked and X-rayed frequently for intimations of trouble, of which the usual warnings are pain, swelling, infection, or maybe all three.

A troublesome wisdom tooth should be removed. This takes longer than an ordinary extraction, but is usually done in the dentist's office under local anesthesia. We have four wisdom teeth to begin with, two each in the upper and lower jaws. It is not uncommon for two wisdom teeth to be extracted at the same time in the office, but simultaneous extraction of all four wisdom teeth usually is done in a hospital under general anesthesia. It may be that the patient requires or prefers hospitalization for extraction of just one or two teeth. This decision may be affected by the fact that most health insurance covers hospital services but not office extractions.

Abscessed teeth may result in serious mouth and jaw infections. An abscessed tooth that may have caused no pain, but in which the pulp has died, is sometimes discovered by X-ray examination. Infection may spread to other parts of the face and even to the neck and brain, resulting in serious illness. Infections disseminated from abscessed teeth require care beyond that of the family dentist. Patients are usually referred to an oral surgeon who consults with the family physician prior to and during the course of therapy.

Lacerations and disfigurements. Fractures, cuts, and dislocations of the face and jawbone are usually due to contact sports, brawls, home accidents, falls, and motor mishaps. Elderly and chronically ill persons are quite prone to falls. Correction requires that involved bones and teeth be splinted and wired by an oral surgeon, usually in a hospital.

Not all facial disharmonies are accidental. A lower jaw may recede or protrude excessively; the upper jaw may overhang too much; or a bad bite may cause distor-

ABSCESS

The usual cause of abscess and infection is a deep cavity of the tooth that often, but not always, gives a warning signal of pain.

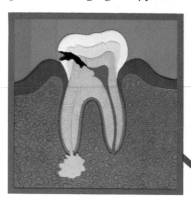

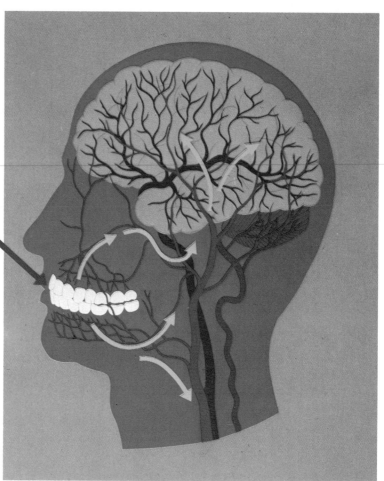

PATHWAYS OF INFECTION

Pathways by which infection originating in an abscessed tooth can spread to parts of the mouth and jaw and to other parts of the head, brain, and neck are shown by yellow arrows. An abscess unsuspected by the patient may be disclosed by routine X-ray examination. Dead and infected pulp tissue in the root canal may cause resorption around the end of the root, which shows as a dark shadow in an X ray. Severe infections require care by an oral surgeon and a physician.

tions, of which the patient is embarrassed and self-conscious. Great cosmetic improvement is attainable, but one should be reconciled to treatments—bone lengthening or shortening, grafting, bite reconstruction, and wiring and splinting—that can be quite long and expensive, depending on circumstances.

Facial rehabilitation may require the combined efforts of a team of professional specialists to get the most satisfactory results. The team may consist of a family dentist and physician, an oral surgeon, orthodontist, plastic surgeon, and others if needed. Unless an accident is involved, the cost must be borne by the patient, since the primary objective is improved appearance.

Denture comfort. Many persons with dentures that click and slip despair of ever wearing them comfortably and consign them to a bureau drawer. Before giving up, however, confide in your dentist who may refer you to an oral surgeon for what is called a *ridge extension*. This is a minor office procedure that is soon completed, after which the patient can wear the dentures immediately. The gums are cut along the outer and inner edge of the denture and are moved back to extend the ridge, which is the area covered by the denture. This gives more surface for the denture to adhere to.

Tumors, cysts, ulcers, blisters, sores, and cracks can occur on the lips or in the mouth and jaws. "Ordinary" ulcers, sores, cracked lips, and blister-like lesions can be treated by the family dentist. He also examines the mouth for suspicious lesions that may become cancerous or already are, and refers the patient to an oral surgeon if he discovers any (see page 183).

CANCER OF THE MOUTH

The percentage of mouth cancer is small compared to cancers of the lung, reproductive system, stomach, and intestines. But when it occurs, it is extremely dangerous, miserable, and disfiguring.

It is well known that a clean, well-cared-for mouth rarely develops cancer. However, certain predisposing factors are known or suspected: chronic irritation of the tongue, lips, and cheeks by ill-fitting dentures, crowns, or bridges; broken teeth and rough or jagged fillings; and smoking or chewing tobacco. Most of these factors are preventable or correctable by timely dental care. Nutritional deficiencies and some diseases (syphilis, scurvy, and leukemia) also affect the mouth and make it more susceptible to cancer.

Ninety percent of oral cancer occurs after 40, and the peak age of diagnosis is 60 years.

Diagnosis. Mouth cancers in their early stages do not often cause pain. Even in advanced stages, they may cause no pain, swelling, or bleeding to warn the patient. A sore in the mouth that does not heal in a reasonably short time calls for examination by a dentist or physician. Regular visits to a dentist give the best chance of early detection, and the probability of complete cure is high if lesions are discovered early.

A condition generally regarded as precancerous is the appearance of white patches in the mouth, possibly *leukoplakia,* although there are many types of white patches. Local treatment and total cessation of smoking may very well reduce the patches. This condition may be quite harmless, but not necessarily so. Indeed, "white" may be a lesser index of mouth cancer than "red." Researchers at the Veterans Administration found, in a twelve-year study, that most early mouth cancers first appeared as red lesions with white specklings. The next most frequent type was red with no white areas. Very few were classified as all white. They also found that the areas most susceptible to cancer were the floor of the mouth, the sides or underside of the tongue, and the soft palate.

DETECTION OF VISIBLE MOUTH LESIONS

Inspection of oral tissues by a dentist to detect possible lesions is an important part of dental care. Self-inspection of the mouth also may disclose abnormalities that should be brought to a dentist's attention (inspect the cheeks, under the tongue, the palate, gums, and side of the tongue). At left, a papilloma (green arrow), usually a benign growth but one that tends to recur unless completely eradicated. At right, a tumor of the gum.

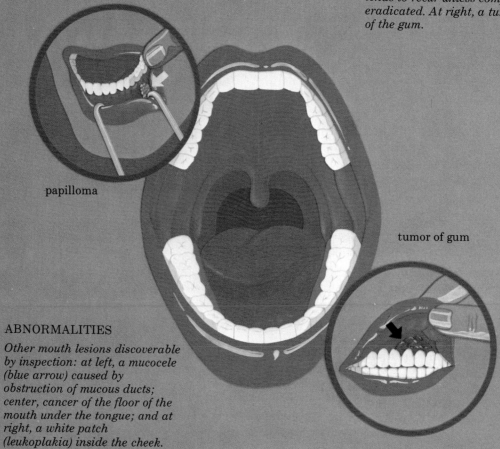

papilloma

tumor of gum

ABNORMALITIES

Other mouth lesions discoverable by inspection: at left, a mucocele (blue arrow) caused by obstruction of mucous ducts; center, cancer of the floor of the mouth under the tongue; and at right, a white patch (leukoplakia) inside the cheek.

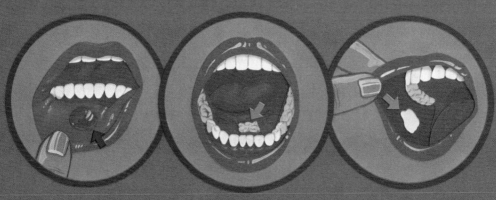

mucocele   cancer   leukoplakia

An oral surgeon can tell if a growth is harmless (benign) or cancerous (malignant) by incising a bit of tissue and sending it to a pathology laboratory where a specialist examines thin slices of the tissue under a microscope and reports his findings. Cancer cells have characteristics that give a positive diagnosis. If the cells are normal, there is nothing to worry about.

Treatment. At present, the only curative treatment of mouth cancer is surgery and radiation, separately or in combination. Drugs may relieve symptoms and reduce pain, thus making the patient comfortable, but they do not cure the cancer.

Surgery may be quite extensive. It may be necessary to remove a major portion of the tongue, lips, or jaw, resulting in rather massive disfigurement and difficulties in eating and swallowing. In many cases, the disfigurement can be reduced by fitting the patient with an artificial jaw or an artificial roof of the mouth. Artificial teeth also can be added to replace those removed by the surgeon.

Radiation therapy is often used to halt the growth or reduce the size of the tumor, but it also damages normal tissue. Treatment of oral cancer is drastic, but an untreated cancer of the mouth cannot be tolerated for long. It becomes extremely painful and interferes seriously with vital functions.

PAIN IN THE JAW

Headaches and toothaches are the most common symptoms for which people consult their doctors. The multifarious causes of headaches—upward of a hundred are listed in medical books—are beyond the scope of this chapter. There is one kind of headache, however, that is often undiagnosed, untreated, or mistreated by one therapy after another, while the underlying source of trouble goes unnoticed.

The headache in question is a dull ache or stabbing pain that is linked to a malady in the mouth. It can feel like a headache, toothache, migraine, sinus infection, or earache, and can even travel through the neck and shoulders. The source of trouble is

a malfunctioning jaw joint—the *tempero-mandibular joint,* or TMJ—which connects the jaw to the head. It is the most complex joint in the body and is acted upon by great forces, as you can feel if you press your fingers, while chewing, upon powerful muscles above the curve of the jawbone in front of the ear.

A principal cause of the TMJ syndrome is tension, often expressed by clenching or grinding of the teeth, especially at night. The patient may not at all be aware of this. Many TMJ problems originate with a bad bite that throws the jaw joints out of harmonious position. Fatigue, emotional tension, and bad bite can give rise to spasms of the jaw muscles, as can poorly fitted dental devices, or even a long session in a dentist's chair. In extreme cases, cartilage at the ends of the jawbone joints may become deformed or eroded.

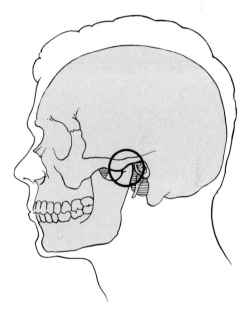

JAW JOINT

The tempero-mandibular joint (circle), which connects the lower jaw to the head, is subject to powerful pressures that sometimes cause pain of mysterious origin in the head, neck, jaw, and shoulders. Tensions are frequently an underlying factor.

Symptoms of TMJ trouble are not very specific, which is why some persons with very real pains in the head, ear, jaws, neck, and shoulders go through many tests and procedures in efforts to get at the root of the problem. The mouth is not ordinarily thought of as a primary source of mysterious pains. If you have such pain, you might suspect that you have TMJ trouble, and ask your dentist about it, especially if you answer "yes" to the following questions:

- Does the pain ease when you open your mouth?
- Is it worse when chewing?
- Are your jaws clenched in the morning when you wake up?
- Do you grind your teeth or clench your jaws when you are upset or concentrating hard?

Treatment. Probably the most important measure is to help the patient to ease tensions—more easily said than done. Tooth-grinding habits may be modified if brought to the attention of a patient who is not aware of them. Or, correcting a bad bite can bring jaw joints into comfortable alignment. Medications and injections into "trigger points" of the jaw muscles also may give relief. In some cases, what is called a *bite plate* may be fitted. This is a removable appliance, fitted to the upper jaw, that keeps the upper and lower teeth slightly separated, thus relieving pressure and muscle spasm so that after some months, the joint functions normally. Surgery is not necessary unless the joint has been severely damaged.

There are other causes of pain in the jaw region—sinus infections, tumors, and teeth themselves. But correct diagnosis and treatment can relieve many patients of distressing jaw pain.

TODAY AND TOMORROW

Fear keeps more people away from dentists than lack of money. Almost everybody over 40 has some memory of dental terror in youth—a drill vibrating and grinding into a tooth, getting red hot; shivering with pain while gripping the arms of the dental chair in agony; the unrelenting jaws of a monstrous forceps; or the ominous medicated scent of a dentist's office. It is truly unfortunate if phantasms of the past deter one from accepting professional services that are vital to personal health, not to mention the joys of eating.

Matters are quite different today. Modern equipment and materials have made a tremendous difference in the practice and sufferance of dentistry. The red-hot drill of yesterday has been superseded by cutting instruments that rotate at ultra-high speeds and virtually eliminate sensations of pressure, heat, and vibration. Heat is generated but is dissipated by a spray of water and air that keeps the area comfortable. The cutting process is rapid, not only because of the speed of the rotating burr, but because its cutting edges stay sharp and do not soon become dulled.

New filling materials are quite remarkable as well. Today there is a whole new family of composite resins containing adhesive materials that often eliminate the need for drilling a tooth. For example, if you break or chip a tooth, it may be restored simply by applying these adhesive fillings and without the need to grind down the tooth for a crown. New insulating materials are used under a deep filling to prevent excessive sensitivity to heat and cold. Acrylic resins of lifelike appearance have replaced the old rubber and vulcanite materials once used for the gum replacement parts of dentures.

Painless injections are achieved with sharp disposable needles that slowly inject a prewarmed solution after a topical anesthetic has been applied. Pressure guns, like those used for vaccinations, are also used for injections. Some practitioners even employ hypnosis to control gagging, nausea, or habitual grinding of the teeth *(bruxism)*.

Electrosurgery used in taking biopsies or removing gum tissue, as in the treatment of periodontal disease, is bloodless; the current seals the vessel ends. Ultrasonic equipment is used to remove tartar and make prophylaxis a quick and painless procedure. If a patient is very nervous and fearful, the dentist may administer nitrous oxide (laughing gas) to wipe out apprehension and any memory of the procedures.

The future. An effective way to prevent tooth decay would be to seal the teeth with a substance that would make them permanently impervious to invasion. Sealants presently used are a valuable part of preventive dentistry, but they can be chipped and cannot be regarded as permanent. Transparent sealants to keep plaques (see page 186) out of the pits and fissures of tooth enamel are under development and have made encouraging progress. These new materials form an actual bond with the enamel and thus provide a permanent seal.

Ultrasound techniques also may find new applications. A pulse of high-frequency sound can be sent into a tooth, especially the root canal, to return a signal that indicates that the sound has encountered a change in texture. Ultrasound is now used for cleaning dental instruments, but its use in patients is limited because of possible injury to the sensitive cochlea of the ear.

Computers are useful in almost all fields of endeavor nowadays, and dentistry is no exception. They are now being used in the differential diagnosis of oral pathology. With the aid of a computer, a dentist may soon be able to judge whether a child should have unerupted wisdom teeth removed in early childhood to prevent impaction problems in adult life.

Bone resorption is a factor in periodontal disease and in osteoporosis. Studies are in progress to determine if electric currents can be used to stimulate the restoration of diseased or injured bone as well as of aging bone, not only with respect to periodontal disease, but with repair mechanisms of older bone. A class of compounds called *thiopene derivatives* seems potentially useful in controlling bone resorption.

Scientists of more than 40 disciplines are now engaged in far-flung dental research. They seek knowledge of how bones and dental tissues grow, develop, self-repair, function, and react to nutrition and environment, to the end that constructive processes may further the advance of general as well as dental health.

Indeed, the modern dentist is not concerned with the teeth and mouth alone. He is frequently the first to see and recognize the early symptoms of systemic diseases. Enlarged gum tissue in a patient with sound teeth may indicate leukemia. Red, swollen gums alert the dentist to the possibility of diabetes. Signs of jaundice and gastric ulcers also may be seen in the mouth. And ulcers, dry mouth, and burning tongue may indicate vitamin deficiencies.

Hormone abnormalities, too, are commonly reflected in the teeth. If an X ray shows certain bone changes in the jaw or skull, the dentist may suspect anemia. Congenital syphilis is marked by notched, narrow-edged teeth *(Hutchinson teeth),* and gonorrhea may be suspected from mouth ulcers and an inflamed pharynx. Future research may prove a relationship between oral infections and tonsillitis, middle ear infection, some types of kidney infections, as well as infection of the lining of the heart, ulcers, and inflammation of the gallbladder.

Indeed, we have come a long way from the frontier dentist with a pair of pliers who could only tell his patient, "Hold still and take it!"

ROUTINE SELF-CARE OF THE TEETH AND MOUTH

Plaque is a destructive enemy of the teeth and their supports. Plaque (technically, *bacterial plaque)* is an invisible thin film attached to the surface of a tooth. It forms from oral debris and bacteria that are always present in the mouth. Sticky masses of bacteria and their waste products form a film that at first is soft, but soon hardens. Tooth decay is produced largely by the action of bacteria on starches and sugars, with production of acids that attack the tooth enamel. Bacterial action in plaque on the teeth and gums is thought to be a predominant factor in periodontal disease.

Newly formed plaque is soft for a day or two and can be removed by toothbrushing and the self-care measures described below. But if oral hygiene is neglected, plaque soon becomes hardened and cannot be removed by brushing. *Tartar* at the base of the teeth and under the gums is an accumulation of plaque that has become mineralized and stony hard. At this point, it can be removed only by a dentist.

Toothbrushing is hopefully a habit you have established and pursue effectively, but a suggestion or two may be tolerated. If you wear dentures, remove them before brushing. Choose a toothbrush that you can maneuver around the mouth and teeth, even baby-size if necessary. Four rows of medium-firm bristles are enough. Tooth powder has greater cleaning action than toothpaste, as the glycerin in toothpaste decreases its cleaning power. A good practice is to brush with powder in the morning and evening and after meals. Before social activities, use toothpaste.

Brushing need not be long and drawn-out. People brush "up and down" and "side to side"; it will not hurt to use both methods. Move the brush in gentle, circular motions across the teeth and gums, making sure that you cover all tooth surfaces. When you move the brush up and down, you should emphasize brushing toward the biting edge of the teeth.

Tongue-cleaning. Get in the habit of brushing your tongue every morning and evening. Brush it from front to back and side to side until there is no coating on the tongue and its surface is pink. This coating, usually a shade of brown to black, is produced by food particles and bacteria trapped on the rough surface of the tongue. This is one of the chief causes of bad breath and bad taste in the mouth. If you gag when brushing your tongue with a toothbrush, try wiping it clean with a wet washcloth wrapped around a finger.

Flossing. Even the most conscientious brushing leaves much cleaning to be done between the teeth, where gums and tooth contours shelter bacteria, plaque, and food particles. These surfaces must be cleaned with dental floss or tape. Flossing is especially important for persons who have periodontal disease or wish to prevent it, and for reducing susceptibility to tooth decay.

Waxed or unwaxed types of floss or tape are equally good, and there are extra fine varieties for persons whose teeth are very close together. Tear off four or five inches of floss and wrap the ends around the index fingers of each hand, leaving an inch or less of floss between the fingers. Slide the floss gently between the teeth (not so hard as to actually cut the gums). Pass the floss back and forth along the tooth surface, slightly below the gum line but not far enough to do damage. Then move the floss across the gum to the opposite tooth surface, sliding it firmly up this surface with a saw-type motion. Repeat several times at each contact area. Flossing should be done daily, or at least every couple of days, to remove plaque that is temporarily soft.

Electric toothbrushes are effective, but should be used with caution. If used too forcefully, they tend to erode gum line fillings and injure gum tissue. An electric toothbrush can be of considerable value for anyone with limited motion of the arms and fingers, since it can be manipulated easily and can reach all areas of the mouth.

Irrigating devices employ a continuous jet or pulsating stream of water, propelled by a small motor or by tap pressure. Their main virtue is to loosen debris between the teeth and wash it away, as well as to stimulate blood flow in tiny capillaries that feed the gum tissue, which improves the general condition of the gums. This "liquid massage" is especially beneficial to persons who have periodontal problems.

Some practice is required to use a motor-driven irrigation device while keeping the "exhaust" within bounds. Ask your dentist to demonstrate how the device works so it will not spray all over the wash basin and clothing. As with an electric toothbrush, if the stream of water and manual pressure are too strong, an irrigator may loosen fillings and even injure the gums. Irrigators are intended to be used in addition to toothbrushing, not as a substitute.

Mouthwashes in a great variety of colors and flavors supply an oral rinse and leave the mouth with a pleasant, refreshing taste. Much the same effect can be accomplished by a homemade wash consisting of a teaspoonful each of salt, soda, and vinegar in a glass of warm water.

Gum massage. Gentle massage between the teeth with a soft rubber cone, attached to a toothbrush or separate handle, helps to stimulate blood circulation in the area. Similar gentle massage can be attained by rocking a soft-bristle toothbrush slowly back and forth at the gum line. This helps to cleanse possible pockets under the gums and to stimulate circulation.

Care of dentures. It is desirable to clean removable dentures after each meal or, if that is not possible, to rinse the mouth. Partial dentures with clasps are particularly likely to collect food particles and debris; they should be taken out and cleansed with a stiff toothbrush. Any of the many commercial denture cleansers will do, as will ordinary soap and water. Dentures may be removed at night and placed in a glass of water or cleanser to prevent their drying out. Even if you wear full dentures, see your dentist at least once a year. Tissues of the mouth change with age, and dentures may benefit from some changes, too.

CHAPTER 7   E. CLINTON TEXTER, M.D.

THE PLEASURES & PAINS OF DIGESTION

> "Some people have a foolish way of not minding, or of pretending not to mind, what they eat. For my part, I look upon my belly very studiously and very carefully, for I look upon it that he who does not mind his belly will hardly mind anything else."
>
> —Samuel Johnson

In this chapter we shall heed Samuel Johnson's admonition to look upon the belly very studiously, and will extend the term "belly" to include the entire gastrointestinal (GI) tract.

More than most systems of the body, digestive processes are infested with euphemisms for politely mentioning unmentionable manifestations of absorption and excretion. "Stomach" is a common synonym for "belly," although their aches are well apart. The terms "bowel" and "intestine" are used if absolutely necessary, but the more forthright "gut" is forbidden — unless someone has a "gut reaction" to an idea, gauged by how the belly feels about it.

It sometimes seems that the digestive system is regarded as a vulgarity imposed shamelessly by nature, which ought to have invented a process of greater seemliness and propriety. But this does scant justice to a quite marvelous tract that ultimately makes it possible for us to play tennis, write a letter, and even to think, by making energy and materials available from the foods we eat.

It is doubtless true that a healthy gut thrives on being ignored, but disorders of the tract are disproportionately frequent in the after-40 age group. Two recent conferences on digestive disease as a national health problem produced some rather surprising data.

Digestive disorders account for the largest amount of time lost from work, are the number one cause of disability absence, and comprise at least one-sixth of all hospital admissions. Their overall cost is 10 percent of the health-care dollar. Approximately 40 percent of all cancer originates in the GI tract. And one well-recognized condition, the irritable bowel, affects more than half of the population at one time or another.

With advancing age, especially of persons who live alone or in retirement homes or who are relatively inactive, there is often an inordinate focus on bowel activity. With less pleasure in eating and possible decline in physiologic functions, including sex, a good bowel movement every day may be a reward to look forward to. Such anticipation is fostered by incessant promotion of products to induce "regularity," implying that life can be wonderful if one takes pharmacologic command of the digestive tract.

Emotions felt in "the pit of the stomach" and other more subtle psychological factors also can intrude upon the processes of digestion. Digestive complaints may even be a symptom or major manifestation of depression.

For all of these reasons, we need to know something about how our bodily systems function in order to provide normal and necessary self-care.

Anatomy of Digestion

Think of the digestive tract as an open-ended inner tube that runs through the body from mouth to anus. It has numerous bulges, flexures, valves, and connections with organs that assist its operations, but substances inside the tube are really outside of the body proper. Nutrients processed in the tract are assimilated through its walls to serve the body *per se:* the principal function of the tract is that of absorption. Its other activities — secretion, propulsion, digestion, storage, and excretion — are subservient to this prime function of absorption.

Mouth to stomach. Digestion begins in the mouth with the chewing of food and mixing with saliva, which contains an enzyme *(ptyalin)* that begins the digestion of some carbohydrates. Next comes a swallow, in which a portion of chewed food is moved to the back of the mouth and down the esophagus or gullet into the stomach. Gravity has nothing to do with it; we could swallow just as well if hanging upside down. The esophagus propels food by wavelike muscular squeezes, constricting and pushing ahead somewhat analogous to milking. This action, called *peristalsis,* also occurs in the stomach.

When filled with a big meal, the stomach is the biggest bulge in the digestive tract; if empty, it is more like a deflated balloon. A normal stomach is an acid stomach, determined by its own secretion of hydrochloric acid, a highly corrosive substance. Millions of tiny glands and specialized cells in the slick lining membrane of the stomach secrete not only acid, but pepsin, an enzyme that digests proteins, as well as mucus and a complex substance that enables vitamin B_{12} to be absorbed.

Since most germs can't stand the acidic environment, the stomach is normally free of bacteria. It has three "bias-belted" layers of muscle that enable it to squeeze, mix, and knead its contents quite powerfully. The resulting mixture is called *chyme,* a thin soup that is made tolerable to delicate structures of the small intestine. A meal remains in the stomach for as long as four hours, but initial emptying begins in about 15 minutes. The bigger the meal, the more rapid the emptying. But since the stomach empties only a fraction of what remains at any one time, the rate slows.

Through a purse-string valve at the outlet of the stomach *(pylorus),* chyme is spurted into the *duodenum,* which lies just beyond. The duodenum is a horseshoe-shaped tube about ten inches long. It is the first part of the small bowel and the port of entry for chemical materials essential for digestion.

Liver and biliary tract. The liver is a solid organ, the largest in the body, that develops as a bud from the primitive digestive tube. The liver is a consummate chemist. Among other things, it manipulates hormones and produces bile and cholesterol. Bile to solubilize fat collects in the gallbladder under the liver where it is stored and concentrated, and normally is emptied with each meal.

The pancreas gland lies high in the abdomen, horizontally from the duodenum. It produces major digestive enzymes for each classification of foodstuffs: carbohydrate (sugars and starches), fat, and protein. It also produces insulin, not related to digestion but to diabetes.

Ducts carrying biliary and pancreatic juices enter the duodenum at about the midpoint of its bend. There, the environment changes from acid to alkaline, largely because pancreatic enzymes are highly alkaline in pH.

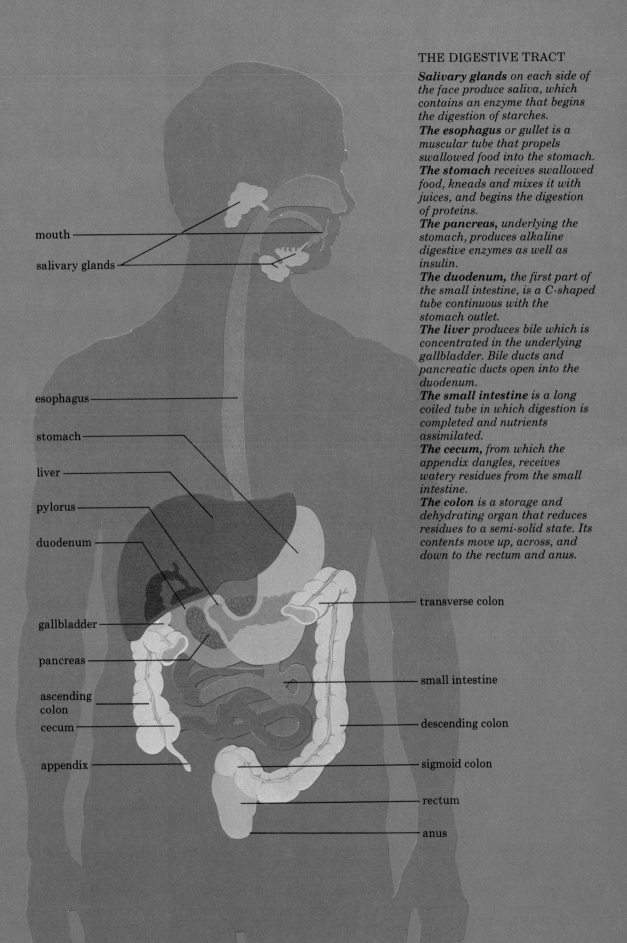

THE DIGESTIVE TRACT

Salivary glands on each side of the face produce saliva, which contains an enzyme that begins the digestion of starches.

The esophagus or gullet is a muscular tube that propels swallowed food into the stomach.

The stomach receives swallowed food, kneads and mixes it with juices, and begins the digestion of proteins.

The pancreas, underlying the stomach, produces alkaline digestive enzymes as well as insulin.

The duodenum, the first part of the small intestine, is a C-shaped tube continuous with the stomach outlet.

The liver produces bile which is concentrated in the underlying gallbladder. Bile ducts and pancreatic ducts open into the duodenum.

The small intestine is a long coiled tube in which digestion is completed and nutrients assimilated.

The cecum, from which the appendix dangles, receives watery residues from the small intestine.

The colon is a storage and dehydrating organ that reduces residues to a semi-solid state. Its contents move up, across, and down to the rectum and anus.

mouth

salivary glands

esophagus

stomach

liver

pylorus

duodenum

gallbladder

pancreas

ascending colon

cecum

appendix

transverse colon

small intestine

descending colon

sigmoid colon

rectum

anus

The small bowel. Somewhat arbitrarily, the small bowel, although continuous, is divided into three parts—the *duodenum,* already mentioned, connects with the *jejunum,* and the latter with the *ileum.* Altogether, the small bowel is about 12 feet long and is coiled in the abdomen. Its all-important function, the assimilation of energy and nutrients from food, is accomplished by a remarkable velvet lining.

The lining contains millions of microscopic *villi,* which resemble minute finger-like protuberances and are so densely packed that their top surfaces have the feel of extraordinarily soft velvet. If all the villi were flattened out, the lining would be seen to have an enormous surface—about the size of a tennis court. Villi are not passive but are active structures, moving and swaying their surfaces into contact with fluids. Glands at their bases secrete juices. Lymphatic channels in the villi carry fat elements to the body, and networks of blood vessels transport digested carbohydrates and proteins to the liver.

One can maintain reasonably good health with only 50 percent of the small bowel functioning. With less than that, however, malabsorption difficulties occur (see page 216).

The colon. Liquid contents of the small bowel enter the large bowel or colon through a valve at the *cecum,* which is neighborly to the appendix. The job of the colon is to reabsorb excessive water, form the stool, conserve electrolytes (dissolved minerals), and serve as a storage chamber. Most of its activity is inhibitory, but once or twice a day, a mass motion moves the contents of the bowel halfway around the colon. The stimulus to a bowel movement is entrance of contents into the dilated terminal portion of the colon (the *rectal ampulla).* Inhibitory waves about ten inches from the rectum normally keep the ampulla empty until the call to stool is heeded.

Arrangements of convenience. The fundamental need for having a digestive tract is absorption of nutrients—the end for which all else is made. Much of the tract, except the small bowel, can be regarded as a convenience system. The colon enables us to empty the bowel once a day or once in three days—whatever physiology dictates. With a stomach, we can eat one or three meals a day without the more or less continuous ingestion necessary for a creature of high metabolic activity, as is the case with the hummingbird, for example.

CHANGES WITH AGING

No one supposes that peptic ulcer occurs regularly at age 43 or gallstones at 51, or that disorders of extreme old age are just as frequent in middle life. Nor is physiological age the same as chronological age. Nevertheless, some diseases become more common in the general population (though not necessarily in us!) after age 40, and many of us will have to cope with them. It is principally these that we shall attend to.

Although the digestive tract ages along with the rest of the body, it has such great reserves that, in the absence of disease, we can generally count on it to serve us pleasurably and well for the duration. Measurements of secretions and activity of the tract do show some slight decline with age, but rarely to the extent of causing any problems. For instance, you will probably have less carbohydrate-digesting enzyme in the saliva after age 60, but you won't know it and no harm will come of it.

Stomach secretions, including hydrochloric acid, also decrease with age. The decrease is sometimes associated with atrophy of the stomach lining, which in old patients may result in lessened production of the factor necessary for absorption of vitamin B_{12}. But this decrease is seldom severe enough to cause anything so troublesome as pernicious anemia. The major enzyme secreted by the stomach, *pepsin,* remains quite stable up to about age 40, falls off between the ages of 40 and 60, and thereafter remains fairly stable at a lower level.

These changes are not firmly correlated with any disease. It is possible, however, that "dyspepsia" in older patients may be related to them. Supplements of acid and digestive enzymes have been advocated, but there is little evidence of their value.

Pancreatic enzymes for digestion of fat, protein, and carbohydrate likewise tend to decrease somewhat after age 40. However, even with advancing years, a normal pancreas is active enough to promote adequate digestion. Indeed, not all investigators agree that there is an age-related decline in pancreas function at all.

The mouth. Digestion may, however, be handicapped where it begins, with loss of teeth or inadequate dental care of conditions that worsen with the years if unattended to (see page 154). Missing teeth, worn surfaces, gum disease, and wobbly restorations all impair the chewing and saliva-mixing of foods, and present the digestive tract with poorly processed material to work on. And undue reliance on a few "comfortable," soft, semi-liquid foods may result in deficiencies of nutrients.

Absorption. There is some direct and indirect evidence that absorption, the ultimate purpose of digestion, is somewhat decreased in older patients. That is, the assimilation of foodstuffs may not be total in older persons.

Overweight is a problem for thousands of people. But studies indicate that, at least in Caucasian patients, it ceases to be a problem by age 70, and after that, the average person is somewhat underweight. One factor may be decreased food intake with age, due to reduced metabolic needs, and lessened acuteness of the senses of smell and taste.

Another likely factor appears to be a decrease in the amount of blood supplied to the small bowel after eating. Approximately 35 percent of your blood is in vessels of the digestive tract at all times. After a meal, blood flow to digestive organs increases about 25 percent more (the diversion has something to do with that nap-time feeling after a heavy meal).

This extra blood to digestive organs has to come from increased pumping of the heart or diversion from other organs. In older persons with decreased efficiency of heart and lungs, abundant blood for digestion may not be available, and this may account for decreased absorption of foodstuffs.

Calcium absorption also decreases with age, as may iron absorption, which is dependent upon acid in the stomach. It is possible that vitamins such as B_1 and B_{12} are less well-absorbed by older persons and that some oral drugs—pills and capsules—are incompletely absorbed by older gastrointestinal tracts. More needs to be known.

The liver. There is some evidence that liver function changes with age, and some microscopic changes in its appearance can be seen. However, the most recent studies indicate that if your liver is free of disease, you can depend upon it to serve you adequately regardless of age. Normally, it does decrease slightly in size, most markedly during the seventh decade, and its associated organ, the gallbladder, is increasingly susceptible to stone formation in middle age and after.

Sagging tissues. As we grow older, we lose some resilience and sturdiness of connective tissue (see page 234). These pervasive tissues support and give shape to structures throughout the body, and degenerative changes are associated with arthritis and a host of other conditions. With respect to the gastrointestinal tract, their laxness is relevant to two disorders that are very frequent after middle age: *hiatal hernia* and *diverticulosis,* which we shall later discuss in detail.

Connective tissues keep the junction of the esophagus and stomach in its proper place. If support is weakened, part of the stomach may protrude up into the chest, a condition called *hiatal hernia.* Similarly, outpouchings like small pockets may occur in the wall of the colon *(diverticulosis).* Both conditions are definitely age-related in that they are much more frequent at middle-life and after than in youth.

CARDINAL SYMPTOMS OF
DIGESTIVE DISORDERS

A great many health problems—heart trouble, kidney stones, eye and ear difficulties, and broken bones, to mention a few—have diagnostic advantages. That is, a physician is usually able to establish the diagnosis with the help of physical findings. But this is not true of many digestive disorders that primarily produce subjective symptoms of which the patient complains bitterly but that may have no physical basis, or none that is readily discoverable.

About three-fourths of the information that leads to a diagnosis of digestive disorder comes from the patient himself; the rest is obtained from physical examination and from laboratory studies. Thus, the ability of the patient to tell the doctor quite specifically where, when, and how his symptoms occur is very important in diagnosis. So is the doctor's willingness to take the time to listen, question, and separate significant symptoms from the trivial.

The mechanism of symptoms. How do symptoms originate? Largely from derangements of normal mechanisms that are ultimately noticed as something that hurts, distresses, irritates, is "different," or departs from the norm. Symptoms may not be very specific or descriptive of what is going on, and may not even appear until some process is well under way.

Almost any gastrointestinal symptom can be indicative of serious disease or of something quite trivial. One doesn't run to a doctor for a transient stomach upset or a bout of heartburn consequent upon overindulgence. But symptoms that persist or are managed week after week by self-chosen doses of over-the-counter medicines—their name is legion—are possible portents that should have the benefit of medical counsel.

We will try to give some information about the nature of various complaints, what should be done, and their significance.

Pain

Gastrointestinal pain is usually caused by spasm, obstruction of the bowel, or some tugging on the *mesentery* (the fan-shaped apron that supports the intestines). Vigorous running produces "a stitch in the side" in some people. It usually goes away with rest, but any pain that recurs and has some relation to activity should be investigated.

Your doctor will want you to describe the pain. Is it cramp-like, burning, steady, severe? Is it located in one place or spread around the abdomen? Some pains radiate to a particular area. The relationship of pain to activity, particularly eating or bowel movements, also gives useful information. Pain that wakes a patient during the night is almost always of organic or physical origin.

Ulcer pain or distress characteristically occurs when the stomach is emptying or is nearly empty. It is generally located high in the abdomen and is relieved by antacids or food. Pain associated with bowel problems tends to be crampy and is sometimes associated with audible bowel sounds.

Pain of gallbladder disease is usually colicky, with tenderness in the upper abdomen. Pain associated with pancreatitis tends to be steady and radiates to the back.

All pain of more than transient duration should be investigated by the medical history, physical examination, and X-ray studies, if indicated.

Loss of Appetite and Weight

An obvious cause of weight loss is poor appetite with insufficient food intake; less obvious are decreased intestinal absorption, uncontrolled diabetes, and occasionally an overactive thyroid gland. Symptoms are especially significant when other problems are present.

The symptoms may indicate an obstructing lesion, an ulcer in the stomach outlet, cancer, hyperthyroidism, or food aversion of psychiatric origin *(anorexia nervosa)*. In alcoholics, weight loss may occur when most of the caloric intake is obtained from alcohol instead of food. The point is, both pain and weight loss can occur in a variety of digestive disorders and may have no localizing features.

Difficult Swallowing

Dysphagia is difficulty in swallowing and is not necessarily painful. The patient is frequently able to recognize a definite area where a mouthful of food seems to stop in its passage from mouth to stomach. The condition must be differentiated from the so-called "lump in the throat" *(globus hystericus)* that is associated with emotional and psychiatric factors and is not indicative of primary disease.

Dysphagia usually points to some disorder of the esophagus: obstruction of its opening, internally or from the outside; diffuse spasm; or motility disorders, such as failure of the valve to open at its end. Dysphagia with significant weight loss is an ominous symptom, highly suspicious of cancer of the esophagus.

Obviously, dysphagia is a serious symptom demanding prompt investigation. Frequently, however, it occurs with eminently treatable conditions such as hiatal hernia, peptic esophagitis, or yeast infections of the esophagus.

Heartburn

Two very common GI-related complaints are "gassiness" and heartburn. Heartburn is so ubiquitous that definition is almost superfluous. Practically everybody has felt the sensation of burning along the esophagus, even rising into the throat, and often accompanied by a sour belch. Run-of-the-mill heartburn is harmless and generally is relieved by taking a half-glass of milk or an antacid. It is almost a normal expectation in the middle and late months of pregnancy, and is only important if it is associated with some organic disease, such as gastritis, peptic ulcer, or hiatal hernia, in which case treatment is directed to the primary cause.

Nausea and Vomiting

These are universal experiences that hardly require any description. "Nausea" derives from a Greek word meaning "sea sickness." Queasiness aboard a rocking boat is not a sign of disease, but a penalty of maritime adventure. Vomiting is a way of ridding the stomach of insults, benevolent in purpose and effect if the incitement is recognized as "something I et" or too much of a good thing.

However, nausea and vomiting may be symptomatic of underlying disease. Nausea may be an early sign of drug intoxication, pregnancy, hepatitis, or a product of alcohol withdrawal if morning hangover is relieved by a drink.

Repeated vomiting is a critical symptom, associated with gastritis, peptic ulcer, alcoholism, some drug intoxications, and disorders such as renal (kidney) failure.

Retention vomiting is the result of obstruction by an ulcer or tumor: the vomitus contains food eaten many hours or even days before. Ejected material that looks like coffee grounds indicates the presence of blood that has been in contact with acid in the stomach. A fecal odor also is significant, and suggests obstruction of the lower small intestine or colon.

The patient's previous history of ulcer or some other problem is important in relation to these symptoms. Diagnosis may entail emptying the stomach through a large-bore tube for chemical analysis of its contents; X rays, if bowel obstruction is suspected; and more vigorous measures if the vomitus contains blood.

Signs of Bleeding

Hematemesis is the vomiting of gross blood, which may be bright when fresh, or black when digested in the acid stomach. *Melena* refers to stools that are black and tarry from blood that has been digested. Both of these symptoms help to locate the part of the tract where bleeding occurs. Hematemesis alone usually, but not always, originates near the junction of the stomach and duodenum. Melena alone generally originates from lesions between the stomach outlet and the adjoining small bowel. The site of bleeding can be determined more precisely by fiber-optic techniques, employing flexible narrow tubes that bend light rays around twists and turns and enable direct inspection of tissues.

Both of these symptoms suggest a disease process that is potentially serious. In fact, any amount of hemorrhage should be considered serious business.

After basic laboratory studies are done, fiber-optic exploration of the esophagus, stomach, and duodenum is performed on most patients with bleeding. Meanwhile, blood, fluids, and electrolytes are given. Washing the stomach with iced saline solution yields important information and, in many instances, helps to stop the bleeding. If these conservative measures do not suffice, surgery may be necessary.

Indigestion and "Gas"

"Indigestion" is a word used by patients to describe almost any distress in the GI tract, thus the word does not identify anything specific. Complaints are mostly of symptoms such as "gas," belching, bloating, abdominal fullness, or flatulence—that is, passing of gas by belching or through the rectum. The symptoms can be terribly distressing, but rarely indicate serious disease. The physician needs a full description by the patient to make a diagnosis.

"Gassiness" is popularly thought to be due to large amounts of gas in the gastrointestinal tract. However, studies indicate that the problem is not the quantity of gas but its delayed passage because of spasm or disorders of muscular activity of the intestines. "Gassy" patients may be unusually sensitive to distention of the bowel, a prime stimulus of abdominal discomfort.

Where does gas come from? One source is unconscious air-swallowing *(aerophagia).* Talking while chewing, hasty chewing, gulping drinks, or taking large amounts of a carbonated beverage all can carry surprising amounts of air down the gullet. Air swallowers may have a large bubble of air at the top of the stomach; belching relieves the discomfort, like burping a baby. If unbelched, air passes into the small bowel and may be trapped in the left side of the colon where it can simulate chest or stomach pain. Symptoms are usually relieved by a bowel movement.

Another source of gas is bacterial fermentation. Food intolerance also plays a role in indigestion and flatulence. Certain foods—baked beans, cabbage, and onions are notorious — produce gas by fermentation. Individual reactions to foods are highly variable and personal—one man's food is another man's gas-maker. Milk products, too, may cause bloating, flatulence, and diarrhea in persons who lack a necessary digestive enzyme. The association of gas and indigestion with particular foods may be recognized by patients or may be discerned from a history of eating habits. In any case, common sense suggests that the wisdom of the body be heeded and that foods that have proved untrustworthy be avoided.

The possibility that symptoms may have an organic cause may be investigated by X-ray studies, a barium enema, or other diagnostic procedures, if indicated.

Abdominal Distention

A sudden or gradual increase in the size of the abdomen may cause no sensation, although usually there are feelings of fullness or pressure with some pain. Abdominal distention, not all of which is of gastrointestinal origin, may be caused by enlargement of the liver, spleen, or uterus, or by an ovarian cyst, obstructed bladder, fecal impaction, or intestinal obstruction.

Distention by *ascites,* an accumulation of fluid in the peritoneal cavity, has serious implications. Fluid in the abdomen may be associated with chronic liver disease, tumors, peritonitis, and other problems. This generally calls for a thorough medical work-up to determine its cause and nature—analysis of the fluid, barium studies, biopsies, and liver studies. Sometimes an exploratory operation is necessary.

THE DISORDERLY STOMACH

We shall now presume to attend to the stomach, a distensible bulge in the upper tract that is delightful when good-humored, but quite otherwise when truculent. For convenience, we will include the esophagus—the swallowing tube that joins the stomach and shares some of its misbehaviors.

Hiatal Hernia

A statistical risk of living to age 40 and after is a 50-50 chance of having a hiatal hernia. The exact incidence is hard to determine. Symptoms may be mild and uncomplained of. But we can be sure that the condition is surprisingly frequent after middle age, although younger people are not immune. Studies in England indicate that about one-third of the general population has a hiatal hernia. In this country, studies of patients referred for symptoms demonstrated that 72 percent had a hiatal hernia, and that its incidence was 52 percent even in patients under age 40.

What is a hiatal hernia? The hiatus is a normal hole in the diaphragm, the big horizontal muscle of breathing, through which the esophagus joins the stomach. Its supporting ligaments may become so stretched and weakened that abdominal pressures force a protrusion or herniation of the junction into the chest. There is some evidence that hiatal hernia also is associated with common hernias in more familiar areas, such as the groin, and this suggests a general aging of connective tissue.

Symptoms. The herniation may cause a burning pain under the breastbone, with *reflux*—regurgitation of stomach contents into the lower esophagus. At times, jets of juices may well up in the throat at the back of the mouth. The herniation may be fixed, but often is of a sliding type, moving more or less easily up and down. As might be

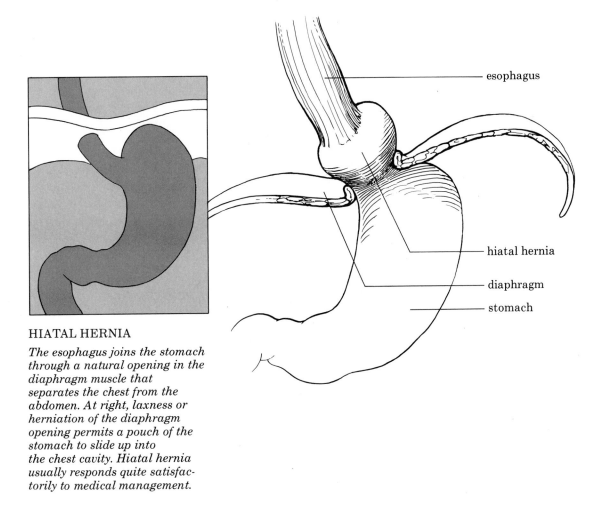

esophagus

hiatal hernia

diaphragm

stomach

HIATAL HERNIA

The esophagus joins the stomach through a natural opening in the diaphragm muscle that separates the chest from the abdomen. At right, laxness or herniation of the diaphragm opening permits a pouch of the stomach to slide up into the chest cavity. Hiatal hernia usually responds quite satisfactorily to medical management.

expected, symptoms are most noticeable under pressure—after meals, while straining or stooping, and when reclining. The condition is often associated with chronic *esophagitis,* inflammation of the esophagus, usually due to baths of acid juices frequently erupted from the stomach. *Heartburn*—a painful or burning sensation behind the breastbone that may radiate to the chest, arms, or jaw—may occur with or without hiatal hernia.

To the patient, the symptoms may indicate "dyspepsia" or "indigestion." Similar symptoms can have a variety of causes. Heart pain, gallbladder distress, hiatal hernia—all can be evinced in an area under the breastbone that is easily covered by the palm of the hand. In fact, some persons who are having a heart attack actually think it is indigestion.

Elaborate tests are not always necessary. The patient's medical history, the quality of symptoms, and their relationship to eating habits can be highly informative. Occasional or even frequent heartburn that is clearly consequent upon too much alcohol or food is rarely alarming and simply may be a price that the reckless indulger is willing to pay.

It may be necessary, however, to identify the cause of trouble precisely or to recognize concurrent disease, in which case X-ray studies of the upper GI tract with special attention to the esophagus would be indicated, as well as, perhaps, inspection of the esophagus with a fiber-optic instrument (see page 231).

Treatment. Hiatal hernia is often tolerated quite well with medical management. This includes judicious use of antacids after meals and before bedtime. It is helpful to avoid tight garments and to elevate the head of one's bed on blocks about six inches high, thus enlisting a little aid from gravity in keeping down the stomach and its contents. Of course, it is prudent not to overload the stomach at any one time.

Intractable, severe hiatal hernia may require surgical correction, accomplished by tightening the ring at the junction of the stomach and esophagus, which keeps the upper part of the stomach in its place.

Antacids are a standard treatment for heartburn when not associated with other disease.

Tumors of the Esophagus

Tumors of the esophagus may be benign or cancerous. Symptoms of a benign tumor are usually those of partial obstruction of the esophagus—discomfort or impediment in swallowing. Diagnosis is made by X-ray studies, with visualization of the esophagus and the obtaining of tissue specimens for analysis. Treatment is surgical.

Cancer is more common in patients with chronic inflammation of the esophagus, as in *achalasia,* a condition resulting from inability of the sphincter at the lower end of the gullet to relax, resulting in irritation from stagnant materials. The average age at diagnosis is 60 to 65 years.

Symptoms of esophageal cancer are similar to those of benign tumors, although they develop more rapidly. There is a feeling of fullness and pressure in the esophagus and increasing inability to swallow, at first for solid foods and then for all foods.

Unfortunately, treatment is not very satisfactory. Surgery may be performed for early tumors, but the spread to adjacent lymph nodes and tissues tends to occur rapidly. Sometimes the patient may be made more comfortable by X-ray treatments. The five-year survival rate is quite disappointing.

Varices of the Esophagus

These are varicose veins of the esophagus, which are highly subject to bleeding. The usual underlying cause is disease of the liver (see page 206). Cirrhosis or some obstruction of blood flow into the liver creates backflow pressures. The first symptom is usually vomiting of blood.

Peptic Ulcer

Quiet stomach? There's no such thing. Comfortable stomach, yes. The stomach is incessantly active, secreting hydrochloric acid, pepsin, enzymes, and a variety of other substances; breaking down proteins; expanding and contracting, squirming, and kneading.

Hydrochloric acid and pepsin, the major digestive enzyme of the stomach, are highly corrosive: gastric juices with an acidity of pH 1 to 2 can inflict a bad burn. In this seething hotbed, surface cells of your stomach lining do not live long. About 500,000 cells are cast off every minute and are replaced by an equal number of newcomers, which, in turn, will soon be shed. In less than a week, this cell layer in your stomach is totally renewed.

Why doesn't the stomach digest itself? Sometimes it does, partly, if protective mechanisms go awry. The result is an ulcer, a raw sore eroded into the stomach wall, sometimes penetrating through it. Locations of ulcers vary, but all are classed as "peptic ulcers."

Duodenal ulcers, located in the duodenum just beyond the stomach outlet, are their most common form. Young people can suffer from them, but the peak incidence is in the 40s and 50s. It is estimated that duodenal ulcers affect 10 percent of the population at any one time, and men three times more frequently than women.

By legend, the ulcer-prone person is hard-driving, conscientious, very ambitious, a deadline fighter, and a tireless worker. This is flattering, but does not account for people of that temperament who do not develop ulcers and perhaps cannot. A physical predisposition is plausible. Many, if not most duodenal-ulcer patients, have a larger than average mass of cells in the stomach lining that secrete acids and juices. Peptic ulcers also tend to be associated with other disorders, such as chronic obstructive lung disease, cirrhosis of the liver, and overactivity of the calcium-regulating parathyroid glands.

Symptoms. The characteristic symptom of a duodenal ulcer is pain or distress that occurs an hour or two after eating or when the stomach is empty, and that is relieved by taking food, a glass of milk, or an antacid. The distress may be like a hunger pain, gnawing, or burning felt in the vicinity of the navel. The pain recurs with regularity over periods of time, with a tendency to recur in the spring and fall. The diagnosis is made from the medical history and symptoms and barium X-ray studies that commonly reveal a punched-out "crater" that identifies the ulcer.

Treatment. The great majority of patients (85 percent) do well with medical treatment. The mainstays of management are: antacids to neutralize stomach acidity, medications that decrease gastric secretion, and avoidance of foods that stimulate such secretion. A new drug, cimetidine, taken four times a day, reduces gastric acidity by about 80 percent in recommended dosage, without serious side effects. This effect helps to prevent recurrences, may make surgery unnecessary in some cases, and can be helpful to persons with inflammation of the esophagus caused by reflux of stomach acids.

Usually it is not very difficult to heal an active ulcer. The problem is to keep it healed over many years of possible recurrence. Ideally, hospitalization during the acute phase is desirable—a week or two for adaptation to a medical program, rest, and freedom from tensions and anxieties that could aggravate the condition. However, innumerable patients do very well in a home environment that is not unduly combative or upsetting.

During the healing phase, which takes about ten days, frequent feedings of bland foods such as milk and crackers are advised, along with rest and prescribed medications. Dozens of ulcer diets have been advocated over the years, but it now seems that after a duodenal ulcer is healed, most patients can eat what they like without permanent over-rigid restrictions on certain foods.

It is prudent to avoid or be moderate about foods or habits that stimulate acid secretion, such as alcohol, smoking, and coffee. A simple measure that seems physiologically sound is to take frequent small meals during the day, instead of one or two large ones, so that the stomach always has something to work on besides itself. It may be necessary to continue medications or antacids indefinitely, as a doctor advises.

One heartening fact: duodenal ulcers virtually never become cancerous.

Complications. A duodenal ulcer may cause swelling around the stomach outlet and obstruct it partially or completely. Vomiting is one symptom; vigorous peristaltic waves traveling toward the navel, another. Diagnosis is made by examination of stomach contents obtained by suction, and by barium-meal X-ray studies that determine the size and location of the lesion. If the obstruction is total, surgery will be necessary.

A serious ulcer complication is *acute perforation,* in which the ulcer penetrates completely through the wall and disgorges contents into the peritoneum, leaving the patient in extreme agony from abdominal pain. Acute perforation is a life-threatening emergency that demands immediate surgery: the perforated area is repaired and steps are taken to combat peritonitis.

Another form of perforation, sometimes called chronic, is not so immediately critical. The ulcer perforates, but nature plugs the "hole in the dike" by causing the perforated area to adhere to adjacent tissues—in effect, corking the opening. The patient may feel pain in the back, or perhaps no pain at all.

Another possible complication is *bleeding ulcer.* Massive hemorrhage may first be indicated by weakness, dizziness, or faintness, and later by vomiting blood or passage of a tarry stool, proving the escape of blood into the intestinal tract. The amount of blood loss varies; if massive, the patient may be in shock. Treatment must be given in a hospital, with preparations for transfusion. Initially, the patient is usually given frequent liquid and other feedings and is encouraged to eat, in hope that bleeding points will self-repair, as is often the case. If hemorrhage continues unabated despite conservative measures, surgery probably will be necessary.

Surgery. Some patients with a severe duodenal ulcer do not improve satisfactorily on medication, rest, and diet, and will benefit from surgery.

One solution is to remove the lower half of the stomach *(partial gastrectomy).* Acid production is mainly incited by this area, and its removal produces a less acid environment, favorable to the healing and prevention of ulcers.

Various symptoms collectively called *postgastrectomy syndrome* may occur after the operation. The most common, which occur soon or immediately after eating, are feelings of bloating, weakness, pounding heart, sweating, and even vomiting. These generally disappear in less than an hour. Distress may be lessened by taking small meals, lying down after eating, and using medicines prescribed by a physician.

Another operation called *vagotomy* does not involve the stomach directly, but certain nerves *(vagus)* that stimulate gastric secretion. Orders to produce excessive amounts of acid are disconnected by cutting the vagus nerves. Currently, operations on a section of the nerves serving only the secreting part of the stomach are under study, and may have expected benefits without the side effects that occur after gastric surgery in some patients.

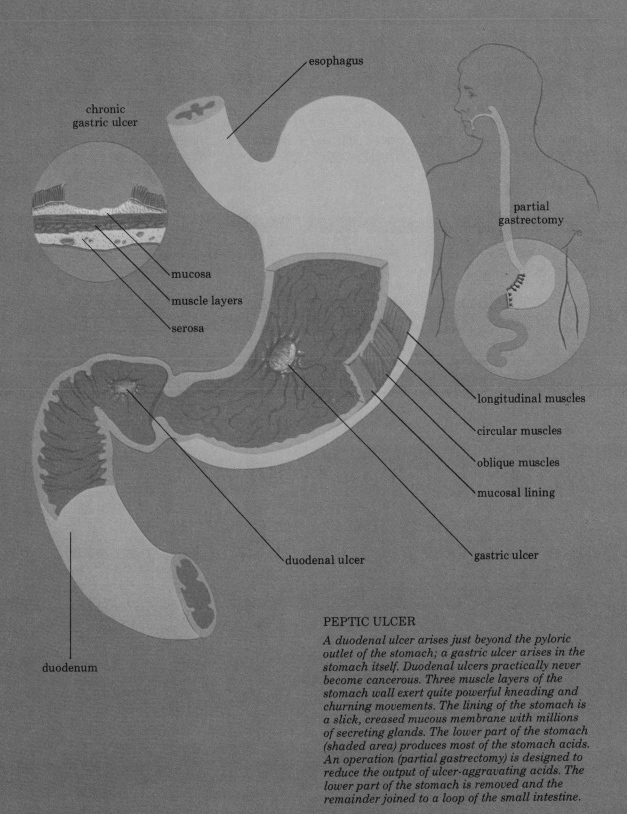

chronic
gastric ulcer

esophagus

partial
gastrectomy

mucosa

muscle layers

serosa

longitudinal muscles

circular muscles

oblique muscles

mucosal lining

duodenal ulcer

gastric ulcer

duodenum

PEPTIC ULCER

A duodenal ulcer arises just beyond the pyloric outlet of the stomach; a gastric ulcer arises in the stomach itself. Duodenal ulcers practically never become cancerous. Three muscle layers of the stomach wall exert quite powerful kneading and churning movements. The lining of the stomach is a slick, creased mucous membrane with millions of secreting glands. The lower part of the stomach (shaded area) produces most of the stomach acids. An operation (partial gastrectomy) is designed to reduce the output of ulcer-aggravating acids. The lower part of the stomach is removed and the remainder joined to a loop of the small intestine.

After the operation. How does one fare after removal of part of the stomach? Quite well, as a rule. The stomach that remains is smaller, but it stretches and adapts in a few months. Digestion proceeds in essentially the same way as before, except that stomach secretions no longer contain an excess of acid. There may be restrictions on diet after surgery, but these are usually temporary, although the prudent patient learns to avoid as far as possible provocative factors such as stimulants, smoking, and nervous tension.

Gastric Ulcer

Stomach or gastric ulcers differ from duodenal ulcers in some respects, aside from their location in the stomach proper. Patients are likely to be older: peak incidence is in the 50s and 60s, suggesting that impaired circulation of blood in the stomach may be implicated. Usual statistics indicate that duodenal ulcers are four times more common than gastric ulcers, but it is more likely that they occur on a more or less equal frequency, especially in the older population. They have no seasonal trend.

In contrast to a duodenal ulcer, the person with a gastric ulcer does not have an increased mass of acid-secreting cells. Gastric secretion is normal or less than normal, although many patients experience inflammation of the stomach lining. One hypothesis is that a laxness of pressure barriers near the stomach outlet, which normally prevent the backflow of its contents, may permit alkaline bile to seep into the stomach where it may be conducive to ulcer formation.

Symptoms are similar to those of duodenal ulcer, but are less distinct. The usual pattern is pain relieved by food. However, if the ulcer is near the stomach outlet, eating may precipitate pain or distress. Loss of appetite and weight also occur.

The longtime course is one of remissions and exacerbations, and the recurrence rate is high. In one series of patients on medical management for six years, three-fourths had a recurrence, generally in the same location as their previous ulcer.

Treatment is similar to that for duodenal ulcer, including antacids, even though the gastric-ulcer patient does not produce excessive acids. Similar complications also may occur.

Most gastric ulcers are benign, but the possibility that the lesion may not be an ulcer but a cancer must not be excluded. Differentiation can be made at least 96 percent of the time by modern techniques. These include X-ray studies, gastroscopic inspection of the inside of the stomach, and tissue specimens and cell washings studied by a pathologist.

Gastritis

Gastritis is an inflammation of the mucosal lining of the stomach. Acute gastritis with burning pain, nausea, and vomiting can come on quite suddenly, but with prompt treatment usually does not last long. Generally there is a discoverable cause, often something that has been swallowed—drugs, caustics, alcohol, toxins, or bacteria, to mention a few—or a reaction to an infection.

Chronic gastritis that persists for months or years has no specific cause, but continued insult by gastric irritants is highly suspect. Alcohol is high on the list, but nicotine, cathartics, caffeine beverages, and salicylate (aspirin-like) drugs cannot be wholly ruled out, nor can idiosyncratic reactions. Gastritis near the outlet of the stomach is common in association with gastric and duodenal ulcers. Symptoms may be mild stomach distress, or severe episodes of vomiting and ulcer-like pain.

Treatment is similar to that for peptic ulcer. A frequent complication is widespread bleeding from minute hemorrhages in the stomach lining, somewhat comparable to a bleeding ulcer. In fact, hemorrhage from gastritis accounts for about one-fourth of all gastrointestinal bleeding encountered in practice. Healing is relatively rapid in most cases, but sometimes surgery is needed.

Atrophic gastritis is a particular variety in which the lining tissue is thinned and normal glands are replaced by other structures. An important type of atrophy is associated with pernicious anemia. The atrophied tissues do not secrete intrinsic factor, a stomach secretion that is essential for the absorption of Vitamin B_{12}. About 10 to 15 percent of pernicious-anemia patients develop gastric cancer. To detect possible cancer in an early stage, such patients should be examined every six to 12 months. Probably the best screening measure is fiber-optic visualization of the esophagus, stomach, and duodenum.

Stomach Cancer

Tumors of the stomach may be benign or malignant, but the great majority prove to be cancers. Fortunately and for reasons unknown, stomach cancer is in absolute decline in the United States.

Initially there are no symptoms, and later symptoms are mostly indefinite: "indigestion" or almost any kind of abdominal discomfort that persists. By the time diagnosis is made, most patients have experienced some weight loss, pain, and vomiting. Massive bleeding is uncommon, but occult blood is often found in the bowel movement.

Investigation of persistent mild symptoms is important for early diagnosis. X-ray examination helps to differentiate cancer from gastric ulcer. Along with gastroscopy and cytology (cell studies), the presence of cancer can almost certainly be confirmed.

Definitive treatment for stomach cancer is surgical—removal of the cancer and as much surrounding tissue as possible. If the lesion involves only the lining tissue of the stomach, the cure rate is nearly 100 percent. But more invasive cancer, even though the lesion is small, has a 5-year cure rate of about 35 percent.

THE PANCREAS GLAND

The stomach keeps us more or less aware of its digestive functions at all times: pleasing fullness after a meal, an occasional discreet burp, or an ache or expulsive protest if we eat something toxic or too much of a good thing. But the pancreas never has a pancreas-ache, and gives no feeling of its presence unless something goes wrong. It is even more essential to digestion than the stomach, but is so unobtrusive that many people don't recognize its importance.

The pancreas has complex functions, one of which is the production of insulin. Another function, which we shall here discuss, is the production of digestive enzymes.

The pancreas gland lies high in the abdomen, in a crosswise position from the duodenum toward the spleen. It has a soft consistency (sweetbreads in a meat market are the pancreas glands of animals). Descriptively, the pancreas has a rounded "head," and a "tail" that tapers toward the left side of the body. Highly alkaline enzymes that split fats, proteins, and carbohydrates flow through ducts into the upper part of the duodenum where they mix with materials moved down from the stomach, for further downstream processing in the small bowel. (Upstream flow of alkaline fluids into the stomach is thought to be a probable factor in gastric ulcer.)

The pancreas presents many problems to the doctor. It lies too deep to be palpated (felt), and there is no way of visualizing it by X-ray studies, as with other parts of the digestive tract. Tests of its function are complex and frequently indirect.

Pancreatic disorders can affect juvenile diabetics and other young people, but to a large extent, the problems appear around and after age 40, following long periods of abuse, particularly by alcohol, and the development of biliary tract disease. Less-common causes are trauma, postoperative inflammation, and perforated ulcer contiguous to the pancreas.

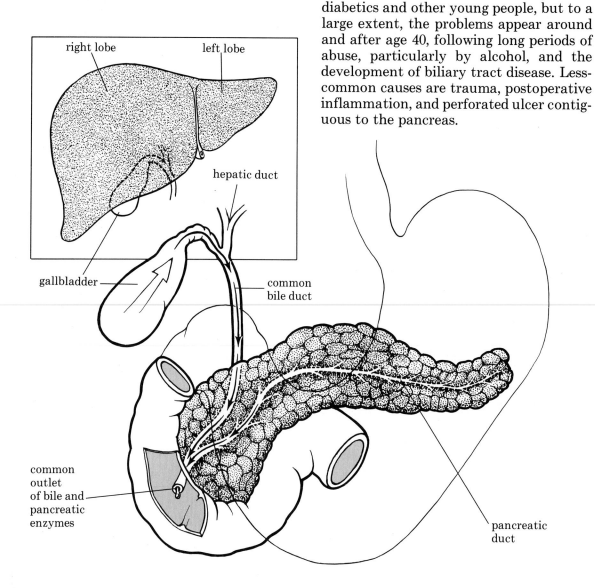

right lobe
left lobe
hepatic duct
gallbladder
common bile duct
common outlet of bile and pancreatic enzymes
pancreatic duct

THE BODY'S MIXING CENTER

Structures and juices essential for digestion converge at the bend of the duodenum. Bile and pancreatic enzymes mix with acidic materials arrived from the stomach, and the environment becomes alkaline. Watery bile from the liver is collected through the hepatic duct, concentrated in the gallbladder, and delivered into the duodenum through the common duct. Pancreatic enzymes drain into the duodenum through the pancreatic duct.

Acute Pancreatitis

The cardinal symptom of acute pancreatitis is sudden, excruciating pain in the upper abdomen, extending into the back. The abdomen is tender but not rigid, and vomiting is severe. The skin becomes cold, clammy, and blue, and the patient may go into shock.

What has happened? Corrosive enzymes have escaped from confining channels in the pancreas into the substance of the gland, resulting in self-digestion of the pancreas and extensive damage to peritoneal tissues. In men, the usual underlying cause is alcoholism; in women, biliary tract disease that obstructs enzyme channels.

Treatment. The object is to put the pancreas at rest and to reduce the stimulation to secretion. Pain is relieved by appropriate medication, and no food or drink by mouth is permitted. Intravenous fluids are then administered to replace blood volume and to help put the pancreas at rest. Removal of stomach acids also reduces the stimulus to pancreatic secretion.

Surgery is not considered unless an abscess forms.

Chronic Pancreatitis

Chronic pancreatitis is similar to the acute form except that attacks of pain may be less severe. The chronic state may be the end result of recurrent attacks of acute pancreatitis. In the most common form (chronic relapsing pancreatitis), there are frequent acute flare-ups superimposed on an already-injured gland.

One of three patients with acute pancreatitis goes on to develop the chronic form. The great majority of patients with chronic relapsing pancreatitis have a history of chronic alcohol abuse or of biliary tract disease. And as the condition progresses, digestion may be disturbed by deficiency of juices, and the destruction of insulin-producing cells may set the stage for diabetes.

Patients complain of recurring attacks of pain, with nausea and vomiting. Treatment includes absolute abstinence from alcohol, agents to suppress pancreatic secretion, and supplemental digestive enzymes. Biliary tract disease, if present, should be corrected, if possible.

Many patients with chronic relapsing pancreatitis do not have a very satisfactory course of improvement, and some ultimately become dependent upon pain-relieving narcotics. Surgery appropriate to the individual patient may be considered, and is helpful in about 50 percent of patients. Some surgeons advocate total removal of the pancreas to abolish recurrent attacks of pain. The functions of the pancreas—production of insulin and enzymes—can then be served by supplementation therapy.

Cancer of the Pancreas

Benign tumors of the pancreas are quite rare. The major problem is cancer of the pancreas, important in older age groups. The peak incidence is in the decades of the 40s through the 60s.

Symptoms are usually those of increasing vague upper abdominal distress. An early diagnostic sign is depression, which may be very significant and the earliest manifestation. Weight loss is particularly rapid in this disease, along with loss of appetite. By the time the patient is seen by a physician, the usual weight loss is about 30 pounds. Jaundice and enlarged liver also are commonly present. Another association of some importance is that of phlebitis with pancreatic cancer.

At present, cancer of the pancreas is an almost hopeless disease. Efforts are under way to improve the prognosis by effecting earlier diagnosis.

LIVER AND BILE

The liver is the largest solid organ in the body, weighing about four pounds. Its size is appropriate to its importance. Few people would guess that the liver has upward of 500 specific functions. A mere fraction of these may be mentioned: the liver manufactures bile, cholesterol, and vitamin A; it stores energy in the form of glycogen; breaks down drugs; detoxifies poisons; manipulates sex hormones; produces blood-clotting factors; and is concerned with iron storage.

The liver and its appendages, the gallbladder and bile ducts, are very frequent sites of medical and surgical problems. Apart from infections, liver disease is a greater threat to older than to younger people. In the 45-to-64 age group, cirrhosis of the liver is the fourth leading cause of death, after heart disease, stroke, and cancer.

Anatomy. The liver lies mostly in the right side of the upper abdomen. Its lower edge can usually be felt below the bottom rib by an experienced hand. On the underside of the lower part of the liver lies the gallbladder, a pear-shaped organ into which bile, secreted by liver cells, trickles through the hepatic duct. The gallbladder is essentially a storage organ for bile. Bile moves through the common duct from the gallbladder into the duodenum where it mixes with food materials, assisting digestion by detergent action on fatty materials.

Blood and its elements are carried to the liver by the vital *portal vein.* The liver disposes of worn-out old red blood cells; conversion of remaining hemoglobin leaves a substance called *bilirubin,* significant in some tests of liver function.

Secretion of bile by the liver is constant, but bile that enters the duodenum is considerably less fluid. In the gallbladder, the volume of bile is concentrated about tenfold. This is discharged with each meal to facilitate digestion and absorption.

Signs of Trouble

Jaundice refers to a yellowish tinge of the skin, mucous membranes, and the whites of the eyes. It is the most common finding in any derangement of the liver, and is frequent with concurrent biliary tract disease. It results from an excess of bile pigments in the body.

The cause of pigmentation may be relatively benign, such as acute hepatitis; an obstruction, possibly malignant; or the result of gallstones. Jaundice is a more serious symptom in an after-40 patient than in a younger one. An obstructive origin is more likely, whereas the most frequent cause in a young patient is viral hepatitis (see the opposite page).

A diagnostic work-up to determine the nature of the jaundice includes liver function tests and, if indicated, X-ray studies and possibly more sophisticated procedures. Normal-colored urine and stools suggest that the jaundice is due to excessive destruction of blood cells; amber (darker than normal) urine with normal-colored stools indicate that the primary disease is in the liver; amber urine with clay-colored stools may signal obstruction in the liver or in the biliary tree outside it.

Drug-induced disease. Liver disease induced by drugs is a large problem, despite increased awareness that certain drugs are potentially toxic to the liver. Toxicity may produce jaundice (or another symptom) from direct damage to the liver, or from indirect interference with one or another of its functions.

Because of the frequency of drug-induced liver disease, it is important that a physician have detailed information about drugs a patient is taking—over-the-counter preparations, prescribed medicines, and even illicit drugs.

Possible liver-damaging drugs cover a wide range, including some anesthetics and anti-hypertensives, oral contraceptives, certain antibiotics, tranquilizers, and others.

Enlarged liver (hepatomegaly) is associated with a large number of possible disorders, such as heart disease, cirrhosis, all varieties of hepatitis, tumors, leukemia and other blood disorders, and obstruction of the biliary tract.

Hepatitis

Any inflammation of the liver is classed as hepatitis. Predominant causes are infections or toxins. Jaundice may or may not occur; frequently the liver is enlarged; and usually there is fever and other systemic symptoms.

Acute viral hepatitis is caused by a virus. Two forms have been identified. *Infectious hepatitis* (hepatitis A) is caused by ingestion of fecally-contaminated food or drink. *Serum hepatitis* (hepatitis B) is caused by transmission of virus from transfusions or contaminated instruments. Some scientists believe that a third form, hepatitis C, also may exist.

Infectious hepatitis mostly affects young people. Serum hepatitis is more frequent in older persons, has a longer incubation period, and may have a more insidious onset.

Because hepatitis B can be transmitted by blood from persons who are carriers, blood donors are routinely screened to rule out those who carry the B virus or other forms. There is significantly less risk of blood-transmitted infection with blood derived from family and friends than with that from commercial donors.

The attack rate of hepatitis is high, and there is some evidence that it is as common as measles.

Symptoms. Classical symptoms of viral hepatitis are loss of appetite, nausea, abdominal pain, malaise, and a flu-like syndrome, followed in a few days by jaundice. Other findings such as pain in the joints and skin rash may be associated with systems other than the liver. Jaundice does not always occur, and in fact may be evidenced by only one in ten or even one in a hundred patients. A high index of suspicion is necessary to establish a diagnosis of hepatitis without jaundice, but non-jaundiced patients are as susceptible to complications as are the jaundiced.

Treatment. Bed rest for three weeks or so, together with a good nourishing diet, is the usual treatment. The doctor checks the recovery of the liver with liver-function tests, watches for relapses or complications, and advises about gradual return to activity.

The great majority of viral hepatitis patients, in the area of 98 percent, recover completely and uneventfully.

Complications. However, a small percentage of patients with viral hepatitis develop a more serious illness, *submassive hepatic necrosis*. They may show signs of liver-cell failure, have increased risk of progression to chronic liver disease, and an increased mortality rate.

During the past ten years, *chronic active hepatitis* has emerged as a leading cause of morbidity and mortality in the hierarchy of liver disorders. Patients with this condition (also called *chronic aggressive hepatitis*) have a high incidence of prior viral hepatitis, persistent signs of liver disease, and abnormal tests over a period of three months.

A liver biopsy is necessary to establish the diagnosis. There is frequent progression to cirrhosis, which is already present in one-third or more of patients by the time diagnosis is established. Fortunately, most patients respond well to corticosteroids, but if the disease is untreated, survival is only four to five years.

In contrast, a variety of hepatitis called *chronic persistent hepatitis* has a good outlook. The course is benign and there is no increased mortality.

It is likely that many patients who develop cirrhosis of the liver without obvious cause have had previous viral hepatitis without the signal of jaundice.

Cirrhosis of the Liver

Cirrhosis is an inflammation of the liver substance, with fibrosis, scarring, and deformities of structure that interfere gravely with circulation of blood and bile. Cirrhosis is a chronic disease with a high mortality rate; progression and complications account for its rank as the fourth leading cause of death after age 45. Cirrhotic patients are not often encountered after age 65, probably because relatively few survive that long.

Cirrhosis may be a sequel to viral hepatitis, drug-induced liver disease, or more rare causes. But the great majority of cases are secondary to prolonged excessive consumption of alcohol.

Alcohol and the liver. Alcoholic hepatitis may be recognized before frank cirrhosis develops, although differentiations may be somewhat hazy. Full-blown cirrhosis can develop as early as three months after a diagnosis of alcoholic hepatitis.

The typical patient is a man of late middle-age who has a history of long-continued excessive alcohol ingestion. You could call him an alcoholic, although the criteria of chronic alcoholism are inexact. However, some associated factors may be recognized: alcohol withdrawal syndromes, continued intake despite career and domestic devastations, presence of alcohol-associated disorders, and high tolerance to alcohol.

Alcohol is metabolized by an enzyme in the liver, alcohol dehydrogenase. Ingestion of more than nine to ten ounces of 100-proof liquor per day (100-proof is 50 percent alcohol) is associated with much higher risk of developing chronic liver disease than with an intake of lesser daily amounts.

A normal man can metabolize about 22 ounces of whiskey in 24 hours, a little less than one ounce of whiskey per hour. To put it another way, he could take a drink containing a 1½-ounce jigger of hard liquor every hour and a half without any sign of intoxication.

Chronic alcoholics have a more rapid turnover of alcohol. One indication of tolerance to alcohol is ingestion of a fifth or more of liquor per day without any evidence of intoxication, although the blood level of alcohol is high. Overuse of alcohol leads to incorporation of fat in the liver, and ultimately to alcoholic hepatitis.

Symptoms include weakness, jaundice, weight loss, fever, and diarrhea. Physical examination may reveal an enlarged liver and fluid in the abdomen. A liver biopsy may reveal coexisting cirrhosis, infiltration, and a peculiar pink-staining material that is usually, but not always, present.

Treatment. Alcoholic hepatitis is a grave illness with a mortality rate up to 90 percent. Treatment is total abstinence from alcohol, a 2,000-calorie-per-day diet high in protein, bed rest, and avoidance of sedatives and other drugs.

Gin-Drinker's Liver

The most common type of cirrhosis of the liver is *portal cirrhosis,* also rudely called "gin-drinker's liver" and alcoholic cirrhosis. Malnutrition is often present, along with alcoholism. At one time, it was thought that the main cause of liver damage was poor nutrition—too many calories from alcohol, too few from food—but it is actually probable that alcohol has a direct toxic effect of its own.

Symptoms. Early cirrhosis may cause no symptoms, and gradual advance of liver failure only vague ones such as loss of appetite, nausea, and abdominal pain. By the time most patients are seen, the major features of cirrhosis are jaundice and accumulations of fluid in the abdomen *(ascites).*

Laboratory and liver-function tests may reveal deficiences of the blood-clotting mechanism and increased sodium retention, with development of ascites and edema or swelling of the legs. A superficial finding characteristic of liver disease is the presence of vascular "spiders" on the chest, face, neck, and arms. These are small, red, "leggy" blood vessels that somewhat resemble the configuration of a spider.

Treatment. By the time the patient has ascites, treatment is directed toward the fluid-swollen abdomen and toward correction of factors that caused the liver disease in the first place. Ascites is managed by bed rest, restriction of sodium and water, and judicious use of diuretic drugs. Salt restriction alone can improve the ascites if the patient is treated long enough. Alcohol is forbidden, and proper diet is prescribed. Intensive treatment for two or three months may restore a fair percentage of patients to an active life.

Complications. A dreaded complication of cirrhosis is massive bleeding from varicose veins in the esophagus *(esophageal varices),* or from similar dilated veins in the stomach. This results from elevated blood pressure in the portal system of the abdomen. The spleen becomes enlarged, and blood tends to shunt around the liver due to obstruction of normal pathways. Elevated blood ammonia may even impair consciousness. Terminal problems in these patients are those of massive gastrointestinal hemorrhage, with or without the stuporous state of hepatic coma.

Other complications can develop. Heart failure may supervene along with kidney impairment, and there is increased incidence of infections. Almost all primary cancers of the liver are superimposed on a previously damaged liver. It is these large overall problems that make chronic liver disease a leading cause of death.

How much is too much? Only a minority of alcoholics in the United States, an estimated 10 percent, develop cirrhosis. Why more do not do so is unclear. Genetic differences, body weight, eating habits, liver enzymes, and patterns of drinking are relevant but hard to pinpoint.

It is possible to be perpetually sober while consuming dangerous amounts of alcohol over a period of years. The quantity of daily customary intake is more significant than an occasional outright binge. Although alcohol is a potential poison, it is not possible to incriminate it without specifying quantity. If it were, water and oxygen, though essential to life, also could be considered poisonous.

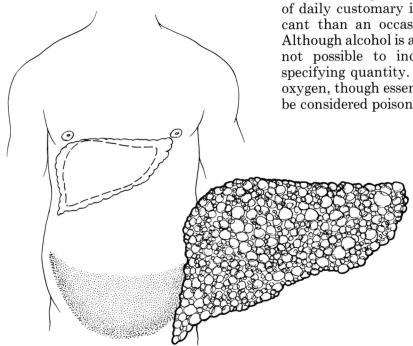

HOBNAIL LIVER

In the most common type of cirrhosis of the liver, the normally smooth surface of the organ becomes studded with pinhead- to bean-size nodules, giving a hobnailed appearance.

Is there a safe threshold of alcohol consumption? Though there are individual differences (a fat person can withstand alcohol better than a thin one), a fair assumption is that a daily intake of more than a half-pint (eight ounces) of hard liquor a day is risky. This is about equal to four or five cocktails or highballs, depending on the generosity of the host, or to a standard bottle of wine.

Certain patterns of drinking, short of excess, are probably kind to the liver, or at least are less harmful. Combine food with drink, don't drink on an empty stomach, and take drinks in diluted forms. Unlike food, alcohol is absorbed directly from the stomach, and straight "shots" of high-proof liquor are hard on the stomach lining. Remember the legendary greeting of the Governor of North Carolina to the Governor of South Carolina, "It's a long time between drinks." Space drinks decently apart, and even insert a dry day or two to give the liver time to recover.

Alcoholic Impotence

Folk wisdom about alcohol and sex was expressed long ago in words about drink spoken by the Porter in *Macbeth:* "Lechery, sir, it provokes and unprovokes. It provokes the desire, but it takes away the performance." Modern physiologists have not undermined this opinion, but have put a good deal of blame on the liver.

It is an old observation that chronic liver disease, usually associated with alcohol, tends to feminize males. Physical signs are enlarged breasts and scantiness or absence of body hair. Feminization can progress to atrophy of the testicles, impaired sperm production, impotence, and sterility. Some investigators believe that alcohol abuse is the most frequent cause of impotence and sterility in the United States, apart from impotence of psychological origin. This reservoir of impotence is huge: an estimated 9,000,000 people in this country have an average daily intake of one quart of hard liquor per day.

The liver has a primary role in chemical conversions of sex hormones, androgens (male) and estrogens (female). In chronic liver disease, intricate biochemical pathways appear to be disturbed so that male hormones are diminished, leaving an excess of female hormones in the blood plasma. It also has been shown that alcohol can induce atrophy of the testicles in laboratory animals. In early stages, the condition is reversible, but with continued high alcohol intake, it is permanent and may indeed be intensified if impotence and loss of sex drive are assuaged by chronic drinking.

Cancer of the Liver

Cancer may originate in the liver or spread to that organ from elsewhere in the body. But the distinction is not very significant, since surgical removal of an indispensable organ is out of the question.

Symptoms. The most common symptoms are weight loss, abdominal pain, loss of appetite, nausea, and vomiting. The liver is greatly enlarged, perhaps the first abnormality the patient notices, as a mass in the upper right abdomen. There is fluid (bloating), jaundice, and tenderness over the liver.

Cancer should be suspected in a previously stable patient with cirrhosis of the liver who is rapidly deteriorating. About three-fourths of liver-cancer patients have underlying cirrhosis of the liver.

Treatment. There is no effective treatment, and response to chemotherapy is poor. The average survival is a disappointing four to eight months.

THE STONY GALLBLADDER

If you are a woman over 40, there is a 50-50 chance that you have gallstones; if you're a man, a 20 percent chance. In addition, the older you are, the greater the likelihood that you have gallstones. But even so, you may never have symptoms, and you may never know it.

Gallstones loom as a problem in middle-life; young people are rarely affected. Overweight women who have had pregnancies ("fair, fat, and forty" is the old cliché) are particularly prone to gallbladder troubles; men, somewhat less so. It is estimated that 15,000,000 people in the population have gallstones, but this is based on extrapolations of incidental findings at autopsies of persons who, for the most part, had no significant gallbladder problems during life and who succumbed to something else. Innumerable gallstones are "silent."

Still, gallbladder surgery is one of the most frequently performed operations in the United States—nearly half a million operations a year. And the gallbladder is a frequent cause of worry to many after-40 patients who, not necessarily correctly, attribute commonplace symptoms such as distress after meals, belching, gassiness, and "biliousness" to its misbehavior.

The gallbladder is a sac, tucked under the liver, that receives bile, concentrates it, and discharges it at mealtimes through the common duct into the duodenum. "Stones" that form in the gallbladder may be tiny, gravel-like particles, numerous small or medium-sized stones, or a single large stone. If a stone tries to "pass," it may move into the duodenum with little trouble, or it may become snagged in the gallbladder outlet or the common duct and cause excruciating pain as the body attempts to push it along.

How Gallstones Form

Chronic *cholecystitis* (inflammation of the gallbladder) is almost always associated with the presence of gallstones. Inflammation does not cause the stones; it's the other way around.

Most gallstones are composed primarily of cholesterol, but a few have a calcium component. Cholesterol is the same substance that is associated with atherosclerosis (see page 86). It is a normal constituent of bile, and in fact gets its name from the Greek word for bile.

Much new evidence has shed light on the complex physical chemistry of gallstone formation. In oversimplified terms, stones precipitate out of materials in a super-saturated solution. Bile cholesterol is held in solution by a chemical structure known as a *micelle,* which enables the conversion of a fat-soluble substance to a liquid-soluble substance. The micelle also has components of bile acids and lecithin. Cholesterol gallstones form when the bile becomes supersaturated with cholesterol—an excess in proportion to lecithin and bile acids. The proportion of supersaturated bile from the liver that enters the gallbladder is a major factor. One might say that gallstones begin in the liver.

The solubilization of cholesterol in normal gallbladder bile is rather precarious and there is little in the way of built-in mechanisms to avert stone formation.

Can Gallstones Be Dissolved?

Patients who keep abreast of medical news sometimes ask, "Can't my gallstones be dissolved?" Newer knowledge of the chemistry of stone formation has indeed led to experimental measures for dissolving cholesterol stones in the living body.

The drug under investigation, which might not be called a drug since it occurs in human bile, is *chenodeoxycholic acid* (CDC). Its action is to "desaturate" cholesterol from bile so, in theory, stones do not precipitate and the bile acts as a solvent of those that exist.

An ongoing cooperative study of one thousand patients at ten treatment centers is evaluating the effectiveness and safety of CDC. Preliminary observations indicate that multiple radiolucent (cholesterol) gallstones disappear in 80 percent of patients treated with CDC for one to three years. Larger stones containing calcium do not respond similarly. Stones recurred in 20 percent of the patients one to three years after CDC treatment ceased. Resumption of CDC brought similar dissolution of stones over a period of about 18 months on the second course of therapy.

Matters of dosage, long-term effects, and safety remain to be resolved, but thus far, no serious side effects have been reported. Recurrence of stones after stopping treatment suggests that patients may have to continue the drug indefinitely, like insulin for diabetes. Patients may weigh this inconvenience against gallbladder surgery, which usually gives permanent relief. It will probably take several years for stone-dissolving therapy to be evaluated and incorporated into medical practice.

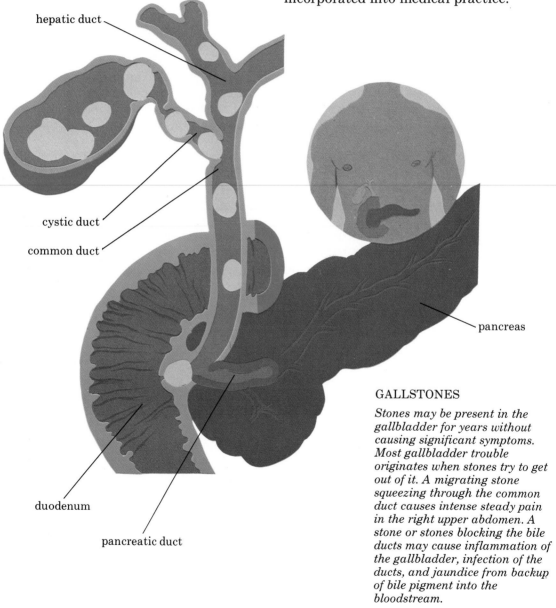

hepatic duct

cystic duct

common duct

pancreas

duodenum

pancreatic duct

GALLSTONES

Stones may be present in the gallbladder for years without causing significant symptoms. Most gallbladder trouble originates when stones try to get out of it. A migrating stone squeezing through the common duct causes intense steady pain in the right upper abdomen. A stone or stones blocking the bile ducts may cause inflammation of the gallbladder, infection of the ducts, and jaundice from backup of bile pigment into the bloodstream.

Symptoms of Gallbladder Trouble

One acute symptom of gallstones is hard to mistake. It is the severe pain of "gallbladder colic," resulting from entrapment or movement of a stone in the gallbladder outlet or in the bile ducts. The classic symptom is intense pain in the upper right abdomen, radiating to the shoulder. The pain is steady, persists for hours, and usually is accompanied by nausea and vomiting. The discomfort often comes on an hour or so after eating and may awaken the patient at night. Jaundice also may be present.

Chronic *cholelithiasis* (stones in the gallbladder) may cause no symptoms at all, at least for a long time; the symptoms result from complications. Tenderness of the upper right abdomen, however, is a clue. Patients typically complain of upper-abdominal discomfort, fullness after a heavy meal, biliousness, bloating, belching, and intolerance of fried foods. But these are very common symptoms with many causes.

Diagnosis. Whether or not gallstones are present is readily determined by *cystography,* an X-ray procedure. In the evening, the patient swallows a tablet containing an iodine compound that will make any gallstones that are present visible on X-ray films taken the next day. Sometimes an additional dose of contrast medium is given the next day to reinforce the visualization.

To visualize the bile ducts, which may contain stones, the dye is administered intravenously. Because the contrast between bile ducts and surrounding tissues is poor, *tomography*—a short-focus X-ray procedure that visualizes tissue in planes or cross sections at different depths—is essential. Stones show as translucencies.

If jaundice is present, other tests are advisable. Eighty percent of cases of jaundice in patients over 65 are of an obstructive character. Is the obstruction within the liver itself, or is it caused by stones, tumors, or strictures outside of the liver? Presumptive impressions are not wholly reliable, but distinctions are important for proper treatment. Newer, highly sophisticated procedures have vastly improved the capability of making accurate diagnosis, modifying the approach to surgical intervention in presumed obstructive jaundice, and permitting alteration of drainage procedures in patients with strictures of ducts outside of the liver.

Is Surgery Always Necessary?

No, not always. Complications—such as a perforated gallbladder that pours pus into the abdomen, repeated attacks of biliary colic, and other conditions recognized by the physician—warrant gallbladder surgery. But the mere presence of gallstones, often discovered incidentally in the course of an X-ray examination, does not invariably mean an immediate operation.

Less than half of all persons with gallstones have symptoms. Many symptoms attributed to a diseased gallbladder, such as intolerance of fatty foods, "flatulent dyspepsia," belching, distention, and reflux of bitter fluid into the throat, are not supported by good medical evidence. Some persons have the same symptoms after gallbladder removal as before, indicating that the gallbladder had nothing to do with them. Abdominal complaints resulting from functional rather than anatomic disturbances are common.

Decisions for surgery should be made with good medical counsel and expectation of benefit. After removal of the gallbladder, there will be no more gallstones, or trouble they have genuinely caused.

Some guidelines of treatment have emerged. For persons with a large, single gallstone, surgery is not recommended in absence of symptoms. The stone is too large to work into the biliary tract. Such persons should be kept under medical follow-up. Patients with numerous small stones that have the potential for obstructing the duct are at greater risk of cholecystitis, but here again surgery is not routinely advocated. Relatively young persons may elect to have their stony gallbladders removed to avert future trouble, or they may choose to remain under medical observation until, or if, surgery becomes advisable.

Surgical risk is somewhat greater in older people, and if their gallstones cause no symptoms, they will usually be treated by other means.

Patients who have coexistent disease, such as diabetes, will usually be advised to have necessary surgery while they are at their physical best, rather than later when risks would be greater. There are, of course, acute biliary conditions for which prompt surgery is not optional but mandatory.

Gallbladder Operations

Gallbladder surgery is major surgery, but techniques have been so perfected that a good outcome is to be expected. The operations are performed under general anesthesia.

The gallbladder may be opened, closed, and left in place after stones are cleaned out of it. This is rarely done, however, because stones may form again. A "red hot," pussy gallbladder merely may be drained and removed later in a second operation after the area has quieted down.

In the usual operation, the surgeon dissects the gallbladder from its base, removes it, and ties off its ducts. At the same time, he examines the main bile duct for the presence of a stone or stones. Preliminary X-ray studies may have shown that a stone is present, or X rays taken at the operating table may disclose it. If so, the bile duct is opened, cleaned out, and sewn shut.

Patients scheduled for gallbladder surgery should be prepared to spend up to a couple of weeks in the hospital. The site of incision up the middle of the abdomen from the navel is rather well-known, thanks to a famous photo of Lyndon Johnson. When you awake after surgery, there will be a soft rubber tube protruding from the space where the gallbladder used to be. Its purpose is to drain fluids oozing from raw surfaces. The tube is gently pulled a little distance from the gallbladder bed every couple of days, and is finally removed in about a week.

Another kind of drainage tube, shaped like a T, is inserted if the main bile duct has been opened. The tube may be kept there until shortly before discharge from the hospital. Sometimes the patient goes home with the tube still in place—it does not interfere with activity.

Living Without a Gallbladder

Bile from the liver continues to seep into the intestines after the gallbladder is removed. Ordinarily the digestive system works perfectly well, and there is no need for special diets after full recuperation from surgery.

Some patients, however, have a so-called "postcholecystectomy syndrome" that is poorly understood. In general, they have similar or the same symptoms that they complained of before gallbladder removal. The absence of bile-concentrating and ejecting properties of the gallbladder may possibly be involved. But in many instances, it means that symptoms result from other problems, such as a disturbance of motility (propulsive digestive actions), which the gallbladder had nothing to do with and which was unimproved and unchanged by its removal.

THE SMALL BOWEL

The small intestine, wound compactly in the upper abdomen, is a rather silent part of the digestive tract. It begins with the *duodenum,* which joins the *jejunum,* which joins the *ileum*—arbitrarily named parts of a continuous tube that is about one inch in diameter in its lower part.

The major function of the small bowel is the digestion and absorption of food. Digestion initiated in the stomach is continued in the small intestine, where foodstuffs are chemically converted into nutrient forms small enough to be transported across the lining tissue of the bowel. Every day about ten quarts of fluid—water, secretions, and liquid foods—pour into the small bowel, which reabsorbs most of it. Disorders of the small bowel are principally inflammatory, obstructive, and disruptive of its capacity to absorb food elements.

Intestinal Obstruction

It can come on quite suddenly: sharp, colicky abdominal pain, cramping, abdominal distention, nausea, and vomiting. These are signs of intestinal obstruction, so intense that medical help is immediately sought. Symptoms may be milder if obstruction is partial, or more insidious if the large bowel is involved.

There is a paralytic form of obstruction, usually after surgical procedures or severe damage to the intestine, in which the bowel cannot propel its contents through it. However, mechanical obstructions are more common: the bowel may telescope into itself, usually a pediatric problem; inflammations may cause strictures that narrow the passageway; or gallstones, other foreign bodies, or small benign tumors may block the tube.

However, the most common form of intestinal obstruction occurs in adults who have had previous abdominal surgery, resulting in obstructive adhesions. It may take years after surgery for adhesions to herniate or form constricting bands, and the patient is more likely to be a mature person than a youngster.

Diagnosis. Abnormal high-pitched bowel sounds can generally be heard. X-ray study reveals dilated loops of small bowel with characteristic levels of air and fluids.

Treatment. Passage of a long tube through the stomach may decompress the bowel and reopen the passageway to some degree. Intravenous fluids and other supportive measures are then given. If the obstruction is mechanical, prompt surgical correction is necessary. The operation varies according to the specific nature of the obstruction.

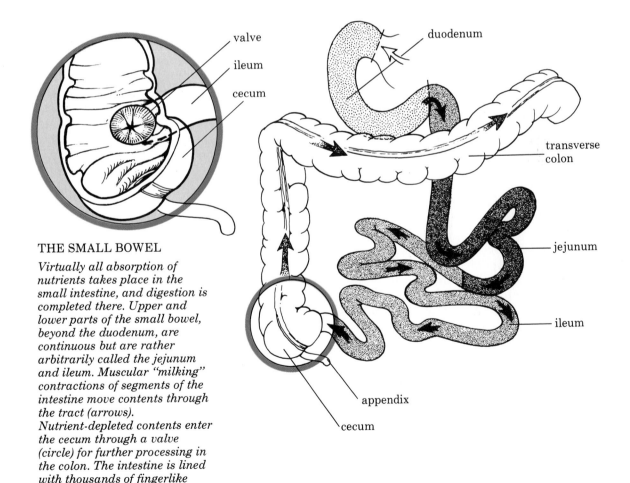

THE SMALL BOWEL

Virtually all absorption of nutrients takes place in the small intestine, and digestion is completed there. Upper and lower parts of the small bowel, beyond the duodenum, are continuous but are rather arbitrarily called the jejunum and ileum. Muscular "milking" contractions of segments of the intestine move contents through the tract (arrows). Nutrient-depleted contents enter the cecum through a valve (circle) for further processing in the colon. The intestine is lined with thousands of fingerlike projections (villi) that greatly increase its surface area.

Tumors

Tumors of the small intestine are infrequent. Symptoms and signs of primary small bowel tumors, whether benign or malignant, are similar. Characteristically, they produce intestinal obstruction with or without bleeding.

Patients with intestinal lymphoma, a tumor derived from lymphatic cells, may have manifestations of malabsorption (see below). Intestinal obstruction also may occur, along with abdominal pain and fever.

Carcinoid tumors are slowly growing tumors, most frequently arising from the small intestine and sometimes the appendix. Their characteristics are somewhere between a benign and malignant tumor. The usual carcinoid tumor arises from the terminal portion of the small bowel and then slowly spreads to the liver and lungs. When this occurs, patients experience flushing of the skin, diarrhea, valvular lesions of the heart, and wheezing. Treatment is not very satisfactory, although anti-serotonin drugs have been used with radiation to decrease the metabolic activity of the tumor.

Malabsorption

This term merely indicates that the nutrient contents of the small bowel are inadequately absorbed into the service of the body. Malabsorption may develop from inadequate digestion of food, from disease of the bowel lining, or from involvement of the small bowel by lymphatic tumors.

Symptoms are consonant with disordered nutrition: weight loss, diarrhea, malnutrition, anemia, and vitamin deficiencies. Bone pain may develop from decreased supplies of calcium and protein, and stools become bulky and foul-smelling.

Malabsorption may be a reaction to virtually all the components of a diet or to only a few; specialized tests can identify its many causes. Celiac disease is common in children; it is called sprue in adults, in whom it is less common. Celiac/sprue is characterized by lesions in the small bowel lining and by sensitivity to gluten, a constituent of wheat and rye. Elimination of gluten-containing products from the diet usually brings remission of symptoms and frequently a return toward normal of the lining tissue of the small bowel.

Milk intolerance. A more widespread—in fact worldwide—form of malabsorption is the inability of some people to digest or split milk sugar (lactose). In these persons, drinking milk in sizable amounts precipitates abdominal pain and diarrhea.

Milk intolerance results from the lack of an enzyme, lactase, that splits milk sugar. From 5 to 10 percent of the adult Caucasian population in the United States have primary lactase deficiency. But in American Negroes, Bantus, and Orientals, the incidence is as high as 60 to 80 percent.

Probably what we see is a cultural adaptation. Peoples who herded cattle and drank milk generation after generation doubtless developed or intensified their secretion of the necessary lactase enzyme and passed the trait along on an hereditary basis. Populations that rarely or never drank milk had no need for the enzyme and lost or never had the trait of producing it.

Persons intolerant to milk simply have to get along with less of it than is usual if they live in the western hemisphere, with its dairy farms, cattle herds, cowboys, and faith that milk is a perfect food that you can't get too much of. Most adults in other parts of the world do not customarily drink a great deal of milk.

Powdered milk produces the same symptoms in the intolerant. In fact, shipments of the product to some countries have been used to whitewash fences rather than to feed the population.

PAIN IN THE ABDOMEN

A number of diseases, some of them more common in older age groups, manifest abdominal pain as one of a great variety of symptoms. For convenience, we will group these diseases under the above heading, although they are unrelated to each other. Acute or chronic abdominal pain is a symptom that calls for careful diagnosis that may reveal some easily correctable condition or identify a complex and more serious disorder.

Regional Enteritis: Crohn's Disease

This is an inflammatory disease of the gastrointestinal tract and is of unknown cause. The inflammatory process is not limited to the bowel lining but extends through the entire wall, and is often accompanied by ulceration, fibrosis, and scarring.

Historically, the disease is linked to the small bowel, since the first report by Dr. Burrill B. Crohn some 40 years ago described lesions of its terminal part. But today we recognize that all areas of the gastrointestinal tract can be involved.

Symptoms depend in large part upon the area of bowel involved and upon the extent and severity of inflammation. Ulceration of the esophagus may cause difficulties in swallowing. Or, pyloric-outlet obstruction can cause pain symptoms like those of peptic ulcer. Intestinal obstruction is characterized by a crampy abdominal pain.

Malabsorption, diarrhea, and weight loss often occur as well. Abnormal connections between loops of bowel or outside it result in further malabsorption, and fistulas (see page 229) and inflammation about the rectum are common. Regional-enteritis patients also tend to have a high incidence of gallstones and kidney stones.

Diagnosis of the disease is made by X-ray study of the small bowel and colon and by tissue diagnosis.

Management. Crohn's disease is frustrating to the patient and even more so to the physician. The course of the disease is unpredictable, and there is no specific treatment, although corticosteroid drugs may be helpful. Surgery is generally delayed until complications develop, and then, multiple operations are usually necessary because of fistulas and draining tracts. The experience of one clinic in treating 200 patients over a 25-year period indicated that an average of 2.3 operations was necessary to rehabilitate the patient.

Disorders of Circulation

Digestive organs are supplied with blood by arteries subject to the same processes of aging, atherosclerosis, and clot formation as vessels that supply the heart and brain. After 40, there is increased susceptibility to gastrointestinal diseases somewhat analogous to heart attacks, angina pectoris, or strokes.

Mesenteric insufficiency. The mesentery is a fan-shaped fold of peritoneum, a membrane that encircles most of the small bowel and supplies blood to the tract. It is attached to the back of the abdomen and acts as a sort of supportive hanger for the intestines. Its major arteries may gradually become narrowed, perhaps causing no particular symptoms, or so choked with blood clots (occluded) that the flow is greatly reduced or completely blocked.

Various events may predispose to constrictions of circulation called "low-flow states"—trickles instead of a good flow of blood. This insufficiency may produce bleeding necrosis of the stomach or small or large bowel, accompanied by bloody diarrhea. This is an ominous event in persons who already have serious heart and lung problems.

Total occlusion of mesenteric vessels *(mesenteric thrombosis)* is an acute abdominal catastrophe. Pain and shock are so severe that the patient collapses. Deprived of blood, the intestine will become gangrenous and die. Immediate surgery is imperative.

Abdominal angina, which merely means abdominal pain, is another syndrome associated with vascular disease. It is due to gradual narrowing of a blood vessel near its opening from the aorta. The usual symptoms are abdominal pain after eating, partial relief of symptoms with restriction of food intake, and weight loss. Characteristically, these patients have malabsorption. Some may not have initial symptoms but lose weight in spite of apparently normal appetite. Medical or surgical measures to correct malabsorption secondary to decreased blood flow are indicated.

(Abdominal pain arising from the colon and other organs is discussed elsewhere.)

LARGE BOWEL TROUBLES

The colon or large bowel is a hollow muscular tube that receives the contents of the small bowel for a little further processing and evacuation. The drawing shows the direction of traffic flow through the abdomen: up, across, and down. Although the colon is continuous, its parts are directionally labeled as ascending, transverse, and descending.

Liquid contents of the small bowel enter the colon through a sphincter or valve at the *cecum,* the lowermost part of the large bowel. The cecum, from which the blind

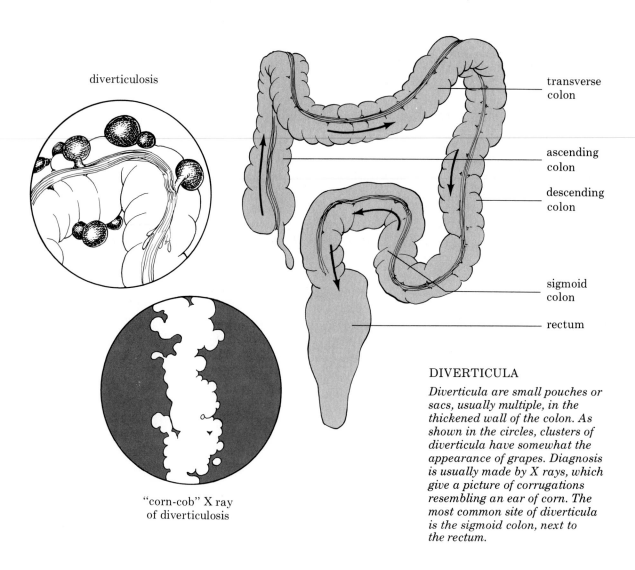

diverticulosis

transverse colon

ascending colon

descending colon

sigmoid colon

rectum

"corn-cob" X ray of diverticulosis

DIVERTICULA

Diverticula are small pouches or sacs, usually multiple, in the thickened wall of the colon. As shown in the circles, clusters of diverticula have somewhat the appearance of grapes. Diagnosis is usually made by X rays, which give a picture of corrugations resembling an ear of corn. The most common site of diverticula is the sigmoid colon, next to the rectum.

pouch of the appendix dangles, is situated low in the right abdomen. The muscular bowel moves contents up the right side of the abdomen, then across to a downward bend on the left, through the descending colon to another bend (the *sigmoid flexure*), and into the rectum.

The colon has several functions, all related to the final disposition of intestinal contents. It serves as a reservoir and absorbs water to produce a normally formed stool. The colon can absorb about twice as much fluid as it is normally called upon to do. If it is overloaded, diarrhea may result.

The Irritable Bowel

(Mucous Colitis; Spastic Colitis)

This is a very common gastrointestinal complaint, affecting 50 to 75 percent of the population at one time or other. The prime age range is from the third to the seventh decade. It has various names, such as *mucous colitis* and *spastic colitis,* but they are quite inaccurate since no inflammatory process is at work.

The classic syndrome consists of abdominal pain without discoverable organic cause, with variations in bowel habits. The patient may complain of constipation, interspersed at intervals with painless diarrhea or normal bowel function. The diarrhea, when present, is mainly in the morning, and the patient feels better in the afternoon and evening. Hard, dry stools may be covered with mucus, or pure mucus may be passed (which is harmless). Symptoms are generally intermittent and are reactive to psychological factors.

Physical examination discloses no organic abnormality. People with the irritable-bowel syndrome appear to have unusually rapid or hair-trigger response to eating, emotional stress, and hormones and chemical agents that are conducive to speedup of gastrointestinal motors. Irritability is probably not limited to the colon, but involves rapid transit through the small bowel and perhaps rapid gastric emptying.

The condition is not serious, but it may be hard to persuade a patient of that. The patient should be encouraged to relax and be reassured that no harm will befall him or her. Sedatives, dietary advice, and agents for symptomatic relief may be helpful, and remedies for constipation (see page 222) can be important.

Pockets in the Bowel

(Diverticula)

If you are over 40, there is one chance in three that you have *diverticulosis,* which isn't as bad as it sounds. Diverticula are small pockets or sacs in the wall of the colon. They cause no trouble and need no treatment unless there are complications.

Young people can be affected by diverticulosis, but the incidence increases with age and probably reflects degenerative changes. The pockets form in the weakened wall of the colon where blood vessels penetrate. The basic abnormality is muscular. In longstanding cases, the colonic muscle is thickened and corrugated. The entire colon may be involved, but the prime locus is the sigmoid colon. Pain in that general area is sometimes described as "left-sided appendicitis."

Diverticulitis is a symptom-causing infection or inflammation of one or several of the pockets. It is characterized by tenderness on the left side of the abdomen, diarrhea, and occasionally fever. The diagnosis is confirmed by X-ray pictures of the colon, which somewhat resembles an ear of corn, with the diverticula being the kernels. Signs of diverticular disease also can be seen on colonoscopic inspection.

Treatment of diverticula and the irritable bowel is essentially the same. It involves the art as well as the science of medicine. The patient must be convinced that the diagnosis is accurate, must have some understanding of the nature of the condition, and must be helped to live with himself as well as with his bowels.

The keystone of the program is the institution of a high-fiber diet (see opposite). Bulk is added to the diet in the form of unprocessed bran, or other forms of fiber such as psyllium seed (Metamucil). Patients with constipation should take laxative foods, such as prune juice, or stool softeners. Patients with diarrhea may be helped by a combination of "quieting" medications, or anti-diarrheal drugs such as Lomotil.

Prevention. A probable factor in producing diverticula is straining at stool. Straining, typical of severe constipation, increases pressures within the abdomen and puts stress on weakened intestinal walls. The same strain-pressures may play a part in hiatal hernia and be harmful to persons with heart disease. In such case, a soft stool is desirable and agents that bind water to produce a softer stool are recommended. Adequate amounts of fiber in the daily diet have a similar beneficial action.

Surgery. Uncommonly, a diverticulum may become so grossly inflamed and swollen that it bursts and intestinal contents seep into the abdominal cavity, causing an abscess or peritonitis. Emergency surgery will be necessary to drain the site and remove the diseased part of the colon.

If inflammation is massive, it may be necessary to remove the colon in stages. A healthy section of intestine is diverted through the skin to form an opening through which intestinal contents pass to the outside. The channel bypasses the inflamed area of the colon, which usually heals quite rapidly. At a later operation, the diseased parts of the tube are removed and the healthy ends are sewn together. At a third operation, the outside opening *(colostomy)* is closed and the intestinal tube is restored to its normal route through the rectum.

High-Fiber Diets

A great deal has been written and discussed, both in medical and lay circles, about the virtues of high-fiber diets. Bran is a convenient and readily available source of fiber. However, there are many other common sources of indigestible fiber (as well as some differences in defining fiber) and variations in composition.

Sir Denis Burkitt has been a main proponent of bran. His studies, reported in medical journals, implicate low-fiber intake with an astonishing number of diseases: hiatal hernia, gallbladder disease, appendicitis, colonic polyps (see page 224), cancer, ischemic heart disease, deep vein thrombosis, obesity, and diabetes. The concept has been promoted as a near-panacea by some persons with something to sell. Many claims remain to be documented, a project that presently engages biologists working with the Food and Drug Administration.

High-fiber intake is probably most sound and reasonable with respect to the health of the digestive tract, the subject of this chapter. In England, extensive studies of patients with diverticula have shown that similarly matched patients without diverticula consumed twice as much fiber.

There is little question that high-fiber intake increases stool weight, shortens transit time through the bowels, decreases pressures in the colon, and produces a stool of desirable consistency.

There seems to be no reason not to encourage individuals to follow a high-fiber program. Experience has shown that the vast majority of patients with diverticula or the irritable bowel syndrome improved on high-fiber intake, regardless of whether their symptoms were predominately constipation or diarrhea. Patients may do well to take a cereal bowl full of a bran product every day, and if constipation is a problem, to increase the bran intake until the constipation is overcome. Similarly, those with diarrhea should continue a high-fiber program to stabilize the condition. Many of these people are so sensitive to lack of bulk in the diet that if they discontinue the bran for two or three days, the diarrhea returns.

Many physicians were taught to manage patients with bowel disorders with a low-residue diet, and not all are convinced of the virtues of a high-fiber diet that departs from accepted treatment of the past. It has been a truly educational campaign during the past ten years to convince dietitians that a high-fiber diet should be a part of the hospital regimen.

Appendicitis

Acute inflammation of the appendix—a useless worm-shaped pouch that dangles from the cecum, the first portion of the large bowel—is commonly thought of as a condition that affects young people. But the belief that appendicitis is rare in the older patient is mistaken. The mortality rate from appendicitis is higher in older people, in part because the condition may not be suspected, leading to delay in diagnosis and treatment.

"Normal" or classic symptoms of appendicitis are pain around the navel or generalized over the abdomen, shifting after a while to the lower right abdomen. Nausea and vomiting also occur. In contrast, in the older patient pain may be slight and not in a typical location, fever may be minimal, and the white blood cell count may not be elevated.

It has been said that appendicitis in the aged is often "missed appendicitis." A high index of suspicion is important in recognizing its symptoms in older persons. The appendix ruptures early in a large percentage of older patients, and there may be coexisting disease to complicate matters.

Early operation lowers the mortality rate, and appendectomy is desirable in low-risk patients. But if perforation has occurred, simple drainage is preferable, followed by appendectomy under better conditions.

Ulcerative Colitis

Chronic ulcerative colitis is predominantly a disease of young people. It may continue into later years, but rarely originates in middle age or after.

Ulcerative colitis is an inflammatory disease of the lining of the colon that produces ulceration and easy bleeding. The cause is unknown. Its principal symptoms are abdominal pain, diarrhea, and rectal bleeding. Some patients have only one attack and the disease does not recur. But in the majority, the disease runs an intermittent course with remissions and exacerbations. In about 10 percent of patients, the disease is continuous and they are seriously ill.

Patients with early or mild ulcerative colitis are treated with medications that prevent relapses or, like steroid drugs, act systemically. Complications may require prompt or eventual surgery, and in severe instances, the large bowel is partially or completely removed.

There seems to be evidence of later incidence of cancer in ulcerative-colitis patients. Out of almost 400 patients followed over a period of 25 years, the incidence of cancer was almost 100 times the expected incidence in the corresponding normal population. This incidence rose rapidly after the disease had been present for ten years. One out of three developed cancer between the tenth and twentieth year of the disease. Pre-cancerous changes may be identifiable on rectal biopsy, and early surgery may be recommended in those patients who are thought to be at great risk of cancer.

Diarrhea

Diarrhea may be defined as the frequent passage of unformed (loose, watery) stools. We have mentioned that diarrhea is present in a great variety of gastrointestinal diseases. If persistent and accompanied by more significant symptoms, a medical diagnostic work-up is advisable.

But a great many surges of diarrhea are transient, not serious, and of fairly obvious origin—the result of "tourist trots," a touch of food poisoning, or the overuse of laxatives. These are self-limiting problems and probably require little or no investigation.

Many people learn to recognize things that precipitate episodes of diarrhea, and they avoid them. A change in bowel habits is common when regular routines are interrupted or when stresses are severe. In these functional disturbances, the diarrhea tends to be provoked by anxiety, is usually worse in the morning, and improves during the day. The diarrhea is not bloody, may be associated with pain, and almost never awakens the patient during the night.

It seems reasonable to add a sufficient amount of fiber to the diet to help the formation of normal stools.

Acute diarrhea is usually of abrupt onset and short duration. It is basically caused by an infectious process or the ingestion of a toxin. Common causes include food poisoning (usually salmonella bacteria or staphylococcus toxins), viral illnesses, chemical poisons, drugs, irritating food or drink, and allergic reactions.

Acute diarrhea usually is relatively benign. Treatment is given for dehydration and abdominal pain. Bloody diarrhea indicates something more serious, and requires immediate diagnostic evaluation.

Chronic diarrhea has numerous causes. The most common are functional disorders (irritable bowel), diseases of the colon and small intestine, and abuse of laxatives.

Certain characteristics of the diarrhea point to one or another cause. There may be no underlying disease—habitual use of cathartics, for instance, can keep the intestines in a constant hurry—but diagnosis may disclose a disorder of which diarrhea is a symptom. Important information is provided by the patient's history, age, diarrheal patterns, relationship to meals, weight loss, characteristics of the stools, and specialized tests as may be indicated. Treatment depends on the nature of the disease that may be discovered.

Constipation

Many persons seem to feel that constipation is the failure of bowel movements to come up to expectations in frequency, color, consistency, or other qualities, and that this failure is a threat to their health. Almost everyone has a rigid concept of his or her evacuative norm; commonly, that a good bowel movement every day is a *sine qua non* of bright-eyed vigor.

The physician's concept is different. There is great variation in habits of bowel emptying. Some persons have a bowel movement after each meal and perhaps on arising in the morning. Others go two or three days without a bowel movement. All of these variations are well within the range of normal.

"Constipation" is a much-used term that is seldom precisely defined. It may be taken to mean infrequent stools, harder-than-normal stools, straining at stool, decrease in stool caliber, or a feeling of incomplete bowel action. Symptoms of loginess, dullness, and zestlessness are commonly attributed to "irregularity."

The type of constipation that truly requires medical attention is exceedingly rare. Habitual constipation of long duration does not require an extensive medical work-up if the patient is otherwise in good health. The most common form, which does not have an organic basis, is classified as simple constipation.

Simple constipation is largely related to insufficient bulk in the diet. Some foods leave very little residue for the intestines to work on. Chemically refined diets of astronauts in space travel reduced bowel action to once in five to seven days, which was not constipation but the result of the time required for material to fill the tract. Such low-residue diets are not uncommon in the United States.

Environmental factors such as a break in routine, prolonged bed rest, and postponing the call to stool also can play a part in simple constipation. Bowel disturbances are frequent problems of flight attendants, particularly those flying long distances overseas. Certain drugs, particularly anti-hypertensive drugs, also can produce constipation.

Simple measures are helpful in simple constipation. Sufficient fiber in the daily diet (see page 220) may restore comfortable regularity. Non-dietary and non-drug bulk producers such as methylcellulose or psyllium seed act similarly. Drinking a glass of hot water with orange juice on getting up in the morning helps to stimulate evacuative reflexes. Laxative juices and foods, such as prune juice or figs, also are helpful and improve fluid intake. There are preparations in pill form that bind water and soften hard stools, thus alleviating straining.

Abuse of laxatives produces false constipation by hurrying materials through the tract without giving the tract a chance to refill. Omitting a daily laxative, without worry if there is no bowel movement for a day or two, frequently restores normal function, to the surprise and pleasure of the patient. There is a legitimate use for laxatives, but ordinarily they should not be taken more often than once in three days.

Severe constipation. Constipation can have an organic as well as a functional basis. Severe constipation (sometimes called obstipation) is a stoppage of the bowel that is not relieved without an external aid such as a cathartic, suppository, or enema. Constipation may be the result of psychiatric disorders, neurological diseases, medical or surgical treatment, and may be associated with inflammation of diverticula and the rectal areas.

Examination may disclose fecal impaction (hard masses of feces that block the tract). Increasing constipation may be the first symptom of an obstructing cancer on the left side of the bowel. Cancer of the right side of the bowel is less likely to produce symptoms. Whenever constipation is of recent origin and fecal impaction is excluded, a thorough investigation is warranted.

Fecal impaction and loss of control of bowel movements are common in older age groups. Many of these persons have little stimulus to have a bowel movement, are not physically active, and may go for days without even an attempt at evacuation.

If a hard bit of stool lodges in the bowel, incontinence will develop and the impaction must be cleared out. After this is done, efforts should be made to prevent impactions by adding fiber to the diet and taking appropriate medications. Laxative abuse is very common in the elderly; more than 30 percent of those over 60 are habitual users of laxatives.

Mobilization is helpful in preventing fecal impactions in the elderly. The key to much of the problem is to try to move these people around and allow them to have normal bowel movements.

TUMORS AND CANCERS
OF THE BOWEL

Both benign and malignant tumors occur in the colon and rectum. They are predominantly found in middle-aged or older people, and are second only to cancer of the lung as a cause of death from malignancies.

Early symptoms are not very specific and may be absent. In general, symptoms that should be investigated promptly are a change in bowel habits, blood in the stools, increasing constipation, and sometimes diarrhea. Anemia also may develop.

Pre-cancerous conditions or suspicious lesions may be discovered early, when prospects of control are excellent, as findings incidental to GI studies for other indications. X-ray findings also may raise suspicions of cancer. *Proctosigmoidoscopy*—visual inspection of the interior of the lower colon—also may disclose abnormalities. The desirability of occasional physical examinations, including proctosigmoidoscopy, is obvious—especially at middle age and after.

Polyps. The colon is a common site of polyps—growths that project into the bowel. Polyps may be flat or rounded, or may hang from a thin stalk. Most polyps of the colon are benign, but there is also the possibility of malignancy.

One of the most controversial areas in gastroenterology is the relationship of polyps of the colon to cancer. What treatment should be given? At present, it is felt that cancerous potential is present if there are multiple polyps of any size, if a polyp is more than two centimeters in diameter, if a polyp is flat without a stalk, if it has a villous (shaggy) pattern, or if there is a familial history of colon cancer.

Removal of polyps is readily accomplished with a colonoscopic instrument that works inside the bowel. No external surgical incision is necessary. This capability encourages efforts to remove all accessible polyps. A newer instrument has been developed for fulguration (electrical destruction of tissue) of very small polyps. The procedure is done under general anesthesia, and the stay in the hospital is only a day or two.

Certain "special" types of polyps are more threatening than the common varieties. "Familial polyposis" is a condition of multiple polyps that occurs in family bloodlines. Persons with such polyps are at high risk of developing cancer. Treatment consists of removal of the entire colon or, in more limited disease, removal of the polyps and continued close follow-up of the patient thereafter.

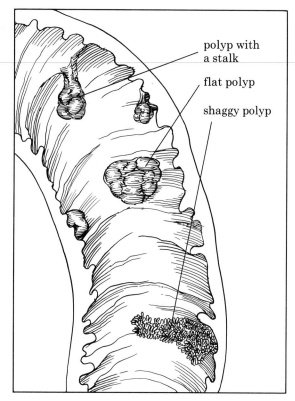

polyp with
a stalk

flat polyp

shaggy polyp

POLYPS OF THE COLON

Polyps are growths that project into the canal of the bowel (and from other membranes, such as the nasal passages). Different forms are shown above. Most polyps of the colon are not malignant, but their removal, which is relatively simple, is thought to be prudent. Small polyps rarely cause recognizable symptoms.

Cancer of the colon. It used to be thought that about half of cancers of the colon could be diagnosed by digital examination, and that 60 percent were within seeing distance of the sigmoidoscope. But more recent studies suggest that cancer is rather evenly distributed throughout the entire colon. The prospects for cure are most favorable in the patient with an early lesion, and there is considerable enthusiasm about the prospect that the incidence of colon cancer can be greatly reduced by removal of premalignant polyps.

Surgery. In principle, operations for cancer of the colon and rectum aim to remove the diseased section of intestine and join the healthy ends together. The extent and location of disease determine what has to be done. Either half of the colon may be removed without a great change in bowel movements. Or, it may be necessary to divert the flow to the outside through a surgical opening in the skin of the abdomen *(colostomy)*. Bowel movements then collect in a bag. With a bit of special training, the patient is able to continue social and business activities in a normal way.

Not all colostomies are permanent. The rejoining of healthy parts of the intestine may require a temporary colostomy that puts the affected area at rest for healing. Later, the colostomy is closed in a second operation and normal bowel movements through the rectum are restored.

Cancer of the rectum. Surgery is the usual treatment of cancer of the rectum, of which there are 25,000 new cases a year. Two new approaches have recently become available: supervoltage radiation and local excision.

The rationale for supervoltage radiation is that results should be equal or superior to those of surgery, that the rectum is preserved and no colostomy is needed, and that failure does not preclude later surgery. Experience with supervoltage treatment is limited but impressive, and is associated with few side effects or problems.

Local excision is a surgical procedure that gives excellent exposure of the interior of the rectum and anal canal, and provides access to the space around the rectum. Structures can be restored later to leave the patient with normal bowel mechanism and complete fecal continence. The surgeon can determine whether the lesion is mobile and removable in this fashion. The technique is most suitable for patients with early cancer, and it is felt that it gives survival rates equal to those of more radical procedures, with no operative mortality and a better quality of life.

Prevention. Certain measures may well help to prevent cancer of the bowel. Absolute proof is lacking, but the odds are certainly favorable. We have already mentioned that removal of pre-malignant polyps very probably decreases the likelihood of cancer. The main obstacle is that the patient must present himself or herself to a physician for physical examination that includes instrumental inspection of the accessible bowel.

Possible relationships of dietary habits to cancer of the colon are much discussed currently. The disease is rare in African people who have high-fiber diets and bulky stools. Theoretically, and plausibly, low-residue diets that are quite common in the United States may lead to sluggishness and stagnation of bowel contents. This could alter the normal bacteria of the bowel and give prolonged contact with abnormal breakdown products that could be cancer-causing. A theory that generous amounts of fiber in the intestines might absorb and eliminate carcinogenic substances has been postulated but lacks definitive proof.

It would seem prudent to include a reasonable amount of fiber in the diet as a matter of habit. If it should happen to stave off cancer, that's an extra plus. But fiber-yielding foods are excellent and satisfying in themselves, even if they do not cure all of the diseases that enthusiasts claim.

NETHERMOST AFFLICTIONS

Complaints referable to the rectum and anus are so common that they have become quite mentionable, even redundantly so in TV advertisements. The cluster of complaints includes pain, discharge from the rectum, protrusion of tissue, itching, and a vague sensation of a mass.

Pain following a bowel movement is usually associated with inflammation such as a fissure, hemorrhoids, or an abscess. Pain radiating toward the anus from within the pelvis, occurring in spasms lasting several minutes, usually has a psychoneurotic basis and no organic cause can be found. Rectal cancer causes no pain until the process extends into tissues about the rectum, at which time there is a boring continuous discomfort.

Tenesmus is a distressing feeling of rectal urgency that may be present in any diarrheal disorder and is often painful. It is associated with spasm of the rectal and anal muscles, and may accompany inflammation of the prostate.

Probably the most common affliction of the gastrointestinal tract is hemorrhoids.

Hemorrhoids

Hemorrhoids, or piles, are dilated blood vessels (varicosed veins) inside and around the rectal opening. A bowel movement dilates the rectum so the stool can pass through, after which the parts return to previous size. With repeated stretching of the canal and the thin walls of blood vessels, weakened veins can become permanently stretched, dilated, and bulging. Clusters of such veins are hemorrhoids.

Technically, hemorrhoids are internal, external, or both. Internal hemorrhoids are situated well up in the canal above the sphincter muscle. External hemorrhoids occur in the skin around and outside of the sphincter. Entirely internal hemorrhoids are sometimes treated by injection of sclerosing or hardening solutions that obliterate the veins. Short-term results are reasonably good. However, the stretched veins commonly run the entire length of the canal and are both internal and external.

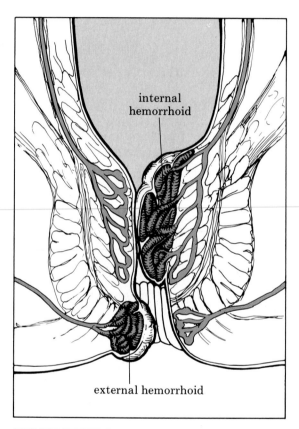

HEMORRHOIDS

Internal hemorrhoids (dilated veins) are situated fairly high in the rectum, above the sphincter muscles. External hemorrhoids are located below and outside of the sphincter. Both internal and external hemorrhoids frequently occur together. Most hemorrhoids respond well to treatment.

Symptoms. Hemorrhoids may hang out of the anal opening, squeezed by the closing purse-string muscle (protruding piles). The protrusion is felt as a mass that can be pushed back into the canal with a finger after a bowel movement. Such protrusion in an older person may be the first symptom of more extensive prolapse of the rectum. Mucus also may be discharged.

Hemorrhoids may become clotted with blood, causing severe pain that can be relieved by surgical excision of the clots. Only a small incision is made under local anesthesia, and no hospitalization is necessary. Often the clot will dissolve by itself. Bleeding that occurs only with bowel movements is characteristic of hemorrhoids, but there also are problems of itching, burning, and maintaining cleanliness.

Treatment. Probably almost everyone has an episode of hemorrhoids at some time or other during a lifetime. Mild varicosities may cause no symptoms at all, or only occasionally when squeezing or straining puts on pressure. Many persons with infrequent mild hemorrhoidal discomfort merely use local ointments on occasion and get along fairly well—without curing the hemorrhoids—as long as no complications befall them.

Chronic hemorrhoids that cause repeated distress or more acute symptoms do require treatment, however. The first step is examination to make sure that complaints of bleeding are actually caused by hemorrhoids and not something more serious. The aim of treatment is to abolish the symptoms of bleeding, discomfort, and itching.

Most patients with hemorrhoids respond well to medical treatment. Often, a doctor will recommend sitz baths—sitting waist-deep in hot water — and, for acute hemorrhoids, suppositories that may contain hydrocortisone. Hemorrhoids are most frequent in constipated populations; straining and passage of hard stools puts a great squeeze on weakened vessels. Also, the rectal area tends to narrow, particularly in older patients.

Thus, bulky formed stools, which are kind to hemorrhoids, are desirable. The patient can do a great deal to achieve this, rather simply, by improving his bowel habits. Enemas and cathartics should be eliminated, or at least spaced far apart. Sufficient fiber in the diet (see page 220) also helps to form a bulky stool that is comfortably passed. Agents that bind water to soften hard stools are discussed under *constipation.*

Hemorrhoidectomy. Chronic hemorrhoids that enlarge and repeatedly cause severe symptoms have traditionally been managed by surgical removal—*hemorrhoidectomy.* The surgeon makes incisions along the veins and stretched membranes and cuts out the veins. This is done under general anesthesia. The next day, lubricating laxatives and frequent sitz baths are initiated in anticipation of the first bowel movement on the third or fourth day. The hospital stay is about a week, followed by a healing period that can be quite prolonged and not exactly pleasant, despite the solace of medications and inflated doughnut-shaped cushions.

In the last few years, there has come some disenchantment with hemorrhoidectomy. One factor is the painful post-operative period and the rather long period of full rehabilitation. Another is the possibility that hemorrhoids may recur—not the same hemorrhoids that the surgeon removed, but new ones originating from other veins in the rectal canal. Other methods of treating minor hemorrhoids more simply can be considered.

Freezing. Cryosurgery—the application of extreme cold—has been used since about 1969 to "freeze off" hemorrhoids. A probe about a foot long is attached to a reservoir of liquid nitrogen that keeps the tip of the probe, or iceball, at a temperature some hundreds of degrees below zero.

Touching the tip of the probe to a hemorrhoid freezes the tissue into a solid icy mass, instantly and painlessly. Nerve fibers of hemorrhoids are destroyed so there is no sensation, and normal surrounding tissue is not affected. Anal skin tags and protruding hemorrhoids can be painlessly removed in this way without an anesthetic. The frozen-dead hemorrhoidal tissue puffs up with fluid that drains copiously for three or four days, requiring that an absorbent pad be worn.

The cryosurgery procedure takes only about 15 minutes and can be done in the doctor's office, thus saving hospital costs and time lost from work. Ordinarily the patient can comfortably resume normal activities the day after.

Rubber-band treatment. Ligation or tying-off of hemorrhoids has been a standard procedure in the past. More recently, a technique of squeezing hemorrhoids to death with rubber bands has come into use, particularly in England.

The doctor grasps a hemorrhoid with a special device that enables him to slip a rubber band very tightly over the base of the hemorrhoid. The tight band shuts off the blood supply of the hemorrhoid, which sloughs off in a few days.

Rubber bands are applied to one or two hemorrhoids at a time so as not to disturb bowel function. If the patient has numerous hemorrhoids, successive treatments a month or so apart may be necessary. It is possible to combine cryosurgery with rubber band treatment. The bands cause some discomfort, but not so severe as the postoperative pain of hemorrhoidectomy, and hospitalization is not necessary.

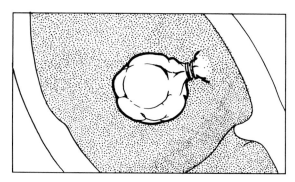

RUBBER BAND LIGATION

A rubber band slipped tightly over the base of a dilated vein with a special instrument shuts off the blood supply and the hemorrhoid sloughs off in a few days. The procedure does not require hospitalization and the patient is usually able to go about his or her daily affairs without a great deal of discomfort.

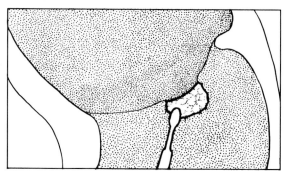

CRYOSURGERY

Extreme cold applied by the tip of a cryosurgical probe freezes and destroys hemorrhoids quite painlessly. Fluids seep from the treated area for several days, requiring temporary absorbent pads. The procedure takes only a few minutes and is commonly done in a doctor's office.

Dilatation. Another treatment of hemorrhoids, pioneered by Dr. Peter Lord, a British surgeon, consists of dilatation—enlargement by hand—of the bowel opening. Its theoretical basis is that constricting bands tighten and narrow the lower bowel so that the purse-string muscle cannot dilate sufficiently for easy passage of a bowel movement; this increases pressure in the ano-rectal area and leads to hemorrhoids.

Dilatation is done in a hospital under general anesthesia. The surgeon forcefully enlarges the bowel opening by hand to a diameter equivalent to eight fingers, and inserts a large foam plastic pack. The stool is kept soft and bulky. The patient continues the dilatation at home, sometimes for many months, by daily insertion of a special dilator. A possible complication of the procedure is splitting of the bowel. Proponents of dilatation and rubber-band techniques feel that the procedures virtually eliminate the need for hemorrhoidectomy and enable the patient to go back to work almost immediately.

Fissure

An anal fissure is a small break in the skin in the region of the rectal outlet. Symptoms are a sharp, burning, aching pain that is worsened by bowel movements and persists afterward. Diagnosis is made by direct inspection.

The usual cause is constipation with passage of large, hard stools that split the skin. Medical treatment includes improved bowel habits, sitz baths, and analgesic ointments. Treatment aims to break the cycle of hard stools-pain-reflex spasm with a high-fiber diet and ointments or suppositories to reduce pain.

Chronic fissure may be treated by anal dilatation, as with hemorrhoids. The anus is dilated to a size of about six fingers. Self-dilatation with a dilator is continued by the patient at home.

Most fissures heal within three weeks, and most patients who attain the natural dilating capacity of a large bulky stool have little or no further trouble. It is important that cathartics not be used in conjunction with stool softeners, since a normal bulky stool is necessary.

Fistula

An anal fistula is an abnormal connection between loops of bowel, or between the bowel and skin around the rectum, through which fecal matter discharges. An opening may be present in the skin, or X rays may reveal a deeper connection. Treatment should not be attempted unless it is certain that regional enteritis is not present.

Treatment of the condition that caused the fistula-forming infection or inflammation may correct the abnormality. If not, surgery is necessary. Most fistulas are located low between the internal and external anal sphincters. The surgeon lays open the fistula by cutting parts of the sphincters to permit the abscess to drain. The wound is then allowed to heal.

Patients have to take baths twice a day and have the wound redressed. A good deal of postoperative care is necessary, and the treatment is time-consuming for patient and surgeon. The patient may have to spend six to eight weeks or more in the hospital. However, this procedure has been particularly rewarding to patients who had previous operative procedures that did not correct the problem.

THE DIGESTIVE TRACT: TESTS & PROCEDURES

Tests most frequently used in diagnosis of digestive-tract disorders are described briefly below. In the past few years, there has been rapid development of numerous other procedures that give highly accurate information of a special nature and add greatly to diagnostic capability.

Gastrointestinal (GI) series. These are X-ray studies of the tract that use barium sulfate as a contrast medium. The barium is opaque to X rays and gives good delineation of structures. For an upper GI series (esophagus, stomach, and duodenum), the patient swallows a barium "meal." For a lower GI series (colon and terminal small bowel), a barium enema is instilled into the rectum and colon. Progress of the barium is observed with a fluoroscope; spot films are taken, and motion pictures (cine studies) are made if indicated.

Cholecystography refers to X-ray studies of the gallbladder, usually for stones. The patient takes a contrast medium by mouth the night before, and X rays are taken the following morning. Intravenous *cholangiography* is a similar technique for visualizing the bile ducts, except that the dye is administered by vein. Dilated ducts within the liver can be visualized by *transhepatic cholangiography,* performed by injecting a water-soluble contrast medium through a long skinny needle introduced through the side of the chest.

Endoscopy is inspection and examination of the interior of a canal or hollow organ with an instrument. Modern *fiber-optic* instruments, in contrast to rigid devices of the past, are completely flexible and easy to pass. With a fiber-optic instrument intro-

duced through the mouth, the operator can visualize and take photographs and tissue specimens of the esophagus, stomach, and the small bowel, and with small catheters can outline the biliary and pancreatic duct systems. The *colonoscope,* introduced via the rectum, enables the operator to visualize the entire large bowel, even the end of the small bowel, and to biopsy it or remove polyps or tumors.

Gastric analysis is the examination of stomach contents for acidity, blood, volume of secretions, pepsin, and cells. Stomach contents are withdrawn for an hour through a plastic tube passed through the nose into the stomach.

Stool examination. The most frequent reason for stool examination is to detect occult or "hidden" blood that is not grossly visible but may be revealed by chemical tests. Microscopic study may reveal protein fiber or increased fat indicative of impaired digestion. Another major reason for stool examination is the detection of eggs or parasites, and cultures for bacteria in instances of infectious diarrhea.

Liver-function tests. In many instances, these tests do not necessarily measure abnormalities associated with liver disease, and are imprecisely related to pathological changes in the liver. Most of these tests require the simple drawing of venous blood and a chemical analysis. Among the substances analyzed are bilirubin, which determines the degree of jaundice; serum proteins, which increase or diminish in certain types of liver disease; and a variety of enzymes that are normally absent or are present in low concentration. BSP or

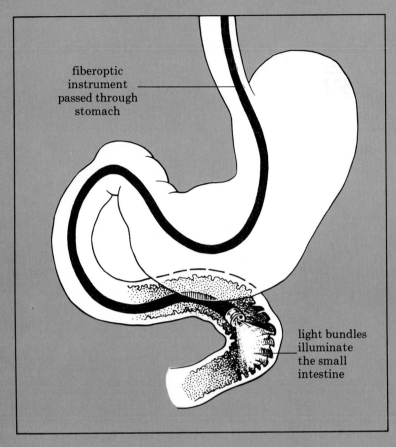

fiberoptic instrument passed through stomach

light bundles illuminate the small intestine

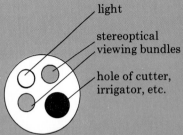

light

stereoptical viewing bundles

hole of cutter, irrigator, etc.

FIBER OPTICS

Flexible fiber-optic instruments, easy to pass down the throat, transmit light around bends and curves and enable direct inspection of interior surfaces. Various refinements permit the operator to take photographs, irrigate, obtain tissue specimens, and delineate the biliary and pancreatic duct systems. A similar instrument, introduced from below, enables the entire colon to be inspected.

bromsulphthalein is a dye that, injected intravenously, is extracted by the liver, giving a measurement of liver blood flow that is a screening test for liver disease.

Biopsy. Techniques for obtaining small pieces of tissue are invaluable in the diagnosis of digestive-tract disorders. The liver can be biopsied with a small needle. The technique is of enormous value, and is necessary to establish diagnosis of alcoholic hepatitis and chronic active liver disease. Biopsies of the esophagus, stomach, duodenum, and colon can be obtained with endoscopic instruments.

Tapping. A diagnostic tap of accumulations of fluid in the abdomen *(ascites)* is frequently of value. A local anesthetic is introduced into the skin, a small needle is inserted into the abdominal cavity, and fluid is drained off for laboratory studies that may give information about underlying disease.

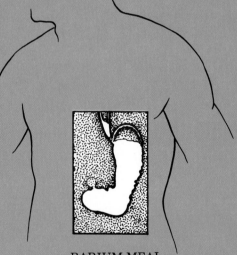

BARIUM MEAL

For an "upper G. I. series," the patient swallows a contrast medium (barium sulfate) that is opaque to X rays. Progress of the "meal" can be followed with a fluoroscope and X-ray pictures can be taken, revealing structures and possible abnormalities of the esophagus, stomach, and duodenum. For a lower G. I. series, a barium enema is instilled into the rectum.

CHAPTER **8**   CHARLEY J. SMYTH, M.D.

YOUR BONES & JOINTS

Bones are as busy as any part of the body. They manufacture blood cells, repair themselves, store and transport minerals, and perform other vital services. Here we're concerned with bones and associated structures as marvelous levers, hinges, and girders that support the body and enable it to move.

The skeleton has a frightful public image. It's drawn on Halloween costumes to scare people. If hidden in a closet, all sorts of scandalous secrets are implied. We would be panic-stricken if we should see our own skeleton creaking toward us, and yet it's all that keeps us from collapsing into an amoebic blob.

About three times your body weight is thrust upon your knee and hip joints when you walk, and more if you run. Your bones and joints have manipulated millions of tons of cumulative weight by middle age. So it's not surprising that diseases broadly labeled "arthritis and rheumatism" should first be recognized around middle life or in later years.

Arthritis is one of man's oldest and most misunderstood diseases. Television and other media advertisements tend to describe it as a minor ailment responding to simple treatment. On the contrary, arthritis is an extremely complex and varied affliction, often severely crippling. It is not a single disease, but more than 100 different conditions that attack joints and connective tissues throughout the body.

"Arthritis" literally means "inflammation of a joint." The word is often confused with an older term, "rheumatism," that has a broader meaning and includes disorders not only of the joints themselves, but of immediately adjacent tissues—tendons, ligaments, bursae, and muscles—that allow motion and provide support, strength, and stability. Injury or inflammation in any of these structures may give rise to stiffness, aching, and pain. Because these symptoms are common to a variety of conditions, regardless of cause, the various ailments are sometimes collectively called "connective tissue diseases."

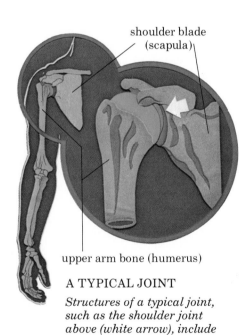

A TYPICAL JOINT

Structures of a typical joint, such as the shoulder joint above (white arrow), include bone, cartilage (blue), joint space, and interconnecting tissues. Freely movable joints are called diarthrodial joints.

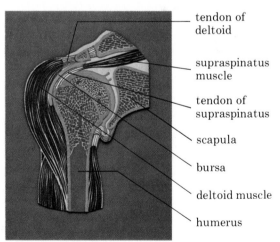

WORKING PARTS

Interacting parts of the shoulder joint are shown above. Tendons attach muscle to bone and transmit movement. Bursae are sacs with lubricating action on parts that move upon one another. Cartilage covers the ends of bones for easy gliding.

Arthritis is not a peculiarly human condition or attributable to conditions of modern life. Dinosaurs had it. Millions of years ago, Pleistocene apemen who probably swung heavy clubs had stiffened joints. Egyptians limped with arthritis prior to mummification. In ancient Rome, the devastating economic effects of arthritis impelled the Emperor Diocletian to bestow the ultimate benefaction: exemption of the afflicted from taxation.

Today, arthritic diseases are the leading cause of crippling in this country. We will all develop some arthritis if we live long enough. Virtually everybody over 60 years of age has enough arthritis to be detectable by X rays. At least 50 million Americans have some degree of arthritis, and of these, some 20 million have disease severe enough to require medical care. Obviously, not all of these millions will wind up in wheelchairs. But the toll in pain, limitation of activity, restriction of choices, and depression is tremendous. Government surveys estimate that the economic cost of rheumatic diseases, in terms of lost wages and medical care, is a staggering $12 billion a year. And that's not to mention money wasted on multiple forms of quackery that promise cures from useless weird devices or exotic medications.

The fact that there is no cure for arthritis does not in the least mean that nothing can be done. What can reasonably be hoped for from treatment, considering the variability of rheumatic diseases, will be apparent in following pages.

To understand the nature of arthritic afflictions, one should know something about the structures involved.

The Physiology of Support

Connective tissue is so pervasive that if all other substances were dissolved away, the remaining connective tissue would be a near-perfect sculpture of the body. These tissues are remarkably varied and adapted to different functions, and are primary supports and protective coverings for the body and internal organs. Specialized functions of connective tissue are suggested by some of the structures in which they occur—in bones, cartilage, ligaments, tendons, and as major components of skin, blood vessels, and joints.

One form of connective tissue is composed of bundles of parallel fibers that have great strength in transmitting pulls in one direction. This form is present in ligaments that tie bones together and in tendons that connect bones and muscles. You can get an idea of their great strength by sitting in a chair, laying one foot on its side over your knee, and pressing with your thumb against the back of your leg a little above the heel. Now bend your foot upward. The hard, almost bony structure that moves under your thumb is your Achilles tendon.

Another form of connective tissue, composed of fibers interwoven like a basket, has great strength in all directions. It's present in capsules that cover organs, as in the layers that hold your eyeball in the shape of a globe.

The principal protein of connective tissue fibers is *collagen,* which in fact constitutes nearly one-third of total body protein. Collagen can be "seen" indirectly as gelatin, produced by boiling collagen.

Cartilage, or gristle, is a firm, slippery, grayish substance at the ends of bones, familiar to anyone who has disjointed a turkey. It's an essential component of joints, but other forms of it occur elsewhere in the body. You can feel cartilage by pinching your ear or the tip of your nose.

The different forms of arthritis begin with some kind of injury, infection, or inflammation. Connective tissue plays a major role in repairing damage caused by a disruption of normal structure, and is an arena for inflammatory and immunologic reactions that protect the body.

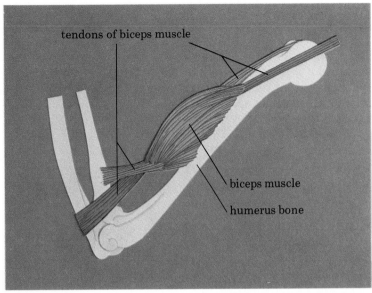

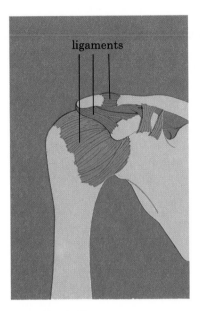

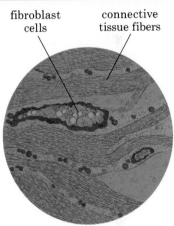

LIGAMENTS

Ligaments, composed of tough strands of connective tissue, tie bones together. A torn ligament causes loosening and separation of parts.

TENDONS

Tendons connect bones and muscles, and enable us to move limbs by muscular effort. In this drawing of the arm, the biceps muscle moves forearm bones.

COLLAGEN

Collagen, produced by fibroblast cells (microscopic view at right), is the protein substance of the white fibers of bone, cartilage, tendons, and connective tissues.

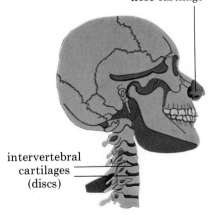

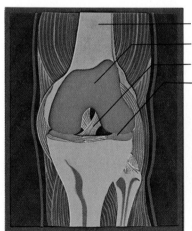

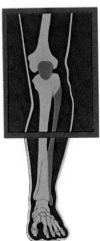

CARTILAGE

Cartilage (gristle) is firm, cushiony connective tissue that covers the ends of bones in joints and is found in innumerable structures, such as the external ear, the tip of the nose, the larynx, the windpipe, the chest cage, and the vertebrae.

SHOCK ABSORBER

Shock-absorbing cartilage covers the ends of leg bones in the knee joint, above and at right. Destruction of cartilage in forms of arthritis deprives opposing bone ends of springy protection against weight-bearing pressures and stresses.

Anatomy of a Joint

A joint is a place where two or more bones come together—almost; in health, bones do not directly touch or rub on each other. Some joints are so firmly bound by tough tissue that they move very little, if at all. Other joints (called *diarthrodial*) are freely movable. Without them we could not sit, stand, walk, run, jump, grasp, lift, or do anything that requires movement. And such joints are the most common sites of arthritic troubles.

To understand arthritis and related diseases, one should know a little about joint structures and how they interact. A typical healthy joint is shown in the accompanying drawing. At first glance, the mechanism looks quite simple: bone ends are held together by a bag-like structure or capsule made of tough fibrous tissue, supported by muscles and tendons. This architecture permits the bones to move up, down, and sidewise. But the cooperative action required to bend a knee or hold a pencil is not at all simple.

Opposing bone ends are covered by a special kind of cartilage or gristle, called articular cartilage. This dense gray tissue is elastic and supersaturated—two-thirds or more of its weight is water. When bone ends are squeezed together, as when you step off a curb, the cartilage "weeps" fluid, which is reabsorbed when pressure is relieved. Your weight, one might say, is water-borne. It is truly a remarkable hydraulic shock absorber and bearing.

The inner surface of the joint capsule is covered by a lining of loose connective tissue called *synovium,* which forms a sac enclosing the cavity. It produces straw-colored, slippery *synovial fluid,* which is an all-important lubricant and a source of nutrients for cartilage. What is called the joint cavity is not an empty space but a cleft containing tissue.

Immediately outside the capsule are the tendons and muscles that hold the joint together and keep it stable, and also transmit power to move the joint at your command. Around and between these supporting structures lie thin-walled sacs or *bursae,* which provide a thick, oily fluid that reduces friction and absorbs mechanical shock. These are the sites of homely complaints such as housemaid's knee, which are not arthritis but hurt just as much.

An abnormal joint can differ from a normal joint in a variety of ways, as will be seen in following discussions.

KINDS OF JOINTS

Some joints, such as the bones of the wrist (near right) and the bones of the skull, are bound so tightly that they move very little or not at all, but they can be injured. Freely movable (diarthrodial) joints permit a wide range of movement within the limits of their structures. Some are gliding or hinge-like joints; others are ball-and-socket joints, like the hip joint at far right, which permits swinging of the leg (white arrows) and some rotary movement.

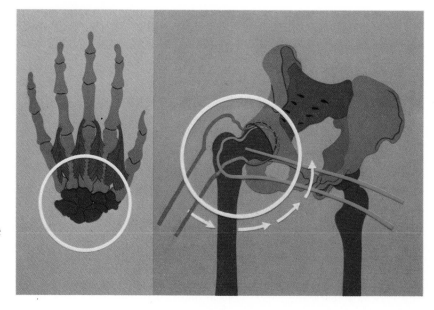

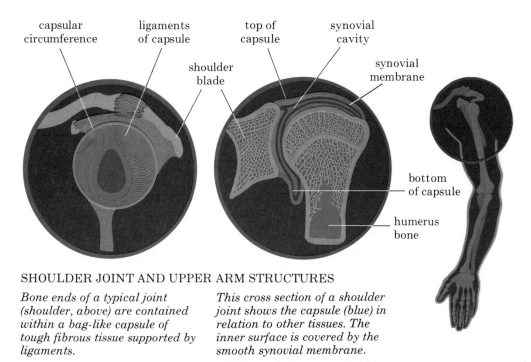

capsular circumference

ligaments of capsule

shoulder blade

top of capsule

synovial cavity

synovial membrane

bottom of capsule

humerus bone

SHOULDER JOINT AND UPPER ARM STRUCTURES

Bone ends of a typical joint (shoulder, above) are contained within a bag-like capsule of tough fibrous tissue supported by ligaments.

This cross section of a shoulder joint shows the capsule (blue) in relation to other tissues. The inner surface is covered by the smooth synovial membrane.

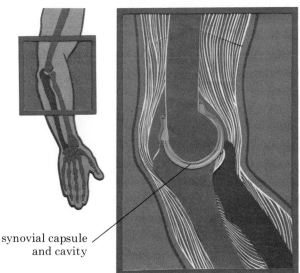

synovial capsule and cavity

ELBOW JOINT

The synovial membrane (red) lines the capsule and encloses the joint cavity, which is not an open space but a cleft containing tissue. Shock-absorbing cartilage is shown in yellow.

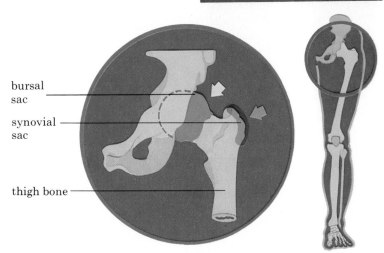

bursal sac

synovial sac

thigh bone

BURSITIS

Bursitis is the painful result of inflammation of a fluid-filled sac called a bursa (green arrow). Bursae lie outside the capsule, around and between supporting structures that hold a joint together, as in the hip joint at left. Bursae produce a thick fluid that reduces friction. The white arrow points to the synovial sac that lines the joints.

OSTEOARTHRITIS

We all earn a touch of osteoarthritis if we exert ourselves commendably for many years. The term "wear and tear arthritis" is more respectful than the one doctors use—"degenerative joint disease." Weight-bearing joints are affected: the lower back, hips, knees, ankles, and feet.

Except for injury, it takes about half a lifetime to acquire significant osteoarthritis, which is usually not recognized until the mid-40s or later. *Primary* osteoarthritis is joint disease without any apparent associated illness. Whether or not aging is a specific cause, osteoarthritis seems to be part of the aging process.

Secondary osteoarthritis results from direct injury to cartilage, as may occur in sports or occupations that impose great stress on particular joints. For instance, the elbows, wrists, or shoulders of a jackhammer operator may be damaged by the constant hammering of the tool, or the knees or feet of football players may be injured by repeated hemorrhage into joints. Certain rare conditions may predispose to secondary osteoarthritis.

Here we are primarily concerned with the primary form, and some heartening things can be said about it. Perhaps half of the 40 million Americans who have detectably abnormal joints are hardly aware of it, beyond a little stiffness when they get out of bed in the morning. The disease is limited to a few joints and does not spread. It is not a systemic disease that involves other organs or tissues. Patients do not seem sick. And gross deformity or widespread crippling is not likely.

Nevertheless, moderate to advanced osteoarthritis can cause much pain, loss of freedom of movement, and limitation of activities on the job or in recreation. Symptoms depend on the joints affected and extent of damage, but affection of the hip joint is the most disabling.

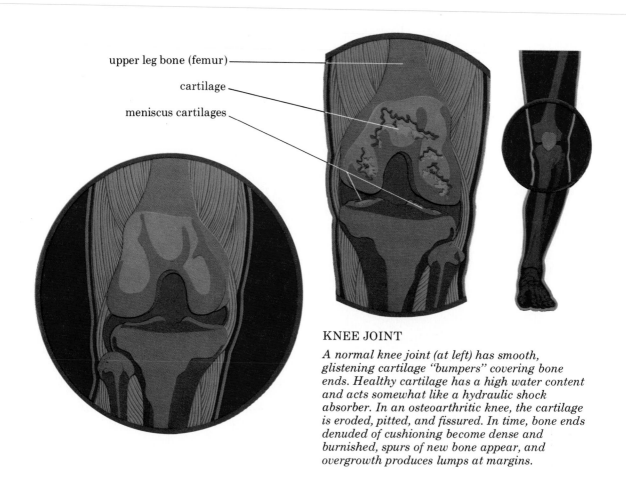

upper leg bone (femur)

cartilage

meniscus cartilages

KNEE JOINT

A normal knee joint (at left) has smooth, glistening cartilage "bumpers" covering bone ends. Healthy cartilage has a high water content and acts somewhat like a hydraulic shock absorber. In an osteoarthritic knee, the cartilage is eroded, pitted, and fissured. In time, bone ends denuded of cushioning become dense and burnished, spurs of new bone appear, and overgrowth produces lumps at margins.

The Osteoarthritic Joint

The target tissue here is *articular cartilage,* previously described, and adjacent bone. Cartilage is first affected when its surface becomes frayed, pitted, or cracked. Ultimately, bone-deep fissures occur and cartilage is destroyed, leaving the bone ends without cushioning. "Raw" opposing bone ends then make contact.

Attempts of bone to repair itself are fruitless, and even harmful. Its ends become overgrown, and very dense and hard, like burnished ivory. Hurtful spurs of new bone appear. The lining of the joint capsule (synovium) may show mild secondary inflammation. Muscles and ligaments tend to contract, giving rise to stiffness, tenseness, and pain. Bone overgrowth enlarges the joint and produces firm lumps at its margins.

Symptoms. Often, the first symptom one becomes aware of is stiffness, soreness, and an aching type of pain when a joint is moved. The joint is peaceful during sleep, lying, or long sitting but protests when moved.

Aching and stiffness tend to wear off quite soon, even to disappear completely, when a joint is put into action. This is often evident on getting out of bed in the morning or getting to one's feet from a sitting position. At first, the knees or hips are uncomfortable and feel unsteady. But after standing and taking a few steps, the affected joint eases up and permits more normal and pain-free walking.

Diagnosis. In the initial diagnosis, the physician depends on a patient's history of mild aching and soreness around joints, particularly upon moving them. The next most common finding is stiffness or inability to move a joint easily or comfortably. In more advanced cases, the joint is obviously enlarged and has firm lumps at the margins, giving a knobby look. The joint may make grating, crunching sounds when manipulated (crepitation). The joint is not red or hot, nor are there constitutional symptoms—fever, fatigue, weight loss, or weakness—findings that help to rule out other forms of arthritis.

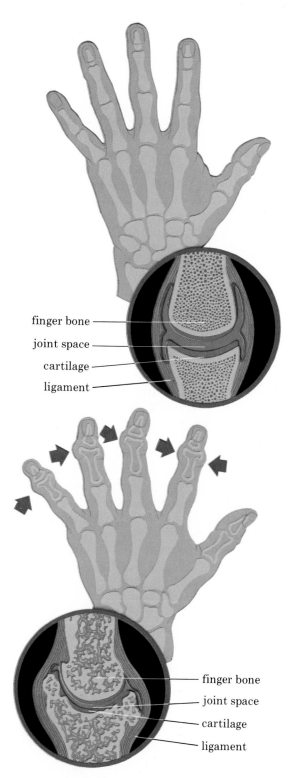

finger bone

joint space

cartilage

ligament

finger bone

joint space

cartilage

ligament

FINGER JOINTS

In the bone structure of a normal hand, finger joints (circle) bend easily and comfortably, and are not stiff, aching, or swollen. The straight configuration of the hand is not distorted. Advanced osteoarthritis often is self-evident from inspection of the hands. The finger joints (red arrows) are obviously enlarged, knobby, angled out of position, and may be immovable.

Treatment

Don't expect cure, but do expect gratifying benefits from treatments that can ease pain, help to keep joints flexible, and prevent progressive disability. Osteoarthritis is a chronic disease and treatment must be continuous for happiest results. One should understand that cartilage has little ability to heal, that the disease is likely to remain in a few joints, and that the widespread crippling that the word "arthritis" conjures up is not probable.

Drugs. The most useful drugs are pain-relievers, of which aspirin is best for most people and most commonly prescribed. Common household remedy though it is, aspirin is rather special for arthritis. It reduces inflammation, stiffening, and aching pain, and helps by blocking the release of enzymes that break down cartilage.

For maximum benefit, most patients require two or three tablets four times a day after meals and at bedtime, with milk or antacids to avoid stomach upset. There are other aspirin-like drugs for persons who can't tolerate aspirin in high doses, as well as more potent medications that require a doctor's supervision because of possible side effects.

Steroids (cortisone-like drugs) are not given by mouth for osteoarthritis. But in special situations, they may be injected directly into a joint to give comfort for a considerable time or to permit exercises to be done without distress.

Exercises, passive as well as those performed against resistance, aim to prevent contractures and keep the joints stable and "unwobbly." Affected joints tend to become fixed in a bent (flexed) position, counteracted by exercises that extend the joint and strengthen flabby muscles. Bicycling and swimming are probably the best exercises for maximum muscle tension.

Heat applications are comforting and preferably should precede exercise. Wet or dry heat, hot tub baths, hot packs, and paraffin treatments (dipping of the hand into melted paraffin that is allowed to harden) are all useful.

Joints must be protected against severe stress and strain. A severe, continuous, round-the-clock stress is *obesity*. Weight reduction that "unloads" the joints may well be the best treatment available—not easily attained, but well worth striving for.

Simple measures. Some very helpful measures are not at all complicated. Among them are:
• Take brief periods of rest during the day, 15 to 30 minutes. Recumbency is best.
• Use a straight chair, and avoid overstuffed furniture.

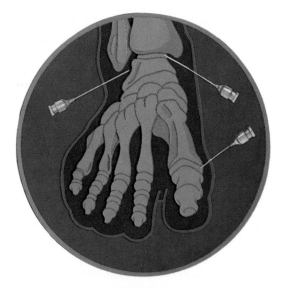

INJECTION TREATMENT

When appropriate, cortisone-like drugs injected directly into an arthritic joint may permit comfortable movement for a period of time. Various arthritic joints respond to palliative treatment by injection; the drawing above shows several sites for the injection of foot joints.

- If the knee joint is affected (as it very often is in older women), a slightly raised chair or bed is helpful.
- Avoid unnecessary stair-climbing.
- If the hip joint is involved, use a walking stick or crutch on the opposite side.
- Specially fitted shoes can also be of great value. Needs differ from patient to patient, but custom-fitted footwear is obviously superior to shoes that can be bought off the shelf. By corrective adaptations to individual conditions, skillful orthopedic design can cushion impacts, restore arches, build up one side of the body to shift the line of weight-bearing, help to stabilize the foot, and reduce limitation of movement (see page 253).
- Heat and exercises, previously mentioned, do not require elaborate equipment, and can usually be done at home by a motivated patient, with the help of an understanding family member if necessary.

Surgery

Most osteoarthritic patients do not need or desire surgery. The disease is not life-threatening and a decision for surgery may be made on the basis of how disabling or distressing a joint problem is to a particular person. An otherwise bearable joint disease might be serious indeed if it threatened one's ability to keep on working at an accustomed job. For instance, limitation of finger movement might not be very bothersome to some people, but of considerable concern to an organist.

Remarkable advances in orthopedic surgery have made possible a high rate of success in banishing pain and restoring joint function. Such surgery is not limited to a particular kind of arthritis. Various techniques—total joint replacement, fusion of joints, insertion of artificial joints, and others—are described on page 248.

HEBERDEN'S NODES

This form of osteoarthritis is almost, though not entirely, limited to postmenopausal women. If well advanced, the condition is obvious from the appearance of the hand, as shown in the accompanying drawing.

The end joints of the fingers, next to the nails, are prominently enlarged. Usually all fingers are affected, with finger ends angled to one side, out of a straight line. The knobby bumps are hard, sharply localized, bony, and unyielding. Tender, knobby enlargements of the middle finger joints (Bouchard's nodes) are not uncommon, and other forms of arthritis may coexist.

As a rule, the nodes become noticeable in the 50s, two or three years after the last menstrual period. The condition is a sex-linked hereditary trait, dominant in women and recessive in men. Ten times more women than men exhibit it.

Intensive treatment of Heberden's nodes is hardly ever desirable. The joints may not look good, and sometimes may hurt a little, but the hand usually retains good manipulative skill. For occasional aches, it's comforting to immerse the hands in warm water for four minutes, then in cold water for one minute, repeating this alternation three or four times, twice a day.

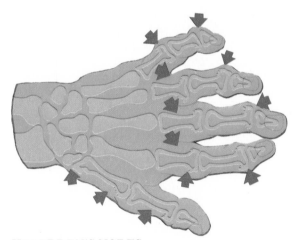

HEBERDEN'S NODES

Enlarged, bony-hard, angled end joints of the fingers are typical of Heberden's nodes, which primarily affect post-menopausal women. Arrows point to end joints and middle finger joints, which also may be enlarged and knobby.

RHEUMATOID ARTHRITIS

Rheumatoid arthritis is potentially (but not inevitably) the most crippling and disabling of arthritic disorders. It is the most common of a closely allied family of rheumatoid diseases that includes psoriatic arthritis, juvenile rheumatoid arthritis, ankylosing spondylitis, arthritis associated with intestinal diseases, and others.

Unlike osteoarthritis, rheumatoid arthritis is a systemic disease that can affect many tissues and organs, but joint inflammation is the predominant complaint. It is a sex-biased disorder, afflicting three times more women than men. It usually begins between ages 25 and 45, but onset after age 50 is not uncommon and many older patients seek medical help because hitherto bearable symptoms have become severe.

Symptoms. Although symptoms may appear suddenly, onset is more often insidious. Often, before joints are involved, there is numbness and tingling in hands and feet, fatigue, loss of appetite and weight, and sometimes low grade fever. Classic morning stiffness persists for more than an hour after arising. The first joints to be affected are usually small ones, as in fingers and toes. Later, other joints in wrists, knees, and shoulders may become involved. Typically, joint symptoms are symmetrical, affecting both wrists, both knees, or both feet. Symptoms may flit from joint to joint, leaving a previously involved joint seemingly normal, but after several months, inflammation usually stays in one or several joints. The parts are swollen, tender, "hot," restricted in motion, and sometimes red.

Changes in the joints. It is generally agreed that rheumatoid changes begin in the lining (*synovium*) of the joint capsule. The smooth membrane is converted into a thickened, shaggy, abnormal structure called the *pannus* (Latin, "a piece of cloth"). It weeps fluid, causing soft boggy swelling, spreads over cartilage surfaces, exudes enzymes that erode cartilage, and replaces destroyed cartilage, resulting in pain on movement. If the disease remains active, areas of pannus may stick together and ultimately bone ends may fuse into immovable junction.

Tissues surrounding the joint (bursae, tendons, ligaments, muscles, and nerves) are commonly affected. Firm, painless lumps (rheumatoid nodules) developing beneath the skin at points of pressure, such as the elbows, suggest fairly advanced disease. A small percentage of patients with severe rheumatoid arthritis may have systemic manifestations in the eyes, heart, blood vessels, lungs, and other organs.

Diagnosis. Physical signs give a basis for diagnosis. In well-established cases, inspection of the hands alone may tell a story. A typical rheumatoid hand, as shown in the drawing, has soft, tender, spindle-shaped swellings of the middle joints of the fingers, and also of knuckles at the base of the fingers. The grip is weak; it's hard to make a tight fist.

Aside from inflammation of joints, there may be changes in the lining membrane of the eye, with redness and pain. Rheumatoid nodules may be present at pressure areas of elbows, knuckles, or heel cords, and along the course of tendons that flex the fingers. The patient may not even be aware of elbow or knee contractures that prevent him or her from extending the arm in a straight line or laying the leg flat on the bottom of a bathtub.

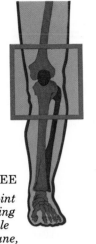

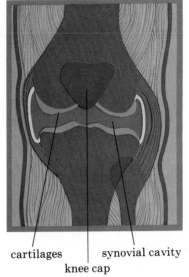

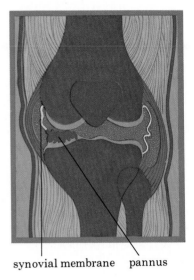

A NORMAL KNEE

A normal knee joint has a healthy lining of the joint capsule (synovial membrane, white line; synovial cavity, blue area). The articular cartilages of the upper and lower leg bones are intact (orange). The triangular bone in the center is the kneecap (patella). The changes caused by rheumatoid arthritis are shown at far right.

cartilages

synovial cavity

knee cap

synovial membrane   pannus

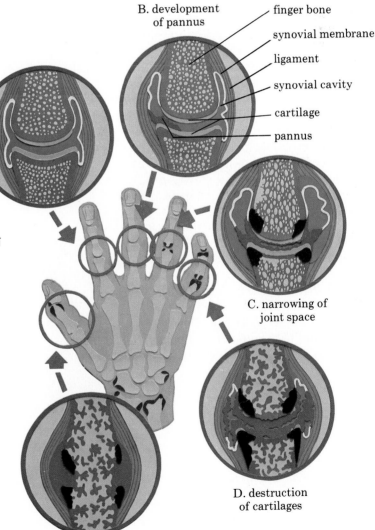

B. development of pannus

finger bone

synovial membrane

ligament

synovial cavity

cartilage

pannus

A. normal finger joint

RHEUMATOID PROGRESSION

In rheumatoid disease, the lining membrane of a joint progressively degenerates into abnormal boggy tissue (pannus), shown in red. Pannus spreads over and begins to erode cartilage and narrows the joint space; fluids cause soft swelling (B, C, D). Ultimately, bone ends denuded of cartilage may fuse immovably (E).

C. narrowing of joint space

D. destruction of cartilages

E. destruction of bones & fusion

Tests. A few laboratory tests help in diagnosing early rheumatoid arthritis. One is the erythrocyte sedimentation rate, which measures the rate at which red blood cells settle out of a prepared specimen of blood. It is almost always elevated in cases of rheumatoid arthritis, but also is elevated in other rheumatic and non-inflammatory disorders. A common finding is a slight anemia. If only one large joint is affected, the physician may withdraw joint fluid to rule out infectious arthritis.

An important diagnostic finding is the detection of *rheumatoid factor* in the patient's blood. This factor is an antibody, present in about 70 percent of patients with classic rheumatoid arthritis, but it's also found in some persons with no joint disease whatever. Unfortunately, the test is rarely positive in the earliest months of rheumatoid arthritis, and may be negative even if the disease exists. Rheumatoid factor is not a likely cause of rheumatoid arthritis, but may perpetuate it.

Course. Rheumatoid arthritis runs a mysteriously unpredictable course that makes both its recognition and treatment difficult. It may become arrested and never reappear. However, ups and downs—remissions and recurrences—are characteristic. The disease may pursue a slowly progressive course with periods of months or even years when there is seemingly no activity. There is tremendous variation from patient to patient in the degree of active joint inflammation, rate of progression, and structural damage.

What is the long-term outlook in chronic rheumatoid arthritis? A primer on rheumatic diseases prepared by the American Rheumatism Association reports that, among various arthritic clinic patients who were followed for many years, about 50 percent are "stationary" or "improved" after 10 years. If there is no improvement by then, there's little likelihood that improvement will occur. Nevertheless, after 10 to 15 years, more than half of the patients remained fully employable, and after 15 to 20 years, those completely incapacitated constituted only 10 percent of the group.

Treatment

Most patients, when told they have arthritis, are prone to depressing thoughts of crippling, limitations in work and play, and humiliating dependency. Let it be said at once that major advances in treatment make this hopeless attitude quite unjustified. Much can be done in most cases to relieve suffering, prevent deformities, and shorten attacks. No single therapy serves all purposes, but a variety of measures, appropriately employed, will reverse many of the manifestations of arthritis.

Well-defined stages of the clinical course of rheumatoid arthritis serve as guides in planning a comprehensive program of treatment. Programs adapted to the course of the disease are described on page 245.

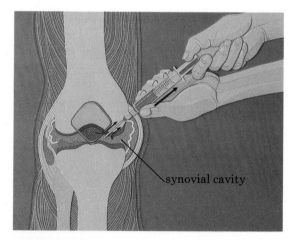

INFECTION

Infection is a possible cause of arthritis, particularly if a single joint is affected. Examination of synovial fluid withdrawn from the joint cavity (black arrows) is a relatively simple procedure for ruling out or confirming the presence of infection.

A Basic Conservative Program

Conservative treatment consistently relieves symptoms and helps to keep affected joints in use. The basic medical program includes rest, emotional support, exercise, heat, support of joints, diet, and pain-relieving drugs. (There is no miraculous "arthritis diet." A balanced diet with adequate vitamins, minerals, protein, and calories does all that diet can do.)

These basic measures do much to decrease inflammation, preserve joint and muscle functions, and prevent or greatly lessen deformities. The physician initiates and supervises the program, but most of the work is done at home.

Many patients with mild disease do very well on the basic program alone. Additional measures may be needed if the major concern is recurrent or sustained disease with severe joint disturbances that seriously restrict activity.

Rest. Never underestimate the healing value of rest. How much rest? That depends on the severity of disease. Patients with mild disease can often continue their regular work or leisure activities if they get nine hours of bed rest at night. In moderately severe cases, additional rest periods of an hour or two during the day may give comfort and permit limited work. Complete bed rest is desirable if weight-bearing joints (hips, knees, or ankles) are so acutely inflamed that walking or standing is impossible or unwise. Special kinds of rest can be given to inflamed joints by splinting and by several other procedures. The benefits of rest can be judged by diminished redness, pain, and swelling, by shortened duration of morning stiffness, changes in weight, and certain laboratory tests.

Exercises. Active exercises are extremely important. Ideally, they should be recommended by a physical therapist.

Emotional support. Emotional stresses do not cause rheumatoid arthritis, but can certainly aggravate established disease. Mental stress is inevitable in coping day after day with the pain and limitations that often are not sympathized with or even recognized by family or associates. Persons who have been self-sufficient before becoming ill may have to accept a dependent pattern of living. The disease may compel a change in occupation, recreation, and social habits. Small wonder, then, if the patient harbors resentments and hostilities that can only worsen his or her condition.

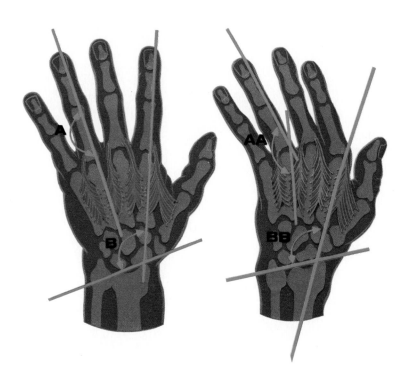

DEVIATION

In normally aligned hand bones, the finger-hand angle (A) is 180 degrees. The wrist-finger angle (B) is 114 degrees. Arthritic changes can cause a deviation in wrist bones (AA becomes 140 degrees, BB becomes 122 degrees). An imbalance of the forearm muscles and tendons attached to the wrist distorts the "grasp" of the hand.

It's not easy for most patients to discuss such matters, but they should know that emotional factors play a role in the treatment and progress of rheumatoid arthritis. An understanding physician can do much to bring repressed feelings, fears, and concerns into the daylight in discussions with patients and family members.

Drugs. Aspirin has both pain-relieving and anti-inflammatory properties and is the most widely used single drug in treating rheumatoid arthritis. But an ordinary "headache dose" will not do the job. The amount of aspirin a patient requires may be enormous—during "flare-ups," up to 100 grains daily. Such large doses may cause stomach irritation, bleeding, or ringing in the ears. Every patient has individual limits of tolerance that must be determined, and modified forms of aspirin or other salicylates may be better tolerated.

Moderately severe arthritis affecting multiple joints with much pain, fever, and weakness may require other drugs when the basic program does not control the disease. Indomethacin and phenylbutazone have been useful in arthritis for some years. Newer drugs become available to the physician from time to time; the pharmaceutical search for better arthritis drugs is very intensive. Some of the newer agents are comparable to aspirin but better tolerated. All are prescription drugs and the physician is watchful for side effects, principally gastrointestinal ones—nausea, vomiting, and abdominal pain.

Relief from inflammatory symptoms may not be evident for several weeks, and even then may not be dramatic. However, the relative safety of these drugs and the benefits that usually come if they're allowed time to work give them real value in treatment of rheumatoid arthritis.

Anti-malarials. Certain anti-malarial drugs (Aralen, Plaquenil) have anti-rheumatic properties and have been used in treating rheumatoid arthritis. Benefits are seldom evident in less than three months, and maximum improvement may take six months to a year. Their use in arthritis has been limited in recent years by the hazards of toxic reactions, principally in the form of permanent damage to the retina of the eye.

Gold salts. Of all anti-inflammatory agents, only gold salts may stop or slow down the disease process of rheumatoid arthritis. These salts are water-soluble gold-containing compounds given by injection into muscles. They have been used for rheumatoid arthritis for nearly 50 years, not as initial treatment, but in patients who have responded poorly or not at all to aspirin and basic measures.

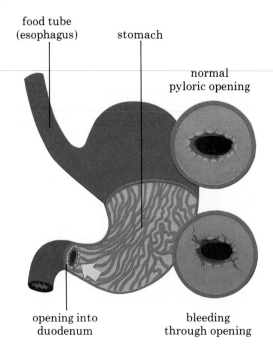

food tube (esophagus)   stomach   normal pyloric opening

opening into duodenum   bleeding through opening

DRUG INTOLERANCE

Aspirin, the drug of first choice in arthritis, may cause gastric bleeding when taken in necessarily large or untolerated doses in some patients, requiring an adjustment of dosage or drug substitution. The drawing shows the normal opening into the duodenum (pylorus), and bleeding through the opening, as seen with endoscopic instruments.

There is no way of telling which patients will benefit. Ordinarily the patient is given an initial small dose. If there is no untoward reaction, weekly injections, slowly increased to maintenance level, are continued for three or four months. No benefit is evident for six to ten weeks. If no benefit is noted after some months, gold salts should be discontinued. But if there is definite improvement, maintenance injections are given once a month, and these may be continued for several years.

Gold salt therapy commits patient and physician to long-term treatment. The patient must be "dependable" and regular in visits—not only to space injections, but because possible toxic reactions to gold are of utmost importance. The most common reaction is a skin rash preceded by itching. The physician makes frequent tests of blood and urine to check for possible toxic reactions in kidneys and blood-forming organs. Most such reactions are minor and easily overcome, and severe reactions are uncommon. If gold treatment is stopped immediately when any reaction occurs, serious complications can be avoided.

Corticosteroids. These potent drugs are close relatives of cortisone, which made headlines in 1949 when crippled, bedridden arthritis patients got up and walked after injections of the wonder drug. Cortisone was briefly hailed as a cure for arthritis. Today, steroids—the collective name for improved cortisone-like drugs—are recognized as a two-edged sword, a valuable tool not to be discarded because it has potential side effects.

Steroids can suppress the manifestations of rheumatoid arthritis in the majority of patients, who may become more active, suffer less pain, and feel more normal—but who later pay a price. Steroids do not alter the natural course of rheumatoid arthritis and they do pose a risk of untoward reactions, such as "moon face" (deposits of fat at the base of the neck), high blood pressure, loss of calcium from bones, ulcers of the stomach, and increased susceptibility to infections.

Steroid doses must be kept at the lowest possible level to partially suppress inflammation, and be maintained for the shortest possible time. Patients considered for steroid therapy are those who have severe unremitting disease with fever, anemia, weight loss, effusions into joints, and crippling deformities, despite adequate use of conservative measures.

Small doses may allow a patient to carry out household duties or to continue at a job—otherwise impossible tasks. For instance, they may enable elderly single persons who live alone, and who would otherwise be dependent on relatives, to manage for themselves. Another use of steroids is to provide "cover" for a few weeks while awaiting the possible benefits of other agents, such as gold.

Hospitalization. The value of four to six weeks of intensive hospital care for rheumatoid arthritis patients who do not respond well to other treatment is well recognized. The combination of intensive physical therapy, care by nurses with special training, and temporary removal from home and work favorably alters the course of the disease. Benefits obtained in hospital units devoted specifically to arthritis treatment have been clearly established.

Rapid expansion of orthopedic treatment procedures is a major benefit of special units within or adjacent to general hospitals. Truly great progress has been made in improving patients' comfort and mobility by corrective surgery combined with physical therapy and drugs. A number of rehabilitative operations (see page 248) are of particular help to the patient with rheumatoid arthritis.

SURGERY IN ARTHRITIS

Surgery has a great deal to offer arthritis patients who are suitable for reconstructive operations and who choose to have them. Surgery almost always eliminates pain. Usually it restores a gratifying range of motion to an affected joint and enables the patient to use the joint comfortably, perhaps for the first time in years. Sometimes the results are spectacular—from wheelchair to walking status in a few days.

In the past, surgery was largely a last resort or a salvaging procedure for severely crippled patients. But today, for patients who can accept surgery within the general framework of medical care, operations are performed much earlier, before severe damage has occurred.

New Joints for Old

Over the past decade, striking advances in inserting artificial joints can largely be credited to a remarkable kind of glue—called methyl methacrylate—used as a bone cement. Instead of hammering pins and bolts into bone, the surgeon carefully shapes opposing bone ends to accept complementary parts—male and female—of an artificial joint made of metal or plastic. The mating ends of the artificial joints fit precisely, and their "anchor" ends are firmly bound to bone by the methacrylate cement. The secure artificial joint permits easy motion and pain is gone.

After the operation. Complications can occur after such operations, and although rare, they can be serious. As with any major surgery, blood clots may occur in veins near the joint, and if these become loosened, particles (emboli) may be carried in the blood to the lungs. Another rare but important complication is infection. Most infections respond to antibiotics, but an intractable one may require removal of the artificial joint. Rarely, too, the parts may loosen, or if the bone is thin, it may break.

Much of the success in joint replacement depends upon physical therapy that is begun before surgery and continued afterward. Exercises strengthen the muscles that bend and extend the joint. The program calls for several hours of diligent work every day for many months.

Improvements in the materials and design of artificial joints come from continued research and orthopedic experience. While the artificial joints described below are representative of those that currently give very satisfactory results, they are not necessarily the last word.

The hip. A diseased hip joint is a great crippler. It can cause continuous pain, restrict the most ordinary activities, make walking or standing difficult or impossible, and even lead to invalidism. The hip was the first joint chosen for total replacement with the then-new bone cement technique developed by Dr. John Charnley of England more than a decade ago.

The hip joint is a relatively simple ball and socket unit, as the drawing of an artificial hip joint shows. After careful shaping of surfaces, the surgeon cements a cuplike half-sphere of metal or plastic into the hip bone, and a shaft-like unit with a ball-shaped end into the upper end of the thigh bone (femur). The ball end of the device fits precisely into the artificial socket and rolls easily as in a normal joint.

Surgery takes two to three hours, and the cement sets rapidly into a permanent bond. Usually the patient is out of bed on the fourth day, and with assistance, may stand the next day.

How long does such a hip joint last? It may last indefinitely; the procedure is too new to know for sure what to expect after 20 or 30 years. Cemented hip joints are still in use after 15 years, which is as long as the bone cement technique has been performed.

Rheumatoid and osteoarthritis patients are well suited for hip joint replacement since they are less likely to put great stress on a major weight-bearing joint than young people who want to play football or climb mountains.

A NORMAL HIP JOINT

The ball-and-socket principle allows the ball end of the thigh bone to glide easily on a bed of smooth cartilage within the socket that holds it. This great weight-bearing joint is subject to osteoarthritis, injuries, and disorders that can cause discomfort, severe pain, limping, and restriction of movement during such commonplace activities as walking and standing.

AN ARTIFICIAL JOINT

Below, drawing A shows erosion of the ball end of the thigh bone and its socket. Drawing B shows replacement by a metal ball end with its shaft in the femur, and an artificial socket into which the ball fits, secured to bone by screws. Newer techniques of joint replacement employ a quick-setting bone cement (methacrylate) to "glue" artificial parts into position, as in the femur (C).

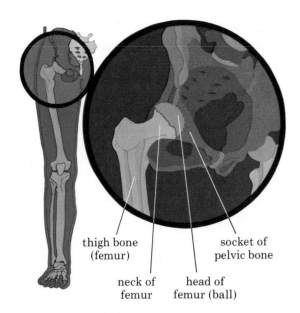
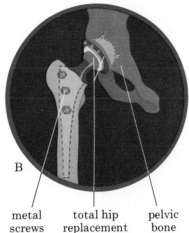

thigh bone
(femur)

socket of
pelvic bone

neck of
femur

head of
femur (ball)

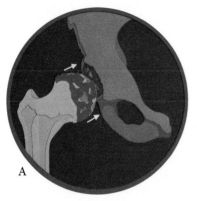

A

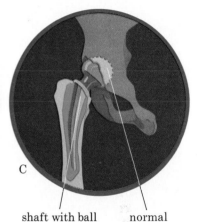

B

C

metal
screws

total hip
replacement

pelvic
bone

shaft with ball
end cemented
in femur

normal
socket

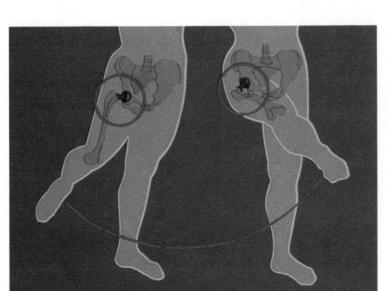

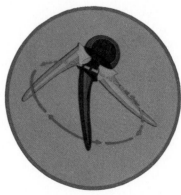

FREE MOVEMENT

At left, an artificial hip joint in action. Successful surgery restores the normal range of pain-free swinging and rotary movement. In circle, the excursion of the prosthesis is shown as an elliptical arc.

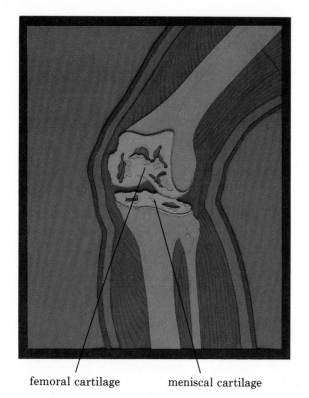

femoral cartilage   meniscal cartilage

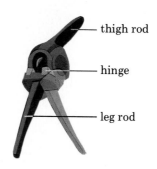

thigh rod

hinge

leg rod

KNEE JOINT

The knee is a vital weight-bearing joint, quite complex in structure, and prone to inflammation and injury as well as arthritis. At left, the drawing shows an arthritic knee with eroded cartilage. The small drawing shows one type of artificial knee joint with hinge action, designed for implanting into the leg bones. The bottom drawing shows an artificial knee joint cemented in place. Several designs have been developed, but the perfect artificial knee joint still is elusive.

artificial knee device   hinge joint

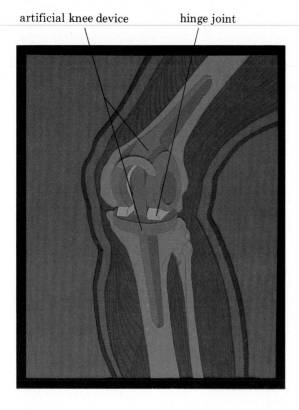

The knee. Headlined operations on athletes have informed the public that the knee is a notorious target of disablement. But non-athletes develop wobbly, painful knees from forms of arthritis and inflammation unrelated to the acute tears of ligaments and muscles that plague football players. "Bad knees" are a frequent and disabling complaint of older women, especially if they are obese (reduction in weight can take a big load off a complaining joint).

The knee joint has been called an "engineer's nightmare." It is much more complex than the hip joint. Four different bones are involved: the kneecap (patella), the lower end of the thigh bone, and the two long bones of the lower leg (tibia and fibula). Ligaments and structures that hold opposing ends in conjunction are quite complicated. Nevertheless, severely crippled knee joints have been restored to pain-free motion by implantation of artificial joints of various design, one of which is shown in the drawing.

Surgery to implant an artificial joint is similar to the hip surgery described above. The new joint is ready for tentative weight-bearing in a few days.

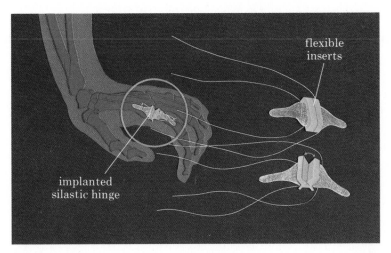

KNUCKLES

Hands or fingers that cannot grasp, bend, write, or sew because of "frozen knuckles" may be restored to good function by the surgical implantation of flexible diamond-shaped silastic "hinges" in the bones of the fingers, or by Dacron-covered inserts that permit free motion of the joints.

The hands. Everyday activities such as writing, sewing, grasping objects, and buttoning clothes can be cruelly handicapped by arthritic processes that immobilize joints of the hands and fingers and weaken muscles. Remarkable restoration of hand function can be obtained by plastic operations on the thumbs, and by silastic implants in the fingers. These flexible diamond-shaped implants permit free motion of joints. After the implanting operation, the hand is placed in a cast for several days and then in a splint for several weeks. Intensive physical therapy is needed to force fingers to bend to the maximum.

Another surgical procedure is the repair and transplantation of tendons that continue from the back of the hand into the fingers.

Arthritic changes may reduce the size of a tunnel through which a big nerve enters the wrist, causing discomfort of the hand and clumsiness in fine movements, especially in women over 40. This condition (carpal tunnel syndrome) is correctable by relatively simple surgery that relieves compression of the nerve.

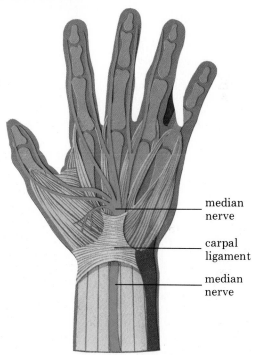

CARPAL TUNNEL

Discomfort and clumsiness in fine movements of the hands result from compression of the big median nerve that extends from the wrist to the hand through a tunnel under the carpal ligament. Arthritic changes may tighten the ligament and squeeze the nerve, but the compression can be relieved by rather simple surgery.

The elbow. The normal elbow joint is not a plain hinge, as it allows some twisting motion. Hinge-like artificial joints have been implanted successfully, but more full-functioning designs are being developed. One design involves implantation of a round-headed stem in the upper arm bone. This fits into a cuplike implant in the lower arm bone, in a ball-and-socket relationship similar to that of the hip.

Usually we do not fully appreciate the structural complexity of joints that automatically permit us to make movements we want them to make—mediated, of course, by brain-directed nerves that serve joint muscles. The ankle is an example of a homely joint so complicated that a completely satisfactory artificial substitute has not yet been devised, although repair of injuries is usually possible.

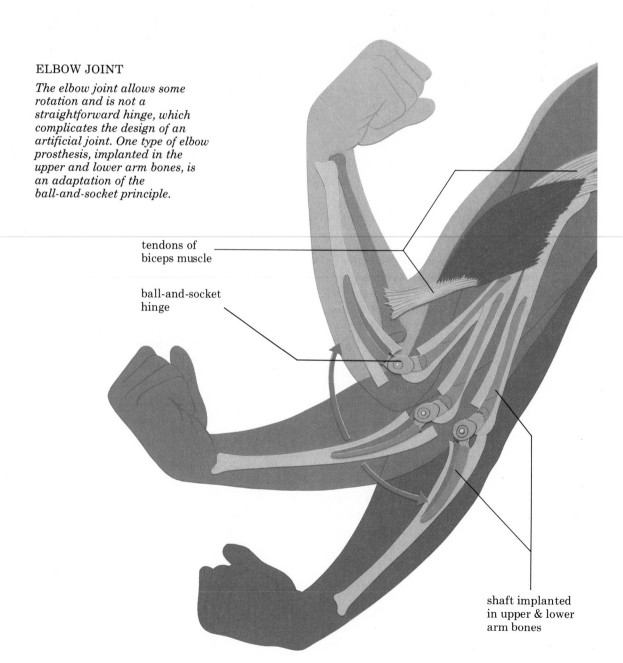

ELBOW JOINT

The elbow joint allows some rotation and is not a straightforward hinge, which complicates the design of an artificial joint. One type of elbow prosthesis, implanted in the upper and lower arm bones, is an adaptation of the ball-and-socket principle.

tendons of biceps muscle

ball-and-socket hinge

shaft implanted in upper & lower arm bones

The feet. The feet contain one-fourth of the body's joints—small ones but with big potential for pain. Osteoarthritis of the weight-bearing joints can distort posture and gait and put abnormal stresses on the feet. Rheumatoid arthritis characteristically affects the feet as part of the disease process.

The drawing shows typical rheumatoid changes: spasm forces bones out of alignment and pulls the toes into a cocked-up position, susceptible to corns. The forefoot spreads, especially at the joint of the big toe where a bunion develops. The head of a long bone between toes and instep (metatarsal) may be forced down into the cushion part of the forefoot, resulting in a callus or even ulceration, with pain at every step.

Surgery is not the first recourse. Simpler measures—warm foot-soaks are certainly simple—may suffice, at least for a time. Many persons gain considerable relief from well-designed footwear, but high fashion must be disregarded. Shoes should be wide enough not to press on painful points, with heels neither too high nor too low. Orthopedic examination may suggest the value of compensating devices such as bars or wedges that shift weight-bearing areas away from painful spots. Shoe linings of spongy polyethylene foam can give a "walking on air" feeling. And custom-built shoes designed around a plaster cast of the affected foot are sometimes, but not always, necessary.

Surgery may be considered, usually when the rheumatic process is more or less at an end point or when the patient is quite unable to stand or walk comfortably without pain, deformity, or instability. Bunions can be corrected, toes can be brought into better alignment, and bony prominences that press painfully on the ball of the foot or the back of the heel can be removed.

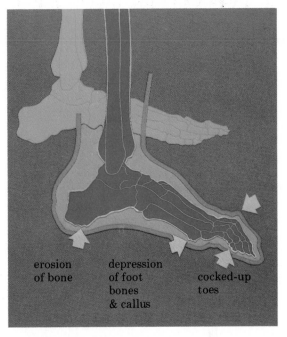

erosion of bone   depression of foot bones & callus   cocked-up toes

FOOT DEFORMITIES

The foot in advanced rheumatoid arthritis shows typical structural changes (background, normal configuration). Spasm pulls bones out of alignment; toes are cocked up. The ball of the foot is callused, painful when bearing weight, and even ulcerated from the downward pressure of the bone above it. Erosion of bone or bony prominences may occur at the heel.

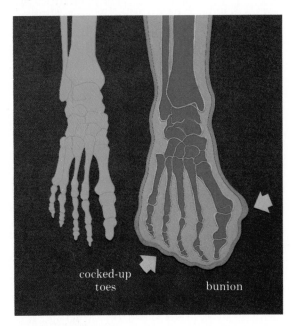

cocked-up toes   bunion

FOREFOOT

The front view shows the bones of the forefoot spread. The malaligned great toe joint is liable to bunion. Osteoarthritis of the hip or knee can throw body weight out of plumb, distorting gait and posture, and putting great stress on the feet.

Synovectomy

This operation removes a diseased joint lining in order to reduce pain and swelling and inhibit the erosion of cartilage. It is most effective when performed before significant destruction of the surface of the cartilage has occurred, and benefits frequently persist for two or three years.

Osteotomy

In this operation, the surgeon makes a division or cuts a section of bone to correct a deformity. It is appropriate when bony parts are distorted from their normal position and is designed to bring them into better alignment. Osteotomy is most often performed on the knees, to line up weight-bearing forces with the supporting structures of the joint.

Fusion

Two joints may become tightly united (ankylosed) through some disease process. A similar fusion of two or more joints can be achieved deliberately by surgical "welding." Small pieces of the patient's own bone are used as grafting material that is packed into place and gradually becomes a united mass. Fusion is most frequently performed on vertebrae of the lower back, sometimes in conjunction with repair of a herniated disc (see the opposite page).

The recovery period from bone graft surgery is quite prolonged. Time in the hospital with a cast is three to four weeks, with another six weeks or so in the cast to allow the new bone to knit solidly. To regain full strength and motion, the patient must build up his back and leg muscles by exercises, usually begun in the hospital, using a therapeutic pool and walking with the aid of parallel bars. Later, walking with crutches and then with a cane, and a long continuation of back and leg exercises are necessary for full recovery.

Joints other than vertebrae (for instance, the hip or knee) can be surgically fused. This alternative to artificial joint replacement, if suitable, may be more acceptable to many patients. Fusion almost always gives permanent relief of pain. However, a welded hip, knee, or other joint may compel a stiff-legged gait, make it awkward to sit in a chair, and impose other disadvantages.

GOUT

The cartoon concept of gout is familiar to everyone. A grossly fat man sits with a leg outstretched on a pillow. Imaginary devils jab pitchforks into the red-hot swollen joint of his big toe while the table beside him overflows with rich foods and bottles of liquor. The implication is that gout is the price paid for riotous and dissolute living.

How accurate is this picture? The tormented victim is almost surely a man (less than 5 percent of gout patients are women). He is middle-aged or older; initial acute attacks are most frequent in the fifth decade of life. Quite possibly he is overweight or heavyset. His big toe joint is probably, though not necessarily, the site of attack. The violence of his pain can hardly be exaggerated, but his torment does not arise directly from years of wanton gourmandizing.

The nature of gout. A gouty person's primary trouble is incapacity for handling uric acid. This substance, which everybody excretes in urine, is derived from *purines,* which are nitrogenous materials contained in many different foods. They are also synthesized in the body, so even if we never ate purines, we would still make a lot of our own.

A gouty person produces too much uric acid, or gets rid of too little of it, or both. Abnormal accumulations of uric acid in body fluids—a sort of supersaturated solution—allow deposits of urate crystals (salts of uric acid) to be laid down in the lining of joints or on the surface of joint cartilage. When this happens, the needle-sharp crystals trigger an explosive inflammatory reaction, with extreme pain in one of the big toes, or in a wrist, knee, or ankle.

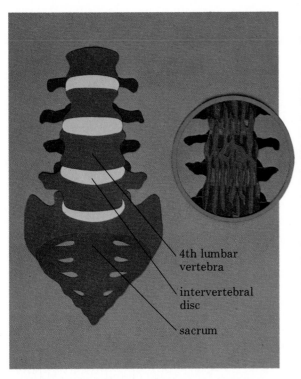

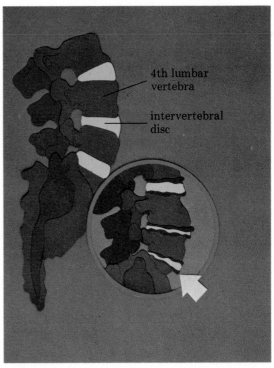

NORMAL AND ARTHRITICALLY FUSED VERTEBRAE

Arthritic disease may cause joints to grow together immovably (ankylosis). Compare the fused bones of vertebrae (in circle) to the normal spinal relationships at left.

The side view shows normal vertebrae with shock-absorbing discs between them. The circle shows degenerative disease of the edges of the lumbar vertebrae (white arrow).

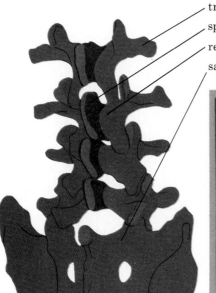

transverse processes
spinous processes (lumbar vertebrae)
rear plate of vertebra
sacrum

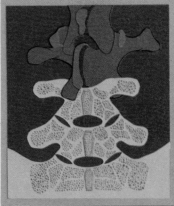

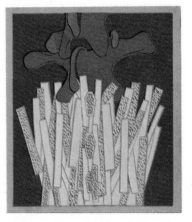

SURGICAL "WELDING" OF VERTEBRAE (SPINAL FUSION)

Shown above is a three-quarter rear view of the vertebral column of the lower back. The powerful muscles of the back attach to the spinous and transverse processes.

In preparation for bone grafting, surface bone is removed from spinous and transverse processes and the rear plate of the lumbar vertebrae and sacrum.

Bone chips from the patient's pelvis are packed over the surface of vertebrae and gradually fuse solidly, leaving the joint stiff but pain-free.

Gout runs in families, and gout-prone persons have a hereditary tendency to produce too much uric acid or excrete too little, or both. This does not mean that every member of a family will necessarily have gout attacks, even though uric acid levels may be high. Some students believe that persons with high blood levels of uric acid (hyperuricemia) have exceptionally high intelligence, a legend rarely if ever disputed by gout patients.

A secondary form of gout, unrelated to heredity, is caused by some other diseases or by certain drugs. Whether gout is primary or secondary, the affected joint looks, feels, and responds to drugs exactly the same.

Symptoms and progression. An initial attack of gout is sudden, affects a single joint, and is unimaginably painful. The joint swells, becomes purplish red, hot, and so tender the slightest pressure is unbearable and even the weight of a bed sheet may make the patient cry out in pain.

Each attack is self-limited and subsides completely in a few days or weeks. Thereafter the affected joint is perfectly normal until another attack occurs many months or even years later. An ancient Greek runner is known to have won an Olympic race between attacks of gout. As time goes on, intervals between attacks become shorter and more than one joint is involved at the same time. Various unusual events in the patient's life may provoke attacks—injury, injection of drugs, operations, or the intake of certain foods.

Without adequate treatment, many joints, especially in the hands and feet, may be crippled and deformed. Urate deposits in the kidneys may cause kidney stones and kidney failure. High blood pressure and heart trouble also may be associated. Deposits of chalky urates called *tophi* may form near the rims of the ears or near joints. Generally these cause no pain, but they may interfere with joint motion if the untreated disease advances.

Diagnosis

Superficially, a gouty joint may look very much like a joint affected by rheumatoid arthritis or infection. Clues that suggest a predisposition to gout are (1) a family history of the disease, and (2) urinary passage of a kidney stone. Recurrent attacks of severe joint pain with long intervening periods of complete freedom from arthritis are highly suggestive of gout.

Urate crystals in joint fluids may be identified under a microscope, and tests may be given to rule out other conditions and to measure uric acid in the blood. Although most patients with gout have high uric acid levels, similar high levels are associated with other conditions such as kidney failure, certain blood diseases, lead poisoning, starvation, psoriasis, and the use of certain drugs.

Pseudogout or "false gout" closely resembles true gout but has a different origin. Pseudogout usually affects older men (mean age, 57 years) who have deposits of calcium salts, rather than urate salts, in the cartilage of affected joints. X rays, as well as the identification of different types of crystals, distinguish the two conditions.

Treatment

The major complications of gout—joint crippling, kidney stones, and kidney failure—have been greatly minimized by treatments that are highly effective if followed faithfully under a physician's direction.

Sudden, acute gout attacks respond promptly to drugs that suppress the specific kind of inflammation caused by uric acid crystals. The oldest of these drugs, known for centuries, is colchicine, derived from the autumn crocus.

The pain in a red-hot gouty joint subsides within 24 to 48 hours if an adequate dose of colchicine is given, but timing is important. Even a short delay in beginning treatment after onset may increase the severity and delay the drug's abatement of pain and swelling. Colchicine has no effect on other forms of arthritis. If it works, the vanquished inflammation was almost surely caused by gout.

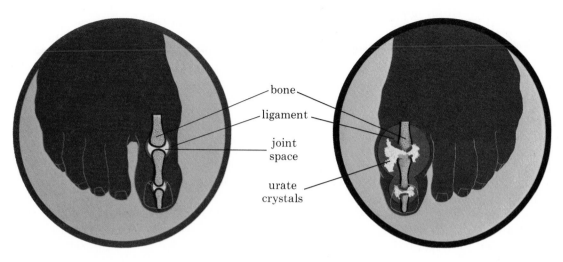

A NORMAL TOE

A normal toe joint has a clearly defined joint space and ligaments. After an acute attack of gout subsides, the joint returns to normal and remains so until the next attack.

A GOUTY TOE

In an acute attack of gout, deposits of urate crystals penetrate the joint space and cartilage, causing swelling and extreme pain, both of which eventually subside.

Unfortunately, the amount of colchicine that overcomes an acute attack is practically the same as the amount that causes stomach upset or diarrhea. Undesirable side effects are so common that other less toxic drugs have largely replaced this time-honored remedy.

Two other drugs for controlling acute attacks are in common use today. Phenylbutazone (Butazolidin) is reliable and effective, and indomethacin (Indocin) also has been used with good results.

Prevention. A plausible way to prevent acute attacks of gout would be to deprive the disease of its "raw material," uric acid, so that urate crystals could not form. This can in fact be accomplished by two kinds of drugs that work in different ways.

A class of drugs called *uricosurics,* or urate diuretics, increases the outflow of uric acid through the kidneys and thereby reduces accumulations in the blood. Two such drugs, probenecid (Benemid) and sulfinpyrazone (Anturane), have a long record of effectiveness, but they act slowly and require continuous daily use to maintain uric acid at a normal level.

A dozen years or so ago, a newer drug, allopurinol (Zyloprim), came into widespread medical use for gout. It acts uniquely upon enzyme systems to cut down the production of uric acid in the body so there's less to excrete. Allopurinol effectively keeps uric acid at a normal level year after year, but has to be taken every day on a continuous basis. Alone or in conjunction with uricosurics, allopurinol can be taken to reduce the size of urate deposits in the tissues in or around joints, bursae, and tendons.

The net effect of drug control of uric acid levels is to greatly lessen, if not abolish, the complications of joint deformities, kidney stones, and kidney damage, as well as the likelihood of acute attacks. The outlook for gout patients who receive adequate care and are willing to take their medicine daily for long periods, even a lifetime, is hopeful indeed.

BACKACHE

Backaches arise from scores of causes, but hurt in much the same places: along and to the sides of the spine, and particularly in the region of the lower back called the lumbosacral area. Vulnerability to low back pain is partly the fault of nature, which gave us 33 separate vertebrae piled atop each other in a double-S curve (viewed from the side). A bewildering interlinkage of muscles, ligaments, cushions, cables, nerves, and joints keeps the "blocks" from toppling and permits movement of the back.

Anyone who goes through life without a bout of low back pain is exceptional indeed. The accompanying drawing gives an oversimplified idea of the complex structures involved in complaints of "lumbago" or "sciatica" or "oh my aching back." And it suggests why it is often difficult to pinpoint the cause of pain if there is no detectable abnormality. In fact, it is sometimes impossible to determine whether trouble originates in bones, muscles, joints, or possibly in deep-lying organs in the back or in the pelvis.

Low Back Syndrome

The most common cause of pain in the lower back is low back strain. Acute strain usually follows an injury that at the time may seem trivial—tripping on a carpet, twisting the foot on a stone, or leaning over a counter to raise a window. Or the injury may be quite severe, as in lifting something heavy, and may feel as if "something gave way." Onset of diffuse pain is usually rapid. Muscles go into spasm and "splint" themselves to prevent painful movement. Certain motions cause stabbing pain and the sufferer may assume an odd posture to avert anguish. Areas of the lower back are tender when pressed.

The condition is benign (though the pain isn't) in the sense that it wears off in a few days while nature heals whatever needs healing. In the meantime, local application of heat is comforting, as is bed rest on a firm mattress with a pillow under slightly bent knees. Sometimes a corset that constrains movement of the back is helpful, but it should not be worn habitually because underlying muscles soon go flabby.

Chronic low back strain is probably the most common form of backache. Usually there is stiffness, some degree of pain on motion of the back, and tenderness to pressure on certain spots. However, pain does not radiate into buttocks, thighs, or legs, as would result from pressure on nerve roots. Symptoms may persist for weeks, months, or years, with repeated flare-ups, perhaps elicited by a sedentary man's violent weekend of sport or a housewife's day spent rearranging the furniture.

Young people who are presumably slender, muscularly active, and in good physical shape are not particularly prone to chronic low back pain. Susceptibility increases as we grow older, heavier, lazier, and as joints begin to wear. The common precondition of chronic strain is flabbiness of back and abdominal muscles, lack of exercise, and bad posture, which put stress on muscles, ligaments, and soft tissues.

The "cure" is largely in the hands of the sufferer: progressive muscle-strengthening exercises, designed to make a strong back out of a weak one. Various "backache" exercises that flex muscles of the back and shoulders are effective. Continued, repeated exercise, gradually increased in duration, can do much to restore normal productive capacity and enjoyment of leisure activities.

Warm-ups. Backaches can be triggered by rushing pell-mell into strenuous physical activity. Take a tip from athletes who warm up before going into all-out action. Loosen tight muscles and relax tensions before exercise, or on arising in the morning, by rotating your arms windmill-like, or bending and twisting at the waist. Or swing a broom, rake, or golf club over, back of, and around your head and shoulders, the way an on-deck batter swings his bat before facing the pitcher.

Have some item of clothing to protect against chill when you relax after becoming soaked with perspiration. A soft breeze playing on your sweaty back can lead to muscle aches.

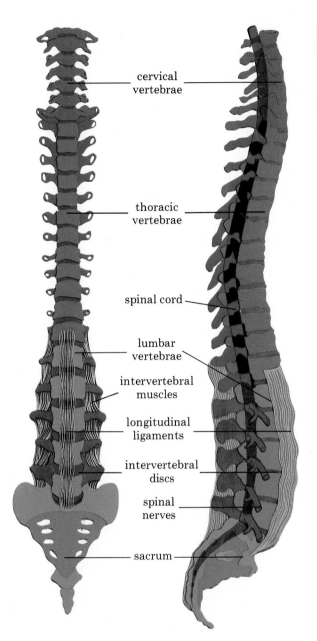

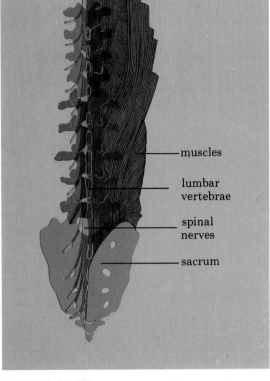

ACHING BACK

The complex interlinkage of structures of the lower back, a few of which are shown in this rear view, indicates why it is sometimes difficult if not impossible to pinpoint a specific source of pain if no abnormalities are detectable.

THE SPINAL COLUMN

This front view of the vertebral column (left) suggests the complexity of the structures that keep its building blocks from toppling. Ligaments tie bones together; back muscles (not shown) attach to the bony projections like cables. Springy discs between vertebrae permit back movement. The side view (right) shows the normal curves of the vertebral column. The common complaint of low back pain originates in the lumbosacral area, shown in green. The spinal cord runs within a protective shell of bone, and spinal nerves emerge between vertebrae.

Disc Trouble

Many kinds of back pain do have clear-cut physical causes. Thorough examination and medical history-taking are obviously important in diagnosis. One rather common kind of back pain with a definite cause is "disc trouble." The condition has a peak incidence around middle age, in part because of degenerative changes.

The injured part of the spine is one or more of the intervertebral discs that act as shock-absorbing cushions between vertebrae. The doughnut-shaped disc has a tough outer ring with a soft pulpy mass (nucleus) in its center. A small tear in the rim permits the pulp to protrude (herniate) into the spinal canal where it can press excruciatingly upon a nerve root. The result is sharp knifelike pain that shoots over the course of the nerve.

Most frequently the rupture occurs between the two lowest lumbar vertebrae L4 and L5 or between the lowest lumbar vertebra and the sacrum just below, as shown in the drawing. You can cover the general area with the palm of your hand laid across the midline just above the buttocks.

Symptoms. Disc trouble often begins with a popping or snapping sensation in the back followed by gripping pain. There may have been preceding intermittent back distress for some time, but the sudden attack is usually provoked by stooping over to pick up a heavy object or by lifting or twisting motions. Sneezing, straining, and leaning forward accentuate the pain. Severe muscle spasm may freeze the patient in a bent-over position. He tends to protect the affected side by leaning the opposite way (listing). Standing or walking may be nearly impossible, but pain usually can be relieved by lying down.

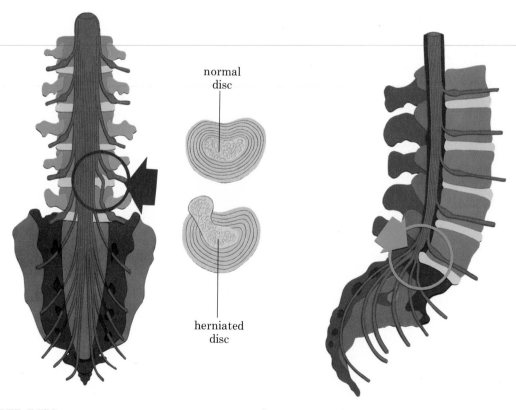

normal
disc

herniated
disc

SLIPPED DISC

Cushiony discs between vertebrae (small drawings) have a tough outer ring and a pulpy mass (nucleus) in the center. The nucleus may herniate into the spinal canal through a break in the ring and press against nerves (blue arrow).

SOURCE OF PAIN

This side view shows a herniated disc pressing against nerves at the level of the fifth lumbar vertebra (green arrow). The trouble-causing disc (or discs) may be identified by the course of pain over the compressed nerve.

Diagnosis. Pain follows the course of the compressed nerve, which helps to identify the disc that is responsible. The physician may detect decreases in tendon reflexes at the ankle, loss of sensation to a pinprick on the outside of the foot, or weak calf muscles. If the protrusion occurs between Lumbars 4 and 5, it can cause numbness, prickly sensations inside the upper leg, weakness of muscles that extend the knee, and a decrease or absence of the knee-jerk reflex. More than one disc may be affected, and ordinary X rays are of little diagnostic help.

Treatment. The initial acute attack may subside but there is a tendency to recurrence. The degree of disability depends on many variables: the amount of pulp extruded, the degree of pressure on nerves, and the number of nerves affected.

Conservative treatment is often highly successful. Basic measures—absolute bed rest, heat, pain relievers, and sedatives —can usually be carried out at home. Bed rest tends to reduce the irritation of nerve roots and reduces symptoms. The herniated pulp does not retract into the center of the disc where it belongs, but tends to atrophy or wither a bit and reduce symptoms. After recovery, a supervised course of progressive exercises to strengthen the back muscles can do much to prevent future attacks.

Surgery. Patients who do not respond to conservative treatment or have repeated attacks may benefit from surgery. Preliminary tests are necessary, such as *myelography* (visualization of the spinal cord after injecting a substance opaque to X rays), and nerve conduction studies. The surgeon removes the herniated disc material along with any degenerated fragments that may be present. Spinal fusion may or may not be done at the same time. Fusion is a technique of "welding" vertebrae together with bone-graft material as cement.

Pain of Many Causes

Low back pain may be an accompanying symptom of a great many diseases or abnormalities. Fortunately, these are less frequent than the common widespread backaches described above. But unexplained persistent back pain calls for thorough examination to detect causes, if possible. Some underlying causes are minor, but some are quite serious.

Pain caused by fractures is usually of obvious origin. Persons with osteoporosis (see page 458) are quite subject to spontaneous fractures; their skeletons are very fragile. Numerous kinds of infections, chronic or acute, can cause disabling low back pain. Ankylosing spondylitis ("bamboo spine") affects the vertebrae and sacroiliac joints. Low back pain is an early symptom of this condition, which is progressive and can eventually lead to a bony union of spinal parts.

Diseases such as ulcerative colitis, regional enteritis, and psoriasis can affect the spine and cause sacroiliac arthritis. Some forms of cancer (breast, kidney, lung, prostate, and thyroid) spread readily to bone, causing fractures and pain. Back pain without any abnormality detectable by physical examination or laboratory tests is an aspect of nervous tension that leads to muscle spasms.

Obviously, back pain that does not wear off in a few days or respond to simple measures calls for thorough examination.

NON-ARTICULAR

RHEUMATISM

Some disorders that cause pain in and around joints are not true arthritis, in that joint structures themselves are not involved directly. Affected tissues are those that surround joints (tendons, ligaments, bursae, and muscles) and disturbances are collectively called non-articular rheumatic diseases. They are not age-limited; young people can suffer from them. But they are common causes of aches and pains in older people, perhaps resulting from a seemingly trivial injury or overstressing an unadapted body, as in the strenuous weekend athlete or the inactive woman who has painted a ceiling.

Bursitis

Surrounding all large joints are small sacs that produce lubricating fluid and act as shock absorbers that cushion the underlying joints and permit muscles and tendons to glide smoothly over bony ridges and turns. Big joints such as the hip and shoulder have several bursae, and some may communicate with the interior of the joint through thin tubular ducts. Repeated injury or a sharp blow may lead to inflammation or "bursitis." Often bursitis is an acute condition that lasts only a few days to a week, but sometimes pain may persist and severely restrict motion of the joint.

Shoulder bursitis. One of the largest bursae is located near the outer tip of the shoulder joint. Above it lies a strong tendon that helps to elevate and rotate the arm. Over the tendon is a bony arch that forms the rounded part of the shoulder tip. The area is easily bumped or overstressed. Injury to the tendon at this bony rim may result in deposits of calcium as part of the healing process. These deposits, from pinhead to bean size, irritate the tendon and the wall of the bursa.

Rupture of the calcium deposits into the cavity of the bursal sac is announced by a sudden burst of severe pain that the sufferer is not likely to forget. Flecks of calcium cast a shadow by X ray. This shoulder condition is called *calcific tendinitis.* Usually the tendon injury results from heavy lifting or strenuous exertion, but the excruciating knifelike pain may come on without any apparent cause and even awaken the patient out of a sound sleep in the middle of the night.

Even the slightest motion triggers pain during the acute phase and the patient keeps his arm rigidly at his side. The shoulder tip is extremely tender. Motion is restricted or carried out very gingerly. Usually the acute spell lasts only a few days, but after it subsides, a dull ache may persist for many weeks. In this chronic state the range of motion is limited, and discomfort is aggravated by overhead raising of the arm.

Pain relief is usually prompt and complete if treatment is given early. Analgesic drugs, X-ray therapy, and diathermy are effective, but all measures fail in some cases. It may then be necessary to remove the bursa and the calcium deposits.

"Frozen shoulder." Another type of shoulder bursitis involves the tendon (bicipital) that bends the elbow. It runs in a bony groove in the upper arm bone in the front of the shoulder. When inflamed it causes pain that is usually less severe and has more gradual onset than calcific tendinitis, but is likely to last longer. Widespread reaction of other tissues around the shoulder may cause them to stick together. These adhesions progressively restrict shoulder motion and prevent its elevation away from the side of the chest—a condition called "frozen shoulder."

If allowed to reach this stage of marked loss of motion, protracted and extensive therapeutic exercises or even surgical correction may be needed. However, if the condition is recognized early, it can be prevented by repeated injections of novocaine and cortisone-like drugs, combined with persistent exercise.

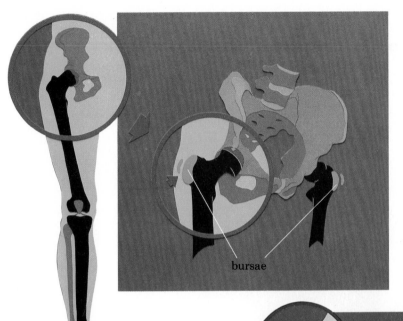

BURSITIS

A bursa is a small sac between parts that move upon each other. The fluid-filled sac produces a lubricant that permits muscles and tendons to glide smoothly over adjacent structures. Bursitis is a painful inflammation of the sac that causes pain and restricts movement. Big joints, such as the hip joint shown at left, have more than one bursa (red arrow).

bursae

deltoid bursa   coracoid bursa

SHOULDER BURSITIS

A large bursa lies near the tip of the shoulder, under muscles and tendons that raise and rotate the arm (bursae shown in green). Injury to the tendon may produce calcium deposits that can rupture into the bursal sac, causing pain so severe that the victim holds the arm as immovable as possible.

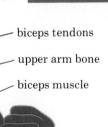

biceps tendons

upper arm bone

biceps muscle

FROZEN SHOULDER

Inflammation of the biceps tendon (yellow arrow) that passes over the head of the upper arm bone causes surrounding tissues to react and stick together. If this condition goes untreated, shoulder motion is limited and the arm cannot be lifted from the side of the chest.

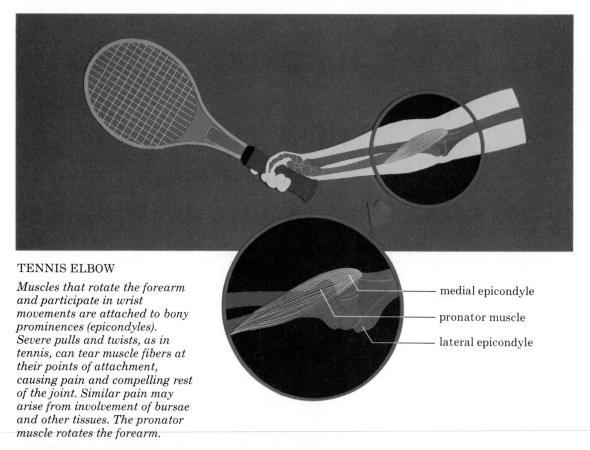

TENNIS ELBOW

Muscles that rotate the forearm and participate in wrist movements are attached to bony prominences (epicondyles). Severe pulls and twists, as in tennis, can tear muscle fibers at their points of attachment, causing pain and compelling rest of the joint. Similar pain may arise from involvement of bursae and other tissues. The pronator muscle rotates the forearm.

medial epicondyle

pronator muscle

lateral epicondyle

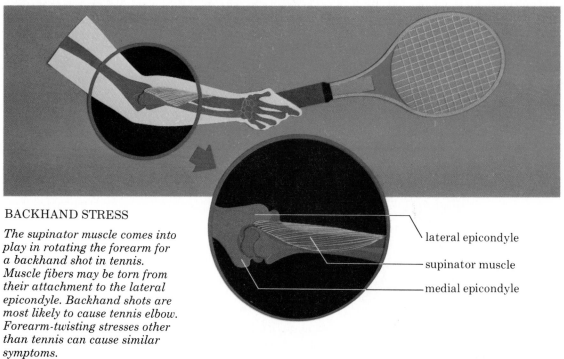

BACKHAND STRESS

The supinator muscle comes into play in rotating the forearm for a backhand shot in tennis. Muscle fibers may be torn from their attachment to the lateral epicondyle. Backhand shots are most likely to cause tennis elbow. Forearm-twisting stresses other than tennis can cause similar symptoms.

lateral epicondyle

supinator muscle

medial epicondyle

Tennis elbow. On both sides of the elbow, the muscles that rotate the forearm are attached to bony prominences called *epicondyles.* Sudden pulls or severe tension may tear the muscle fibers at these points of attachment, resulting in an inflammatory reaction.

Motions used by a tennis player in swinging a racket are especially prone to tear these muscles from the membrane that covers the knobs of bone at the elbow—hence the term "tennis elbow." Less athletic activities such as twisting a screwdriver can do the same thing.

The pain may come on slowly, but is usually abrupt in onset and compels some rest of the affected joint. Discomfort usually lasts only a few days but may continue for weeks and be very disabling. Injections of local anesthetic with or without cortisone-like drugs, or the use of oral analgesics, are usually effective. The healing process is, of course, impeded if the joint is repeatedly stressed.

Fibrositis. Connective tissues surround and hold together muscles and tendons and separate the capsules of joints. "Fibrositis" is a nonspecific reaction of these soft tissues, causing stiffness, aching, and tenderness. The cause is not known; the tissue fibers are not truly inflamed, as the suffix "-itis" would suggest.

In the neck and upper back, where symptoms of fibrositis are common, it is thought that the aches are nearly always referred pain from joints of the neck or upper spine, not due to primary soft tissue disease. Diffuse muscle aches and pains of the same type are seen during acute infections such as influenza. Localized tender areas or "trigger spots" are frequently present in fibrositis.

Many persons attribute nagging low backaches and aching between shoulders and neck to exposure to drafts, sudden changes in temperature, excessive humidity, or cold damp weather. Folklore holds that when someone's rheumatism gets worse, it forecasts a change for the worse in the weather. Scientific proof that abrupt weather changes cause aches and pains is lacking, but the relationship is so commonly observed by patients with many types of arthritis that we tend to believe that perhaps there is some physiological basis for the phenomenon.

Treatment of fibrositis includes the injection of trigger spots with local anesthetic that may break the pain cycle and give prolonged relief. Various forms of heat (lamp, electric pad, hot water bottle, and sauna), massage with minor manipulation, and stretching of the neck or back also can be effective.

Inflammation of any tissue or organ is identified by the suffix "-itis" at the end of its name. Thus, *bursitis* means inflammation of a bursa; *arthritis,* of a joint; *myositis,* of a muscle; *tendinitis,* of a tendon; *neuritis,* of a nerve; *fascitis,* of fascia; *capsulitis,* of the joint capsule; and *osteomyelitis,* of bone.

EMOTIONAL ASPECTS
OF RHEUMATISM

A common but frequently unrecognized cause of pain in and around joints is muscle spasm resulting from emotional stresses and nervous tension. The pains are just as real as the discomforts caused by true arthritis or fibrositis. The patient does not just imagine that he has pain; he actually experiences it. But it originates in unconscious actions of the mind that cause the body to respond.

This is a very difficult concept for most patients with "psychogenic rheumatism" to appreciate, yet it is very important that the mechanism be recognized and distinguished from forms of arthritis that can progress to disablement. These rheumatic symptoms do not result from any abnormality of the joint or surrounding tissues and they never produce crippling or loss of function. They are not treated like cases of true arthritis.

The psychogenic type of rheumatism occurs in persons of susceptible emotional makeup. For instance, a formerly stable person who has undergone a great emotional shock or a series of stressful events becomes more and more upset by minor stresses and has difficulty in coping with the ordinary demands of living. A connection between pains in joints and muscles and tension-producing circumstances is almost never apparent to the patient and his or her family, however.

The physician recognizes that the patient's symptoms are vague, fleeting, variable in location, and often extremely intense. The complaints do not fit the pattern of any organic illness. Thorough physical examination, X rays, and laboratory tests show nothing abnormal.

Without help, the patient may more and more avoid meeting with and resolving the everyday demands of life. He or she may retreat into "arthritis" as a way of life, a self-defeating solution of conflict.

Most patients with psychogenic rheumatism cannot recognize a relationship between emotions and "arthritic" pains that are real and severe. As far as they are concerned, they are not nervous or upset in any way. When an association is suggested by a doctor, the response is often "are you telling me that I'm just imagining all this pain?"

No, the pain is real, not imagined. To accept its origin, the patient needs understanding counsel. So, often, does his or her family. Commonplace examples of how the body is unconsciously influenced by the mind can help to make psychogenic processes understandable and nothing to be ashamed of. Embarrassment, for example—a purely emotional event—causes tiny blood vessels to open up and heat and redden the face; we blush. Sudden fright quickens the pulse rate, raises blood pressure, makes the heart pound. Some emotions make the tear glands flood; we weep. In a similar way, continuous stresses can affect the blood vessels serving muscles and joints and alter the functions of secreting glands.

There is, too, the happiest of assurances: the worst disasters of crippling and deformity that the word "arthritis" can conjure up will never befall the patient with psychogenic rheumatism.

PROSPECTS FOR TOMORROW

Causes of most of the common forms of arthritis remain unknown, but significant advances have been made in understanding the underlying mechanisms of rheumatic disorders. Research gives hope for more effective methods of treatment and prevention of these widespread diseases. The following is a brief review of some current directions of research.

Osteoarthritis. This is the most frequent form of arthritis in middle-aged and older people. Degenerative changes in joint structures have previously been described and illustrated (see page 238). Current evidence indicates that these changes result from biochemical stresses that injure cells in the cartilage called *chondrocytes.*

When injured, these cells release enzymes that destroy protein fibers that make up the matrix of soft elastic tissue covering the gliding surface of the end of the bone. Attempts to repair the damage result in inadequate and abnormal bone growth. The rate of breakdown eventually exceeds the ability of cartilage cells to repair themselves.

Current research seeks knowledge that may be effectively applied to control osteoarthritic changes: how fibers of collagen (see page 234) are formed, the nature of cartilage ground substance, the chemical regulators of cartilage breakdown and repair, and the action of drugs upon the functions of chondrocytes.

Rheumatoid arthritis. The possibility that rheumatoid arthritis is caused by infection has intrigued investigators for years. Current evidence suggests that in rheumatoid arthritis and SLE (systemic lupus erythematosus, a closely related disease), viral agents may provoke a series of untoward events in the immune systems of the body. The immune system destroys or neutralizes substances that are foreign to the body, but at times it also reacts harmfully against normal body substances.

A good deal is known about cellular and blood-carried mechanisms that produce inflammation in joint-lining tissues, in rheumatoid arthritis and SLE. It has not been possible to culture a virus from patients with arthritis, so the theory that viruses are a primary cause of joint inflammation is still a hypothesis. The tremendous magnifying power of the electron microscope has revealed tiny elements that look like virus particles inside the blood vessels of patients with SLE, but this evidence is not yet confirmed.

If a viral origin of arthritis could be proved, and if the disease could be induced experimentally in an animal, possible means of prevention—for instance, by a vaccine—might be found. So far there is no model or counterpart in animals to assist such development. However, research on SLE has been greatly aided by the availability of an animal model, the New Zealand mouse, which undergoes pathologic changes similar to those in the human disease. Studies of patients and animal models suggest that both genetic and infectious (viral) factors play a part in causing the disorder, but investigations are incomplete.

New drugs. The search for more effective and less toxic arthritis drugs is intense and continuous. One group of promising drugs for treatment of rheumatoid arthritis and SLE is classed as *immunosuppressive agents.* These drugs came into use to prevent the rejection of a transplanted kidney as a foreign agent. The drugs—azothioprine (Imuran), cyclophosphamide (Cytoxan), and others—suppress the reactivity of the immune system and thus enhance the probability that a transplanted organ will be accepted by the patient's body.

How do these drugs give benefit in rheumatoid arthritis and SLE? Not by killing the virus (if it is a virus), but probably by suppressing inflammatory reactions. Whatever the mechanism, the drugs do work and show promise, but will have to undergo thousands of tests to determine benefits and safety before they will be approved for general use.

D-penicillamine has been used experimentally in treatment of rheumatoid arthritis, but its use has been limited by side effects. Some of these are nuisances—nausea, vomiting, and diminished sense of taste—while others are more serious: albumin in the urine, and reduced clotting ability of the blood. Because of potential toxic effects, frequent blood counts and examinations of the urine are necessary.

If arthritis and rheumatism are such widespread and disabling diseases, why has there been relatively little research progress in finding causes and cures? The diseases are complex, and basic studies can only be carried out by highly trained, diversely specialized personnel. Funds for arthritis research have been limited, but nationwide efforts are under way to finance research in these diseases which are not dramatic killers, but insidious destroyers of dignity and quality of life, and, as such, are very costly to society.

EMOTIONS & SEX IN MATURITY

Only now is our society learning what many people over 40 have always known: that the middle and later years bring not only special problems but special enrichments. As in the earlier phases of life, there is continuing change. Therefore the later decades can present an open venture. And at no other time does emotional well-being play so strong a role in general health and vitality.

The majority of people now live longer than the Biblical three score years and ten. Despite public talk of our living in a youth culture, we are increasingly a society of the mature. The birth rate continues to fall, and life expectancy to rise. The proportions of people over 40 and over 65 have more than doubled since the turn of this century, and the trend will continue. Growing technology and affluence will keep raising the demand that life be not only prolonged but enhanced.

The number of middle-aged people with elderly parents also will keep growing. This may turn out to be beneficial in many ways. Most people prefer to put off thinking about later life until it arrives, rather than plan for it. Through their relationships with their elderly parents, middle-aged men and women may come to understand the emotional, social, and sexual aspects of aging — and thus be better prepared for their own futures.

Better preparation is increasingly possible because of research into the emotional and social aspects of aging now under way in medicine, psychology, psychiatry, gerontology (the study of aging), and geriatrics (the study and treatment of late-life disorders). Such knowledge opens more avenues to health and fulfillment in the second half of life than were thought possible even a few decades ago. Certainly it shows that the realities of full maturity need not fit old, pessimistic stereotypes.

Grim cliché presents aging as a gradual, gray descent into feebleness, solitude, inactivity, and loss. There are real problems in aging, but most people who understand and adapt to them need not lose involvement in the world, achievement, pride, companionship, love, and sexuality. Age, once seen as an inevitable disease, can be one of life's finer surprises.

Unfortunately, our society still fails to prepare people for a healthy, active later life. Coping with age is usually left to individual trial and error. In fact, physicians often complain that the weakest spots in their professional training are aging, sex and marriage problems, and emotional and psychosomatic disorders. As we have said, psychosexual factors influence general well-being more and more as years pass. The best health insurance for later life is to join one's physician in cultivating a knowledge and awareness of these matters.

THE MIND AND EMOTIONS IN NORMAL AGING

The Nervous System

Since the nervous system organizes our thoughts, emotions, and behavior, its aging can affect our mental well-being. As many people enter middle age, they start worrying about mental aging in themselves and older relatives. Forgetting a telephone number is a normal lapse at 20; at 50 it may arouse fears of creeping senility. Slow sexual response, which is a normal occasional event in young adulthood, may make someone 50 or 60 despair of remaining an adequate love partner. Fortunately, many common ideas of middle-age slump and late-life enfeeblement are far worse than reality; and deficits, if they do occur, are often treatable.

Aging happens at different rates in various individuals, and in different parts of the body. One's hearing is most acute at age ten; from then on, it's all downhill! A major-league pitcher may be "too old" at 25 because of a strained tendon, or at 35 because his legs tire after a few innings of peak professional effort—and he may feel for a while that "my life is over." Age is relative. When discussing it, one must always ask, "Too old for what? For how long? Under what conditions?"

The nervous system, like all body tissue, shows slowing and wear with time, but less than many other parts of the body. As late life approaches, brain and nerve cells consume less oxygen; as a result, they transmit and process information a bit more slowly. This slowing may begin in middle age, but it rarely becomes marked until the seventh or even the eighth decade.

The other major age-change of the nervous system is in memory. There are at least two kinds of memory, *short-term memory* (STM) and *long-term memory* (LTM). STM handles new information for up to about 15 minutes; then the information is lost or is stored by LTM. Aging brings a slight decrease in STM, finally up to some 15 percent in a healthy old person. However, LTM remains stable or even sharpens. As we will see later (see page 281), this change in STM-LTM balance may serve a biological purpose for our species and be as much of a gain as a loss.

The net result of these changes is usually small. Most scientists and other observers have long claimed that we reach the height of our mental powers well on in middle life. Hippocrates, the father of medicine, put the pinnacle of life at the middle fifties. Modern psychological testing generally is a bit more optimistic. The ability to learn and to solve problems increases in most people until about 60. In many, it not only holds up past that time but keeps growing. It is no accident that those who run most enterprises, from small organizations to governments, are usually in their fifth, sixth, or later decades of life. They have mastered the complexities of decision making and human relationships. Experience and normal good health prevent "too old" ever from arriving for many people.

Old dogs and new tricks. The ability of the middle-aged and elderly to keep learning is vitally important in professional retraining, creating new life-styles, and developing leisure and avocational interests. Dr. Kenneth Soddy, former director of the World Federation for Mental Health, says that even in old age there may be forward strides in intellectual mastery and acquisition of new skills, such as learning languages, painting, playing musical instruments, writing—and, if one wishes, a second career.

Some mental slowing and STM loss are inevitable, but we have noted that changes are rarely striking in a healthy person before very advanced age. If neurological and mental function are affected by age or illness, in oneself or an older relative, these steps can help compensate:

• Consult a physician and take every possible step to ensure general good health, with special emphasis on the circulatory system and nutrition.

• Be sure that deficits in sight and hearing aren't contributing to problems in reading, comprehension, and sustained mental effort.

• If emotional or practical problems create depression, seek medical and/or psychological advice. Depression slows mental functions.

• Allow slightly more time for complex intellectual efforts and provide more memory "cues."

The last point may be important in pursuing professional and avocational interests. After 60, many people show a slight drop in time-controlled IQ tests; the pre-60 scores return if time limits are removed. People do not know less after 60; it is simply that in mental as in physical efforts, doing something may take a bit longer. Solving complex problems often involves juggling several new bits of new information; the normal small decrease in STM may make this a little more difficult and tiring. If one becomes aware of occasional but recurring instances of "forgetting things," much work efficiency may be restored by keeping facts and figures directly before one at the desk or work place to cue one's memory.

People with elderly friends and relatives also should keep in mind that neurological slowing in the late decades, especially slowing of speech, may give a false impression of mental impairment.

Finally, one should know that the best way to reach a mentally alert and productive later life is by preparing for it. The more we use memory and intelligence throughout life, the better they survive aging. If minor mental changes do occur, they often can be balanced by accepting the challenge of compensating for them.

MIDDLE AGE

Middle age once belonged to a privileged few, and they didn't always enjoy it. Until quite recently, only a small minority of the world's people lived till age 40; chronic ills and psychic chill plagued many who did. Shakespeare wrote in his later thirties about entering the autumn of his life!

Now most Americans reach and surpass middle age. Compared to middle-agers of previous generations, they are fit, active, and youthful—truly in the prime of life. Furthermore, people now marry earlier and have fewer children, so they reach the postparental years sooner. Sociologist Jessie Bernard points out that this is "a brand new phenomenon in human history . . . its potentials for happiness have hardly been explored." What needs explaining is why middle age is so often considered a crisis, and sometimes becomes one.

Middle-Age Stress and Crisis

Middle age is usually defined as the years between about 40 and 60. By 40, people have begun to notice lower peaks of strength and endurance, perhaps grayer or thinner hair, changing body contours, and minor ailments that cause preoccupation with health, digestion, and sleep. Aging itself may become a preoccupation. In fact, middle age is as much a state of mind as of calendar years. It may begin as early as the late 30s and extend well past 60. A great deal depends on whether it is felt as a problem or a fulfillment.

One stereotype shows middle age as a comfortable, settled state, with domestic and career routines that fit like a well-worn shoe. One allegedly becomes mellow, sedate, conservative, even stuffy and dowdy. A more hostile cliché makes the middle-aged frustrated prisoners of their jobs, families, and society—bitterly resigned, drowning anxiety in alcohol and pills, and unable to understand and communicate with their children or each other. There are just enough people who fit such pictures to keep the stereotypes alive. Fortunately, not everyone finds mid-life a crisis, and even many who do can emerge with greater self-love and satisfaction. We will look at some problems the middle-aged face, problems they may create, and some positive alternatives.

Many events crowd together in mid-life that make men and women review and reassess their lives. Children separate from home, parents become elderly, youthful looks fade, the climacteric arrives, and youthful aspirations are measured against real achievement. One compares oneself to contemporaries in appearance, health, worldly achievement, and success as a spouse and parent. This usually creates some uncertainties and self-doubt, which the majority of people eventually overcome. A person who reviews his life and, realistically or not, doesn't like what he sees, will suffer regret, guilt, and self-depreciation. He reacts in rebellion, slumps into resignation, or vacillates between the two states. In short, he suffers middle-age crisis.

Woman's crisis. The loss of youthful appearance probably hurts women's pride and confidence more than men's. Menopause (see page 441) can provoke grief, desperation, and a sense of having lost femininity and self-worth. Unfortunately, this may happen when a woman's husband is at the busiest stage of his career; perhaps he gives her less attention, and their sex life is routine or deficient.

A middle-aged woman can, of course, continue to win warmth and a sense of desirability. But if she loses her self-confidence, she is in for trouble. She competes with female rivals, real or imaginary, perhaps anticipates rejection from her husband, and shrinks from love and sex. Or she may try to deny that she is aging; she struggles into girlish clothes and behavior patterns, feverishly flirts, and seeks sexual affairs.

She has probably based much of her feminine pride on being a mother. Now her children fight parental control, leave home, and marry. With husband busy and children gone, household obligations diminish. If a woman has no interests outside her home, her existence seems very bleak.

If a woman's marriage was not rewarding, and she invested most of her love in her children, their departure can create a powerful case of the "empty-nest syndrome." The empty house may first bring a rush of freedom, says Dr. John Oliven, but then "a feeling of letdown, a sometimes irrational sense of being discarded. With her vitality no longer consumed by multiple daily problem-solving, even minor somatic symptoms tend to move into the center of awareness . . . they seem the only way to obtain concern from her loved ones. Fear of cancer, of recurrence of a previous mental illness, perhaps problems of job security, disappointment in a child, or absence of interests or hobbies outside homemaking—all can magnify the burdens which the middle-aged woman feels herself carrying."

She may feel that she has outgrown her marriage or that it has become intolerable. More women than in the past seek divorce, some with brave visions of finding a new identity, new assertiveness, a rewarding career, and renewed love and sexuality. Some are successful; others find themselves alone and frustrated or reliving the problems of

> ## "MOST SCIENTISTS CLAIM THAT WE REACH THE HEIGHT OF OUR MENTAL POWERS WELL ON IN MIDDLE LIFE."

their first marriages. Early divorce or widowhood can force a woman to launch herself anew in life with few resources and little experience, bearing many problems of both youth and middle age.

The woman who remained single and worked or who maintained a career through married adulthood faces many of the problems that preoccupy men in assessing their lives, especially the concern over whether one has met youthful goals.

Many of these problems may be swept under the rug as "change-of-life troubles," but not everything that happens in middle age results from menopause. It is not hormones that make a woman see her life as a disappointment, the future as a shrinking promise. Middle age involves a major transition, and it is one of a woman's most vulnerable periods—to doubt, upheaval, and disturbed relationships. It is a time to beware of hypochondria, depression, anxiety, abuse of alcohol and drugs, and psychosomatic ills that can become chronic.

Man's crisis. Men face some of the same problems, and others as well. There is no "male menopause," no marked change in hormone levels and reproductive capacity (see page 310). A man does, however, begin to notice that he has passed his peak in physical strength, sexual excitability, and perhaps in looks. He compares himself to his peers in body, mind, and career, and in social and family life. If disheartened, he condemns himself and fears the future.

The "mid-life blues" can strike strongly in early middle age if a man carries many relentless responsibilities — children to put through college, a wife experiencing her own mid-life problems, or the support of elderly relatives. Though his job probably demands more than ever, he may feel that his career has peaked, that he lives and labors on a treadmill; he also may feel that his family takes him for granted. His obligations seem to prohibit any change he wants to make in his life. As Professor Richard Kerckoff puts it, "Too many people own a piece of you and you can't say no to any of them." Society suggests that it's too late to change things, so a man may feel regret, helpless frustration, and rage.

Life at home can seem gray and constricting. The man's wife may have assumed management of the house, the children, and their social life. As a result, he feels emasculated, a domesticated "walking wallet"; sex becomes routine, and sometimes a chore. He may flee into busyness and use fatigue as an excuse for withdrawing. Just as some women use their households and children as alibis to avoid intimacy with their husbands, some men use their careers to escape marriage, sex, and paternal commitment.

Work and career, however, also may present problems. Perhaps a man has reached or can foresee the limits of his career and has a sense of failure. Missing the electric edge of youthful hope and ambition, he despairs. If he works for a long time at one organization, it may become a second family; if it moves or collapses, he mourns just as if he'd lost a loved one.

Success does not guarantee freedom from work-related problems. A driving, increasingly successful man has less time than ever to spend with his wife, who now especially needs his love, companionship, and support. Some job situations are like the proverbial jungle, and the stress takes physical and emotional tolls. Furthermore, a competitive and highly controlled man usually finds it difficult to admit and cope with feelings of fear and dependence. He plays tin soldier, hiding his conflicts and his softer side. This only sharpens his problems and makes it more difficult to relate to family and friends with easy warmth.

A man also may face a rather common but . little-discussed difficulty, "success phobia." Failure can be a painful but familiar way of life; success sometimes poses equally great emotional threats. The playwright Ibsen spoke of those "wrecked by success." It usually imposes responsibility and competitive pressure, to which even the emotionally resilient must adjust.

To a person with neurotic conflicts, a promotion or other success can bring depression, anxieties, or psychosomatic ills. He may fear rejection by insecure and envious friends and relatives. To understand success phobia, one should imagine someone who feels under pressure to produce a stupendous encore for a potentially hostile audience. Many women admit fear of being inadequate, unloved, and targets of retaliation if they assert themselves. Men often have the very same fears, but tend to deny them.

Denial of aging. Men, like women, may try to deny aging, creating youthful facades and seeking extramarital reassurance. Unfortunately, even minor incidents can thrust a desperate sense of aging on psychologically vulnerable men—one night of impotence, the need for glasses, a petty social or professional rebuff. Some men quickly withdraw sexually and emotionally. Others slip gradually into depression and restless dissatisfaction. They denigrate themselves, worry about minor lapses of memory or health, and find new tasks frightening or even paralyzing.

Another defense against aging is "middle-age rebellion." An extramarital venture may restore old levels of emotional and sexual vitality. Perhaps a man decides that he has changed deeply since he made his present commitments to spouse, career, and daily life. He seeks not only divorce but radically different work and life-style. This may be a genuine renovation or a frantic spin into unreality: sometimes a better life is found, sometimes old, deep-seated insecurities and conflicts reappear after the rush of excited change is spent.

Job problems often lead to problems at home, and conflicts at home can have echoes at work. Both spouses should be alert to this. They also should recognize that men's middle-age stress and crisis can lead to anxiety, depression, psychosomatic ills, self-destructive changes in behavior, the abuse of alcohol and drugs, and may predispose the heart and other organs to disease.

Both men and women often keep middle-age insecurity a gnawing secret; even admitting its existence seems like accepting defeat. But what is kept secret resists solution. If not resolved, the emotional problems of middle-age crisis, such as depression and psychosomatic illness, may go on for many years or throughout life. If poorly resolved, they may leave a person emotionally and sexually beaten. Resignation is a sorry alternative to what can be the prime of life.

Many people work through the problems of middle age on their own. Often individual or joint counseling brings better and faster solutions. The crisis period will put great demands on a husband or wife. Nagging, moralizing, and retaliation are fruitless; it is patience, understanding, support, and communication that help.

Healthy Middle Age

Middle age need be neither stuffy nor painful, let alone a crisis. Recent research suggests that for the majority of people, middle age is in fact a most gratifying time of life. Most people's health is still good. They are more affluent and secure than ever before. As middle age proceeds, their obligations are likely to decrease and their incomes continue to rise. The middle years are the most productive ones for most people in the arts, professions, and many crafts and businesses. After a few decades in the school of life, they have gained in knowledge and self-assurance. To them fall the positions of leadership and a feeling of earned authority.

The middle aged may not feel totally in charge of life, says Professor Bernice Neugarten, but they know that they are decision-makers in "a society which, while it may be oriented toward youth, is controlled by the middle-aged." The successful middle-aged person, she says, often describes himself as no longer driven but the driver, a person in command.

Menopause is a deep crisis for relatively few women. The empty nest commonly produces not unhappiness but relief and freedom. Most men do not suffer paralyzed misery because they aren't going to be President. Middle age has its difficulties, but perhaps fewer than many other times of life.

This is a time to review and re-assess the past and future. Many people, perhaps most, start adulthood with grand aspirations based on little experience. Reality may fall short of or exceed those aspirations, but not often in the ways one expected at 20. Therefore middle age usually involves some figuring out of "Why I'm not exactly where I expected to be," even in people the world thinks worthy of pride and contentment. Besides, experience has affected one's standards and goals. Now one consciously sets new standards, redefines oneself, and establishes new aims. This is a gradual process, and many people are torn for a while between a variety of conflicting feelings and self-images—fear and confidence, regret and self-acceptance, anxiety and freedom.

> **"THE SUCCESSFUL MIDDLE-AGED PERSON OFTEN DESCRIBES HIMSELF AS NO LONGER DRIVEN... BUT THE DRIVER."**

A woman's middle-age course is strongly influenced by family events—when her children mature, whether she must contribute to the family's income, whether older relatives must be looked after. Some have used household or job to avoid the mutual dependence of a committed marriage; in middle age they must confront this disturbing fact. However, the women who seem to suffer most from middle-age crisis are those with no interests outside marriage and home, and no preparation for life beyond them. As family and household tasks diminish, women can gradually shift to new activities that give them a feeling of involvement, competence, and practical resources. Perhaps only vague guilts and fears have limited their aspirations until this time.

Some women seek social, church, or volunteer activity, a return to school, or new avocations. More now return to part- or full-time employment or to education for a profession, while their children still live at home. About four out of ten middle-aged wives are now employed, twice the number of three decades ago. A woman who already has job skills or has always worked meets far fewer problems on the job market than one who has never worked and lacks occupational training.

Jobs, children, and in-laws. A man also examines job, family, and other commitments. He may find that a competitive job consumes more time and emotion than he ever expected; he must choose whether to pursue it single-mindedly or to redirect energy back to family and avocations. Or perhaps he realizes that he is not actually "married" to his job, as he and his wife have felt, but to exaggerated feelings of ambition and perfectionism. Or he may learn that he has always driven through life with one foot on the brakes because he lacked confidence or feared his own assertiveness; free of such limits, he can resume his education, start a second career, and strike out on his own professionally. Some people decide that no amount of money is worth a career's stress and emotional isolation, while others reach out in new ventures, drawing on unsuspected reserves of courage, energy, and inventiveness.

Middle age also brings changing relationships with one's parents and children. Seeing a parent grow old compels awareness of one's own aging. It can produce powerful guilt and resentment, especially if the relationship was ambivalent or not very warm. If such a reaction is powerful, it signals a need to explore the relationship. Eventually the exploration may provide to both sides the gift of a new, clearer, and richer bond.

One's own child may continue for some years to need a varying balance of independence and occasional support. Sometimes children hang on to the home; they must be given a loving, gentle push to venture out and live their own lives. Others need to step away for a while in outspoken rebellion. If the door is lovingly left open, the two generations may finally form a new and better tie, with less conflict and ambivalence. This sometimes happens when a grown child temporarily returns home or needs help and understanding because of emotional, marital, or practical problems.

The middle-aged may acquire in-laws. With their children and children-in-law, they must be warm and accepting and relax old controls, giving help and advice only when asked to. Sometimes a premarital "in-law" situation arises, when a young-adult child lives outside marriage with a partner. Whatever parents' moral convictions or social conventions may be, they should remember that lectures and moralizing achieve little, and that in arguing they may create lasting resentments in their children —and in their future children-in-law! Understanding and open communication are especially needed when the child's partner or marriage is of another social background, religion, or race.

Time for themselves. Once a couple have raised their family and established careers or other life patterns, they can give more time to themselves. In fact, for the first time since adolescence, they can think of themselves first. Some people are content to more or less follow the paths they've already marked out. They may do so with greater joy as their new privacy and leisure allow them a blossoming of intimacy, love, and sexuality.

Many others find change and innovation in almost every aspect of life. They may change residence; engage in new sports, reading, and travel; become involved in church, neighborhood, and political activities; or learn languages, musical instruments, arts, and crafts. They renovate old friendships and make new ones. Such a many-faceted expansion of life is becoming common as our society's picture of middle age changes from sedate to exploratory. This not only provides people with pleasure and vitality but prepares the way for a satisfying later life.

Middle age, then, is a time of transition in which reflection can lead a person to realign his sights and enrich his life. He can best achieve this through self-examination and by sharing his ideas and feelings with his spouse, friends, and if necessary with a counselor. The result is often new opportunities or a happier acceptance of the changing present.

LATER LIFE

Like middle age, later life is continually being extended and enriched. Studies show that there is no typical older person, no typical way of aging. And there is no dramatic point at which one ceases to be one's accustomed self and becomes "old," as if exchanging one identity for another. In fact, for many people, the passage from middle to late life may go almost unnoticed.

Some change, of course, is inevitable. Men must finally admit that they no longer can rely on their physical strength and endurance as they once did; women who are widowed or with disabled husbands may have to take on what they once considered masculine tasks and responsibilities. Yet throughout life, as the poet Goethe said, "Age takes hold of us by surprise." At 20, 40, 70, one looks in the mirror and thinks with amazement that one is now that many years old. There is, fortunately, a child in one's heart, which keeps hope alive. As the body changes, one's self-image changes gradually and reluctantly.

People who persistently refuse to face aging may pay a price. Daily realities will force them to recognize and envy the health, energy, achievement, and happiness of the young. Their denial of age ultimately makes them more vulnerable to pain and disappointment. If they have not worked through assessments of their aspirations and real lives in middle age, they will have to do so belatedly.

Older and happier. Despite the real problems of aging, the older are happier, as a group, than the young. Oliver Wendell Holmes said, "To be 70 years young is sometimes far more cheerful and hopeful than to be 40 years old." A large study made for the National Council on the Aging found that more than half the people over 65 said they felt as happy as when they were younger; a third said they were now living their best years. "Granted, life could be happier for 45 percent of older people, but an even higher 49 percent of those under 65 feel the same." Expectations and life assessments were also revealing: four out of five older people looked back over their lives with satisfaction, and for every one who found late life worse than expected, three found it better.

Older people report fewer feelings of anxiety and inadequacy than the young and middle-aged. They seem increasingly likely, as years pass, to have come to terms with life. Such findings are hardly surprising. The old have experienced some of the worst and best of life, in themselves and from others. They have survived, and they tend to see their age itself as an accomplishment to be proud of. They have less than ever to lose, and are no longer desperate to prove themselves to the world. Psychiatrist Leopold Bellak writes:

"If you have been 'successful,' you have learned that all success is limited, and limited, too, in the amount of pleasure it can give. If you haven't been signally successful in the eyes of the world, you may have come into the even more gratifying freedom of doing things—your job, or play or other diversions—for their own sake, rather than for the secondary results of money or power or recognition." Free at last to be oneself, he says, free from the tyranny of opinion, parents, teachers, employers, overpowering drives, "you can enjoy a special sense of freedom that borders on adventure."

This is far from the fearsome picture of hopeless old age, rigid and crotchety and depressed. Later life does have special changes and emotional problems, and they can be severe; fortunately, many are avoidable or can be remedied if understood by older people and their families and friends.

Personality

There is debate about whether aging brings personality changes, but opinion is shifting toward a qualified no. Class reunions dramatically show that personalities become more distinctive, so that people find they have less in common except chronological age. The alleged mellowness, rigidity, and other characteristics of late life are far from inevitable.

It is true that emotional peaks may flatten or occur less often in the latest years, depression is more common, and lifelong mental habits are hardly likely to vanish. Some other tendencies have been studied. From as early as the 40s on, many people view life more cautiously, without the bold confidence of youth. The world, as psychologist Bernice Neugarten puts it, seems "more complex and a bit dangerous." This change may reflect life experience as much as an altered personality.

Other studies reveal that after 40, many men accept their emotional and nurturing selves more easily, and many women feel less guilt about aggressive and egocentric impulses. This change, too, can be interpreted as greater self-knowledge and self-acceptance rather than automatic character change. It may be part of what is sometimes called mellowing in certain people.

There is a theory that with aging, people normally and inevitably disengage from life, and the world disengages from them. Physical changes, retirement, apparent differences from younger generations—all make an aging person withdraw his emotional investment from the world about him. He looks to the past for satisfaction, and the world looks to his children.

This disengagement theory is doubted or only partly accepted by many experts today. Even some who accept it say that basic personality doesn't alter with time, and many common later-life changes have better explanations. Being gloomy, quarrelsome, crotchety, or childish can result from specific problems in coping with illness, loss, and change. Therefore they are often reversible.

Depression (see page 283) is common in later life because it follows disillusionment and loss—of loved ones, security, status, or a sense of purpose. It can cause sadness, withdrawal, hopelessness, preoccupation with one's body, and exaggerated or psychosomatic ills. Like unhappy people of any age, a depressed older person may express inner hurt by erecting a defensive shield of critical and hostile reactions; this pushes others further away, increasing his isolation and pain. If loss follows loss, he fearfully digs in his heels against investing emotion in new friends and activities, in an attempt to avoid further pain.

A long period of grief, illness, or isolation can make an older person slip into an uninvolved, chronically depressed way of life—the ultimate disengagement. This is tragically prevalent among solitary older people without adequate private resources; our society fails to help most of them live worthy, dignified lives. For the more fortunate, with friends and relatives and even moderate funds, there can be help. With understanding, attention, perhaps counseling, medical treatment, and some changes in life-style, much apparent psychological aging may be reversed.

Other emotional events of later life can be consequences of disability and dependence. Then, as at any age, the pain and frustration of chronic ailments can make a person quarrelsome or tearful. Some ailments have known psychological effects; for instance, hearing loss often creates a suspicious or even slightly paranoid turn of mind. Reduced mobility can bring out buried cravings for dependence, creating such childlike behavior as clinging to others and using fearful complaints to demand their care.

Feeling helpless and dependent can easily make one feel anger, guilt, and self-depreciation. In many people it also gives rise to insecurity and even desperate fear. That is why failing to receive a phone call or some small accustomed service can produce frustration and self-pity—actually, fear of being at the mercy of others' attention.

Selfishness can also rise from such insecurity; this accounts for some aged people's apparent self-preoccupation, and insistence on gratifying their own needs yet ignoring others'. Becoming garrulous may be their way of holding people's attention and relieving loneliness. Repetitiousness, says Dr. Bellak, "is like sticking to a well-known path when one is scared of getting lost in a wilderness."

Certainly these characteristics never appear in many people, even at very advanced ages. The point is that if some of them do, they may reflect normal and familiar emotional reactions, not unreversible personality changes. Attention to the causes may take years off the person's age.

> "**T**O BE 70 YEARS YOUNG IS SOMETIMES FAR MORE CHEERFUL AND HOPEFUL THAN TO BE 40 YEARS OLD."

Later-life personality problems may not be products of later life, but continuations of earlier patterns. Some people have always coped well with life, and they use their late years constructively; they remain vital, flexible, and aware of their own strengths and weaknesses. They continue to enjoy activity, friendship, and love, and above all, self-esteem. Others have always shown anxiety, hypochondria, suspiciousness, and rigidity, and in later life they may do so a bit more. The person who was always an angry, anxious complainer ceases to be a young grouch and becomes an old grouch. The person who was always involved with others only reluctantly is now free to disengage from much of the world. Defensive, obsessive-compulsive people who always sought the narrowest sort of security, may have planned well for everything in later life except their own freedom and leisure. Their small capacity for pleasure and their avoidance of emotional involvement then take a greater toll than ever. Passive-dependent people, who always stayed childlike, may now become like old children.

Psychologists Henry Maas and Joseph Kuypers recently reported on a group of people who had been studied over 40 years of adult life. They found no pattern of personality change caused by aging, retirement, divorce, or widowhood. They affirmed that aging does not flatten individuality but enhances it. The only consistent influence on emotions and life-style was maintaining health. Barring disaster and severe illness, these people showed in later life the same strengths and vulnerabilities they had had as young adults. This does not mean they didn't change, but that their personality development was not cramped or dictated by aging itself.

This study, say Maas and Kuypers, disputes the popular myth of inescapable decline in old age. Most of their subjects led rewarding and diverse lives in their eighth decade. Some had experienced major improvements in life-style and satisfaction. The minority who were troubled were not suffering from age:

"In early adulthood these men and women were in various ways at odds with others and themselves or too constricted in their involvements. Old age merely continues for them what earlier years had launched. Finally, even when young adulthood is too narrowly lived or painfully overburdened, the later years may offer new opportunities . . . we have found repeated evidence that old age can provide a second and better chance at life."

Retirement

Retirement as we know it today is a new phenomenon. In the past, people worked until they no longer could, no longer had to, or no longer wanted to. The age 65 was somewhat arbitrarily set in the 1930s for legislative reasons as the time to stop work, and in some jobs it is now 70. But people vary greatly in their desire and ability to stay at their work. Sixty would be an ideal retirement time for some people, 75 for others; for some, a reduced work schedule without retirement is best.

The approach of retirement has different meanings to various individuals. To some it seems a well-earned end to labor, routines, and responsibilities imposed by others. To others it is a frightening portent of old age; a loss of status, from producer to nonproducer; a loss of independence; a loss of needed income; and a threat of a lowered life-style. A man will lose the occupation that gave him a social role through adulthood; "retiree" seems a poor replacement for his identity as lawyer or salesman or bricklayer. If he is a compulsive worker, he faces loss of his primary daily coping mechanism. If his domestic life has been unhappy or drab, he will lose his escape hatch—challenges and ventures away from home, daily social contacts, and routine involvements with people. In short, he will lose his "second family" and "second home." Perhaps, worst of all, he may feel that he is ceasing to be useful and needed, and he loses self-respect.

The anticipation is usually worse than reality, even for a person who faced retirement with depression and helpless resentment. This is especially true if he was self-employed or in a profession that permits continuing on a part-time or free-lance basis. Some companies, schools, and other institutions are now making provisions for this or for optional later retirement. There are even companies now that hire only retirees; since older workers are, as a group, patient and reliable, this has been useful to both parties.

Even some who must break completely with their occupations are surprised at how satisfying their lives can be. Many vigorous retirees turn their energies to volunteer and community work, hobbies, sports, family activities, further education, and second occupations. Even people of advanced age or with some degree of disability take pleasure in reading, walking, gardening, community affairs, hobbies, and the arts.

Plan to enjoy it. Study after study shows that regardless of whether people looked forward to retirement, those who planned for it, both practically and emotionally, tend to enjoy it most. Some look forward only to lying in a hammock, and for a minority this is apparently satisfying. But many retirees find after a while that they are bored, bewildered, and depressed. The same dissatisfaction strikes many who long hoped to do things they hadn't had time for while working; they rush zealously into hobbies, travel, or sports, but the elation passes, and soon they find themselves just treading water.

People must, of course, get used to living without externally imposed schedules and adapt to changes in status and life-style. But the greatest problem may be a lack of deeply rooted interests that will survive the immediate post-retirement dabbling phase. Middle age is the time to cultivate interests that can enrich later life. Sitting and watching the world go by satisfies some people, but most need activity, relationships, and a sense of accomplishment. It is in middle age, says writer Simone de Beauvoir, that one should commit oneself "to undertakings that set time at defiance." Then the late years do not leave one an empty vessel, deprived of its one old cargo.

All of this probably applies to most women who have had long-term jobs or careers. There has been very little study of retirement's effects on professional women, but since many women embark on careers later than men or interrupt work during the child-rearing years, they may want to continue working later in life.

Although many women joke about how irksome it may be to have their husbands constantly about the house after retirement, their lives are usually little changed by it. If the marriage has been hostile or unsatisfying, the couple can be thrown together with a jolt. If they have difficulty adjusting to their new life together, counseling may benefit both of them. Some companies and organizations now offer pre-retirement counseling and include the retirees' spouses.

It is usually the loss of children, husband, and other relatives from women's daily lives that is crucial to late-life readjustment. Some women, widowed in late middle age, make new and satisfying lives, find new friends, and take pride in their productiveness; they may remarry or find satisfying, self-sufficient new ways of life. But for most women in the second half of life, interests and involvements beyond marriage and home are crucial to happiness (see below). As with men, the best preparation for later life takes place in middle age, so that loss in one area of life doesn't leave one impoverished.

Health, Involvement, and Activity

There is no question that good health, economic security, and preparation give one the best start toward a happy later life. And as we have said, being free to do what one wants, not what one must, doesn't help those who haven't cultivated interests. While rocking-chair disengagement suits some people, the happiest older people are usually the active ones. Well-meaning friends may urge a person to take it easy, not take up challenging involvements; they may be asking him, in effect, to spend the rest of his life killing time. Change and loss are realities of later life, but one must have the courage to invest emotion in new people and activities, seeking companionship and a sense of worth, rather than slip into depressed isolation.

Many older people are quite aware of this. In increasing numbers they become very involved in social and political issues, especially those that concern their own age group. Adult education has become one of the most rapidly expanding services in our society, yet the resources don't keep up with the demand. And although it is less likely today than in the past that three generations of a family will live in one house or in close proximity, the role of grandparent is still an important one. The older members of a family can be accepted and accepting confidants and teachers of the young, and offer help and involvement with their own adult children—always, of course, being careful and tactful in their respect of the middle generation's rights to privacy and final child-rearing authority.

Escape from boredom. One of the worst enemies of later life is boredom. Boredom is not merely the absence of something; it is an active disorder. Research has shown that long hours of work and pressing responsibility produce less emotional and physical illness than monotonous, unsatisfying labor. The natural hunger of body and mind for stimulation, activity, and satisfaction can be ignored only at the cost of depression, irritability, and ailments.

When a person has insufficient outlets for his energies and skills, say Drs. Doris and David Jonas, his brain is like a motor being revved in neutral. "Heat and noise are generated but not movement." But the mind and body were not meant to be raced in neutral; just as boredom may explode as violence in young people, it may create quarrelsomeness in the elderly.

It is hardly surprising, say the Jonases, that once a bored older person focuses on symptoms and disabilities, these become "a new center for his life and the only barrier between him and renewed boredom." Relatives and friends wonder why he has become crotchety and something of a complaining hypochondriac—especially since he may swing back into full vigor if there is a real emergency! His real problem may be that his inactivity, his lack of purpose and participation in life, are "like using a high-powered battery that could activate a locomotive to run a toy train."

It is not the further prolongation of life that will create a problem in the future, but failure of some older people to use life. "To grow old," said Goethe, "means to begin a new occupation." The task—potentially a joyful one—of the elderly is to carry out an occupation provided by human evolution but sometimes forgotten in urban, industrial society. Only the human species preserves all its older members as long as possible; societies may fail to do this only when they teeter chronically on the edge of group survival. We depend on accumulated knowledge, for we are the only creature

that survives by learning as much as instinct. "In man," say the Jonases, "the aged contribute to the survival of their group by their becoming the repositories and the passers-on of the group's experience and wisdom."

It is not mere custom or altruism, but sound social survival, to draw on all the assets older people can offer. They are the links of continuity, connecting past, present, and future. They are natural teachers, advisers, leaders, and sources of tradition. The Jonases suggest, in fact, that the greater relative strength of long-term memory (see page 270) in later life helps the elderly fill this important role, preserving the most vital and deeply valued human experiences from generation to generation. It will be a major step toward greater health for individuals and society when as many older people as possible can exercise their special abilities fully in their private and public lives.

EMOTIONAL HEALTH AND ILLNESS

There is a childhood illusion that remains embedded in many adult minds: that eventually one's life becomes stable, settled once and for all. This child's view of grown-ups ignores their energies and fears, their passions and doubts, their capacity for change. It is as unreal as the idea that age must be a grim decline. The middle and late years, like all times of life, bring particular problems, strengths, and changes, which must constantly be brought into a new, productive balance.

Age brings knowledge, experience, greater confidence and mastery over life, and sometimes wisdom. Even someone who doesn't consider his life broadly fulfilling has seen himself endure, learn, and change. At the very least, he has survived the responsibilities and crises of adulthood, which is sometimes no small feat. He need only think back to the relative insecurity and naiveté of youth for reassurance of just how far he has come.

Age also brings the loss of loved ones, changes in appearance and physical capability, and times of inner pain and fatigue. The first step in maintaining emotional health is knowing the pitfalls that can damage it. We will look first at the commonest neurotic symptoms and mechanisms, especially those prominent in the second half of life. Such knowledge suggests many ways to maintain emotional health.

The Neuroses

A neurosis is an emotional disorder that can cause mental pain, physical discomfort, troubled relationships, or chronic practical problems. It is not so acute that it cuts a person off from reality or requires hospitalization.

Sigmund Freud, the creator of psychoanalysis, was once asked to define mental health. "The questioner," comments analyst Erik Erikson, "probably expected a complicated, 'deep' answer. But Freud simply said, *Lieben und arbeiten*' ('to love and to work'). It pays to ponder this simple formula; it grows deeper as you think about it. For when Freud said 'love,' he meant the generosity of intimacy as well as genital love; when he said love and work, he meant a general work productiveness which would not preoccupy the individual to the extent that he might lose his right or capacity to be a sexual and loving being."

It is sometimes difficult to decide whether or how people are neurotic. People have been labeled "sick" merely because others found their behavior unfamiliar or unpleasant. Many psychiatrists are increasingly reluctant to use diagnostic tags that can be made tools of social conformity. Still, there do exist many kinds of emotional *dis-ease* and dysfunction—when pains and problems consistently seem greater than their causes, and there are chronic difficulties in feelings, friendships, love, marriage, sex, work, practical matters, and physical health.

Common signs of neurosis are persistent and exaggerated fear, suspicion, and rage; recurrent nightmares; sexual dysfunctions; self-destructive behavior (chronic alcoholism, gambling, or drug abuse); psychosomatic illness; very prolonged guilt, grief, or remorse; compulsive behavior; apathy and fatigue without physical causes; feelings of depersonalization (feeling emotionally dead or zombie-like); and suicidal preoccupations. The neurotic person sabotages friendships, love relationships, and work. He often seems to create pain and "bad luck" for himself by his rage, discouragement, self-concern, or unrealistic stinginess or extravagance.

In short, the neurotic, faced with life's usual problems, manages to end up regularly on the short end of the stick. A witness may be tempted to impatiently tell him, "Be reasonable, get a grip on yourself." That misses the very nature of the problem, for neurosis is not consciously chosen, its sufferings are real, and they usually puzzle and frighten the neurotic himself. That is because they result from old mental habits and distorted perceptions, many acquired in early life and still lurking beneath conscious thought.

The child within us. To understand this, one must step inside the mind of a very small child. He is full of grandiose self-love yet helpless in a world of giants. The ways he is handled and spoken to make him secure or insecure, timid or defiant, in a primitive way he has no words to express. He has no adult sense of time: if a parent withdraws love and sends him to his room, he fears it might go on forever—he could starve to death! He thinks not logically but magically: if he is angry at his mother and she has an accident, he fears that his thoughts caused it. If he is ashamed because his feelings are chaotic and angry, he may try to conceal or "make up" for them by being faultlessly clean and neat.

Growing up, we become too sophisticated for such thinking. We learn that thoughts can't kill, that solitude isn't forever, that clean fingernails aren't proof of a loving heart and clear mind. But like all of our past, magical and irrational thoughts don't disappear, but are overlaid by later experience. Like the pea under the princess's mattress in the fairy tale, they may change the surface of later life and experience in seemingly mysterious ways. They may even emerge fully in their primitive forms at times of stress.

So with an effort of imagination, one can understand the neurotic; he is acting, in exaggerated ways, like the small child buried in us all. His unwitting attempt to solve life's problems with unrealistic mental mechanisms makes him like everyone else, but more so.

Consider someone raised by very strict and irritable parents, who learned in childhood that his every word or move may offend. He habitually goes through each day as if it were a minefield; the resulting safety from rebuke and rejection is small comfort. If he also was expected to meet high standards of achievement, he has a further problem: he feels he must succeed yet remain "nice." He may stumble over his own feet every time he nears competitive success—and blame circumstances every time. Thus he fulfills the commands to compete and to be obedient (nonaggressive). He resents feeling compelled to live this way, so ripples of conflicting anger, fear, and self-contempt are set off whenever he feels he should assert himself. He is chronically "nervous" and may find relief in the sedation of alcohol. Eventually his drinking takes a severe toll on himself and his family, creating new problems in turn. Like most neurotic solutions, alcoholism is an uneconomical "cure" for inner hurt.

Or consider a girl with a cold and distant mother, who carries through life an enormous need for the warmth she never got enough of. Knowing her need is childlike, that an adult can't just be cuddled by the world, she hides her yearning beneath a facade of active intelligence, charm, and efficiency. But when she becomes close enough to another person to feel safe and "just be myself," she reverts to the affection-starved little girl inside, so needy that she is unable to give. Her exasperated husband wonders, "Where's the girl I married? Now she just wants to cuddle and isn't interested in sex, and the littlest thing makes

her accuse me of not loving her." If the husband also has buried dependency needs, their similar demands may create a deadly, unspoken competition for who can win the most care.

Often a combination of insight and emotional support reduces neurotic problems; sometimes counseling or psychotherapy is needed. We will describe some of the commonest neurotic symptoms and mechanisms—of necessity, one at a time. But one should remember that most people show not one clearcut neurotic mechanism but several, in various degrees and combinations. They may be anxious and depressed, guilt-ridden and compulsive, or addictive and depersonalized. Fortunately, easing one symptom often opens the door for change in another.

Depression

The word depression tells exactly what happens to its victims: they feel pressed down by inner pain and bleakness and by life's daily demands. Anyone who feels overburdened by problems, real or imagined, may lose sleep, energy, hope, and mental and physical appetite. He demands sympathy, becomes helplessly dependent, or feels set-upon and bitter. Depression ranges from a mild, temporary reaction to neurosis to severe mental illness. It is one of the commonest emotional problems of middle and later life, for it often follows loss of any kind—of loved ones, status, strength, beauty, or hope. The loss leads to irrational blaming of others or of oneself; the latter causes feelings of worthlessness. "Having the blues" is also a normal part of chronic illness, and sometimes of convalescence.

It would be alarming if someone didn't show sadness after loss or misfortune. Depression is neurotic when it is prolonged and disproportionate. Often the first signs are becoming glum, sluggish, overwhelmed by ordinary tasks, and having difficulty concentrating. Emotional bounce and sexual interest fade. The victim then may have trouble falling asleep and getting up in the morning, suffer headaches and constipation, and feel a vague but unshakable hopelessness.

When others encourage him, he may be temporarily cheered, but he soon responds irritably or with greater withdrawal. Like a child separated from his mother, says psychiatrist Walter Bonime, the depressive becomes greedy for love, frustrated, angry, and guilty. By his hand-wringing and sadness he seems to cry out for help, yet he argues help away. This doesn't mean he enjoys his sit-down strike against life: he cannot pull himself out of it. Unfortunately, his gloom is contagious and eventually very demanding, and it can demoralize an entire household.

If someone becomes aware of long-lasting or deep depression in himself, he should seek professional help. If he notices it in a loved one, he should gently but insistently urge treatment, despite the sufferer's apathy, complaints, or sense of helplessness. Chronic and severe depression are probably the most common and destructive mental problem of middle and late life, and can lead as far as psychosis and suicide (see page 290). Depression is also one of the most easily treated emotional problems, so one should not hesitate to go for help. Often a physician can help relieve mild forms of depression with sympathetic understanding and antidepressant drugs; counseling or psychotherapy also may be called for.

The roots of depression are sometimes complex, but mild and transient bouts often result from loss and unacknowledged anger. Consider a man who finds his mother-in-law visiting not for the announced weekend but for a month. To accommodate her, sleeping and living arrangements are changed. He and his wife have little privacy for intimate talk, lovemaking, and shared activities. He feels it is selfish and silly to be angry over his loss; he is too grown up and reasonable for that. But he does harbor buried resentment, and in controlling that emotion he controls others. His mind begins to act like a switchboard trying to screen out an unpleasant call; it shuts down many circuits lest the offending message find an open line. He becomes a victim of inertia, fatigue, insomnia, and perhaps headaches or backaches. He may even visit his doctor, wondering whether he needs a rest, a change of scene, or perhaps vitamins.

Such depression usually lifts when he recognizes his anger. He is perhaps right in thinking he shouldn't necessarily act out the anger, but he is very harsh on himself in saying he shouldn't feel it. Like many people with neurotic symptoms, he is much tougher on himself than he would be on anyone else. He would probably tell a friend in a similar situation, "It's natural to feel irritated; try to figure out a solution that's fair to everyone, including yourself." False "nice-guyism" over marital, family, and work situations lies behind much temporary mild depression. Women may be more prone to this than men, for they tend from early life to put a high value on being lovable and accommodating. Brief counseling often gives quick relief.

Anxiety

Anxiety means fear, but it has added meaning in psychiatry. If a person sweats, trembles, vomits, has palpitations, can't breathe, feels dizzily overwhelmed by dread—*and* he is about to be attacked by a tiger—he is quite normal. He is showing the fight-or-flight reactions of any creature whose life is threatened. But if he reacts that way to a look at a party, a word at the office, an elevator or airplane ride, a walk to the corner store, then his unrealistic fear is called anxiety. He may sense that his agony of anticipation makes no obvious sense, but it remains, as if he were tricked by mirrors into expecting the roof to fall on him.

There is, of course, a hidden logic to anxiety. Often the anxiety-ridden person fears losing mental controls and "going crazy." Buried feelings threaten to erupt from within him—rage, sexuality, or other impulses he disapproves and fears will be uncontrollable if let loose.

Acute anxiety (anxiety attack, or panic) is very painful and demoralizing. Anxiety also can exist as a persistent sense of impending doom or as a low-grade, pervasive mental "static" that may be dismissed as "just nervousness." In acute or chronic form, anxiety makes life a misery, bringing nightmares, exaggerated fears for one's own and others' health and safety, and psychosomatic ills from palpitations to gastrointestinal upsets.

> **"MIDDLE AGE IS A TIME OF TRANSITION IN WHICH REFLECTION CAN LEAD A PERSON TO REALIGN HIS SIGHTS & ENRICH HIS LIFE."**

Anxiety may flare up temporarily because of separation from a loved one, change of residence or job, or changes in close relationships. When more than temporary, it is usually part of a complex problem. The term anxiety neurosis is used when panic is the chief symptom, but anxiety is generally a signal of internal conflict rather than an ill in itself. In the form of entrenched phobias and hypochondria, it is a common and taxing problem of middle and later life.

Fortunately, many anxieties respond well to treatment, especially to a combination of counseling or psychotherapy and mild medication. Victims of anxiety should not use alcohol, tranquillizers, and other mood-altering substances as a prolonged self-treatment. The source of the anxiety may persist, while the "cure" creates additional problems.

Phobia

There is a difference between having a phobia and having a neurotically phobic personality. A phobia is a specific irrational fear—of flying, of insects or snakes, of heights, or of closed or open spaces. Isolated phobias are common and may not seriously affect people's lives; if they do become problems, they sometimes can be treated by counseling or behavior-modification therapy. The phobic neurotic, however, lives within a web of phobias, like an animal always poised for flight, and is robbed of a normal, rewarding life. This is a rather common and damaging neurosis of middle and late life, especially in women.

The true phobic fears being mugged or raped, or becoming sick and helpless in public places or when alone; she fears closed and open spaces, crowds and solitude. Finally a blanket of fear produces "street phobia"; the victim is afraid to leave home, sometimes even when accompanied. She may lose her job and stop visiting friends. If she can name no specific threat, she still feels vague anxiety about illness or death. She also may be a hypochondriac and suffer such psychosomatic ills as palpitations, dizziness, diarrhea, and colitis. The phobic's demands on her family become enormous; they must take her everywhere and pick her up, keep her company, and try to quiet her unremitting fears.

Family and physician are likely to offer rational reassurance and finally may become impatient, lecturing the phobic about malingering—especially if they see that despite her fear of heights she doesn't jump, and that in an emergency she may temporarily shed her terrors. They should remember that she is genuinely ill and requires treatment. Unfortunately, getting her to accept this is difficult; her very illness is that she denies having emotional problems. The phobic says, in effect, "Nothing's wrong in my mind, it's the outside world that is full of awful things"—*denying* and *projecting* painful emotions rather than facing them. If she does consult a doctor, her first reaction may be denial: "When I walk too far, I get little palpitations, but otherwise I'm all right."

Treatment is often a long, difficult effort with a psychotherapist. The alternatives are worse. The phobic's family, friends, and physician must try to keep her fearful isolation from becoming a way of life; yet they must tactfully avoid frightening her even further, since she "would rather die" than admit her mental anguish. The family also must prevent her controlling their daily lives with her illness. Gently, lovingly, and firmly, they should emphasize, for her good and their own, that she seek professional help in eventually conquering her fears.

Hypochondria

There are many jokes about people who fear that every gasp is a heart attack, every pimple the first stage of cancer. It is no joke to the hypochondriac or her family.

The hypochondriac, like the phobic, is often a middle-aged woman; and like the phobic, she projects her mental conflicts—not onto the outside world but onto her own body: "My mind is healthy, it's my body that hurts." Not surprisingly, phobia and hypochondria may coexist in one person.

Psychiatrist Charles Socarides points out that we all fear illness and may exaggerate it. "Many quite normal people have mild episodes of hypochondria, especially after a death in the family, when depressed, or after guilt-producing behavior. Most people, normal or neurotic, recover from their fears if a doctor reassures them. The true hypochondriac is basically different; he has proceeded from the *fear* of illness to the *fact* of illness. He truly believes, despite all evidence to the contrary, that he has cancer or some other disorder, and suffers awful bouts of terror."

The hypochondriac easily provokes impatience, but the results can be tragic. Family and physician may be so used to hearing her cry wolf that they ignore symptoms of real physical disease. There is another danger. Some guilt-ridden hypochondriacs find in painful therapies a craved-for "punishment." They may fall into the hands of quacks or even of licensed physicians who resort to extreme or unnecessary treatment, including surgery.

The hypochondriac is less likely to cling to an exploiter's costly, even damaging treatment if she receives sympathy and care from her family and regular physician. They must use tact, for to deny her emotional problems may cause her to indignantly dismiss as a quack the doctor who responsibly suggests psychiatric help! One must check out her physical complaints and offer reassurance without agreeing to her unrealistic fears. Eventually it may be possible to involve her, if not in psychotherapy, at least in psychological counseling.

Paranoia

Paranoia is commonly thought of as a fear or belief that one is plotted against, spied on, and threatened by abuse, attack, or rape. Delusions of this kind reflect severe mental illness. Mild paranoid thinking, however, is more subtle and occurs sometimes in most of us. It is often noticeable in neurotic personalities.

Paranoia can be thought of as a projection of unacceptable thoughts onto other people—putting in their mouths the words one can't bear to say oneself. Imagine someone normally good-looking who retains a hidden adolescent fear of being too fat. When he hears people laugh behind him on the street, he may not assume that they share a joke unrelated to him, but wonder whether they're laughing at his appearance. Instead of saying to himself, "I'm ugly," he says, "*They* must be laughing at my looks." In this light, paranoid fantasies of attack can be understood as an inability to admit angry thoughts: "I'm not angry, the people around me are." Fantasies of rape can be translated, "I don't have nasty sexual thoughts, but all those men on the street do." Life sometimes justifies paranoid thinking just enough to reinforce it!

Mild paranoid thought can appear when people feel under stress, unable to cope with their problems, unlovable, or inadequate. They may suspect that their spouses are unfaithful or that coworkers and neighbors intend to harm them. If paranoia becomes powerful or frequent, it is a sign of emotional difficulties that require professional attention.

Obsessive-Compulsive Neurosis

An obsession is a thought one can't let go of; a compulsion is an action one can't help repeating. There are many common, everyday examples—the compulsive who steps over cracks in the pavement, the obsessive who mentally reargues for hours a minor squabble in a store.

A highly obsessive-compulsive person has trouble dropping worries and busywork. He may return home several times to make sure he turned off the gas; he may worry so much about trivial problems that he neglects important ones. He tends to be rigid and perfectionistic, capable of sacrificing the ship's safety to keep its fittings polished.

Like anxiety and paranoid thinking, obsessive-compulsive behavior occurs to some extent in most people and is rarely a neurosis in itself. However, it may become severe when a person has strong feelings of guilt and inner chaos; then it takes a toll in spontaneity, warm personal relationships, and creative work, and indicates a need for counseling or therapy.

Abuse and Addiction

The wide use of alcohol, diet pills (amphetamines), sleeping pills, and other mood-altering substances has made drug addiction and abuse one of the greatest threats to physical and mental health in our society. The toll is high among the middle-aged and elderly. Some mental-health professionals are in disagreement about whether certain problems should be considered addiction, habituation, abuse, psychological dependence, or mislearning: the question is academic to addicts, or abusers, and their families. The results are mental pain, physical illness, disrupted relationships, and social penalties. The self-destructive drinker, eater, smoker, or drug abuser runs the risk of a shortened, pain-ridden life. Some researchers believe that most addictive behaviors stem from similar basic personality problems, involving a basic lack of trust, self-love, security, and strong personal identity.

Typically, the addict or abuser denies the extent of his dependence: "I could give it up if I had to." Often family or friends must insist, with loving firmness, that heavy alcohol consumption, drug use, smoking, obesity caused by compulsive eating, and similar problems are beyond control and require treatment. Several kinds of therapy have helped many of the addicted and habituated, from heavy smokers to alcoholics to chronic pill-takers. Mutual-help groups such as Alcoholics Anonymous work quite well for many people. Sometimes therapy for addictive behavior requires the spouse's involvement in joint or group therapy. The response may be, "But I'm not the sick one!" At such a time, the real proof of caring is to share the process of recovery.

Psychosomatic Illness

Psychosomatic illness is a physical disorder caused by stress and emotional conflict. Unlike the imaginary disease of the hypochondriac, it is quite real and requires physical treatment. Among ills frequently caused at least partly by emotional conflict and stress are peptic ulcer, spastic colitis, chronic lower-back pain and stiff neck, headaches, asthma, insomnia, hemorrhoids, skin rashes, frequent or chronic colds, diarrhea, constipation, irregular heartbeat, and chest pain.

Some common phrases reflect clearly how the mind *(psyche)* expresses conflict through the body *(soma)*. Sometimes the nervous system, like an overloaded electrical system, "dumps" excess emotional reaction on some part of the body. For instance, we show that we feel we are carrying intolerable burdens by saying "Oh, my aching back!" In many psychosomatic illnesses, the body expresses the thought literally, through lower-back pain. People sometimes say unpleasant situations make them feel "itchy"; itching skin does appear as an expression of depression (a *depressive equivalent*). Dr. Robert Felix and Morton Hunt write: "The particular psychosomatic illness a patient develops often has a symbolic significance. The gasping and wheezing of an asthmatic, in the midst of an anxiety-provoked attack, is not unlike the wailing and sobbing of a frightened child trying to summon his mother. Similarly, the immature adult with stomach troubles, who requires special feeding and attention by his wife, may unconsciously be forcing her to give him a kind of mothering that he never grew up enough to do without."

It is often difficult to know whether an ailment is partly or fully psychosomatic in origin. If it remains chronic or recurs, and there is any suspicion of a psychological element, the emotional sources must be explored with a qualified mental-health professional if cure is to be lasting.

Guilt and Sadomasochism

Many neurotics suffer exaggerated feelings of guilt. Some openly cover themselves with accusations. Others, more subtly, express guilt as thinking of the ball always being in their court; they leap to take responsibility for things beyond their control, especially everyone else's feelings and comfort. And others, though seemingly angry, stern, and resistant to criticism, are their own harshest critics. In a variety of ways,

many people carry a load of self-imposed *shoulds* and *don'ts* that would tax a saint. Sometimes one can hear in their words and tone a highly critical parent whose voice was *introjected*—absorbed and considered part of themselves: "Be nice ... stronger ... polite . . . don't be greedy . . . don't be dirty . . . ."

Hidden anger and guilt lie behind much sadism and masochism. In the strict sense, these mean, respectively, sexual pleasure in hurting others and in being hurt. Both may exist in one person. The sexual sadomasochist is relatively uncommon, but the needs to emotionally hurt others and to be humiliated are common in neurotic personalities.

The masochist always manages to have his toes under other people's feet. Often he is depressed, something of a Sadsack; his very expression may act like a standing accusation or a "Kick Me" sign—inviting the attention of his opposite number, the sadist. His great distinction in life is being more hurt and hopeless than anyone else— what has been called "victory through defeat." Thus masochism can be a way of enlisting sympathy, demanding attention, and manipulating people. But if the masochist could enjoy the results, he wouldn't be a masochist!

The sadist, who makes others squirm in pain, failure, and embarrassment, may vent his neurotic drive on family, friends, and employees, and perhaps rationalize it as just or necessary. At his worst, he is physically violent or a relentless manipulator. He doesn't always enjoy the result of his triumphs; they may bring guilt and isolation from people whose love he needs. Like a child in a tantrum, he may have a glimmering of the nature of his behavior and wish someone would stop him.

One might expect the sadomasochist to rush for treatment, but this is too seldom true. His neurotic pattern, however painful, has long been his way to cope with life. If not happy, he is at least on familiar ground. Furthermore, sadomasochism is sometimes among the most deceptive and complex neurotic patterns. A person who is masochistic in one situation may be sadistic or very controlling in others, and neither party in a relationship may recognize the subtle interplay of emotional power plays.

Guilt and sadomasochism are often entwined with anxiety, depression, and other neurotic symptoms. Breaking such patterns may require tenacious self-examination through psychotherapy. Often this is possible and very helpful in marriage-counseling sessions. If effective, these therapies can bring an individual or couple new strengths, rewards, and flexibility in dealing with each other and with life in general.

Personality Neuroses and Character Disorders

The terms personality neurosis, character neurosis, and character disorder are variously used to describe emotional problems caused by distorted personality development.

The term character disorder is usually used for the person also called a psychopath or sociopath. Such a person seems never to have developed warm emotions and a conscience. Unlike the sadist, he feels little active satisfaction in inflicting pain or using people. He suffers no guilt or remorse afterward. Emotionally frozen, he is unable to love, and often is unable to feel at all. He uses, abuses, or manipulates people rather than forming relationships with them.

Some people with mildly sociopathic personalities are charming, clever, and socially adept; their very lack of conscience and empathy can help them toward success in business or politics, if not in relationships. Some, however, abuse alcohol and drugs and chronically perform antisocial acts, from sex offenses to violent crimes. The old term psychopath has become unpopular because it was sometimes misused to brand nonconformists and people from various social backgrounds as mentally ill; but the term sociopath does still suggest that this recognizable character type ignores some of society's fundamental values. The extreme sociopath passes the boundaries of neurosis and may be judged psychotic.

One reason the sociopath has been put in a separate category is that unlike the psychotic, he seems in touch with reality, and unlike the neurotic shows little emotional conflict or suffering. The neurotic's mental apparatus could be compared to a car with a part or two malfunctioning, the sociopath's to a car that never had certain parts to begin with. However, the unusual case of the sociopath who does respond to psychotherapy shows that great anxiety and conflict may actually lie beneath the hard, cool surface of character disorder, as if covered by thick ice.

Character neuroses, or personality neuroses, exist when personality development has created strong neurotic traits. For instance, someone who became very compulsive in early life may remain overneat, zealous about order and spotless perfection, and emotionally tightly controlled. If one suggests he is neurotic, he disagrees and points out that he is "successfully" married, a parent, holds a good job, has never had a breakdown or been in trouble with the law, etc., etc. He goes through life as a "Marian the librarian," seeing his neurotic trait as "the way I am." True, he has no dramatic symptoms; he is a case of moderation in excess. He pays a price in restricted emotional life, lacking joy, spontaneity, creativity, and initiative. And if circumstances make his way of coping with life inadequate, his neurotic trait does become an obvious emotional problem. Like the sociopath whose shell of ice cracks, he then shows open neurotic conflicts.

Almost any neurotic trait can be involved in character neurosis. The highly hysterical person, who overreacts to everything with wild intensity, may pass for excitable or even vivacious. Hysteria tinges all his feelings—he is hysterically happy, hysterically angry, hysterically frightened. The hysterical quality tends to blot out what he says to people; they react more to his overwhelming whirl of excitement than to the words. When life demands great control, the vivacity may become an inadequate shriek and show how vulnerable he is to the wide range of life's demands outside a protected environment.

Obviously, character neuroses are difficult to deal with, since they may be treasured and defended as part of one's identity. Once the person with a character neurosis does admit that his perfectionism, overcontrol, hysteria, or other traits can be deficits as well as virtues, he may respond to counseling or therapy.

Suicidal Thoughts and Behavior

Whether suicide reflects emotional disturbance depends on many social and individual factors. Some societies consider suicide normal or even obligatory in some circumstances, such as public disgrace. We tend to see it as a sign of pathology (except perhaps in cases of painful terminal illness). Certainly many people who commit suicide or court death by self-destructive behavior would be diagnosed depressed or otherwise emotionally disturbed even were they not suicidal.

Preoccupation with suicide often reflects buried rage or despair. Probably the commonest interpretation of suicide is that it is an act of thwarted rage turned upon oneself; suicide is often associated with deep depression, a condition also often involving bottled-up anger. Thoughts of suicide may be a symbolic way of saying, "I am carrying so much emotional pain inside that I'd rather die than bear it." Common also is a fantasy of rising, like the immortal phoenix, in triumph over people made sorry that they didn't care and give more; this childlike fantasy ignores the fact that the dead aren't around to reap others' imagined sorrow.

Many people fear or think obsessively about suicide yet do not act. This has created a cliché that those who talk about it never follow through. It is a false and dangerous idea.

Some people threaten suicide until others are exasperated and disbelieving, and then do it. Some make several suicidal gestures, then act in earnest; others make what they intend as only a gesture but succeed by accident. Some kill themselves without anyone having sensed a warning.

The suicide rate is highest in this nation for people over 50. This may result from the increase of depression in the later years. Although study of suicide is becoming intensive, there exists no single formula for warning signals, causes, and treatment. If a person has suicidal preoccupations or sees them in a friend or relative, therapy should promptly be sought. Suicidal threats and gestures never should be taken lightly. Sometimes relatively brief counseling can improve the situation; if the problem is serious, an alert family and effective therapist may literally save a life.

Fear of Death

The fear of death is universal; never to have thought of and feared death is a denial of reality, and it naturally lurks in life reassessment. But chronic, debilitating anxiety about dying is often a symptom of other, hidden anxieties—of solitude, abandonment, or helplessness. It occurs in anxiety, depression, and hypochondria. Nagging death fears also may arise in people who have survived severe heart attacks and other life-threatening crises. Counseling often relieves such fear and aids a return to normal life.

Grief and Mourning

Grief and mourning are especially powerful when a loved one's death was sudden, but they occur even after a long terminal illness. The initial reaction is shock, disbelief, and attempts to deny what has happened. After this numbness come grief, preoccupation with the deceased, and a host of confused, confusing emotions.

The griever thinks about the dead person, even talks to him as if he were still alive. If he bore unresolved resentments, there are guilt and self-accusation: "How could I have helped prevent his death? Why wasn't I more loving all those years? I have no right to be alive." Alternating between anxiety and depression, he harps on the past, idealizes the dead person, clings to other people, or isolates himself through irritability. Eventually there emerges a childish but very human feeling of rage at being deserted: "How could he die and leave me alone?"

These reactions are not only normal but necessary. Having invested one's feelings in a person, one feels his death as the death of part of oneself. One wonders, "How can I live without him?" The stages of grief and mourning allow one to accept the present and to continue with life, finally free to reinvest love and interest in the present. It is not morbid or unhealthful to express one's feelings during the process. If people say to "snap out of it" at an early stage, they shouldn't necessarily be listened to; it may be *they* who have a problem—an inability to face death and deep feelings.

Failure to work through grief and mourning produces neurotic symptoms and psychosomatic ills. Some people try to avoid pain and conflicting feelings after a death, but they eventually fail. "Every psychiatrist," says Dr. Leopold Bellak, "has seen people suddenly become depressed a month or a year after the shocking death, suffering from delayed mourning." A woman whose husband died of a heart attack may appear at her doctor's office months or even years later, suffering chest pains symbolic of unresolved emotions.

Friends and relatives sometimes have difficulty dealing with the bereaved. Grief is pain—its resolution, a huge effort. The griever may seem ill, exhausted, restless, full of sighs, and afflicted by unpredictable bouts of rage, despair, and bitterness. Loss of security and having new responsibilities don't make things easier. The best help is to listen, sympathize, understand, and give practical aid. The question is, for how long?

Mourning requires various times for different people, depending on their personalities and the kinds of losses they suffered. Some people mourn for many months or for years, says Dr. Bellak, "under the mistaken impression that this constitutes evidence of a very special love and devotion." Certainly when grief goes on for years rather than months, it shows failure to surmount some stage of grief. This may result from excessive anger, self-pity, guilt, or depression. Often a friend or clergyman can help; if not, counseling or therapy often improves the situation.

Neurosis and Health

After reading about neurotic traits and mechanisms, a person may look at himself and those around him, wondering, "Are we all neurotic?" He has thus shown an important sign of emotional health—being aware of emotions instead of avoiding or denying them, even if they are momentarily disturbing. We all sometimes become mildly depressed, anxious, or compulsive; project emotions; or express them through our bodies. If knowledge of the emotions teaches anything, it is that none are bad in themselves, and they can all be used positively.

For instance, narcissism, or self-love, is a two-edged sword. In excess, it makes one a domineering scene-stealer who turns everyone else into an audience. Since the world won't fully agree with the narcissist's glowing view of himself, he will suffer disappointment and anger. But a healthy degree of narcissism lends confidence, the ability to survive setbacks without bitterness, and the sheen that helps make one attractive and successful.

Depersonalization, the loss of a sense of self that can appear in depression, is frightening. It makes a person feel like a zombie, a nobody; it seems like mental death. Yet such numbness is a necessary temporary self-protection mechanism when tragedy and grief strike. The hysteric, who seems as excited over the loss of a button as the loss of a friend, and cannot stop the widening spiral of his reactions, might benefit from a greater capacity to briefly turn off inner turmoil.

Every mental mechanism and trait, then, has its uses; it is having too much or too little, or using it in the wrong situation, that gives it a neurotic quality. Being a bit obsessive-compulsive has advantages in the work world; it makes one conscientious and thorough. Being strongly obsessive-compulsive makes one rigid, constricts creativity and spontaneity, and takes much of the fun out of doing anything well. A little imaginative suspicion or even mild paranoia doesn't hurt when buying a used car or assessing very competitive environments; it does, however, destroy close relationships. A touch of narcissism helps one sell oneself on the job market and the social scene, but it may make a parent act like a spoiled child.

The neurotic, we have said, is like everyone but more so, in ways that work against him. He needn't necessarily think in terms of wiping out his problematic qualities, even if that were possible. If those qualities are used in appropriate amounts and in the right places, they work harmoniously to create a flexible, diverse, and strong personality. To deny them diminishes the capacity to grow through adversity rather than be impoverished by it.

The Psychoses

Organic mental disorders result from physical illness or injury, especially of the brain (tumors, alcohol poisoning, etc.). Sometimes they result from the wear and tear of aging, such as arteriosclerosis of the blood vessels of the brain.

Functional disorders rise from emotional conflict rather than physical illness. The two categories are not always neatly separate, for mind and body continually affect each other—for instance, stress may induce alcoholism, which in turn causes emotional symptoms.

Psychoses, or severe mental disorders, can badly disable a person in intimate and social relationships, work, and behavior, and make him seem out of touch with reality. People may live with neuroses, but psychoses usually force a person or his family to seek medical aid or hospitalization. Organic psychoses are more common at later ages. Most functional psychoses can appear at any age, but a few are especially common in middle and late life.

Acute Depression

Severe depression, or melancholia, can have physical or emotional causes or both—illness, bereavement, or prolonged stress. Depression ranges from mild, temporary neurosis to long-lasting or suicidal psychosis. Two kinds of severe depression tend to appear or worsen in mid-life, *involutional depression* and the *manic-depressive syndrome*.

Involutional depression is more common in women than in men, and it most often appears around ages 45 to 55, at times of bereavement and stress. Though it may coincide with menopause, it apparently is not caused by the climacteric. The first signs may be tearfulness, fatigue, apathy, and irritability. The depressed person is unhappy and can't make decisions; she has trouble sleeping at night and can't get going in the morning. Attempts to cheer her fail; she is convinced she is a failure in life. Prolonged unhappiness may lead to such physical symptoms as headaches, gastrointestinal upsets, and dizziness.

Beneath such complaints lies deep mental pain. Her hopeless boredom, pessimism, and sense of worthlessness become an anguish—sometimes so awful that suicide seems the only escape. In full-blown psychotic depression, there may be delusions of persecution.

A man is likely to develop involutional depression a little later in life, around 60 to 65. The symptoms are basically the same—apathy, despair, anxious agitation, insomnia, imagined illnesses, and loss of sexual interest. He may suspect that his wife is unfaithful and intends to leave him, and that his business associates are conspiring to cast him aside.

We do not know why such depression arrives; changes in the body's hormone balance or metabolism may play a role, and there should be a physical examination to rule out organic causes. But important personality factors are probably decisive. Severe depression often assails rigid, perfectionistic people when they cannot meet their own overstrict standards. Faced with built-up pressure—including, perhaps, normal aging—they break rather than bend. Dr. Leonard Cammer says that in some cases, "The alteration in hormones at the menopause is just the stress in point, and the person can no longer maintain stability."

> ## "ONE OF THE WORST ENEMIES OF LATER LIFE IS BOREDOM."

For a man, the final stress may be retirement or disabling illness. Psychiatrist Leon Salzman gives as an example a successful 62-year-old lawyer who had had to slow down because of a heart attack. By his own account, the lawyer was a perfectionist who would settle for nothing but the best from himself. When his colleagues tried to ease his work load, he felt inadequate. His sexual activity diminished. He felt increasingly worthless and despairing, and began to fear that his wife would abandon him and that his firm would drop him (though he had helped to found it). "At this point, " says Dr. Salzman, "his depression was still mild, but it was clear that it would not be long before he might be involved in suicidal preoccupations or even in possible attempts at suicide."

Such depression makes life miserable for the sufferer and his family. Untreated, it may last from a few months to a few years, become permanent, or lead to suicide. With proper treatment—often a combination of psychotherapy and medication, and in some cases electric shock therapy—the worst may pass in as little as four to six weeks.

The manic-depressive syndrome occurs equally in men and women and tends to appear with a bout of depression around age 30 (though sometimes a decade earlier or later). Then periods of depression alternate with manic phases — emotional "highs" of overexcitement and euphoria. During the latter, the person seems supercharged, too excited to eat or sleep. He is awhirl with enthusiastic plans, and angrily impatient if anyone tries to slow him down or suggests that he see a doctor. This may continue for weeks or months. Unfortunately, the manic state may end as abruptly as it began, plunging the person back into despair. As in involutional depression, there is sometimes the possibility of suicide.

The full cycle, from depression through mania and back down to depression, may take six months or even six years. Some patients do not show an even cycle, but suffer chronic depression with brief, extreme lows. In middle age, the manic phase may become less frequent and severe, leaving only depression.

Sometimes this disorder clears up and does not return. Antidepressant medication may help to relieve the lows, and tranquillizers to reduce the highs, but these drugs often have a dulling effect. In recent years, some carefully selected patients have responded well to treatment with a compound of lithium, a light metal. It improves 80 percent of hyperexcited patients within weeks. Such treatment, however, must be chosen, administered, and followed up with great care, for lithium can have severe side effects.

Involutional depression and the manic-depressive syndrome have long been among the worst scourges of mental health in the second half of life. Various combinations of psychotherapy, medication, and physical treatment now offer increasing help. Psychiatrist Charles Socarides comments, "One should not underestimate the powerful effect that just talking to someone has in some of these cases." The chief preventive measure is alert sensitivity to one's own and other's feelings. Each person, his relatives, friends, or physician should spot the onset of unusual highs and lows and seek medical help before severe illness develops. Of course everyone has highs and lows; some people are relatively placid, some energetic, some changeable. But when a person starts heading into what for him are unusual peaks or valleys of emotion, it is best to consult a physician, if only to relieve one's concern.

Schizophrenia

Schizophrenia is one of the commonest psychoses, and among the most difficult to treat. It usually develops in adolescence or early adulthood, but it can continue or worsen in mid-life. When it does appear for the first time around age 60 or after, it is called *paraphrenia.*

Schizophrenia is actually a range of related disorders of thought and feelings. It commonly involves withdrawal from people, ideas of persecution (paranoia), delusions of grandeur, extreme anxiety, and disconnection from reality. Many old schizophrenics seem suspicious, eccentric, and socially withdrawn. Such a person—more often a woman than a man—is typically jealous and quarrelsome, incapable of warm relationships, and perhaps a religious extremist or fanatic. Eventually she may suspect she is being spied on, that her thoughts are controlled by radio equipment, or that she is victimized by threats or imminent sexual assaults. Finally her behavior may become socially unacceptable, and she cannot cope with daily realities, so she is hospitalized.

Many researchers suspect genetic or chemical factors in schizophrenia, but there are equally strong arguments for environmental and family influences. As in some cases of depressive psychosis, a genetic predisposition may exist, and the forces of upbringing and life events determine whether the person's strengths or vulnerabilities dominate. There are patients who do not respond well to treatment, but schizophrenia is sometimes improved or controlled through medication, electric shock, and psychotherapy.

Senility

Senility is a broad term that includes many conditions, some of them treatable. Any suspicion of senility should provoke not despair and inaction but a full, immediate medical and psychiatric evaluation.

In the narrow sense, senility is a brain disorder *(senile brain syndrome)* of late life that brings general mental deterioration. This rarely happens until after age 70 and more often in women than in men. Its onset is gradual. The Group for the Advancement of Psychiatry gives these five basic signs that may suggest organic senile psychosis: impaired orientation, memory, intellectual function, and judgment, and changeable or shallow emotional response.

Typically the patient becomes forgetful, loses interest in life, and may return to childish behavior and responses ("second childhood"). She is touchy, perhaps whimpery and angrily impatient over trifles. She sleeps fitfully and may wander about the house at all hours. Sometimes she is confused about her surroundings and even the people she knows best. Finally there may be severe depression, tantrums, irrational fears, feelings of persecution, and refusal to eat. At its worst, senile psychosis requires hospitalization; the patient may be incontinent, unable to feed herself, and often unconscious.

Obviously such changes reflect severe physical deterioration, yet it is surprising how medical advice, proper nutrition, and attentive care may slow the process. Senility is not necessarily a hopeless downhill slide. There is particular hope for the many people whose senile behavior is not caused primarily by brain degeneration.

Hardening of the arteries that supply the brain *(cerebral arteriosclerosis)* deprives the brain of oxygen and nutrients; the result can be gloominess, fits of weeping or laughter, and confused thought or speech. This condition, unlike brain-syndrome senility, may develop rapidly and clear up for periods of time, and leaves the personality structure relatively intact.

Many victims of cerebral arteriosclerosis also have a history of high blood pressure *(hypertension)*. Hypertension and arterial weakness may combine to create stroke—a leak or break in a blood vessel in the brain (see page 115). The outcome depends on how much brain tissue is destroyed by the bleeding, clotting, and loss of circulation. Extreme symptoms are partial paralysis, tremors, speech disorders, mental confusion, and sensory defects.

Unfortunately, some families feel that such symptoms always mean irreversible mental damage. They do not know that some people reach partial or even full recovery after treatment and rehabilitation. Damage to the brain's speech center can create an exaggerated impression of mental impairment. An apparently senile patient, suffering from slurred speech, confusion, and depression, may respond well to medication and rest.

Other illnesses can create apparent senility, and many are treatable. Some disorders of the kidneys and liver; high fever from infectious disease; heavy-metal poisoning (e.g., lead poisoning); alcohol poisoning; some disorders of nutrition, metabolism, and the hormone system; and a number of common medications—all can produce weakness, apathy, depression, mental confusion, and delirium.

One also must bear in mind that an older person returns to normal less quickly after physical or emotional stress. When illness, emotional loss, or prolonged stress tests an older person's capacities, anxious relatives should hesitate to interpret a slow return to stability as "softening of the brain." At such times, medical checkups are called for. Often rest, warm care, and mild medication bring a full cure.

The apparently senile patient, then, should never be automatically written off by family, friends, physicians, and social agencies. Some are actually suffering most from loneliness, isolation, and a sense of uselessness, and therefore from severe depression. Even victims of organic deterioration often can be helped to some degree.

Striking proof is reported by the eminent psychiatrist Dr. Karl Menninger. He tells of an experiment with 88 senile psychotic patients at Topeka State Hospital, in Kansas, most of whom had been there longer than ten years. A doctor and a team of cheerful young health professionals and social workers gave the patients individual attention and took the trouble to perform such small services as playing music, turning on the television sets, and bringing in pets. At the end of the year, only one of the 88 was still confined to bed. Twelve had left the hospital to live with their families, four to nursing homes, six to live on their own, and four to become self-supporting members of their communities again.

In a special report to the U.S. Senate Special Committee on Aging, Dr. Menninger stressed that what seems to be senility may be merely a temporary physical or emotional problem. Tragically, many older people, once diagnosed senile, are given up on by their families and communities. Then the diagnosis of senility becomes a self-fulfilling prophecy; the patients' deterioration continues instead of being stopped or reversed.

MARRIAGE AND AFTER

Marriage, like love, work, and child-rearing, presents changes and challenges over the years. Yet in marriage many people have trouble accepting less than perfection. Perhaps nowhere else in life are their expectations so high, their needs so great, and their frustrations so painful.

In some marriages, probably very few, conflict is almost absent, and satisfaction keeps ripening over the decades with little incident. But only in children's books is life one unbroken satisfaction. Psychiatrist Don D. Jackson, interviewing what he considered average couples, found that 80 percent had at some time considered divorce. This does not necessarily speak poorly of their relationships. Psychologist Carl Rogers points out that in a successful marriage, both partners grow through the years, and growth involves periods of conflict, even crisis. If the stormy times are surmounted, the result can be greater intimacy and happiness.

Origins of Marital Conflict

There is a widespread idea that spouses automatically become bored and impatient with each other over the years. If age did always tarnish marriage, the result would be universal resignation or rage. Since that isn't the case, one must look beyond clichés of inevitable staleness.

Severe conflict is commonest during the first decade of marriage; so are infidelity and divorce. Some couples work through early marital problems. Others merely stifle them during the busy child-rearing years; then in middle age, when they are alone with each other again, old submerged conflicts resurface. Their "middle-age" marital difficulty is really the fruit of long-standing problems that were ignored.

A marriage may have been built on shaky ground, without love and commitment in either or both partners. Some people marry from fear of loneliness, to please their families, to get away from home, for economic or emotional security, after disappointments in love, or to find a substitute parent. In such cases, resentment and guilt can keep growing over the years. Some people's expectations of marriage were so low from the beginning that they created an atmosphere of negativism and mistrustfully fended off warmth when it was offered.

Other marriages begin with expectations of rising romantic love and relentless togetherness. In fact, the couple anticipate an idealized and unchanging relationship; any real marriage would eventually disappoint them. Having believed that romantic love should surmount all obstacles, they feel at mid-life that their normally human marriages are failures. Then a "now or never" desperation makes them yearn to fulfill thwarted adolescent dreams.

Blueprints of behavior. Many people begin marriage with mental blueprints for Husband, Wife, Couple, Parent, Family. Unfortunately, these are often ideal imaginings or old childhood images of Mommy and Daddy. These may be unconscious or silently taken for granted; the other spouse may be totally unaware of his "failures."

These blueprints may also change when suitor becomes spouse, when children arrive, and during other transitions in life. The girl who expected a "strong" husband who would "take care of me" may start treating her husband like the first caretaker she had—her mother. This is especially destructive if her mother was cold or hypercritical.

The opposite also occurs. Psychologist Clark Vincent writes, "Time and time again, I have counseled women who chose a husband because he was 'so considerate' when he was courting, only to reject him after marriage because he looked to his wife for her opinion instead of telling her what to do and making her like it." Many a husband expects the vivacious, enticingly independent girl he courted to become a sedate and passive wife. He himself may eventually become passive yet demanding, expecting her to nurture and pamper him in every way, yet to remain an exciting lover.

Other problems are brought to marriage and sharpen with time: ethnic and social differences; sexual dysfunctions; different ideas of masculine and feminine roles; continuing dependence on parents or siblings; mental or physical illness; alcoholism; drug abuse; the idea that marriage automatically creates trust and commitment. Trust and commitment must be earned and re-earned throughout life.

People bring to marriage all their strengths, weaknesses, and idiosyncrasies. Marriage rarely changes them. Personalities, we have said, tend to become more distinctive with age. By mid-life, characteristics once found charming—flirtatiousness, orderliness, clinging—can become points of chronic conflict. So can differences in being demonstrative, disciplined, playful, empathic, nurturing, hostile, or dependent. Neurotic traits, such as depression, exaggerated competitiveness or passivity, and low self-esteem, can be extremely damaging.

It is an old truism that one cannot have contempt for oneself and be genuinely warm to others: one cannot love without self-love. By self-love, we mean not brassy egoism but realistic regard for one's own worth and rights. People to whom life seems a series of well-deserved bad days cast a pall of depression and guilty apprehension all around them. They often are defensive, suspicious, and critical. Their unconscious or even outspoken attitude to a spouse is, "If I'm worth so little, you must be worth even less to want me."

Many people without self-love become martyrs and "grievance collectors." They treasure and recount every hurt, failure, and rejection they meet or imagine. Actually, they are competing with those around them, getting attention by being less happy and more in need. They become artists of fatalism, implied accusation, well-timed fatigue and illness, and of sad sighs indicating that they are so fine they can rise above the pain their spouses cause them. By always suffering and putting themselves down,

they demand reassurance and protection; eventually they provoke outbursts of resentment that seem to justify their air of pain. Since these maneuvers are often unconscious, they are very effective, and very destructive to a marriage.

Almost as exasperating as the professional martyr is the person who yesses a spouse to death. There are no fits of depression and pain; this is not a pseudo-martyr but a pseudo-saint. Such a person says yes but remains emotionally unresponsive at heart, and tomorrow will blithely do the opposite of what was agreed on today. The other partner becomes angry, only to be told with a smile, "Oh, you always fly off the handle over trifles, even when I agree with you." Fake "niceness" can push the partner to chronic resentment, rage, and in some cases divorce.

Just as destructive, of course, are browbeating, bullying, tantrums, and abuse. Some people are more like prosecuting attorneys than spouses; they accuse, nag, convict, and demand atonement. Some are showing in marriage the hostility and negativism that pervade the rest of their lives. Others are fierce perfectionists; they see nothing wrong in judging others as harshly as they judge themselves. Some people with chronic bad tempers are deeply troubled; they feed on their anger, using it to bury underlying anxiety or depression. There are also angry disaster-seekers, who need to blow off steam by creating and surviving crises. Having done so, they proceed more or less cheerfully with life, leaving their spouses to wonder what the storm was really about, and whether to take more seriously its intensity or its transience.

One of the commonest marital problems is destructive competition. The winner's imagined prize is a sense of control over himself and his spouse. Competition may be about who makes decisions or who is better morally, socially, as a spouse, or as a parent. At its most simple and obvious, it is, "I can do anything better than you." The contest may consist of a chronic cry, "You can't take the limelight away from me!" It may be always having the last word. Unfortunately, the bitterness of the fight leaves no true winners.

Many people who become locked in such competition grew up in families where one parent seemed to control, manipulate, or belittle the rest of the household. They live in terror of being dominated the same way by their spouses. Many are compulsive score-keepers, always afraid of being outdone, overpowered, or ignored—in the words of psychiatrist A. D. Jonas, so busy worrying about the portions on other people's plates that they can't enjoy what's on their own.

One-upmanship. The techniques of competing and one-upping are numberless. Among them are: heckling and scene-stealing; answering a complaint with a complaint; refusing to listen or respond; demanding attention and concessions with a "weak heart" or other pseudo-ailments; using sex as a reward and a punishment; and withdrawing into sullenness or apparently neutral distance. Many people, unfortunately, let their marriages become battlegrounds before they recognize their behavior as competitive manipulations.

Growing Together or Apart

It is often said that a husband's or wife's halo is doomed to fade, and that daily familiarity kills attractiveness, dignity, and respect. To this one must answer that it depends on the couple and how they mature individually and together. We are not the same people at 50 as at 20; we have experienced life's difficulties, and can appreciate the strength and compassion they have demanded from a spouse. It is possible to feel increasing trust, affection, and companionship. Also, as Dr. Olga Knopf recently wrote (at age 87), "people who have spent a lifetime together see each other not only as they are but also retain an image of how the other looked in the early days, like a double exposure that hides to a large extent the tell-tale signs of the passage of time."

Unfortunately, many couples fail to anticipate, notice, or counteract changes in their relationships. Increased intimacy may make them more and more like brother and sister; sometimes this interferes with their remaining lovers. If they began marriage with a Hansel-and-Gretel relationship of exaggerated mutual dependence, they may fail to allow each other enough physical and psychic privacy. The result is a paradoxical mixture of clinging, resentment, and imprisonment. If one partner in such a marriage wins far more success and confidence than the other—say, by achieving high status and recognition outside the home—a serious rift can open between them. The partner who feels left behind may withdraw in anticipation of rejection.

One of the commonest relationship changes is really a change in perceptions. Around marriage age, the woman saw herself as more emotional than the man, comparatively flighty or unstable. She considered him solid and disciplined, someone who would help her give shape to her life and contain her occasional sense of inner chaos. The man, on the other hand, enjoyed the way her emotion brought his own feelings alive, awakened his tenderness, humor, and responsiveness.

After years together, the picture changes. She sees his "strength" as mere emotional constriction; he sees her "spontaneity" as emotional displays used to manipulate people. Both may be right, or partly so. Sometimes this pattern is reversed; an expressive man marries a controlled, withdrawn woman. In either case, the partners come to resent and resist the very qualities that first drew them together.

External events and pressures also pull couples apart. Financial difficulties, caring for disabled relatives, a spouse's chronic physical or emotional illness—all strain patience and sometimes affection.

The woman may become so involved in household, job, or both that she slights her marriage. If domestic commitments totally eclipse her other needs and aspirations, she will probably resent her husband and her life with him. On the other hand, involvement in a job or career may provoke guilt in her, regardless of her husband's reaction. These and other pressures may make her forget or refuse to make her husband feel not only needed but appreciated and loved.

Many spouses drift into complete division of responsibility and authority. A wife who leaves all nondomestic matters to her husband, and a husband who gives up his voice in home concerns, are creating potential conflict. Ultimately, no one wants to be voiceless in any major aspect of life. The wife should remember not to undercut or appropriate her husband's authority at home. He must be able to turn off some of the competitiveness of his work day and participate in his home, not take over in it or merely board there. Neither spouse can live the other's experience—the pressures of job and home—but each can appreciate the other's problems and labors, and share some of the concern and pride. Failing to extend empathy to a spouse's daily efforts can quietly erode a marriage.

Sexual age-changes (see page 307), if not understood, become disruptive; sexual compatibility is then replaced by sexual conflict or dysfunction. There are some troubled marriages in which sex remains unimpaired, but more often sexual rifts reflect depression, hostility, conflict, or complex marital difficulties. If allowed to continue, sexual conflict or dysfunction usually deepens and breeds further conflicts.

Extramarital Sex

Conventional wisdom says that sexual dissatisfaction leads to adultery. That is sometimes true, but it hardly explains all extramarital sex. A few decades ago, Kinsey found that one married woman in four and one married man in two had experienced extramarital intercourse; today the figure may well be a bit higher. For the majority of these people, it was rare or sporadic; for relatively few it was frequent or part of long relationships. Nevertheless, adultery is especially feared around mid-life, when women lose their youthful looks but some husbands grow in attractiveness and assurance; it equally concerns men uncertain of themselves and of their wives' stability and satisfaction. For every person who does engage in extramarital sex, there is probably another who thinks about it or was prevented only by circumstances.

Whether sporadic or a way of life, extramarital sex has a variety of motives and effects. To some men and women, it is a groping for new hope when frightened by aging, when dissatisfied sexually or otherwise at home, or when determined to break old inhibitions. For some it is an isolated experiment or adventure. When, as sometimes happens, it is an act of revenge, it can cause more guilt than pleasure.

Some people find extramarital acts unforgivable under any circumstances, on religious or moral grounds. Such principles are beyond argument. We must note, however, that many experts on sex and marriage know cases in which such experience did not damage and even ultimately helped the person or the marriage. For some it proves—as only testing reality can—that the grass really is or isn't greener elsewhere. Sometimes it restores failing self-confidence. It sometimes awakens new sexual or emotional capacities that are then brought back to the marital relationship. Some people learn through adultery that it is not an answer to marital conflict, and they are finally compelled by this knowledge to stop running away from domestic problems and work them out.

A small number of people maintain long, extensive extramarital sex lives, secretly or openly. Some couples agree to this for one or both partners, sometimes as a life-style, sometimes as a pragmatic way of maintaining a distant or unsatisfying marriage. However, such arrangements are rare, and a secret "double life" is ultimately burdensome to most people, both practically and emotionally. Of course, adultery may lead to genuine emotional and sexual fulfillment outside marriage, and thus to divorce. Yet infidelity is not the most common reason for divorce.

When adultery is discovered, it usually causes rage and a sense of betrayal. Sometimes it does bring on the marriage's gradual or sudden death. But if the infidelity was brief and circumstantial—caused by the married couple's separation, fear of aging, severe emotional pressures—the marriage may survive despite a stormy period of pain, guilt, and recrimination. With time and understanding, the marital rift may be closed by basic love and commitment.

When adultery does reflect sharp (though sometimes hidden) marital conflicts, the aftermath actually may be helpful. The impulses, fears, and troubles that caused it will be forced into the open, and perhaps understood and resolved. This forces an overdue dialogue that airs grievances by both spouses. It sometimes becomes clear that the "injured" spouse was really pushing the other toward infidelity, knowingly, unknowingly, or as a test of love and loyalty. If there is still a potential for commitment, the difficult marital reassessment may finally create a better, more empathic relationship. If the marriage was emotionally bankrupt, the couple will face the fact and perhaps make fresh starts on their own.

Sometimes infidelity—like money and attitudes toward children or in-laws—is really a symbolic issue expressing general disenchantment. Many dry or troubled marriages don't produce such dramatic conflicts. People can grow apart slowly, through a long vicious cycle of mutual withdrawals caused by little omissions, hurts, and inconclusive disagreements that "aren't really worth fighting over." Weary from pain and anger, the couple simply cease to love and feel committed to each other; they have no relationship, only a set of defensive barriers against further disappointment. At this point, they are actually lucky if something forces them to reevaluate their lives individually and together.

Marital Evaluation

Even in satisfying marriages, mid-life often brings rediscovery, reevaluation, and readjustment. Interestingly, men and women tend to differ in their views. Several studies show that middle-aged men, as a group, tend to say they are happier with their marriages than women, praise their spouses more, and are more satisfied with their sex lives than in the past. Women tend more to speak of disappointments, to criticize their husbands, and to be less satisfied with their sex lives than in the past. Perhaps women enter marriage with greater expectations. There are so many possible interpretations of this that we only report it, as something couples might keep in mind.

Both men and women do, however, tend to be more satisfied with their marriages in mid-life than during the child-rearing years. Even many who suffer the "empty nest syndrome" (see page 272) eventually feel more free and content. This doesn't square with the old notion of progressive marital disillusionment. Probably most couples have ambivalent, changing feelings about each other and about marriage over the years. They learn that much of life isn't what they expected—sometimes better, sometimes worse, but different. Most entered marriage hoping for a happy, trusting collaboration. When it meets or exceeds their preconceptions, they glow; when it falls short, they wonder what or whom to blame.

The first step in marital evaluation is to stop trying to place blame. This is difficult even in minor squabbles, let alone when there are accumulated pains and resentments. If a couple in conflict cannot reach a clear evaluation they agree on, they should seek professional help in doing so. One cannot categorize and discuss all types of marriages in this short space, but these are some of the very common ones:

The Satisfactory Marriage. Despite occasional problems, disagreements, even crises, the couple find most important aspects of their marriage rewarding, and they both want it to continue.

The Moderately Conflicted Marriage.
The couple have an underlying reserve of love and commitment, but their relationship is disturbed by quarrels and frustrations. They may be fighting over only a few important, easily identified issues. These are the couples that most often reach counselors' offices, and many are helped. The worst thing they can do is write off their conflicts as "the usual ups and downs" and slip into growing hostility or resignation.

The Silently Conflicted Marriage.
There is little open fighting, but little or nothing positive in the relationship. The couple may call their marriage a good one, but only they think so. They deny emotion and conflict, living in frozen truce. If both are very hostile, they may become partners in snarling at the world and thus direct much of their anger outside the marriage. If loners, they may continue reasonably well as long as they don't spend much time together; it helps if both have absorbing interests. Even such spouses, however, may sometimes feel the lack of warmth and nurture at home.

The Severely Conflicted Marriage.
This consists largely of open or indirect fighting, from violent arguments to sustained mutual withdrawal. The couple may teeter on the brink of divorce for years, yet the marriage may be fundamentally sound or savable. As in moderately conflicted marriages, there may be specific, remediable problems—sexual dysfunction, exaggerated dependence, or habitual competition. Sometimes one partner seeks professional help because of his or his spouse's temper, drinking, extravagance, sex problems, or vindictiveness. If both spouses make serious reparative efforts, the outlook may be good for positive change in their lives and perhaps their marriage. If they refuse to work at understanding and change, one or both may become mentally or physically ill, seek divorce, or reach the stage of negative marriage.

The Negative Marriage. This is a closed system of anger and dissatisfaction that neither the couple nor a third party can alter. They live separate lives under one roof or become relentless accusers and complainers—finally communicating only through anger, sarcasm, manipulation, and psychosomatic ills. They have no moments of pleasure, love, or joy. Only social and practical hurdles, religious edict, or lack of courage and hope keeps them from divorce.

A couple cannot evaluate their marriage by putting a check mark beside a category in such a list. They must examine themselves, each other, and their relationship. They must try this alone, together, and if necessary with professional help. If they find that they habitually fall into quarrels or dreary distance, they should observe when, how, and why. This effort at evaluation can in fact be the first step toward marital repair and renewal.

Repair and Renewal

Even many marriages that seem hopelessly flat or conflict-ridden can be rejuvenated by determined effort. There is no hope if each spouse waits in resentment and stubborn pride for the other to change. Nor can they merely complain, passively hoping for a better life. A couple must admit that problems exist, and that in even the most one-sided marriage, both partners have contributed to the difficulties.

No one is victimized for long unless he permits it. Every domestic dictator needs a professional martyr to permit or incite him. Every nag needs a partner who will put up with him or nag back. Every alcoholic needs a spouse who plays into his illness, however unknowingly or reluctantly—especially by joining in the drinking or by acting like a scolding yet forbearing parent. The sadist and masochist are always secret collaborators. There are few *I* problems in marriage; mostly there are various kinds of *we* problems.

Exploring such subjects is bound to bring argument, even fighting. These are not, in themselves, signs of a bad marriage. Too many people consider expressing anger a brutal or unladylike act, and fear it will make them forever unloved. They chronically smother or deny their anger, but other people sense it anyway; it tends to show in coldness or misplaced quarrels the next day or even years later. Quarrels are destructive only when they can solve no problems, fights destructive only when they are about false issues or become so chronic that they block all other communication.

"There is a place in the best of marriages," said Dr. Don Jackson, "for occasional bluntness or even rudeness. Occasionally, even an out-and-out fight may be in order; as long as it falls short of homicide, it will probably leave both spouses refreshed." People who have had trouble showing resentments can find in this advice the start of a curative process. They will probably observe that much of their anger is over not having expressed their real needs.

Couples must learn when and how to assert their needs; to express them is neither ugly nor destructive. Unfortunately, many chronic marital arguments have "hidden agendas," and contain counter-complaints, baiting, and cherished resentments. A good way to start changing this is with an agreement to express dissatisfaction when it is felt, not to nurse it and take it out on the partner later. One can do so honestly yet without being so hurtful that one provokes secondary fights and never settles the original issue.

For this to work, the complaints must be specific and reasonable, and each spouse must be willing to consider and accept criticism or personal differences—and to act. "Do it now" is a good motto for marital readjustment—complain now, express love now, argue now, give now. This is especially important in resolving mutual competition

> ## "ALL RELATIONSHIPS REQUIRE CONSTANT CHANGE, LEARNING, & READAPTATION IF THEY ARE TO REMAIN HEALTHY."

and withdrawal. The matter of who makes the first move must cease to be an issue in genuine conciliation and renewal. This sounds simple enough, but most of us fear that showing anger, need, or affection makes us emotionally vulnerable.

Competition and emotional manipulation can be approached the same way. When felt or suspected, they should be aired, so that conflict is nipped in the bud. If efforts to resolve anger, competition, and manipulation keep leading to even worse arguments, the couple should consider the possibility that they actually prefer the electricity of battle to contentment. Or perhaps one spouse has a temperamental need to blow off steam regularly, and has ways of finding pretexts for doing so; he can become aware of this, and his spouse can stop rising to the bait. If conflict becomes a way of life, and all attempts at resolution only escalate their arguments, a third party is needed to help them identify and deal with their problems.

What does a spouse want? Spouses should also try to give not what they themselves like giving but what their partners want, and when it is needed. A wife may need to feel not that she is a good housekeeper but that her eyes are still lovely or her opinion still valued. A husband may need to know that he is not only depended on but also admired or desired.

Couples should seek a good balance of intimacy and independence. Unfortunately, some people feel rejected or abandoned if their spouses do anything at all without them, even if they prefer different hobbies, music, or food. It is unjust and useless to resent another's tastes, no matter how baffling they seem. This is increasingly important as middle-aged and elderly couples have more leisure for a variety of activities. Furthermore, a couple with similar interests needn't always pursue them together. Most people need both companionship and privacy, and the particular balance of the two is not a barometer of love.

Understanding this means accepting that two intelligent and honest people can perceive the same situation differently. This is a major step in maintaining or reestablishing intimacy and mutual respect. Sometimes a couple cannot agree on who said what 30 seconds earlier, let alone the inherent interest of poker, amateur astronomy, church work, or baby-sitting with grandchildren. It can be the wisdom of later life to accept human differences without always judging them or taking them personally. Sometimes it is less important to decide what is right than to accept people with respect or compassion.

Emotional messages. Such understanding helps in applying one of the major advances in psychological and marital counseling, the study of verbal and non-verbal communication. A great many emotionally laden messages are not sent or received consciously, but they are nevertheless clear and effective. Consider this hypothetical case:

A husband comes home from work, loudly tosses his coat on a chair, and plops down with a "Whew." Without a word he has proclaimed that he is tired and demands the household's sympathy and attention. His wife gives a fleeting but noticeable sigh, pastes a tolerant smile on her face and says, "How was your day?" She has indicated that she is just as tired and in need of attention as he, and one-ups him by being more "considerate." A bit guilty, he asks in detail about her day.

Within 15 seconds they are locked in polite competition for who deserves more sympathy and attention. Neither is aware of this, but through dinner and into the evening, they feel a vague cloud of discomfort and irritation. The hidden game—"I need love but I'm nicer than you"—can continue that night in bed and the next morning over breakfast. Some couples carry it on for decades, not understanding why they often blow up at each other over trifles.

Sometimes communication becomes tangled because people use verbal shorthand for painful or complex emotions. When a spouse says, "You only think about yourself," it may really be a way of saying, "I hurt because I need you to make me feel loved and worthwhile, but I'm too proud to ask." If the partner answers the statement—denying, counter-accusing, or apologizing—the fight will escalate. One must answer not the *words* but the *message.*

Hidden issues. Some marital quarrels, in fact, arise when a person accurately senses a hostile or belittling message beneath friendly words. When a husband says, "Now, don't worry your head about the accounts," or a wife says, "Remember to take your scarf and gloves this time," the partner may snap back, like a child at an oversolicitous parent. The hidden message, of course, is some variation of "You don't even know enough to walk in out of the rain by yourself."

Sometimes a spouse receives a statement inaccurately; misinterprets fatigue or depression as a personal rejection; or reads in meanings out of fear or insecurity. Consider another series of damaging exchanges:

A man must go away for two days on a business trip; he tells his wife quite accurately that he will be busy from morning to night, and it would be no fun for either of them were she to go along expecting a joint vacation. Perhaps she is chronically jealous or he has had guilty fantasies about meeting women away from home. When he speaks, he is a little more emphatic and detailed than usual; or perhaps he is the picture of studied casualness. His wife, despite the considerate and realistic words, senses wariness—an indirect signal of "I can't tell you everything."

Especially if she is insecure, she offers cheerfully to go along anyway, to care for him and make his trip easier. Her fixed brightness of voice and slightly rigid smile communicate her fear and anger. Picking up her message—"I can't trust you"—he answers accusation with accusation: he makes a "harmless" joke about her getting in the way of his socializing. He is telling her that if he's going to be accused in advance, he may as well do something to earn it. Now she becomes openly angry, and he earnestly asks "why!"

Many people who feel their marriage is stale or "just not working" may learn through observing their communication that there are indeed hidden issues—often involving neurotic mechanisms such as those described in the earlier section on Emotional Health and Illness. It helps every marriage when the partners realize that we cannot avoid communicating—by choice of words, tone of voice, facial expression, timing, hesitations, even by silence. Too often people do not "send" what they mean and misinterpret what they "receive." With insight and practice, a couple can clear much of the static and contradiction from their exchanges.

All relationships require constant change, learning, and readaptation if they are to remain healthy. While effort and determination are prerequisites for avoiding and resolving conflict, they are sometimes not enough. Specific therapy and information—about communication, sexuality, and personal and interpersonal difficulties—are sometimes the vital added factors that enable a marriage to become flexible, enriched, and enduring.

Divorce

The divorce rate has been rising for people of all ages; today about one couple in 15 who enter middle age will end their marriage. Fewer people now are held back by religious prohibitions or social stigma. The legal barriers are being reduced in many states, and the trend is likely to continue. Therefore a couple who feel hopelessly deprived of marital satisfaction are more likely than ever to consider ending their tie.

Perhaps the marriage was never satisfying, but social, economic, and parental commitments seemed to outweigh individual fulfillment. Sometimes mid-life crisis brings a sense of waste and anger over a minimally rewarding marriage. The couple may realize that they have irremediably grown apart, become mired in resentment, or reached an unbearable stalemate. This is especially painful when one partner wants divorce more than the other; he or she may fear being labeled a reprehensible deserter. Sometimes this is true, but sometimes it is the more neurotic, destructive spouse who clings to a sterile marriage—less from love than from inability to face reality and change.

Many states' laws provide for a couple to separate and have time to try reconciliation before divorce is final. This imminence of divorce and a taste of living alone may force a belated facing of problems, sometimes their resolution, with or without the help of professional counseling. However, trial separation also can lead to further estrangement. Individual counseling or therapy is often useful when a person bent on divorce is really using the marriage as a lightning rod for other pressures and conflicts, including fear of aging.

Some people, realistically dissatisfied with their marriages, are capable of better relationships; divorce can offer them a fresh start in life. They should, however, be quite convinced that this is the case, and that they are not acting out problems that will recur in later relationships. Regret and repeated marital problems sometimes follow precipitous divorce.

The majority of mental-health professions are, as Dr. Don Jackson put it, for marriage but against relationships that continue to damage people's well-being. Some couples resign themselves to conflict-ridden or destructive mateships only because they fear the emotional, social, or practical consequences of divorce. The price is likely to be growing unhappiness and loss of a feeling of worth.

Decision to separate is rarely reached without difficulty and pain. People considering the step should be aware that such professionals as counselors and attorneys may help reconstitute a marriage or make the break cleaner; sometimes, unfortunately, they escalate hostility and promote unnecessary bitterness. Their advice, like that of friends and family, should be listened to open-mindedly but critically. If divorce does occur, both parties should know all the legal and practical consequences beforehand.

Divorce often brings a mixture of relief, fear, loss, exhilaration, and guilt. There is usually a period of shock and then of recovery and change while new life patterns are developed. This process lasts months or up to several years. No matter how justified or necessary the divorce seemed, it may provoke feelings of guilt and failure. Furthermore, the break must be explained to children, family, and friends. Some of these may take sides instead of offering as much understanding and support as possible to both former spouses. There are problems of alimony and the support of two households, especially if the man remarries and the woman does not.

When most people hear of the end of a marriage, they say, "I'm sorry to hear it." Often they need not be. Divorce allows some men and women to blossom for the first time in their lives. The great majority of divorcees remarry, and happily (see page 307). With good fortune and good judgment, ex-partners may be able to see their marriage as a source of much good feeling rather than bitterness and regret. They may come to eventually accept that they, once loving and fulfilling to each other, have grown apart—perhaps to the ultimate benefit of both. We will discuss below the possibilities of making a new life when single during middle or later life.

Widowhood

Women tend to marry men older than themselves, and they live longer; therefore more of them end up bereaved of a spouse. Many women, aware of this, go through what Professor Bernice Neugarten has called mental "rehearsal for widowhood." But even if a spouse's death was expected, it brings a period of grief, mourning, and readjustment (see page 290).

If the spouse had to be nursed through a long or painful terminal illness, the survivor may experience a residue of resentment and guilt. This in no way reflects on the marriage. Dr. Robert N. Butler points out that guilt, depression, and other emotional problems are often severe not only for those deprived of a wonderful relationship but for survivors of bad marriages:

"Where the relationship has been grim and complicated by dependency or anger, unresolved and often unarticulated, the grief may be intense and the possibilities of picking up the pieces and renewing oneself are vastly reduced. Thus the tranquil widow or widower must not be seen as a callous survivor relieved by the death of a spouse, but rather as a compliment to the marriage itself."

After working through grief, widows and widowers examine and reorient their lives. The woman may be left with financial and practical problems, the man with difficulties handling daily details once assumed by the wife. A readjustment must often be made socially, seeking the company of family and friends to escape overwhelming loneliness. One must try to resist the temptation to sink into depression and resignation; happiness is not gained from clinging to the past out of guilty "loyalty" or fear of change and risk.

Some people come fully into their own after widowhood, especially women who have submerged their interests and drives over many years. They become involved in rewarding careers, hobbies, volunteer work, or family and social relationships. Thus they avoid two of the greatest spoilers of later life, isolation and unwanted idleness.

The difficulties of widowhood can be severe. Couples should realistically plan together for the eventuality of either partner being left alone; false delicacy in such matters is no favor.

Being Single

A small number of people never marry; by the time they reach middle or late life, most have worked out life patterns for themselves. The widowed and divorced face many new problems. Besides having to adapt practically and emotionally to being alone, they must cope with uncertainty and seek life changes. They may wonder how to feel and behave. Must the widowed act sad and pious? Should divorced men stress their youthfulness? Are divorced women seen as "fair game" by men or as threats or failures by married women? The mature single person may have to learn not to see himself through others' eyes—or as he imagines others see him. He can probably learn to expect acceptance after a while for being his real, quite human self.

The single also wonder at what point to either indulge or try to overcome fears of getting close to a new partner, to again risk hurt by separation or death. Some want companionship but aren't ready yet to build new love relationships. Those who do wish new partners may feel uncertain, afraid of rejection. There is a set social role for the single young adult; to the extent that patterns exist for the mature and single, today they are more restricting than they are conducive to a renewed life—leftovers from a time when people were old at forty. How should the mature single person make friends, have dates, find love and sex, and construct a new way of life?

A good first step is to share the experience of divorce or widowhood with others who have been through its difficulties. If living alone is uncomfortable or a burden, and one doesn't wish to move in with relatives, one can double up with a friend for a while. Despite fears of social or sexual failure, people should try to reenter life, counting on their accumulated life experience—especially their courage, compassion, and humor—to help them. They will find many people who share their situation; social groups exist for the widowed and divorced, and there is a sort of underground social network. A great deal depends on whether one lives in a small town or big city, has a small or wide social circle, and on family and neighborhood and community. Most important, probably, is the will to return to healthy appetites and fulfillments in every aspect of life.

Both men and women continue to have sexual desires when alone in the second half of life, though society pretends they do not or even should not (see page 307). Some people deny such desires to themselves because they are depressed; because they, too, disapprove of such feelings in themselves; or because they lack opportunities for a gratifying sex life. The obvious solutions, unless remarriage is prompt, are nonmarital coitus and masturbation. Each, we have noted, provokes deeply rooted guilt in some people. Nevertheless, either can be a source of gratification, tension-release, and a continuing sense of effectiveness. Remaining sexually active helps sustain one's sexual capacity (see page 309). If a marriage or love partner is eventually found, having kept this capacity helps one snap back quickly to regular sexual activity.

Remarriage and Other Options

Despite talk about the death of marriage as an institution, most people would rather live with its problems than without them. About four out of five people who divorce in middle age remarry, the majority in lasting and satisfying unions. Many of the widowed also remarry, though women are here at a disadvantage. Single elderly women far outnumber single older men, and women have increasing difficulty finding partners as the years pass—though some are successful at it.

In second marriages, each spouse marries the other's past to some degree—a former spouse, children, in-laws, friends, and triumphs and failures shared with others. Sometimes adult children are delighted at the happy remarriage of a parent, but some are still unable to see their parents as loving and sexual beings with a right to their own lives. They also may be upset for financial reasons; the new couple must often make complex arrangements providing for each other and their children, sometimes to no one's full satisfaction.

As in the past, some older people enter a "straw marriage"—a marriage in name and law only, without a sex or even a love relationship, for practical reasons. And unfortunately, an increasing number of older couples live together without the legal marriage they would prefer; often remarriage would bring loss of alimony, widow's pensions, certain Social Security benefits, and other sources of income. These are inequities one can hope will disappear.

We have dwelled briefly here on the problems of remarriage and some of its alternatives. A second (or third or fourth!) marriage does not present many of the problems of youthful marriage; its conflicts and rewards are those of continuing marriages. While the spouses must beware of bringing too many ghosts into their relationship, they have the benefit of bringing all the experience, fortitude, shrewdness, and compassion won from previous years of marriage. The best testimony to this is the comparatively higher rate of gratification and staying power in remarriages.

SEX AND AGING

It seems almost silly to have to say it, but one must: we never outgrow the needs and desires of youth—to be intimate, to touch and be touched, to give and receive love with the voice, hands, skin, genitals, the entire body. Age mellows but cannot dim the pleasures of sexual love, and its affirmation of one's sense of self, of effectiveness, of maleness and femaleness. Despite some physical changes, one's later sex life tends to follow the patterns of earlier years unless fear and negativism get in the way.

Only recently have the middle-aged and elderly insisted that society recognize them as sexual beings. The subject of later-life sex was strictly tabooed until the mid-1960s, even among health-care professionals. The idea that sex survives youth still upsets many people, as the mature may painfully learn from the reactions of family and friends. Our society goes on believing, as Dr. Frances J. Braceland puts it, that what is virility at 25 is lechery at 65—and, we should add, that what is feminine in young women is absurd, greedy, or unseemly in mature women. Dr. Braceland says that sex is a "timeless drive throughout life even into the eighties and nineties."

Myths that harm. Many myths hamper later-life sexuality. One is that wrinkles and the loss of fertility dictate a retreat from full womanhood. Another is that men normally lose their sexual drive and powers in middle age, especially if they are erotically active—as though sex were an easily depleted reserve. Another is that the middle-aged and elderly don't miss sex if deprived of it, and care more for other, less "animalistic" things. Finally, there is the myth that sex is animalistic.

The "animalism" myth reverses biological fact. Most animals are sexually active only a few days or weeks of each year; they reserve sex for procreation. Humans are unique in nature for being sexually excitable and active around the year and through most of life. In our species, sex serves psychological and social purposes, not only reproductive ones. It binds people in pleasure, affection, and trust while they raise offspring through the longest childhood in nature. This pleasure bond continues to hold them together in cooperation as they grow older.

It is humans, then, not animals, that are pervasively sexual throughout life. With fine efficiency, nature makes human sexuality a source of pleasure, self-esteem, and enriched companionship at all ages. Even religions that stress the procreative aspect of sex praise physical love as a way to heighten intimacy.

Age Changes

Those who write, lecture, or counsel on human sexuality have found that two of the commonest questions they encounter go something like these:

"I am 44 and my husband 46. He has hardly made love to me for a few years. Is he homosexual or is it just normal aging?"

"My wife and I are 55. For the past five years she just hasn't wanted sex. She says maybe it's the change of life. She says I'm too old to really want to anyway, that I'm acting foolish. Am I abnormal or is she?"

Such questions show confusion about the basic facts of mid-life and later sexuality. One's sexuality does change somewhat with age, though rather differently in men and women, and knowing about the shifts helps explain whether a situation reflects health, dysfunction, or normal aging. We will look at sexual aging in women and in men, the question of how much sex is "normal," and the ways men and women can synchronize their sexuality over the years.

Aging in Women

The most obvious and most discussed change in women is menopause, the permanent end of menstruation and fertility. The word climacteric is often given the same meaning, but we will use it for the broader event of mid-life sex-related change, of which menopause is only a part.

Menopause (see page 441) usually occurs in the middle to late forties, give or take a few years. Popular myth once made it one of life's nastier physical and emotional crises, but it causes two out of three women little or no distress. Medical opinion increasingly supports the view of the late sexologist Isadore Rubin: "The most negative and fearful attitudes toward the damages of the menopausal period are found in women who have not yet experienced them."

Some women make "change of life" a scapegoat on which to load a variety of problems, from fading youth to marital, social, and career frustrations. They and the minority who suffer marked physical symptoms have perpetuated the idea of menopausal crisis.

Some women do feel major or minor menopausal discomforts, such as flushing, fatigue, headaches, vague pelvic pain, nervousness, and irritability. Certainly women who look forward to menopause with dread should seek pre-menopausal counseling — from a gynecologist to understand the physical facts, and if necessary, from a psychological or psychiatric counselor to cope with her emotional reactions. Those who suffer during or after menopause also can seek counseling and, if their physicians approve it for them, steroid-hormone replacement (see page 445).

Emotional effects. Menopause, like most hormonal changes, has a variety of effects on sex and the emotions. Women who always had a great fear of unwanted pregnancy may feel liberated by menopause; in fact, the end of pregnancy phobia may release their sexual interest and responsiveness fully for the first time. This erotic blossoming is sometimes helped by the fading of such pressures as raising small children and working to contribute to the family income.

For other women, menopause creates fear of something psychoanalyst Helene Deutsch calls "the closing of the gates." Single women, even those who say they have never wanted children, may feel regret or grief. Some women, with or without children, equate fertility with femininity; to them, menopause threatens to end womanhood itself. Some of them yearn for a final pregnancy.

Unfortunately, some women feel that menopause also closes the gate to sexuality, especially since it comes when they feel their loss of youthful appearance. If they were always indifferent to lovemaking or dissatisfied with it, menopause gives them a respectable excuse for retreating from sex altogether. If they were very narcissistic and judged their worth by men's erotic interest in them, they may seek reassurance in new sexual affairs. Others, looking forward to a life that seems sterile in every way and anticipating rejection by their husbands and other men, "quit" love, sex, and femininity before they can be "fired."

Such sexual negativism can be reinforced in several ways. Gynecological disorders, more common in middle age, may add to feelings of feminine and sexual inadequacy. Some women were raised to feel that sex after youth is shameful, silly, or at best undignified. Society jokes not only at "dirty old men" but at "dirty old ladies." Refusing to see the middle-aged and elderly, including oneself, as sexual people is often a carry-over of childhood reluctance to see parents and other "old" people as fully human and sexual.

There is no reason for sex to end with menopause. Rather, there is every reason for it to continue, for it adds to physical, emotional, and social well-being. We have said that the great enemy of later life is less age itself than despairing isolation. A loving and sexual person remains vital and will not accept isolation as a condition of life.

Hormonal changes. The end of menstruation reflects a change in the body's hormone balance, especially a decline in steroid hormones. This shift causes minor changes in sexual response after 50 and more noticeable ones after 60. Sexual arousal and orgasm take a bit longer than in youth. The vagina may become smaller and less elastic, its walls thinner. After 60, vaginal lubrication may take a few minutes to appear, and even during pleasurable stimulation, it is less plentiful. Because of these changes, the thrusting of vigorous coitus can cause vaginal pain or general pelvic discomfort during or after intercourse, and a burning sensation while urinating for some time afterward.

More rarely, orgasm causes painful contractions of the uterus. Vaginal pain *(dyspareunia)*, urinary burning *(dysuria)*, and painful uterine spasm should be checked by a physician; usually they can be relieved by hormone (estrogen) replacement. The man should be aware that vigorous thrusting and prolonged manipulation of the clitoris may now cause irritation.

There is a fascinating psychological side to these changes. In their landmark research on sex and aging, Masters and Johnson found women in their 60s and 70s who still produced vaginal lubrication and showed little vaginal shrinkage, even without hormone replacement. These were the women who had remained sexually active most of their adult lives—coitus (or if that was not possible, masturbation) once or twice a week. Less active women (those who experienced coitus or masturbation once a month or less in the decade after menopause) had difficulty accomodating the penis when they did try.

Masters and Johnson conclude that in sex, as in most mental and physical activities, one stays healthy by staying active. Or as the old saying goes, "Use it or lose it." Even at advanced ages, say Masters and Johnson, a woman needs only general good health and an interested, interesting partner to continue a gratifying sex life.

Other researchers agree: women with active and happy sex lives before menopause are less likely to let physical love dwindle afterward. Furthermore, many women lose some of their old sexual inhibitions during their 30s, 40s, and even later. Their greatest problem in middle or late life may be losing their partners or their partners' interest. Why this happens, and how it can be dealt with, will be clearer after a look at aging in men.

Aging in Men

It is becoming popular to speak of "male menopause" and "men's mid-life crisis." Actually, there is no dramatic, short-range change in a man's sexual or reproductive potential at any time after puberty. Rather, there are gradual changes, some of which correspond with female climacteric but not with menopause.

Physically, a man's sexual capacity peaks during his teens. Minor changes, usually almost unnoticeable, occur for about two decades; more obvious ones happen from the late 30s through middle age. By 50, a man may desire coitus about half as often as during his teens (the difference is more or less in various men). Between 50 and 70, he gradually finds that erection takes minutes rather than seconds; that orgasm and ejaculation, though as pleasurable, arrive more slowly and are briefer; that semen is expelled less strongly; that after orgasm, erection fades faster; that it takes longer to become sexually responsive again. From middle age on, he may not always feel the need to ejaculate during coitus, even though he is capable of it; he may be fully satisfied afterward. Reproductive power may slacken but does not usually stop, as it does in women at menopause. Most men in normal health can remain both potent and fertile into advanced old age.

Many of these changes have the same cause as female climacteric—a drop in the body's steroid hormones. These probably decrease slowly from early middle age until about the early 60s. A small number of men feel such steroid-starvation symptoms as fatigue, weakness, irritability, impaired concentration and sex drive, and spasms of the prostate gland during orgasm. Steroid-replacement therapy often gives relief. Despite popular beliefs, hormone replacement doesn't raise sexual drive or capacity in most normal, healthy men. "Aphrodisiacs," alleged hormone preparations, and mail-order devices to aid or prolong sexual performance range from worthless to dangerous.

Crisis of confidence. The man who notices small, gradual decreases in his sexual vigor and sees his youthful appearance fading may suffer a crisis of self-love and confidence. Society is sympathetic to a woman who resents and laments aging, but it gives aging men contradictory instructions. It says they should age into grandfatherly, sexless dignity, yet it gives winking praise to those who don't; it urges the preservation of youthfulness, yet it laughs at men who try to hide or deny their years.

It is not surprising, then, that men's reaction to normal age changes isn't always consistent or rational. Some men feel conscious or unconscious urges to deny aging, sometimes by trying to prove they can still attract young women. Others may be surprised and ashamed at how strongly they resent their loss of youth, and be torn between fighting and accepting change. Others not only accept aging, they gloomily resign themselves to it; as a result, they age sooner than they must.

Many men face great demands in their family lives and careers between 40 and 60. Some accept, with good or ill grace, that they may have risen as high professionally as they ever will. But since they are at the height of their careers, their jobs may consume more time and energy than ever. They also must contend with changing family needs, from children's departure and higher education to their wives' age-related problems. All of this is bound to affect their sex lives. Some men find sex a tonic after a tough day at work or a pressure-filled weekend at home, but usually such conditions are not aphrodisiacs. And many men, throughout their lives, mistakenly tend to judge their masculinity and worth by their sexual performance.

How Much is "Normal"?

When Alfred Kinsey's pioneering studies of sex behavior appeared, it was a common joke that even his critics rushed to look themselves up in his charts. This desire to know what is "normal"—by which we mean both average and healthy—is natural. Few of us know the facts of many other people's sex lives, so we have no standard for our own sexuality or our partners'. The curiosity may become nagging at times of sexual change, such as adolescence and middle age—especially if our own or our partners' sexuality isn't what we expected.

The ideas "average" and "healthy" must be kept separate. Human beings have an enormous range of sexual activity, influenced by genetic inheritance, upbringing, health, social class, education, ethnic and religious background, and other factors. If a mathematical average is used as a standard, it becomes an unrealistic tyranny. There are men and women of good mental and physical health who want sex once or twice a day, others who want it once a week or less. What is healthy for any person is what, under the best circumstances, makes him or her feel most fulfilled.

This enormous human sexual variety is difficult to grasp and accept, even for doctors and psychologists. We tend to assume that "oversexed" means "more than I want," and that "undersexed" means "less than I want."

Male and female patterns. It is almost as difficult for men and women to understand their basic differences in sex behaviors. Men's sexual patterns tend to be consistent, even rigid. A man who feels the need for three orgasms a week is likely to obtain them, if not through marital intercourse then through extramarital intercourse or masturbation. A woman may enjoy sex three times a week, but if divorced or widowed, she may go for months or years with little sexual activity—and then be happily remarried to a man who wants sex every day. Women do have their own sexual needs, but these are far likelier than a man's to fluctuate because of circumstance and emotional events.

Aging reduces both men's and women's sexual frequency, but usually in proportion to their earlier activity. People who were sexually vigorous in early adulthood are likely to be relatively vigorous in middle or late life. The inactive tend to become less active. A few decades ago, Kinsey found that the commonest (again, not necessarily the "healthiest") sexual frequency of white American males at 50 was somewhat more than once a week; at seventy it was a little less than once a week. Certainly coitus once or twice a week is not unusual in healthy men and women in their 60s and 70s. Kinsey interviewed a man of 88 who had intercourse with his 90-year-old wife anywhere from once a month to once a week.

Sex drive is not a fixed, mechanical instinct, but the product of physical, psychological, and social forces. What most distinguishes mid-life sexuality from youthful sexuality is its great susceptibility to emotional and social pressures. Fatigue, depression, mental and physical stresses, lack of a regular sexual partner, too much food or drink, even a weekend of overstrenuous recreation, can erode sexual desire and vigor in the second half of life.

Healthy later-life sexuality depends on understanding and accepting change. Dr. Charles Socarides notes that from the 50s on, excitement may pass and leave a man feeling almost as if orgastic release has happened. Therefore he suggests, "If you are getting ready to do it, DO IT, for the impulse may not arise again for a while."

A man knows that now it sometimes takes him longer to reach orgasm or that his ejaculation is weaker, especially when he is preoccupied or tired. He may then judge himself a failure, sexually over the hill. His anxiety and preoccupation can create fear or obsessive worry; these feelings create more trouble the next time he attempts coitus. Such a snowballing reaction to minor or temporary sexual reductions is one of the commonest sources of impotence (see page 318). Similarly, anxiety or depression, over sexual or nonsexual matters, may make a woman uninterested in sex and unresponsive in lovemaking, so she begins avoiding coitus as an unpleasant experience. Maintaining sexual compatibility as aging occurs demands knowledge and communication by both partners.

Men and Women Together

Adjusting to sexual changes can be surprisingly pleasureful. As one gets older, one can indeed get better. First, both partners must understand their own and each others' changes without fear, shame, or secrecy. Mutual sympathy and support during the climacteric and later years is the crucial first step in continuing sexual fulfillment. It is good to remember, though, that while support helps, gloomy commiseration is destructive. To say, "I know just how you feel, it's awful!" creates an atmosphere of glum helplessness. Although the message seems sympathetic, it invites sharing the misery rather than seeking positive solutions.

Specifically, the man should not allow practical and career matters to blot out his sexuality; his partner can help by good-naturedly reminding him when he does. He should refuse to be intimidated by his own changes. To remain sexual is not being a "dirty old man," and reacting more slowly than at age 20 is not a failure. If a man has based much of his self-esteem on his sexual prowess, he may find even slight or temporary sexual reductions ego-shattering. He withdraws from sex to avoid feeling defeat and humiliation—by picking quarrels, claiming fatigue, using age as an excuse, or just retreating in silence. His partner must understand his spoken or unspoken fears. If she takes his withdrawal as a personal rejection and withdraws in turn, they will be stalemated.

The man must extend the same considerations, especially if his wife deeply fears aging and climacteric. By attention and warm interest, he must keep her sense of attractiveness alive, reminding her with compliments and constructive suggestions that she is never too old to be lovable and loving, and that he still wants her as a partner in every sense. Her sexual withdrawal may reflect fears about herself, fear of rejection by him, or even confusion about how she should see herself and behave. By gestures of courtship and appreciation—even, literally, a second honeymoon—he can reassure her that she is not merely a familiar sexual outlet of diminishing glamour.

The woman may have become absorbed in her children, household, social life, or job, forgetting that her mate still must be aroused and made interested in her—especially if he begins to physically require a little extra stimulation to reach erection and orgasm. She should remember that men don't turn on automatically year after year without enticement by women. Instead of seeing his changes as signs of failure in him or herself, she should offer extra erotic attention. and imagination. If gynecological or other health problems temporarily restrict coitus, she should not retreat totally from lovemaking out of a feeling of inadequacy. This can be done by limiting but not ending coitus, if that is possible, and by using substitutes for coitus. This also applies, of course, to illness or disability in the man.

Sexual monotony brings boredom, resentment, and withdrawal in both partners. It is common in couples who have led mechanical, repetitious sex lives. They may have done this because they found sexual variety repulsive or immoral—or merely because each was too embarrassed to take the initiative in sexual experimentation. Boredom, like a sense of failure or disappointment, is usually communicated in subtle ways despite every attempt at concealment, and it poisons the relationship in and out of bed.

Sexual boredom turns to active resentment when a man finds he is barely potent with his wife but quite potent with other women, and when the wife learns she is responsive not to her husband but to other men. Some people do find lasting fulfillment with a new partner, and certain sexual and emotional differences are irreconcilable. However, it is a common impression among counselors that excitement rediscovered with a new partner tends to subside after a while, often to the old marital level: changing partners doesn't always mean changing the dance. Therefore couples should explore their sexual dissatisfactions before cutting the tie between them.

Physical changes, health problems, and sexual boredom all make middle age a good time to expand and vary lovemaking. Most couples now have more time, leisure, and privacy from children than ever before. If life has given them more confidence and self-esteem, they can feel free of the inner need to be good performers in bed, to become more accepting of themselves and each other. Maturity can liberate them from imagined standards of erotic excellence, to discover new pleasure, tenderness, and variety.

> **"MUTUAL SYMPATHY & SUPPORT IS THE CRUCIAL FIRST STEP IN CONTINUING SEXUAL FULFILLMENT."**

The different sexual patterns of men and women, a source of conflict early in many marriages, can now be a positive force. In early adulthood, many men have an urgent need for frequent, rapid orgasms; over the years, they slow down. Drs. Helen Kaplan and Clifford Sager say, "Old males become more like women in their sexual behavior in that fantasy and ambience become more important in lovemaking, and there is less preoccupation with orgasm."

While this takes place, a contrary change is happening in many wives. They become less inhibited, more accepting of their own sexual urges and pleasure, more playful and aggressive. They are ripe to enjoy the greater variety and stimulation needed by many husbands after decades of marriage.

Helps to sexual harmony. The man's slowing and the woman's deinhibition are not the only changes that can make a middle-aged couple more harmonious. They are now free to make love in the morning or after dinner, without worries about pregnancy or interruption. Longer and more varied foreplay is easier now that their sexual response is a bit slower, the man less driven to orgasm. If they have never experimented with a variety of coital positions, they can do so now. Some marriage counselors and sex educators suggest that husbands and wives read books on sex techniques together—not only to find new possibilities but to begin communicating more about sex. In middle and late life, it is necessary as never before to be able to say "slower" or "faster," "more gently" or "a little harder," "like this," or to use a guiding hand.

Such flexibility, growth, and communication are vital if sex is to continue satisfactorily when one or both partners have a health problem (see page 325). Various coital positions reduce or increase the depth of vaginal penetration, the tightness or relaxation of the vaginal walls, and the areas of internal touch and pressure. For instance, if the woman keeps her legs flat and close together, deep penetration is impossible, but the grip on the penis is firm; this may be important for a woman with deep vaginal discomfort or over-relaxed vaginal walls, and for a man who requires increased stimulation to maintain his erection. In the past, even many gynecologists and urologists did not give patients specific advice in such matters. Now it is easily available in many doctors' offices and in numerous books and magazines.

Such coital variations as woman-on-top or facing-side-by-side are used by an increasing proportion of mature people. So are such noncoital activities as oral-genital sex and mutual masturbation. Some people have had lifetime discomfort about these acts; if their feelings are deeply rooted in social upbringing or religious conviction, violating them can't improve a relationship. But if only unfamiliarity, fear of doing something badly, or worry over shocking one's partner has prevented sexual exploration, middle age is a good time to take the attitude that one has little to lose by trying something new! If this makes either partner uneasy, honest but tactful discussion, perhaps with the help of a marriage or sex counselor, may help bring new interest and liveliness to a sexual relationship.

SEXUAL CONFLICT
AND DYSFUNCTION

Some couples have always enjoyed sexual compatibility. Some, despite occasional conflicts, haven't suffered major problems. Others share a long history of sexual discord or see it arise in their middle or late years. Masters and Johnson estimate that at least half the married couples in the United States experience some degree of sexual dysfunction. The problem may be a minor but persistent clash about how or how often to have intercourse; it may be a troubling dysfunction such as the man's impotence or the woman's inability to feel pleasure.

Sexual dissatisfaction was once a matter of secrecy and fatalism. That is no longer necessary. Sex counseling has advanced dramatically, and education, therapy, or counseling can bring positive sexual changes, even in the later years.

Sexual Conflict

We have said that there are few one-sided marital problems; even if only one spouse is troubled, the other must respond or adapt. And leaving a problem unspoken doesn't stop it from having effects. In sexual as in other marital conflicts, the husband and wife should begin communicating clearly and try to identify the nature of their conflict, rather than be sidetracked in passionate accusation or self-blame.

Sometimes myths and lack of information cause conflict—say, if one spouse believes age destroys sex, or that certain common practices (such as varied coital positions) are perversions, or that failure to march in the vanguard of sexual revolution is neurotic. We live amid an explosion of sexual information and misinformation. Sometimes the mass media, through shallow reporting, create unrealistic ideas and expectations. Many popular books on sex (including some by psychologists and physicians) are riddled with inaccuracies and prejudices; some outdated and misleading books are still reprinted and widely read.

Conflict also rises from the sexual problems and insecurities people bring to marriage: feeling physically inadequate; fear of being "undersexed" or "oversexed"; guilt over masturbation; anxiety over dreams or fantasies of homosexual or other deviant behavior; being inhibited because sex is "sinful"; inability to enjoy sex except with strangers, prostitutes, or people one dislikes; nagging worries that one should have experienced more sexual variety before marrying; fear or shame over resuming a sex life after the end of marriage; or insecurity about adjusting to new partners. A sexually healthy person without much premarital experience may not realize through years of sexual conflict that the spouse has serious problems, and thinks, "There must be something wrong with *me*."

Sex conflicts can grow from different ethnic, religious, and cultural backgrounds. There are also important influences of parents, neighborhood, and growing-up experience; these may be taken for granted as "the way I am" or "how men and women are." For instance, a wife may have "learned" from parents, teachers, girl friends, and movies that men are spontaneously aroused, a woman need only await their excited approach, and taking the initiative makes her unfeminine, even contemptible. But her husband's background (family, folklore, sexual experiences) may make him expect frequent "green lights" and even passionate initiatives from women. Each partner waits in vain for the other to make the first move and misinterprets the other's inertia as lack of love. By the time they discuss the situation, it is with bitter accusations.

Such conflicts may start early in marriage, persist as rankling resentment and withholding, and finally burst into the open after years or decades. A thoughtful, honest discussion might allow a couple to sympathetically understand the different attitudes they brought to marriage and begin to close the gap.

In some cases, the problem is deeper and more serious. A man or woman may have never truly liked or accepted sex, but masked the aversion through the early phases of marriage. Eventually age or illness is used as an apparently legitimate exit from an always unwelcome scene.

Others find that sex, once pleasureful, becomes dull, a burden, or a resented obligation, for reasons conscious or unknown. If one partner turns off, the other may fight or retreat in hurt. The marriage then turns into a grim adversary relationship. One possible response is extramarital affairs.

Sex as a weapon. Long, serious conflicts about sex are often part of larger marital problems. Like money and child-rearing, sex is a convenient and devastating weapon when hostility is in the air. We have mentioned some of the things that can drive a wedge between husband and wife (see page 296); almost any of them, from diverging life-styles to one partner's depression, may cause or reflect sexual discord. Let us take a brief, hypothetical case:

A woman of 50 has weathered her loss of youth and fertility, but not without some sense of mourning and hollowness. For decades she was a flirtatious attention-getter; all that, she feels, is now behind her. She has few interests outside her home, but her children have grown and left. A change of residence has deprived her of family and emotional ties.

Her husband, to the contrary, is more involved than ever in his work and the social life it involves. Winning greater success and security, he seems to grow in confidence and new enthusiasms. He sporadically tries to involve her in his increasingly venturous life-style; this includes some sexual variations they have never tried. Perhaps he wants to try coitus in a kneeling position, entering from behind; she goes along a few times, embarrassed and secretly angry, wondering whether he is learning such things from other women. She is resentful, he is miffed. Their sex life, which had become routine, is turning into a battle of wills. He insists, she refuses. They reach the classic standstill:

He: "If you really loved me, you'd do it."
She: "If you really loved me, you wouldn't insist."

Obviously this couple's sexual conflict involves larger problems of coping, singly and together, with new stages of life and marriage. He is more active and outgoing than ever, she more isolated and unfulfilled. He wants to assert himself and play, she feels unloved, uncertain. They find it too painful to touch the main conflict, which is complex indeed; they seize the sexual conflict, which is handy and specific, as a symbolic issue.

There are reasons for this particular sex act to represent their larger problem. She, like many women, was raised to feel that sex, in and for itself, is shameful, but that love redeems it. She has always kissed and embraced, then proceeded to coitus with no break in mood. As a young woman, she preferred to think that because of love she was "carried away"; sex was something that *happened to* her, not something she *did*. Coitus without close face-to-face contact seems not making love but a cold, "animalistic" act—a matter of "mere" body-to-body. Her husband, like many men, can more easily accept sex as a pleasure in itself; love heightens it but isn't needed to legitimize it. Coitus from behind has aggressive overtones to him, and it expresses his more assertive, experimental state of mind; to her it seems a loveless act at a time when she doesn't feel lovable.

Consider a couple whose problem is similar, but with the roles reversed. The woman finds that with the years, freer of domestic demands and youthful insecurities, her sexual interest and response quicken. Relieved of old inner commandments to be "ladylike," she takes sexual initiatives more often, tries subtly and then directly to engage her husband in more frequent, varied lovemaking. She would like to try being on top in coitus; she has performed oral sex on him and wants it returned. Yet the more she encourages her apparently amiable but stolid husband, the more he backs off. First he is surprised, then irritated, then locked away in polite unreachability. Finally he claims with an icy smile that he is too old for such foolery, and so is she; he avoids her almost completely in bed. She is left between anger and tears, wondering whether all men wear out so fast or whether he was right in saying she has turned into a "sex-crazy old lady."

She has always been more emotionally expressive than he. He has always been somewhat controlled, withdrawn, and conventional. With maturity, she expresses herself more freely; he, feeling that his career, his whole life, has leveled off short of his expectations, is defensively tight-lipped, despite his veneer of geniality. The woman taking sexual initiative seems assertive and therefore masculine to both of them. In her more expansive mental state, it is a liberation, but it assaults his already eroded sense of masculinity. The same is true of his being on the bottom in coitus; to him it seems a threatening act of male passivity. In his fantasies, "servicing" a woman orally makes him feel that he is her slave. This couple find that their sex conflict turns into a symbolic war.

The commonest sexual conflicts are about how often to have sex, how to do it, the woman's orgasmic response, erotic boredom, and inhibition. Such apparently trivial matters as who makes the first move, who is on top, whether coitus is for nighttime only, whether to engage in oral sex, can take on stubborn importance. Even small variations in sex behavior may have enormous psychological meanings, and when these meanings coincide with marital conflicts, sex becomes a source of corrosive hostility.

Resolving Sexual Conflict

When sexual conflict exists, the first step toward resolution is for both spouses to admit it. This is painful, for it seems an admission of failure or inadequacy. It appears easier to evade such problems, dismissing them as temporary year after year, or calling them inevitable or not worth making into issues. In the long run, this is no kindness to oneself or one's partner, for hidden conflict festers. If a couple make genuine efforts, perhaps with the help of a professional third party, resolving sex conflicts can be a cooperative venture that builds love, trust, and pleasure.

Once conflict is admitted, one cannot gain by accusation, self-accusation, fatalism, or retaliatory sexual bookkeeping ("I did this, you owe me that"). When a couple explore their conflicts, they may find that many issues have lain between them, undiscussed and often misunderstood; attitudes and expectations rooted in sex-role ideals, social background, personality—all can be huge, silent barriers. When these are uncovered, people find it easier to give and receive love and sex. They demythify sex acts, freeing them of symbolic meanings that prevent erotic rapport. Most sex acts are demeaning, enslaving, or animalistic only if one sees them that way.

A couple should seek sexual knowledge individually and together. Few people are willing to admit blind spots; no one likes to be thought ignorant or naive about sex. Unfortunately, very few people's sexual knowledge is complete. A couple should know their own anatomy, physical processes, and the existence of a variety of sexual techniques. Manual-like books about sex turn off some readers, but the better ones are useful and may suggest variations that help a couple accommodate to sexual differences. Once spouses can freely discuss what they read, think, and feel about sex, they have already conquered a great obstacle to fulfillment—taking full responsibility as givers and receivers of pleasure and love.

One should neither ignore the advice of friends nor accept it uncritically. This is also true of books and professional advice. Seek advice but always consider going for a second opinion, even a third or fourth if necessary, until truly helpful information and advice are received.

Some sexual difficulties, we have said, reflect complex marital problems, but a couple needn't wade through all their conflicts before improving their sex life. Resolving sex problems doesn't bring instant happiness, and in some cases it isn't possible; but reducing sexual conflict can take pressure off a relationship and be a first step in resolving nonsexual conflicts.

SEXUAL DYSFUNCTION IN MEN

Premature Ejaculation

Premature ejaculation is reaching orgasm before or very soon after sexual penetration. It may be a problem from the start of a marriage but not reach the crisis point until middle age. The husband has probably tried for years to delay himself by counting backward, pinching himself, instructing his wife, "Don't touch me until the very last second." Finding that these tricks don't work, he may try alcohol or barbiturates to slow his response, and anesthetic creams or other mail-order aids that range from useless to potentially harmful.

The man sometimes retreats sexually, out of shame and guilt. After years of sympathy and attempts at cooperation, his wife becomes resentful. Finally, full of pent-up frustration and rage, she may seek professional counseling or insist that he do so.

Decades ago, some experts believed that childhood and adolescent masturbation caused prematurity, through the habit of seeking orgasm without thought of a partner's response. Today this is widely doubted. The life histories of many premature ejaculators do include hurried or traumatic youthful experiences with prostitutes, years of petting to orgasm, and penile withdrawal *(coitus interruptus)* as a contraceptive gesture, but these are not necessarily *causes*. Often there are complex fears and hostilities toward sex and the sex partner.

Most males reach orgasm quickly in youth; physical aging and sexual experience may give them more control. If a mature man regularly reaches climax before entry or after only a few strokes, there is almost no question that he has a problem, and so does his wife. One reasonable rule-of-thumb definition of prematurity is inability to satisfy a fully responsive sex partner at least half the time. Sometimes it happens only with certain partners—only with the wife or only with extramarital partners.

Psychotherapy has helped some premature ejaculators, but by no means all. Therapy techniques developed by Semans, Masters and Johnson, and others reportedly have high success rates. Such therapy is brief but intensive, and it involves both husband and wife. It can be fitted into a larger program of marriage counseling or individual psychotherapy.

What is premature? We must note that experts have argued for decades about how soon is premature. No stopwatch definition takes in the variety of human sex response. In any given case, one must ask, "Premature for whom?" and "Is it a problem?" Some couples don't consider early ejaculation a problem. If the wife lacks enthusiasm about sex, she won't complain about her husband's speed. They are missing many of the joys of sex, but they aren't likely to try to change the situation.

A small number of men are unusually sensitive and speedy. This might be praised as passionate responsiveness in a woman but called selfish in a man. There are two reasons for this double standard. One is that after orgasm a woman can go right on with coitus and satisfy her partner, but most men cannot—though they can, of course, use noncoital means. The other is our society's increasing emphasis on female orgasm, and on men's responsibility for it. (Men with higher education are more likely to feel responsible for women's orgasms; men without higher education tend to feel that a woman's orgasm is largely her own responsibility.) If a man is unusually sensitive but neither spouse has a physical or psychosexual problem, they can adapt to each other with a little imaginative effort (see page 313). This is also true when the wife requires prolonged stimulation.

Retarded Ejaculation

Inability to reach orgasm can happen occasionally or become permanent. Like premature ejaculation, it sometimes occurs only with certain partners. When it is a more than rare event, it provokes anxiety and discomfort. The correction of retarded ejaculation without physical causes (illness or drugs' side-effects) requires psychotherapy or counseling.

Low Sex Drive

Some men find their sexual interest declining or disappearing at times of stress, depression, or long-term sexual deprivation; when the situation changes, sexual interest usually revives. It is a different matter when males go through adolescence and adulthood without much sexual interest, though they may be capable when aroused.

Sexual interest and capacity vary widely. In a small number of men, sexual interest or capability is low because of physical conditions. It is also possible that some people are constitutionally not highly endowed sexually. However, human sex drive is not a simple instinct, and psychological causes of low libido are commoner. In fact, some men find that as emotional and practical circumstances change, their sexual interest reaches higher levels, even as late in life as their 50s or 60s.

If there is any concern or anxiety about what seems low sexual interest, a physical checkup should be sought. If no organic problem exists, exploration with a counselor or therapist may clarify and, in some cases, change the situation.

Impotence

Impotence, the inability to achieve or sustain erection, is the commonest major sex dysfunction of men. It has happened to many men once, a few times, or for short periods in their lives. Emotional conflict, stress, fatigue, depression, too much alcohol, illness, or certain drugs may be immediately responsible. As an occasional event, it need cause no alarm. When chronic, it can devastate a man and his marriage.

Men tend to judge their fundamental success and human worth by their sexual competence—for obvious biological reasons, more than women do. A woman who dislikes sex or her sex partner can usually still have coitus, bear children, and not question her femininity. A man suffering the same degree of sexual conflict cannot just "lie there and bear it"; unable to achieve erection and intercourse, he fails in basic male functions.

Impotence can occur at any age, but it is increasingly common after 50, as sex drive becomes more vulnerable to fatigue and psychological influences. Even if it occurs only with certain partners or in certain circumstances, it is disturbing. In fact, long-term impotence often begins with one or two minor incidents, which start a downward spiral of fearful anticipation and successive failures. The man feels threatened by one failure, so he sets out the next time determined to succeed, yet fearing another disaster. Anxious, self-conscious, he responds slowly, becomes even more anxious, and fails again. This cycle is repeated until impotence is chronic.

Men with erective problems sometimes retreat into sexless, hang-dog depression, especially if their wives are critical, belittling, and domineering—both in and out of bed. In such cases, joint marital and sexual counseling is called for.

Some chronically impotent men may have backgrounds of other sex problems, general and sexual insecurity, domineering parents and wives, and a variety of neurotic conflicts. The most common immediate triggers of impotence, say Masters and Johnson, are boredom with one's partner, preoccupation with money and career, mental or physical fatigue, mental or physical illness in either spouse, too much food and drink, and fear of sexual failure. They believe too much alcohol is the commonest cause in middle age (see page 398). They also point out that many men with erection problems have consulted doctors or counselors, been told to accept impotence as the wages of sin or as normal aging (even at 40 or 50!), and resigned themselves to this often correctable condition.

Psychotherapy has helped some impotent men. The methods of Masters and Johnson and some other behavior-oriented therapists have good records when used by well trained professionals; they can be used within the framework of broader psychotherapy or marriage counseling. All treatment, of course, should begin with a physical checkup.

One case described by Masters and Johnson has many typical elements. Mr. and Mrs. A. were 66 and 62 years old, had been married for 39 years, were in good health, and had had a satisfactory sex life until five years earlier. At that time Mr. A. retired and took his wife abroad for what turned out to be a hectic vacation. Constant sightseeing left them chronically tired, but because they were away from home and routines, they had coitus more often than usual. Mr. A. began to notice that it was taking him longer to reach erection. His concern increased until finally, just before the vacation ended, he was unable to achieve sexual penetration.

Back at home, Mr. A. found that erection was slow and then failed entirely. After several months the couple consulted their physician. He said that such impotence strikes all men with aging, and nothing could be done. They also learned that some of their friends had had similar problems and not improved. Mr. A. was deeply depressed for several months but recovered. He and his wife accepted his impotence as normal and incurable. They lived in resignation for four years.

Fortunately, they began to wonder again whether this must be their fate. They sought several more professional opinions; all were negative. Still they refused to accept no as an answer, and finally were referred to Masters and Johnson. They were having coitus again within a week. Masters and Johnson report:

"When they could accept the fact that it naturally took longer for an older man to achieve an erection, particularly if he were tired or distracted, the basis for their own sexual inadequacy disappeared. Some six years after termination of the (intensive) phase of therapy, this couple, now in the early 70s and late 60s, continue coital connection once or twice a week."

SEXUAL DYSFUNCTION IN WOMEN

Frigidity

The word frigidity is used loosely and often inaccurately. In the stricter sense, it is chronic inability to reach orgasm through coitus. Even by that definition, it includes many kinds of dysfunction: absence of any pleasure during intercourse *(sexual anesthesia)*; painful coitus *(dyspareunia)*; vaginal spasm that prevents coitus *(vaginismus)*; lack of sexual desire; and probably most common, orgasmic failure *(anorgasmia)*.

In the past, many women were raised to pretend they didn't enjoy sex. Now many feel forced to pretend that they always do. In either case, they may keep sex dysfunction secret for years, fearing that they are unliberated failures or that their desire for a more satisfying sex life is abnormal, immoral, or shameful. Fortunately, more women now seek knowledge and help, and improvements in treating sex dysfunctions mean that they needn't be fatalistic.

Vaginismus and Dyspareunia

Vaginismus is spasm of the vaginal muscles that makes sexual penetration impossible. It can develop from anticipation of pain and calls for a physical examination. Often, though, it rises from neurotic fears and inhibitions; these may be produced by a strictly antisexual upbringing, perhaps in a zealously religious home. Occasionally the cause is the trauma of rape. Sometimes the husband suffers impotence or premature ejaculation; severe sex dsyfunction in either spouse can spark sexual problems in the other.

Dyspareunia, or painful coitus, ranges from mild vaginal irritation after intercourse to acute pain from penile thrusting. In middle-aged and older women, it may reflect steroid starvation (see page 445)

or damage from pelvic infection, surgery, childbirth damage, or endometriosis. A thorough medical examination is a must.

The diagnosis must be thoughtful and precise, for such pain may be psychosomatic or neurotically exaggerated. There are also women who use pain to disguise sexual revulsion; if alleged headaches and fatigue wear thin, they complain that coitus hurts—and may believe it themselves after a while. Only a brutal husband continues if his wife flinches, winces, or cries out in pain. A woman and her physician—with the help of a gynecologist and if necessary a psychiatrist—should explore every possible cause of persistent dyspareunia or vaginismus, so that they neither perpetuate a neurotic problem nor overlook physical illness.

Vaginismus and dyspareunia, like impotence, can end a couple's sex life. Both conditions have been treated effectively by several kinds of therapy, which may call for both spouses' participation.

Lack of Sexual Interest

Some women seem fundamentally indifferent to sex. They may feel affection for their husbands and even enjoy coitus when it occurs, but if it were up to them, sex would never come up. This may frustrate and anger their spouses. Like men without sexual interest, they may lack strong sexual endowment or suffer from skewed personality development; there are mental-health professionals who might argue either way. If sexual uninterest hampers a relationship, one should explore the idea of inhibited response rather than write off the situation. Sexual indifference does occur in some women whose highly moralistic homes taught them to bury erotic impulses, leaving an apparent blank where there might be a positive sexual attitude.

There are other, obviously destructive kinds of sexual indifference—women who are utterly self-centered, who are hostile to their husbands, who reject femininity, or are bound by puritanical guilt. In any of these cases, counseling or therapy may reveal and at least partially free unexpected sexual interest and capacity.

Female Orgasm

Sometimes female orgasm is dramatic, sometimes rather quiet. Since it doesn't always have obvious external signs (such as ejaculation in the male), it has been clouded in mystery and myth. Some women aren't even sure whether they've experienced orgasm. We would guess that most such women have not, at least not fully—perhaps some have reached low-intensity orgasm, such as strongly orgastic women may feel when tense or tired.

Orgasm usually involves some four to six rhythmic spasms of many pelvic muscles, with a peak of pleasure and of total body tension, followed by a sense of release. Many people have believed there are two kinds of female orgasm, one centered in the clitoris, one in the vagina. The research of Masters and Johnson showed no *measurable* differences between orgasms reached by stimulating the clitoris or the vagina. Many women (and some researchers) maintain that they do feel differences, so unmeasured or subjective differences may exist.

Why should women but not men commonly have orgasmic irregularities or problems? Male orgasm, linked to ejaculation, is necessary for reproduction; it exists in most if not all higher animals. Female orgasm isn't needed for reproduction; it is a relatively new experiment of nature, probably existing in only certain higher species. It seems to be a pleasure incentive for forming long, satisfying bonds between child-rearing partners. The potential for orgasm, perhaps even for multiple orgasm, probably exists in almost all women. But biologically it isn't rooted as firmly as male orgasm, and social and emotional influences can block it. The majority of American women experience orgasm at some time in their lives, but not regularly.

The recent conviction that female orgasm is healthful, even necessary, has brought many women greater pleasure and fulfillment. It has also made orgasm a sometimes tyrannical standard of sexual and emotional health. There is still controversy about whether anorgasmia is pathological. For some women and their partners, it may not be a problem or not a major one. We feel that if it distresses a woman or her partner, it is a problem indeed.

Some anorgasmic women, if not physically frustrated, are disturbed by the idea that they are "frigid." Furthermore, their husbands may feel deprived of excitement, a sense of mutuality, and faith in their own sexual competence. Today it is often the husband, feeling rejected or frustrated, who urges an anorgasmic woman to seek professional help. It is always worth exploring.

Loss of Orgasm

Sometimes women who usually reach orgasm find it impossible. The reasons are often those that cause occasional impotence in men—illness, certain medications, fatigue, depression, worries, a quarrel, or too much alcohol. Occasional anorgasmia rarely creates serious problems; few women feel threatened by it, as men tend to be by impotence.

Some women find that they reach orgasm only with a certain partner, in special situations, or through special techniques or fantasies. This may present no problem; a woman may enjoy coitus without orgasm and shouldn't feel inferior because of that. But if lack of orgasm creates conflict within the woman or in her relationships, she should explore the matter. If, for instance, she can reach climax only with men who use or abuse her, but not with a man she claims to love, or by masturbation but not with a partner, the orgasmic limitation probably reflects larger conflicts.

There may be physical causes for loss of orgasm; if these are ruled out by examination, emotional ones must be sought. An obvious source is the husband becoming perfunctory, indifferent, domineering, demeaning, or cruel. Another is the wife thinking he has, through misunderstanding or neurotic exaggeration. A woman also may lose orgasm if she feels that her husband has failed her expectations; if she is not committed to the relationship; if early-life fears of sex revive; or if depression and insecurity become severe. Loss of sexual response can lead a couple to stage-by-stage mutual withdrawal, just when they should keep their love life from becoming perfunctory and boring. Such problems can often be helped through individual therapy or joint marriage counseling.

Lifelong Anorgasmia

A woman may desire and enjoy the intimacy, body contact, and erotic pleasure of coitus, yet never reach orgasm. If she doesn't feel overstimulated and deprived, and if her husband isn't disturbed, this is a problem only in the eyes of some beholders. There is, however, a chronic problem for the woman who reaches a high pitch of excitement but can't attain climax. She becomes tense, unable to sleep—according to Dr. John Oliven, "progressively morose and irritable or else hypochondriacal and depressive. Over the years she may lose her sense of well-being, become bored, restless, feel overburdened and increasingly lose her capacity for tenderness . . . there is a tendency to mobilize the most unfavorable facets of the underlying personality."

If she pretends orgasm, she may find herself in a trap, resenting her partner if he sees through the act, but feeling contempt if he doesn't. She may try extramarital affairs to see if she can find satisfaction with other men (and perhaps in retaliation for being orgasmically "deprived"). Sometimes this works, but often it doesn't; even if it does, she may or may not be able to bring the fuller sexual response back to her marriage.

Some dissatisfied women don't really crave orgasm so much as they feel cheated. They are, says Dr. Oliven, "practically sick with chronic resentment and chronic outrage, because they feel deprived of what they believe themselves rightfully entitled to (or there may be) a compulsive perfectionistic or a chronically worrisome personality; this woman experiences chronic chagrin at not having a perfect reaction, mainly because she had read or heard that it is abnormal—unhealthy, unfeminine, unliberated—not to have an orgasm." This is a problem for general psychological counseling as much as for sex therapy.

There are several reasons why orgasm may be stifled in women who genuinely desire it. A psychological block caused in youth by rape or by exaggerated fear of pregnancy can take on a stubborn life of its own. Complex problems involving anger, passivity, power, dependence, guilt, and distorted self-image are sometimes involved. In many cases, perhaps a majority, childhood and youth were one long preparation for unresponsiveness.

Many anorgasmic women grew up in homes where sex was mentioned rarely, and then as something sinful or disgusting. This "silence-and-sin" syndrome has deep, long-lasting results. Just as damaging are teachings, direct or implied, that "sex is only for making babies" or "just for men's sake." Such very rigid or passive attitudes also may color nonsexual matters; some sexually unresponsive women seem passive and emotionally underdeveloped, others overcontrolled, moralistic, and wary.

Furthermore, women learn from social stereotypes that sex and self-assertion are male monopolies. They feel that expressing sexual urges and reaching out for play and pleasure are at best unladylike, perhaps downright mannish. The women's liberation movement seems to help some women accept their sexual and assertive selves. It also may give certain women ideological justifications for their hostility to men and to heterosexual trust.

Whatever a woman's background, says Dr. Oliven, "Probably the commonest cause of orgasm failure is chronic unconscious self-inhibition of the capacity to love and let go unreservedly during the sex act. The inhibitants are congealed negative emotions such as fear, shame, or hostility."

The letting go is crucial. Body and mind are more vulnerable and uncontrolled during orgasm than at any time except sleep. Mistrust of one's partner, fear of one's own emotions, and fear of losing control work against orgasm. Women may struggle for climax and find that the harder they try, the less they succeed; they are like insomniacs who repeat with rising tenseness, "I *will* relax!" Most therapies for anorgasmia explore the individual's apprehensions and teach physical and mental relaxation in sexual situations. Orgasm is not *made* to happen but *allowed* to happen.

In many cases, both spouses lack sexual experience and knowledge; shyness and shame keep both from the relaxation and abandonment that lead to orgasm. Often the wife justly blames her husband's erotic clumsiness for her anorgasmia. If he suffers impotence, very low sex drive, other psychosexual problems, or alcoholism, she isn't likely to rush headlong into orgasmic delight. Many husbands understand little about female response. They may be ineffective out of ignorance or selfishness, or they may themselves be inexperienced, fearful, or guilty. The wife may not feel able to make such distinctions; she is too busy resenting what she considers his blithe orgasmic success, and instead reacts with mixed feelings of inadequacy, anger, envy, and contempt.

Treatment of Anorgasmia

The obvious solution is for both partners to take responsibility for their own responses and each other's pleasure. In a classic study, spouses were interviewed separately, and many men said they tried hard to please their wives, yet many of their wives complained that the husbands didn't know or care what pleased them. Plainly, effort is not enough; couples must clearly express sexual needs and preferences. Where anorgasmia is long-standing, the chances for success are greater if the couple have advice from a specialist in sex and marriage problems.

If a woman has never reached orgasm, she and a professional advisor should decide whether to set climax as an immediate goal. She shouldn't assume that because she is past youth, she is past help. Usually between one-third and two-thirds of women treated for various kinds of "frigidity" solve their problems. The standard procedure is to check for physical problems, decide whether individual therapy is called for, and often to involve both spouses in counseling about sexual problems and, if necessary, marital problems.

One should be careful not to settle for offhand, simplistic solutions, which unfortunately are still offered by some health-care professionals—to take a drink, sedative, tranquillizer, or antidepressant, to enjoy a vacation and "just relax," or not to expect much "because everyone gets older." Alcohol and mood-altering drugs can bring relaxation, but they can also dull sexual response. Using a vibrator or other devices to learn orgasm through self-stimulation may help some women but have negative results for others; further research is needed. Meanwhile, such decisions should be made with the help of a competent specialist.

Sexual Variations and Deviations

By sexual variation we mean a practice, other than the most conventional forms of petting and coitus, that is used by many people, and which today is thought compatible with psychosexual health. By deviation we mean a minority practice that, at least for some people, reflects psychosexual dysfunction and conflict. The distinction is not always clear; definitions have changed, and some are still being argued. Only decades ago, some authorities called masturbation and oral-genital sex perversions. The majority of men and a very large number of women have done both these things, with no known ill effects. Today they are considered variations and are recommended by many experts on sexuality. (In fact, they were quite common even when called unhealthful and perverted, but people talked about them less.) The great variety of coital positions are considered variations. Anal intercourse is practiced by a substantial minority of people; more experts now than in the past regard it as a variation. Sadomasochism, exhibitionism, fetishism, and some other practices are considered deviations, reflections of inner conflict or of neurotic psychosexual development.

Some individuals and religious groups frown on certain variations and deviations on moral grounds or out of deep personal feelings. Everyone is entitled to his principles and preferences. But to the extent that sex is viewed medically and psychologically, and becomes a matter of research and therapy, variations must be thought of as questions of individual ideals and esthetics, and deviations as questions of health. Science, society, and the law increasingly tend to view sex acts between consenting adults as personal choices, not subjects of legal constraint.

If one sexual partner wants to try sexual techniques or variations but the other does not, expressions of distaste can only create bitter clashes. Honest, empathic discussion may lead to understanding, perhaps to agreement one way or the other. If not, the mediation of brief counseling often helps.

We will not discuss the rare and extreme sexual deviations—transvestism, peeping, sexual sadomasochism, etc. These may bring severe social penalties; because they reflect neurotic conflict, they usually involve inner suffering. If such problems arise in one's family, condemnation will only frighten, isolate, or antagonize the person. One should offer attempts at understanding while firmly urging professional treatment.

Homosexuality. By far the commonest deviation is homosexuality, or erotic attraction to people of one's own sex. A surprising number of heterosexuals have had a few homosexual experiences; still more have occasionally had homosexual thoughts or dreams. As occasional events, these need not cause alarm. If they are either persistent or disturbing, counseling should be sought.

Homosexual experimentation or brief involvement can happen at any age, out of curiosity or as a sign of inner stress and conflict. This is most common in adolescence, but it can happen later in life. Some heterosexual married men occasionally feel driven by stress to seek homosexual contacts. Some women, after a bitter divorce, prefer another woman's companionship and sexuality. Often such experiences are brief, and heterosexual life is resumed; sometimes they set new patterns. Short-term or sporadic homosexual acts may or may not be felt as an emotional problem, but if they become publicly known, they may be a problem indeed. Counseling or psychotherapy often helps the individual clarify such behavior.

Preferred adult homosexuality is a subject of great controversy and changing attitudes today. Some mental-health professionals do not consider it an illness, others say it is invariably pathological. We must point out that most homosexuals are secret homosexuals, the men not effeminate, the women not mannish. Many are decent, productive members of their communities—some, in fact, accomplished and distinguished—and on the whole no more neurotic than many of their heterosexual neighbors. We do believe, however, that homosexuality often involves emotional conflict, not only sexually but socially and emotionally. Good general adaptation to life is probably more difficult and less common among homosexuals than heterosexuals—not only because of social pressures but because the sexual preference seems usually to rise from emotional fears and defenses.

The person who reaches middle age with a long-standing homosexual preference isn't likely to change his or her sexual orientation (though there are a few striking exceptions). A homosexual who has problems in relationships, work, or emotional areas may be helped by a sympathetic counselor or therapist, regardless of his sexual orientation.

THE SEXUAL EFFECTS OF ILLNESS, SURGERY, AND MEDICATION

Most laymen and even many doctors pay little attention to the common ills and treatments that can affect sexuality. Too few are aware that many widely used drugs, such as those employed to relieve anxiety and high blood pressure, often have sexual effects. They may assume that heart attacks, diabetes, disablement, prostate surgery, or hysterectomy will leave them forever disabled as lovers. Patients often avoid asking about sexual rehabilitation, and sometimes doctors fail to offer advice. Ignoring the subject can be devastating to a relationship, inflaming new or dormant problems and depriving a troubled couple of pleasure and intimacy. There are several reasons for this problem.

• Our society remains uncomfortable with sex, aging, and illness and disablement. It is doubly uncomfortable with these things in combination. Silence often surrounds such subjects as sex during illness, after surgery, or despite certain medical conditions.
• Only quite recently have physicians been taught to consider sexual health a part of general health, and to try to preserve sexual function as part of any medical treatment. Sometimes the doctor, preoccupied with a patient's survival or maintenance, does not think about sexual health.
• Some patients and doctors are embarrassed by the subject. Others firmly believe in myths or think they already have the truth and ask no questions. And the patient and spouse, especially in cases of serious illness, often feel it is trivial, selfish, or inconsiderate to "add" sex to the problem they face.

Of course, the problem is not added, it is there even when silent, and it is never shameful or trivial. When illness drives sexuality from a relationship, the couple pay a price in warmth, intimacy, fulfillment, vitality, and sometimes part of the will to live and be well. Therefore a patient and his family should never hesitate to ask about the sexual implications of any illness, medication, or surgery at the earliest appropriate moment. In this as in no other aspect of health care, it is often up to the patient and his loved ones to take the initiative in recognizing problems and seeking information and help.

General Health, Diet, and Medication

To maintain sexual vitality, one must keep a high level of general physical and mental health. Often general disability—for example, a combination of arthritis, fatigue, and mild depression—reduces or ends many older people's sexual activity rather than aging *per se*. As Alfred Kinsey and his colleagues said, "good health, sufficient exercise, and plenty of sleep still remain the most effective of the aphrodisiacs known to man."

One occasionally hears bursts of optimism about special diets or vitamin supplements to maintain or increase sex drive. It is true that some severe dietary deficiencies probably reduce sexuality, but normally nourished people needn't worry about them. Obesity does not change sex drive except perhaps in rare cases, but it may require certain coital positions for adequate penetration.

A few drugs occasionally increase sexual excitement and response, but only as an unpredictable side effect. Antidepressants, by dispelling low spirits, may restore even long-blocked mental and sexual vitality. However, people hoping that "aphrodisiacs" or hormones will bring sexual or general rejuvenation will be disappointed. There is no known aphrodisiac in the popular sense, only some substances that may cause itching, burning, or irritation of the genitourinary tract. A small number of people suffer hormone deficiencies, but hormone-replacement therapy usually helps restore whatever was, for them, normal sexuality. Faddy "hormone" and "rejuvenation" regimens are at best doubtful, and some may be harmful.

Impairment by drugs. A great many drugs reduce sex drive, potency, or the ability to reach orgasm. Some drugs have one or all of these effects in many people, some in relatively few. Unfortunately, many such drugs are widely used, and patients rarely are warned of their sexual impact.

Because of several physical health risks, oral contraceptives ("the pill") are not recommended for women over 40, but some women in early middle age do use them. Among the pill's possible effects on behavior are difficulty or inability to reach orgasm, and a state of agitated depression. A woman taking the pill who notices slower sexual response and a persistent cranky, depressed mood should discuss with her physician the possibility of other types of contraception.

The most widely prescribed drugs with potential sexual effects are among those used to reduce anxiety, tension, depression, and high blood pressure. Some of these (tricyclics, reserpine, guanethidine, phenothiazine, and others) can dull sexual response in both men and women. Some also can cause *retrograde ejaculation* (dry orgasm and milky postcoital urine). Certain antidepressants occasionally have a paradoxical effect, increasing depression and thereby dampening sexuality.

Sometimes another tranquillizer, antidepressant, or antihypertension drug can be used; sometimes a trade-off must be made, relinquishing the edge of sexual response for other benefits. But anyone taking such medication should report changes in mood and sexual response to his physician.

Another substance that alters mood and behavior, alcohol, plays a large role in mid-life emotional and sexual problems. Sometimes a drink is helpful in relaxing and enjoying sex, but large amounts reduce sexual response. Dr. John F. Oliven wrote:

"An occasional anxious-inhibited, or profoundly fearful or depressive individual may use drink as a coping device, to disinhibit himself, to assuage his obsession with fear, or to remove himself from the reality of an unlovely wife or from the awareness of some secret disaster. But sooner or later he may actually need alcohol to make love, and when that happens chances are that he is also well on his way to being an alcoholic. The chronic alcoholic is often impotent."

Sex and Heart Conditions

Men and women who have suffered heart attacks wonder if the exertion and excitement of sex are dangerous, even potentially fatal. The fear of death can cripple or destroy their love lives. Their spouses are almost as fearful; they may become overprotective and treat the recovering or recovered patient like an invalid—that is, as sexless.

About a decade ago, three cardiologists studied men who had had heart attacks one to nine years earlier. Most of the men were under 50; as was then common, almost none had received detailed advice from their doctors about sex. Only a third of the men had returned to their normal sex lives, and 10 percent had become completely impotent. The sexual reaction had no relation to the man's age or the severity of his heart attack. It depended on his state of mind.

Even today, some physicians fail to discuss sex with cardiac patients. Often patients are too embarrassed to ask. There is still too little evidence for cardiologists to draw on, and most of what exists is about men, although heart attacks are increasingly common in women. Many doctors and patients make decisions based on their own experience or guesses. There is, however, more knowledge than a decade ago, and a new attitude is emerging among informed physicians.

Cardiologists now widely agree that many people who have suffered coronary attacks can resume sexual activity within a few months. A common rule of thumb is to wait 90 days; few physicians suggest waiting less than six weeks. An increasingly common belief is that a person should return to sex whenever he can safely and comfortably resume mild to moderate physical activity. Implanting a pacemaker imposes no sexual restrictions on a patient other than those that are usually set for cardiac recovery.

Patients with acute angina are, naturally, advised to avoid sex for a while and then resume unless it causes palpitation, shortness of breath, fatigue, or other discomforts. It may help angina patients to use nitroglycerine before coitus.

The high blood pressure and rapid heartbeat of coitus may come as much (or even more) from excitement than from physical exertion. Coitus can cause a heart attack, but only rarely. Doctors are now concerned that the emotional tension caused by abstinence may eventually be more dangerous than sex. Dr. Eugene Scheimann believes that "A healthy night of sex is nature's tranquillizer, reducing stress and creating a general feeling of relaxation and well-being." For the cardiac patient, that is exactly what most doctors order.

Sexual rehabilitation should begin with the patient and spouse discussing the matter with the physician. All three of them should understand the process of return to sexuality, talking out the emotional as well as the physical problems. The impatient, driving personality common among male coronary victims often reacts to restrictions impatiently; the physician and spouse can help him deal with this. He also may feel frustration and anger about new physical limitations, fear of sexual failure, and visions of invalidism or death—with sexual problems ranging from impotence to retarded ejaculation. Most such problems respond well to treatment, such as brief counseling, so they should be aired with a physician, a psychological counselor, or both. Some cardiac patients may have been having health or sexual problems before the attack; continuing to shroud them in silence is destructive.

There are many ways to reduce the cardiac risks of sex. First, avoid fatigue. It may be a good idea to have coitus in the morning or daytime rather than at night. A brief rest beforehand may be more important than rest afterward.

Second, avoid physical and mental stress by cultivating a slow, savoring, and relaxed sexual style. Do not rush strenuously. It may be wise to avoid coitus after a large meal, while wearing constricting clothes, or under other conditions of possible stress. Begin with gentle foreplay and avoid any sense of hurry. Use coital positions that don't demand supporting the body on the arms for a long time—*isometric* (pushing against a stationary object) effort may strain the heart. Side positions are helpful this way, as are some woman-astride positions (for the woman cardiac patient, these do not demand isometric support of the body's weight). Coitus interruptus and long-delayed ejaculation are hazardous. Irvine H. Page, of the American Heart Association, has said:

"When intercourse is followed by the normal feeling of relaxation and peace of mind, it is altogether beneficial. On the other hand, a state of sustained though mild sexual excitation, whether followed by intercourse or not, can only result in a steady tension, which is especially undesirable for the management of hypertension."

There is no final evidence on another important point, but it is a common impression among doctors that when heart attacks do occur during coitus, it is more often with a new partner—because of haste, fear of discovery, effort to give a "good performance,"—pressures less likely to operate with a familiar bedmate.

We have noted that many drugs used to control anxiety and high blood pressure can reduce sexual response. A cardiac patient should be aware that such relaxing drugs, by making erection and orgasm somewhat more difficult, can trap him into prolonged sexual labor—the very state the drugs were meant to prevent. If a man or woman finds it necessary to strain in order to respond or to reach orgasm, possible psychological reasons should be explored, as should the question of alternative medication.

The aim of sexual rehabilitation is always to restore the sex life that existed before the heart attack; the only rule for frequency and style of coitus seems to be moderation. Moderation, of course, is relative. No frequency is harmful for couples who are accustomed to and enjoy it.

A final point. Dr. Nathaniel Wagner, one of the few physicians who has written at length about sexual recovery in cardiac patients, points out that a heart attack may leave a person feeling that even masturbation threatens his life. Yet after the acute phase of heart attack has passed, sexual interest often reappears, perhaps even when the patient is up and around in the hospital. Dr. Wagner says:

"For many male patients the return of sexual arousal is a welcome sign of rehabilitation and the potential for a normal life. Interviews with patients indicate that it is not uncommon for the cardiac patient to masturbate while still in the hospital. This masturbation can be seen as an extraordinarily positive event from the point of view of continuing sexual life . . . . Despite the obvious advantage of masturbation over coitus for the resumption of sexual activity in cardiac patients, this matter has been neither studied nor discussed."

The advantage to which Dr. Wagner refers is that during masturbation a person can concentrate on and regulate his or her own level of sexual arousal, without concern about a partner's needs. Dr. Wagner has done some preliminary research and concludes, "Physicians should consider discussing the therapeutic use of masturbation as a method of reentrance into sexual activity for cardiac patients (if they) do not find the concept wrong from an ethical or moral point of view."

Gynecological Surgery

It is sometimes forgotten that hysterectomy (see page 452) demands dealing not with an ailment but with a woman, her marriage, and her family. The physical and psychological implications should be understood before the operation.

Simple hysterectomy, the removal of the uterus, has no effect on sexual drive or pleasure. Sometimes it shortens the vagina a bit, but not enough to interfere with coitus and orgasm. "Radical" hysterectomy removes not only the uterus but other pelvic organs, sometimes including the ovaries; if menopause has not yet arrived, it now takes place. As in normal menopause, estrogen-replacement therapy may ease unpleasant symptoms.

Neither simple nor radical hysterectomy reduces sexuality, but losing the womb may cause fear, grief, and helpless anger. Some women feel unfeminine and asexual; some fear premature aging or becoming masculine in appearance. Such fears are groundless. The worst result of hysterectomy in the middle or late years is psychological. A woman may translate her feeling of "I am less a woman" into a retreat from love and sexuality.

It is natural to mourn the loss of any part of the body, but in a woman past the childbearing years, prolonged reactions to hysterectomy are symbolic rather than rational. The sexual results of such surgery are neutral or positive for the majority of women. Naturally surgery removes the condition that called for the operation, so general health and pelvic discomfort are usually improved. In one survey of women who had undergone hysterectomies, 40 percent said marital relations were unchanged, and 38 percent said marital relations had improved.

One of the keys to a positive sexual outcome of hysterectomy is support and reassurance from the husband. It must be given before and after surgery—especially if there is postoperative depression, with the woman feeling barren, incomplete, or undesirable. Reassurance and the resumption of pleasurable coitus will help restore self-love, morale, and responsiveness.

Women often fear even minor genital surgery, such as treatment for prolapsed uterus, a common later-life operation. Most such procedures have no negative sexual results, and some are a help. Again, psychological support and the resumption of a normal sex life raise the chances for full physical, emotional, and sexual recovery.

Mastectomy

The removal of one or both breasts, usually for cancer, is a terrifying and demoralizing prospect. The surgery has no direct effect on sexual function, but it assaults a woman's sense of her body, beauty, and femininity, and she may anticipate rejection by her husband. If there is already tension, discord, mistrust, or dissatisfaction in the marriage, mastectomy may bring further strain.

In a good relationship, the marital problem usually isn't great. Several prominent American women have recently made public their experience with mastectomy. Their example may help other women weather the event and see that it doesn't reduce femininity or sexuality, nor need it hurt a loving relationship. If counseling is not offered before and after surgery, the patient should seek it. Talking with women who have successfully adjusted after such surgery is especially helpful.

Male Genitourinary Surgery

In late middle age and after, many men suffer swelling, infection, or a tumor of the prostate gland (see page 390). This is painful and may require surgical removal of part or all of the prostate. The great majority of men resume normal sex lives after prostatectomy, but this operation often causes exaggerated fears. Coitus is usually allowed, in fact encouraged, six weeks after the operation. Four men out of five produce less semen or show retrograde ejaculation, but this doesn't significantly change their sex drive or pleasure. Many of those whose potency is disturbed are victims of their own self-fulfilling prophecies. The outcome usually depends on the patient's prior sex life, his attitude, and his doctor's support.

One reason for widespread fear is that prostate surgery usually happens when men are concerned about aging in general, and sexual aging in particular. If they were sexually inactive and fearful before surgery, they may indeed be impotent. It does not help if the surgeon, as a protection against malpractice claims, asks a patient to sign a statement saying he is aware that the operation can cause impotence. Fortunately, many physicians today also inform and support the patient about returning to normal sexual function, rather than leaving him with unspoken anxieties.

There are several techniques of prostate surgery, and some may carry slightly greater risk than others of damage to nerves in the genital region. A patient should discuss this with his surgeon. In the minority of patients (usually those with prostatic cancer) whose sexual response is permanently affected by surgery, some degree of sexual function can be restored. Estrogen is sometimes used along with surgery to treat prostatic cancer; it reduces sex drive only temporarily.

In some cases of prostatic cancer, surgeons also must remove one or both testicles. Contrary to popular belief, this doesn't necessarily destroy any sexual function except fertility. Normal or nearly normal sex activity may continue for many years. As in other surgical procedures, post-operative sexuality depends largely on prior sex life, attitudes, and expectations.

In recent years, voluntary vasectomy has become an increasingly popular method of contraception (see page 398). In some cases, fertility can be surgically restored, but one should not count on reversal. Therefore doctors hesitate to perform this operation on men who request it impulsively, under unusual stress, when depressed, or after a history of emotional instability.

It is often said that vasectomy has few or no effects on sex drive or potency, but there has been some controversy over this. Despite an initially rational approach to the operation, some men feel castrated afterward, and there are difficulties for themselves and their wives. Although vasectomy may well be without major physical or psychological effects on most people, further research is needed.

Diabetes

Severe diabetes can interfere with orgasm in both sexes and with potency in men. The reason is not yet clear; the disease may damage nerves controlling sexual reflexes. If this happens, it is usually early in the course of the illness. The amount of sexual impairment varies from slight to severe. Some men show retrograde ejaculation but no other problems; others become impotent. Some women lose the capacity for orgasm. Often the damage is permanent, but sometimes drug therapy improves or cures it. We must stress that diabetes does not necessarily create sexual problems, even when acute. In fact, some doctors suspect that such sexual impairment sometimes results less from diabetes than from anxiety or depression over the illness and from general poor health care.

"Ostomies"

Colostomy, ileostomy, and some other kinds of surgery (see page 225) leave people with embarrassing physical disfigurements that can threaten their sex lives and marriages. In one study, half the patients who had such operations gave up intercourse entirely, some because they had become impotent, some because of their partners' aversion. Such surgery does sometimes damage nerves governing sexual response, but more often the sexual aftermath is psychological. Ostomies damage a person's body image and create shame and fear of others' reactions.

As in other postsurgical problems, a good emotional and sexual relationship may well survive, a bad one worsen. If the patient and spouse abandon sex, it is often because they received little or no pre- and postoperative counseling. When someone learns such surgery is necessary, the couple should seek counseling together and follow it up after surgery. Some physicians and psychologists give help very effectively. Talking with people who have created satisfying social and sexual lives after an ostomy is especially reassuring. There are now societies of such people.

Paraplegia and Major Disabilities

Spinal cord injury is not the commonest ill, but neither is it rare. Partial or total paralysis can occur in various parts of the body after strokes, automobile accidents, gunshot wounds, and some kinds of life-saving surgery. If one adds to paraplegia and hemiplegia such handicaps as those caused by stroke, blindness, and multiple sclerosis, a significant part of the adult population must be counted as disabled.

We give paraplegia special attention here for the same reason as many medical schools today—to show dramatically that even a severely disabled person remains a loving and sexual person. If the paraplegic, bound to a wheelchair, can remain sexual, so can most other people, regardless of age or health problems. Even those who have lost sexual sensation find that modified forms of lovemaking help restore their sense of worth, fulfillment, and effectiveness.

Today the paraplegic can expect an almost normal life-span. With help from various aids, he may be able to walk, drive, and work. With knowledge and medical advice, he can remain happy that he still has his old sexual feelings and needs. Up to 80 percent of cord-injured men can achieve erection by one year after injury. Few can reach orgasm or ejaculation, but they do enjoy sex—some, if not for physical pleasure, for the intimacy they retain with their spouses and the pride in still being able to satisfy them. Those capable of spinal-reflex erection, which may last several hours, are quite able to pleasure their partners!

Some of the severely disabled, for whom coitus is rarely or never possible, maintain a loving exchange of sex with their spouses through embracing, mutual masturbation, and oral-genital intercourse. Thus they can keep alive physical intimacy and a sense of sexual and human effectiveness. There are sometimes specific mechanical problems in sex for the disabled; a couple should discuss these frankly and in detail with a specially trained physician.

Other Health Problems

A number of major and minor health problems can affect sexual drive and capacity. Obviously a stroke can interfere with mental and physical functions, including sex; full or partial rehabilitation is sometimes a realistic hope. Severe cerebral arteriosclerosis occasionally causes uncharacteristic sex behavior, such as public exposure, peeping, or even sexual advances to family members or strangers. These are symptoms of temporary mental disorganization, not sexual deviation in the usual sense. Multiple sclerosis can cause impotence, as can advanced kidney malfunction and severe, untreated hyperthyroidism. Temporal lobe epilepsy may greatly increase or lessen sex behavior.

One could make a long list of less common conditions that sometimes effect sexuality. The important point is that in any physical or mental disturbance, sexuality may suffer—either from the illness or as a result of treatment. Much of this loss of sexual fulfillment is unnecessary. The patient and doctor can usually work together to make sex not a casualty of illness but a positive force that helps restore health and self-confidence.

THE DEVELOPED SENSES: VISION

A familiar way of recognizing that someone's eyes have grown older is to notice that he or she holds a newspaper at arm's length for reading. There is nothing abnormal about this. At 40 we have reached the bifocal age, or are about to. If we want to sew, read, or see things close up, we'll have to wear glasses, or squint and maybe develop crinkly crow's-feet at the corners of our eyes.

Other changes in the eyes come slowly with the years, and some visual complaints not strictly related to age become more common as people grow older. These matters all will be presented with assurance that, with available help and reasonable alertness to symptoms, a great deal can be done to preserve good vision.

The Seeing Brain

The eye is part of the brain—an extension to the outer world. Before birth the primitive brain develops a prominence called the optic vesicle, which elongates to become a ball at the end of a stalk. This ball then folds in on itself to become the eye, while the stalk becomes the optic nerve, which is really a brain tract rather than a nerve.

The eye is not static but incredibly busy. Fluids course within it. Bright or dim light causes the pupil to change size in a split second. The lens gets thicker and thinner according to what we look at. Chemicals surge and ebb as we go in and out of darkness. Torrents of nerve impulses race to

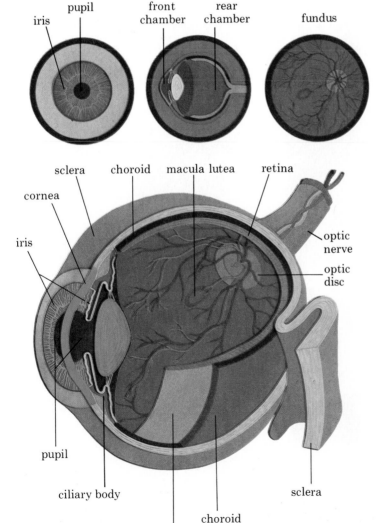

pupil
iris
front chamber
rear chamber
fundus

sclera
cornea
iris
choroid
macula lutea
retina
optic nerve
optic disc
pupil
ciliary body
sclera
choroid
retina

ANATOMY OF THE EYE

The sclera enwraps the eyeball, and in front forms the transparent cornea that admits light. The choroid layer of the eye is rich in blood vessels, and in front forms the iris, which gives the eye its color; the pupil is a circular hole in the iris. The retina is a tissue-thin light-receiving coat. At the optic disc, retinal fibers connect with the optic nerve. The ciliary body changes the shape of the lens for focusing, and furnishes watery fluid (aqueous humor) to the front chamber of the eye. The larger rear chamber is filled with a transparent jellylike substance, the vitreous. The fundus is the rear portion of the interior of the eye. The tiny macula is the receptor for color vision and detailed seeing.

and from the parent brain. Millions of receptors in an area the size of a baby's fingernail turn light waves into colors. It's awesome to realize that the working parts of the eye—which can transform electromagnetic waves into the image of the face of a loved one—are contained in a globe about the size of a table tennis ball, with sensory extensions to the back of the brain.

A little knowledge of the eye parts that work together helps in understanding changes in vision and diseases that may occur as the seeing machine grows older. The drawing on page 333 identifies structures of the eye that will be referred to later in the text.

The eye has three layers. The outer layer contains the *cornea,* the transparent window of the eye, which is continuous with the *sclera,* the white of the eye. The sclera is an extremely tough tissue that holds the eyeball in shape.

The middle layer *(choroid)* is the nourishing coat of the eye, rich in blood vessels. In the front of the eye it forms the *iris,* which gives the eye its color. The *pupil* is the central opening in the iris.

The inner layer forms the tissue-thin *retina* upon which rays of light fall, as upon film in a camera. Light rays are projected in a well-defined image, upside down, on the retina. Nerve endings in the retina collect the light "message" at the optic nerve head and send impulses to the back of the brain, where we actually "see."

Optic nerves from both eyes join at the base of the brain and, by complex routes, conduct impulses from the right side of each retina to the right half of the brain, and from the left side of each retina to the left half of the brain. If the left side of the brain is damaged, as by a stroke, sight on the right part of the field of vision may be impaired although the eyes are normal.

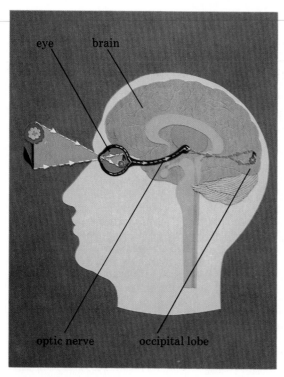

ROUTES OF SIGHT

Rays of light from an object (flower) pass to the back of the eye (white arrows), create an inverted image on the retina, and excite nerve impulses carried to the occipital lobe at the back of the brain, where the flower is perceived as a right-side-up object.

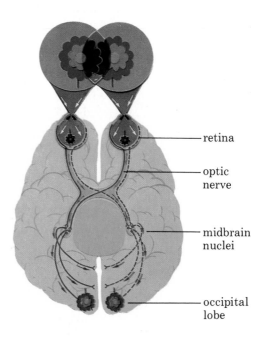

THE SEEING BRAIN

The pathways of seeing are traced in this bottom view of the brain. Nerve impulses from each half of each retina (green arrows) travel along the optic nerve, crisscross to midbrain nuclei, and follow complex nerve tracts to the occipital lobe where impulses are transformed into vision.

A small area of the retina, about as wide as the end of a thin lead pencil, is called the *macula lutea* (Latin for "yellow spot"). This tiny spot is packed with nerve endings called *cones,* so named because of their shape. It is responsible for vision in normal light and everything we see in fine detail—reading, writing, or threading a needle. It is also where we see colors, which only the cones can detect.

The rest of the retina contains mostly nerve endings called *rods.* These serve us for night vision, recognition of coarse details, and movements seen from the "corner of the eye." You can see how your rods work by seeking out a dim star on a dark night. Look directly at the star and it disappears. But move your gaze a little to one side and the star reappears.

The macula has no blood vessels and depends for nourishment on diffusion from nearby vessels. It is thus vulnerable to degeneration and is often the first area to suffer in aging of the retina.

The *crystalline lens* of the eye is a transparent tissue that gets bigger and stiffer as it gets older (see page 353).

The space in front of the iris and lens (anterior chamber) contains a watery fluid called *aqueous humor* that nourishes the cornea, which has no blood vessels and thus can be transplanted. The larger space behind the lens (posterior chamber) is filled with a transparent gelatin-like substance called *vitreous humor.*

Six muscles wrap around the eye and move it in any desired direction, directed by nerves coming from the brain. Injury or inflammation of these nerves may cause paralysis of one or more muscles, resulting in *double vision.* It may be necessary to block one eye for months until the nerve repairs itself, and it may take six months to determine if a nerve has regenerated.

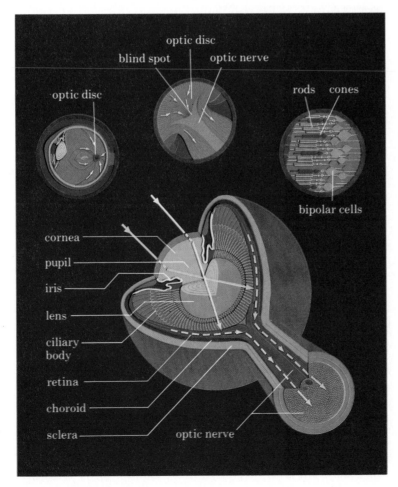

HOW WE SEE

The anatomy of vision is shown here in an unusual cutaway rear view of the eye. Light rays pass through the cornea, pupil, and lens, and project on the retina to excite nerve ends. The dotted yellow and white arrows show the pathways of nerve impulses along the optic nerve on their way to the brain. The small drawings at top show the blind spot where the optic nerve enters the retina, and the arrangement of light receptors in the retina. Cones are nerve endings that serve for colors and fine details; rods, for coarse, colorless vision in dim light. Bipolar cells are connected with the cones and ramify within the retina.

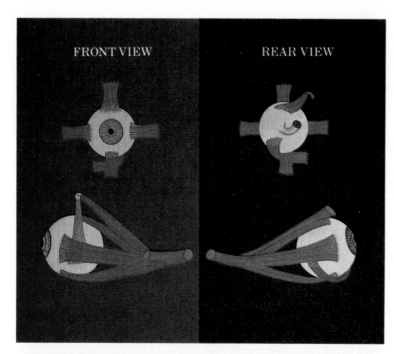

EYEBALL MUSCLES

Each eye has six muscles, externally connected to the eyeball as shown. Directed by a complex network of nerves from the brain, the muscles hold the eyes straight, rotate them, and turn them up, down, inward, or sideways. The two eyes must work together, like binoculars, so that images seen by each eye will be perceived as one image (fusion). Imbalance of eye muscles may result from nerve injury or other causes. A slight imbalance is not uncommon.

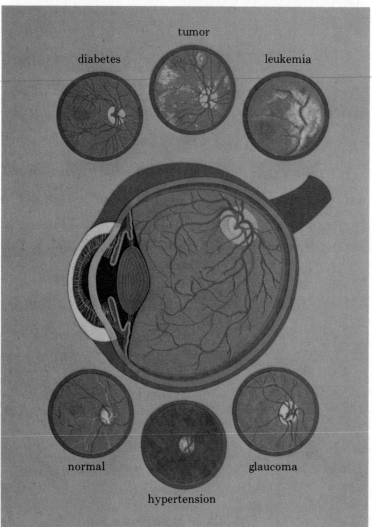

CLUES TO DISORDERS

Signs of diseases, not necessarily eye diseases, may frequently be detected by inspection of the back of the eye (fundus) with an ophthalmoscope. Some diseases manifest themselves by changes in blood vessels and structures of the fundus. The small drawings show representative changes that may be abnormalities characteristic of certain disorders. Thorough eye examination can be an aid in diagnosis, but is not a substitute for a general medical examination.

Eye Examinations

An eye examination, especially after 40, is not an end in itself. Ideally, it should be part of a complete medical examination. The eye can give important information about bodily states quite unrelated to vision. For instance, the back of the eye *(fundus)* is the only place where pulsating blood vessels can be viewed in their natural working state under high magnification. Indications of various diseases—diabetes, brain tumor, leukemia, high blood pressure, multiple sclerosis, and others—may be detected by looking into the back of the eye with an ophthalmoscope.

However, even if an eye examination shows no evidence of disease, it does not rule out its presence. A general physical examination is still necessary. Usually, only long-standing cases of diabetes are picked up by eye examination. A patient must have had diabetes for at least ten years before any evidence of it shows in the fundus.

Most persons seek an eye examination in expectation that glasses or contact lenses will help them to see better. Generally they are not concerned about possibly serious eye disorders that an examination might disclose. Almost everybody needs glasses after 40, if only for reading or close work, and a routine fitting examination provides a chance to discover unsuspected disease.

It is well to be alert to some symptoms that call for competent examination of the eyes:
• Rapid changes of refractive error (frequent changes of glasses; fuzziness of objects previously seen clearly; seeing better without glasses that were previously satisfactory)
• Sudden blurring of vision
• Showers of dirty spots before the eyes, as if sand were thrown in the face
• Flashes of light seen in dim illumination
• Colored haloes around bright lights
• Sunburst-dazzle of oncoming headlights
• A red eye.
These symptoms do not necessarily indicate serious trouble, but they suggest it would be prudent to find out more. Their relationship to specific disorders will be discussed later.

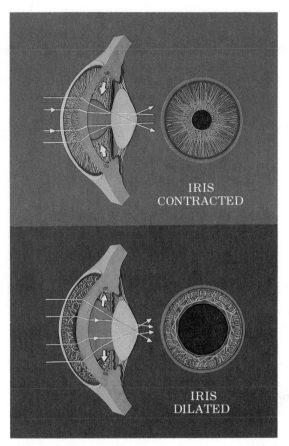

IRIS CONTRACTED

IRIS DILATED

AUTOMATIC EXPOSURE

Like the diaphragm of a camera, the muscular iris constricts and expands to quickly adjust the size of the pupil to the intensity of incoming light. The lower drawing shows light rays from a dim source that cause the iris to open wide, thus enlarging the pupil to admit as much light as possible. Bright light causes the iris to contract, narrowing the diameter of the pupil to diminish the brilliance of incoming light. Orders to dilate or constrict the pupil are sent out by nerves in the retina.

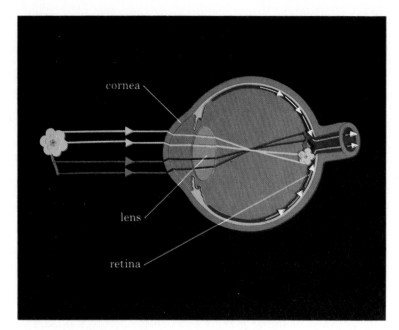

cornea

lens

retina

NORMAL REFRACTION

Light rays from a distant flower (green and yellow lines) are shown coming to focus on the retina in an upside-down position. The rays are bent (refracted) by the cornea, and again by the lens, to bring the image into sharp focus.

GLASSES AND CONTACT LENSES

In a perfect eye, parallel rays of light coming from a distance of 20 feet or more are brought to exact focus on the retina without effort. Incoming light is refracted (bent) perfectly by the cornea and lens of the eye. The most common reason for wearing glasses is to correct refractive errors. That is, a corrective lens in front of the eye bends light waves to bring them into sharp focus. There are three major kinds of refractive errors.

Nearsightedness (myopia). The eye is too long for its optical system. Rays of light from a distance come to focus in front of the retina, resulting in a blur. Close objects, however, focus easily on the retina; reading is effortless. The condition is corrected by concave lenses, identified in a prescription as (−) or minus.

Most nearsighted persons wear corrective lenses long before middle age. Myopia begins quite early and tends to stabilize in the late teens or 20s.

Farsightedness (hyperopia). The eye is too short for its optical system so that light rays focus in back of the retina, causing a blurred image. Farsightedness is corrected by convex spherical lenses, designated in the prescription as (+) or plus.

A farsighted person may get along without glasses for quite a while. Distance vision is often good, and by "straining to see" he may bring close objects into sufficiently good focus to postpone the wearing of glasses. This is very tiring to the eye, however, and no longer suffices when the lens of the eye loses some of its focusing power in the 40s and after. If the eye is very farsighted or if its focusing power is weakened by age, prescribing a convex lens is the only solution.

Astigmatism. If the front surface of the cornea is not perfectly round, but is shaped like an egg or a football, light rays are distorted. This is called astigmatism because light rays do not focus at any one point. Astigmatism can occur in nearsighted, farsighted, or otherwise normal eyes. It is corrected by plus or minus cylindrical (barrel-shaped) lenses.

An "add" is the amount of plus sphere added to distance correction so one can read comfortably through a bifocal. If you wish, you can interpret your own prescription.

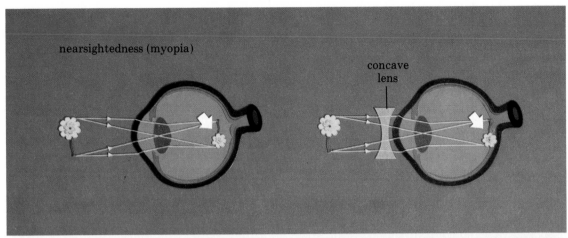

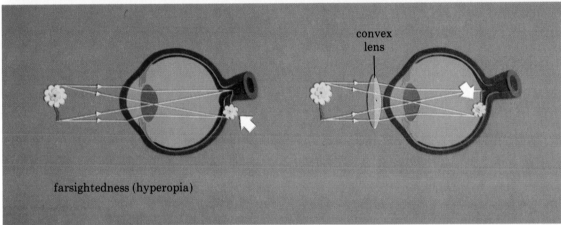

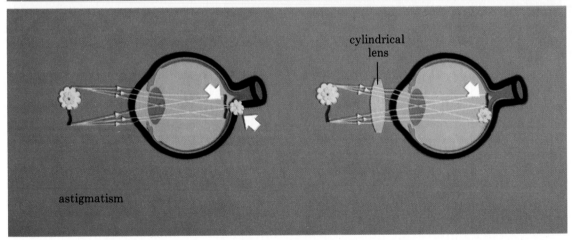

REFRACTIVE ERRORS—NEARSIGHTEDNESS, FARSIGHTEDNESS, AND ASTIGMATISM

Light rays from a distance converge in front of the retina of a nearsighted eye, resulting in a fuzzy image (close objects are seen clearly). A concave lens in front of the eye brings the image into focus. The lens makes the wearer's eyes look smaller, depending on degree of correction.

In a farsighted eye, the image from near objects falls behind the retina. This is corrected by a convex lens in front of the eye. A moderately farsighted person may be able to read or see quite clearly in fine detail, but this requires considerable effort, with complaints of "tired eyes."

Irregular curvature of the cornea is the cause of astigmatism. Rays of light, as if reflected from a wavy pane of glass, are bent more in one diameter than another. Part of the image is correctly focused but another part is not. Astigmatism is corrected by a cylindrical lens.

Joining the Bifocal Brigade

Around age 40, a process called *presbyopia* ("old sight") is under way in your eyes. It is painless—in fact, normal—and so gradual that we are hardly aware of it except that the eyes may feel unusually tired, strained, or uncomfortable after prolonged desk work or reading.

What happens is that the crystalline lens of the eye becomes less accommodating, to say the least. "Accommodation" is a technical word for the ability of the lens to change its shape—from thin to fat and in between—to bring whatever we look at into focus on the retina. In time, it loses flexibility and stiffens against the efforts of internal eye muscles to change its shape. It needs help. Changes that occur in the lens with aging are described more fully in a discussion of cataracts (see page 353).

The focusing power of a child's eyes is astonishing. He can look at a book a few inches from his eyes, shift his gaze to a TV set a dozen feet away, glance out a window at a distant horizon, and see everything clearly. But he, too, like millions of predecessors, will grow to a certain age when he has to hold a magazine at arm's length to read it, and distance vision may or may not remain good. He will become a presbyope.

What can be done about presbyopia? There are several alternatives. One is to do nothing as long as possible. No harm will befall the eyes. Some occupations—driving a bulldozer, riding on a ranch, construction work, harvesting crops—require little or no close-seeing. In a crisis, such as inability to read a phone number in a dim booth, one can seek help from passers-by. Unfortunately, our civilization does impose a few near-vision demands upon almost anybody, if only a tussle with job application or income tax forms.

Another choice· is to be fitted with "reading glasses," focused for about 14 inches. These can be carried in a pocket to put on when close work is necessary. But objects seen at a distance through reading glasses will appear fuzzy.

Then there are "half glasses" that can be worn all the time if distance vision does not need correction, or only when needed for close work. The half-lenses are focused for near points and the wearer simply peers over them to see at a distance. Half-glasses have a certain colonial quaintness that appeals to some.

Most patients choose bifocal glasses. Benjamin Franklin invented bifocals for convenience and "Poor Richard thriftiness." He put the top half, the distance lens, and the bottom half, the reading lens, into the same frame. Thus a single pair of glasses afforded a full range of vision.

Regular bifocal glasses have a thin, visible dividing line between the upper and lower segments. The lower or reading segment may occupy the entire lower half or, more often, only a part of it. Small segments are positioned a little off-center, closer to the nose, because the eyes turn in slightly when looking at near objects.

The size of the reading segment is a matter of comfort, which should be discussed when glasses are ordered. A person who does a great deal of close work may appreciate the broader sweep of a large segment, while one whose need for close seeing is occasional, may need only a small segment.

Learning to Like Bifocals

Adaptation to bifocals is a learned motor skill, like driving a car. Some people adapt to bifocals in a day or two while others take months. At first, one is annoyed by the dividing line and shifts of focus as the gaze is lowered and raised. In time, the brain corrects this perception.

Farsighted persons usually adapt to bifocals faster than the nearsighted. The reason may be that nearsighted persons have an escape hatch: they can often see well at near points by removing their glasses. Indeed, very fine print may seem magnified when they take off their glasses, because lenses for nearsightedness reduce the visual image to some degree.

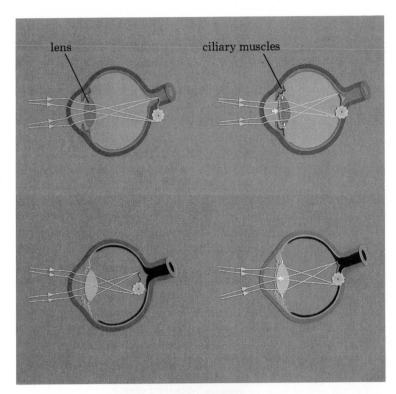

ACCOMMODATION

Accommodation is the ability of the lens of the eye to change its shape (fatten or flatten) to bring close or distant objects into focus. The closer the object, the more accommodation is required. At left above, the image from an unaccommodated lens falls behind the retina. At right, the lens accommodates by becoming fatter to focus the image. The dotted line on the lens shows its normal limits. The lens also can flatten itself to accommodate to an image that falls short of the retina. Changes in lens shape are controlled by ciliary muscles. Eyes that cannot accommodate comfortably and effectively may tire easily and could benefit from corrective lenses (see page 338).

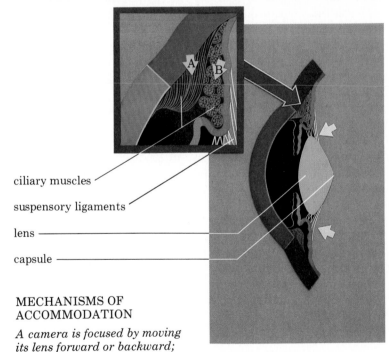

ciliary muscles

suspensory ligaments

lens

capsule

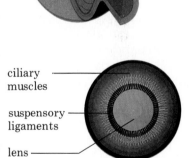

ciliary muscles

suspensory ligaments

lens

MECHANISMS OF ACCOMMODATION

A camera is focused by moving its lens forward or backward; the human eye focuses by changing the shape of its stationary lens. The lens is slung by ligaments to a ring of radiating (A) and encircling (B) ciliary muscle fibers that manipulate the lens. When the A group of ciliary muscles contracts, the suspensory ligaments pull forward and the lens flattens. Then the B group contracts, the suspensory ligaments relax, and the lens becomes thicker and more curved. Ordinarily, the ciliary muscles are most active when we focus closely on objects nearer than 20 feet.

THE LENS AFTER 40

The drawing shows the front of the eye as viewed from inside, with structures that effect accommodation. As the crystalline lens grows older (say, 40 years or more) it becomes less elastic. In time, it loses its power of thickening so that no amount of effort by ciliary muscles can bring fine print into sharp focus. This normal age-related change is called presbyopia.

Must bifocals be worn all the time? Not necessarily. If one has good vision for distance without glasses, bifocals can be worn just for close work. If not, distance glasses can be worn for walking and switched to bifocals when reading or writing. When one has learned to walk with bifocals, they can be worn all the time.

Some patients refuse to wear any bifocal that has a visible dividing line, feeling wrongly that it proclaims old age. Invisible or blended bifocals are available, but are more expensive. An alternative is the Kryptok, a fused bifocal with a very inconspicuous dividing line. It is the least expensive bifocal, but optically not as free of aberrations as the more visible types.

Frames. Properly fitted frames make a big difference in getting used to bifocals. Glasses that slide down the nose and have to be continually pushed into place are annoying and inefficient. Some wearers prefer a frame with an adjustable bridge. Such a frame has wires connected to pads that rest on the nose, an organ of variable size. By bending the wires, an optician can raise or lower the bifocals to their most comfortable and efficient position.

If bifocals are too low, one has to throw the head back to read, risking stiffness and pain in the neck. Bifocals that are too high get in the way when viewing objects at a distance. If glasses are adjusted so the lenses barely clear the lashes, the bifocals are more likely to be well tolerated than if the lenses are pushed far out from the eyes.

Contact Lenses

Patients often ask, "Can I wear contact lenses?" The answer is usually a qualified yes. A few conditions (allergies, glaucoma) may make contact lenses inadvisable. But in some other circumstances they are uniquely valuable, as after cataract surgery (see page 360).

Before 1950, contact lenses were designed to cover the whole cornea and rest on the sclera or white of the eye. These scleral lenses could be worn only for a few hours before vision became blurry. The cornea would become swollen and cloudy, and the lens had to be removed.

Finally it was realized that the surface cells of the cornea receive oxygen from tears. The large scleral lenses trapped the tears and when the oxygen in them was used up, the cornea began to swell and become cloudy.

Today, almost all contact lenses are of the corneal type. They are tiny, thin, light plastic lenses that cover only a part of the cornea and float on a thin layer of tears. With each blink, the lens moves, allowing circulation of tears underneath it. Oxygen continues to reach the cornea, which remains clear. It is not unusual for patients to wear contact lenses all day; however some patients with hard contact lenses take them out for an hour or two in the middle of the day to give the eyes a rest.

Hard and soft contacts. Conventional contact lenses are made of hard plastic that holds its shape in the eye. Soft contacts, which came into use in the 1970s, are made of water-absorbing plastic that acts like a sponge. Each type has advantages and disadvantages.

Soft contacts tend to be more comfortable than hard contacts, not popping out as easily and feeling less like a foreign body in the eye. They may buckle with each blink, causing momentary blur, but this does not cause a problem unless there is significant astigmatism, in which case a hard contact serves better.

To wear contact lenses comfortably, the eye must have enough tears to float the lenses. This is particularly true of hard lenses. Patients with very dry eyes may not even be able to wear soft lenses. Soft lenses may be worn, left out for a few days, then be worn again. Hard lenses should be worn consistently or not at all. Soft lenses cost more, require more meticulous care, are easily torn, and are less durable.

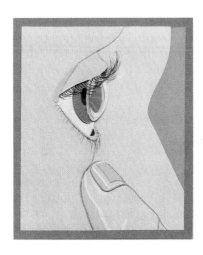

CONTACT LENSES

Modern contact lenses cover only a part of the cornea, the transparent window of the eye, and are remarkably improved over early lenses that covered the entire white and could only be worn for a short time.

CONTACT LENS REMOVAL

Usually a contact lens can be removed easily by tugging sharply at the outer corner of the eye while blinking the eye shut. Bend over a towel or a cupped hand to catch the lens.

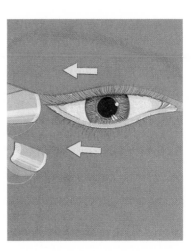

Contacts for Presbyopes

Persons over 40 who wear contact lenses will usually not be able to read or see things closely with them. The most frequent solution is to wear glasses focused for reading distance over the contact lenses.

Hard bifocal contact lenses of various types are available, but in all cases, the patient must first be fitted for and learn to wear a single-vision hard contact lens. No one goes directly into bifocal contact lenses, which constitute only a small proportion of contact lens prescriptions.

It is possible, though not common, to wear contact lenses focused for reading or arm's-length distance only. There might be special motivation, as in the case of a political candidate who refers to notes in making a speech, but wishes to present an image of vigorous youth. To keep the faces of his audience clear, he could wear a lens on one eye focused for distance and on the other eye focused for near vision.

People who are nearsighted are more likely to wear contact lenses successfully than those who are farsighted. Nearsighted lenses flare out at their margins, so contact lenses sag less in myopes as the blinking lids keep raising the lenses by their peripheral flange. Also, glasses for nearsightedness produce a minified or smaller image on the retina. If you look at a printed page through a spectacle lens for myopia, you will see that the image is smaller (the wearer's eyes also look smaller). A contact lens enlarges the image and improves vision, especially with strong corrections. Side vision is also better than with glasses.

Can a contact lens get stuck in the eye? Not really. Occasionally an effort to remove a hard contact lens from the eye may fail, but there is no reason to panic.

First, determine whether the lens is still centered on the cornea. If you can look across the room and see clearly, the lens must still be in place. If it is not, the image will be quite blurred. If the lens is still in place, repeat the removal procedure, tugging sharply on the outer corner of the eye while blinking the eye shut at the same time. Do this while bending over a towel or a cupped hand. If the lens does not pop out, you can try one of two methods:

1. Use an eyecup filled with eye-irrigating solution or even boiled water. Throw the head back and blink the eye under the fluid. This should loosen the lens, and when the head is bent forward, the lens should fall into the eyecup. Several attempts may be necessary.

2. Fill a sink with warm water and immerse the face in it, blinking and allowing the lens to fall into the sink.

On the other hand, if vision of the eye is very blurred, the lens is no longer on the cornea. It may have fallen to the floor during the attempt at removal. Someone with good vision and patience will have to search the area, inch by inch. Tinted lenses are easier to find than colorless ones.

Another possibility is that the lens may have slipped into the upper or lower fornix, the recess between the eyelid and the white of the eye. The fornix is a blind cul-de-sac or pouch. There is absolutely no danger that a lens can slip in so far that it cannot be recovered, or that it can poke through and wander in the body.

To remove a lens from the fornix, you can massage the lens into place on the cornea through the eyelid, then proceed as usual. Or you can use a suction cup, which looks like a miniature plumber's helper. This works better if the suction cup is wet.

If all measures fail, the eye should be examined by an eye doctor. There have been rare instances where a lens was left in the fornix and worked itself into the substance of the eyelid, forming a lump and a chronically irritated eye.

The medicine cabinet should always contain a plastic four-ounce squeeze bottle of sterile eye-irrigating solution, which can be bought without a prescription. A tight lens can sometimes be loosened by squirting a stream of fluid into the eye. The solution can also be used to flush out mucus, irritating chemicals, and foreign bodies if they are not too adherent to tissues of the eye.

Could I go blind from a contact lens?

Like most things in life, contact lenses involve a small but inescapable risk. But serious complications almost always arise from failure to obey instructions, sloppy hygiene, or both.

Soft contact lenses are more amenable to off-and-on use than hard contacts, but it is always desirable to wear contact lenses according to a precise schedule, and essential with hard contacts, which most patients use. Wearing time should be increased gradually, according to instructions from the fitter, who usually checks initial progress over a four-week period.

To wear a hard contact two or three hours a day all week and then 16 hours on a weekend is to invite some terribly uncomfortable (but temporary) symptoms. This "overwearing syndrome" includes pain, sensitivity to light, and watery swollen eyes that are almost impossible to keep open.

Contact lenses must be kept scrupulously clean. The hard lenses should be soaked overnight in a special soaking solution and tenacious deposits removed with cleaning solutions. Before insertion into the eye, the lens must be prepared with a wetting solution that permits tears to wet it (plastic normally repels water). The practice of popping a lens into the mouth before placing it in the eye is terribly dangerous and can lead to blindness if a corneal infection results.

Care of soft contacts is even more exacting. Soft lenses act as a sponge to absorb any medications or chemicals dropped into the eye. Cleaning and wetting solutions intended for hard lenses should never be used with soft lenses as they may be concentrated and burn the eye. Special salt solutions are used for storing soft lenses. A significant cause of discomfort from soft lenses is the buildup of protein deposits from tears that can irritate the eye. These can be dissolved by soaking the lens overnight in a proteolytic enzyme solution once a week. Tablets for preparing such cleaning solutions are available.

Soft lenses must be sterilized once a day. Most commonly, this is accomplished by heat in special sterilizers supplied by the manufacturer, but methods of cold sterilization are under development.

FACT AND FICTION
ABOUT GLASSES

Will glasses weaken the eyes and make one dependent on them? If you are nearsighted, any effort to exert yourself to see better can only make you more nearsighted. The only way to improve distance vision is to wear proper lenses. If you have been reading without glasses, as many nearsighted people do, you may find that reading with new glasses is more difficult because you have to exert focusing effort.

If you are farsighted but manage to get by without glasses, you may find that if you wear glasses all the time you can no longer read as well without them.

If you have a significant amount of astigmatism, you may see more clearly by squinting, but you will do better to wear glasses. No matter how much you wear them, you will see as well as you did before when you take them off.

Can "eye exercises" avert the need for glasses? Despite claims that eye exercises lessen the need for glasses, it is doubtful that a patient can improve his or her visual acuity in that way.

Variations in focusing power can occur with changes in general health and vitality. A person suffering from grippe or undergoing major surgery may have fatigue in reading, which disappears in a month or two when he regains his strength.

The decrease in focusing power that occurs with age is caused by increased stiffness of the lens so that it is more difficult to mold to a more powerful shape. This cannot be changed by exercise.

Will wearing the wrong glasses ruin the eyes? No. Once you have reached visual maturity (after age six), wearing the wrong glasses may make you feel tired and uncomfortable but no physical damage to the eyes will result.

Will failure to wear prescribed glasses damage the eyes? In general, no. However, a nearsighted person who does not wear the proper glasses is more likely to show *exophoria,* a latent tendency for one eye to turn out. This may occur only when one is tired, but later it may happen more often. In long-standing cases, the eye may drift out and stay out. Not every myope who refuses to wear glasses has this trouble, however.

Resistance to breakage. In the past, eye injury or blindness sometime resulted from glasses shattered in accidents. Now all glasses must be "impact resistant" by order of the Food and Drug Administration. Lenses are tested by dropping a steel ball on them from a specified height. Impact-resistant glass is slightly thicker and heavier than ordinary glass. No lens is actually shatterproof, as any lens will break if the impact is forceful enough.

A glass lens can be made impact resistant by heating it, then chilling it quickly. This creates a hard "skin" on the surface of the lens. If this surface layer is scratched, the lens loses its resistance to impact. It may even collapse or "implode" and break up spontaneously. Scratched case-hardened lenses should be replaced. Fortunately, when a case-hardened glass lens does break, it forms crumb-like particles and not the hazardous sharp slivers created by breaking conventional glass. Glass lenses can also be chemically treated to resist impact.

Plastic lenses are lighter in weight, thinner, and more resistant to impact than glass case-hardened lenses. They cost more and are slightly easier to scratch; however, a scratched plastic lens does not lose any of its resistance to impact.

Tinted glasses. Patients often ask about a slight tint for their glasses. Normal eyes have so much adaptability to changes in light that a mild tint contributes little to comfortable seeing in bright light. As we get older, we adapt less well to darkness and need all the light we can get at night. A mild tint in glasses, plus the tint of an automobile windshield, may reduce light perception on a dark moonless night to the point of causing an accident.

Variable-tint glasses that turn darker in bright light have recently become available. These lenses darken to a No. 3 (moderately dark) tint in the sun. They are helpful to persons who are very sensitive to ordinary light, but the lenses do not get dark enough to be a substitute for sunglasses. Variable-tint lenses also darken under fluorescent lamps, but not under incandescent bulbs.

Sunglasses should exclude at least 80 percent of the light, but many commercial sunglasses do not screen out enough light to give protection in bright sunlight, such as over water or on the beach. A variable sunglass that starts at a moderately dark tint and becomes very dark in sunlight also is available.

Night-driving glasses. Many older patients ask if they can get a tinted glass to wear for night driving because they are dazzled by oncoming headlights. There is no glass that can help, and tinted glasses only make matters worse. Dazzling by headlights is often caused by imperfections within the eyes, such as early cataracts.

The best advice is to make sure that the windshield and glasses are scrupulously clean. The driver should look to the side of the road and not try to outstare oncoming headlights.

If you intend to drive back from a day at the beach, it is helpful to wear dark sunglasses during the day. Exposure to bright light reflected from the sand can impair night vision needed to drive home safely after dark.

Recent research indicates that exposure to excessive light may be more harmful than previously believed and that the margin of safety may be smaller. To play it safe, avoid exposure to very bright sunlight at the beach or over the water by using dark sunglasses and a cap with a visor or a hat with a large brim. This may have some value in forestalling the development of cataracts or retinal disease.

GLAUCOMA

The word "glaucoma" stirs panic in many patients who learn they have it. Some even believe it to be a form of cancer, perhaps misled by the suffix "—oma," which occurs in words for types of cancer (carcinoma, melanoma, etc.). Glaucoma is a condition of abnormally high fluid pressure within the eye. It has nothing to do with cancer or with high blood pressure, which is a regulation disorder of another system.

Yet glaucoma is an all-too-common cause of blindness occurring in adults, the more tragic because prompt and proper treatment can usually preserve good vision and halt an onward course toward blindness. There are congenital forms of glaucoma, but the common kinds are age-related, affecting middle-aged and older people for the most part. Glaucoma is unusual in people under 35, but mass screening surveys have shown that about one person in 50 has a suspiciously high pressure that warrants further medical investigation.

Obstructed drainage. Certain structures of the eye associated with glaucoma are called "angles" by doctors. One may think of an angle as a funnel that accepts fluids at its mouth and permits them to flow through. If the sides of the funnel squeeze together so that fluids cannot enter, the angle is said to be "closed." If the funnel mouth is open, the angle is said to be "wide," but fluids can be blocked by debris at the end of the funnel.

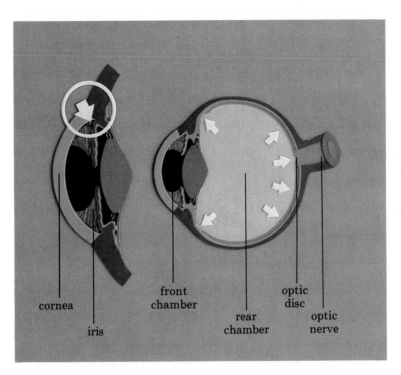

SITE OF GLAUCOMA

The arrow points to the angle at the junction of the iris and cornea through which eye fluids normally drain. A closed or obstructed angle impedes drainage and causes buildup of pressure inside the eye. The cross-section drawing shows areas where high pressures can damage the eye, and if not controlled, destroy the optic nerve.

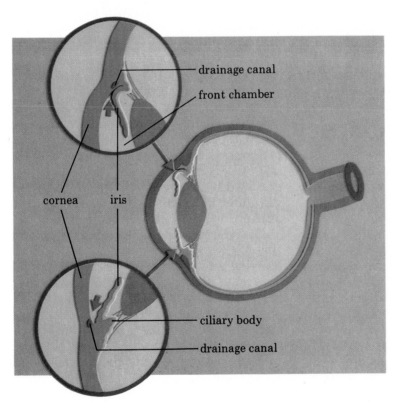

EYE DRAINS

The top drawing at left shows the closed angle at the cornea-iris junction (green arrow) that obstructs the normal outflow of internal eye fluids. The bottom drawing shows a normal open angle. Fluids that cannot escape create abnormal pressure within the eye (glaucoma), gradually destroying sight unless pressure is relieved by eye-drop medicines or surgery.

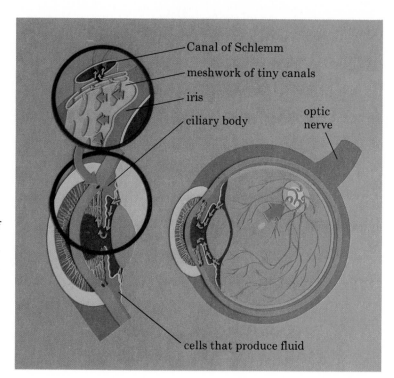

Canal of Schlemm

meshwork of tiny canals

iris

ciliary body

optic nerve

cells that produce fluid

DRAINAGE CANALS

This detailed drawing (leftmost) shows the normal drainage route of aqueous humor through a meshwork of tiny canals to the Canal of Schlemm, through which the fluid exits and is absorbed by veins. The drawing of the whole eye shows "pocketing" of the optic disc (green arrow) due to excessive pressure in glaucoma. Vision becomes tunnel-like as pressure progresses.

Fluid is continually secreted into the eye and drained from it. The aqueous humor, which fills the front (anterior) chamber of the eye, is secreted by the ciliary body, located behind the lens and behind the root of the iris. The fluid, which nourishes the lens and cornea, flows through the pupil to the angle at the side of the front chamber. There it filters through a meshwork into a tiny canal that encircles the eye.

The various types of glaucoma arise from different disturbances of the fluid inflow-outflow balance. Dammed-up fluids exert relentless pressure upon the end of the optic nerve and retinal cells and vessels, ultimately destroying them. Typically, the eye's field of vision narrows insidiously, becoming more and more tunnel-like. Nothing can restore any degree of lost vision, but timely treatment is effective in forestalling catastrophe.

Acute (Angle-Closure) Glaucoma

This is the most dramatic form of glaucoma. It occurs in eyes with a very narrow space in the angle of the anterior chamber between the iris and the cornea. This narrowness may be genetic and can be aggravated by changes with age. Dilation of the pupil may cause obstruction of fluid outflow by the accordion folds of the iris.

A sudden acute attack can cause pain in the eye, headache, nausea, vomiting, and blurring and redness of the eye. The episode may be precipitated by stress, such as grief from a death in the family. Pain may be so severe that the help of a doctor is immediately sought. But often the attack subsides spontaneously, so that by the time the patient reaches the ophthalmologist, pressure of the eye is back to normal.

In such case the doctor may do a provocative test to see whether the angle can close under certain conditions. The most common test is to dilate the pupil, either with drops or by sitting the patient in a dark room. If an attack develops in the office, it can be broken up by treatment.

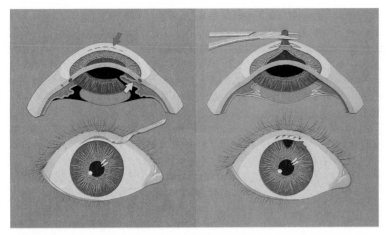
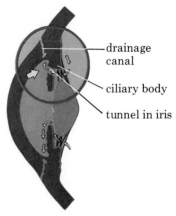

GLAUCOMA SURGERY

At top left, the purple arrow shows the line of incision in the cornea to gain entry to the front chamber of the eye and access to the iris and closed angle (yellow arrow). Below left, the incision in the cornea is viewed from the front of the eye. At top right, a

small piece of the iris is drawn through the opening in the cornea and snipped off (iridectomy). The front of the eye after surgery is shown below. The incision is closed; the tiny triangular nick is a hole at the top of the iris.

RESTORED DRAINAGE

The bottom half of the drawing shows normal circulation. In the circle, a surgical tunnel through the iris (heavy arrow) unblocks a closed angle and reestablishes drainage. Usually both eyes are operated on, even though one eye may seemingly be unaffected.

Treatment. Once a diagnosis is made, the best treatment is surgery. An *iridectomy*—an operation in which a small portion of the iris is cut out—should be done as soon as the eye has become quiet. The effect is to equalize pressure behind and in front of the iris so that it tends to fall away from the cornea, relieving the block at the angle.

The surgical cure rate for acute glaucoma is close to 100 percent if diagnosed promptly and operated on at the proper time. The rule is that once the diagnosis of angle-closure glaucoma has been made, iridectomy should be done on both eyes. Persons who have had an acute attack in one eye are extremely likely to have an attack in the companion eye.

Recently, researchers have been able to make a small but functioning opening in the iris by repeated burns with a laser beam. However, some damage to the underlying crystalline lens may result. This method is still experimental and so far has not replaced the iridectomy.

If repeated attacks of angle-closure glaucoma have resulted in adhesions and damage of the angle, medical treatment (see below) may have to be continued after iridectomy. What happens is that iridectomy has converted the glaucoma into a chronic form and made the occurrence of acute attacks unlikely.

Chronic Wide-Angle Glaucoma

Persons who have this most common type of glaucoma have wide enough angles, but pressures build up within the eye when the filter meshwork of the drainage system resists the flow of fluids. The situation can be likened to a drain clogged by grease or particles. Age seems to play some part by piling up cellular debris and modifying delicate structures.

Symptoms. The sinister thing about chronic wide-angle glaucoma is that in its early stages there are no symptoms. Pressure may be elevated for a long time before the patient is aware of anything wrong.

Suggestive symptoms are frequent unsatisfactory changes of glasses, occasional rainbow-like haloes around lights, and gradual lessening of side vision. A red eye may be a sign of glaucoma, but there are other causes. The glaucomatous process may be well under way by the time symptoms are noticed. Blind areas develop in the field of vision, but these are not close enough to central vision to be recognized. By the time the patient gets an eye examination, large parts of his visual field may have been wiped out and he may have only tunnel vision, like looking through a telescope.

Detection. Actually, there are signs of early glaucoma that are easily detected, but not by the patient. Quick, painless measurements of intraocular tension are routinely given by ophthalmologists, optometrists, general physicians, and in mass screening projects in many communities. Such tests are advised for everybody over 40, and the trend is to extend them to younger people.

If high pressure within the eyeball is discovered, additional tests will be done by an eye doctor to confirm a diagnosis of glaucoma and evaluate its nature, the extent of damage, and the general condition of the eye (other diseases may coexist). Detection of an abnormally high intraocular pressure is not enough to make a diagnosis of glaucoma. Many eyes are structured so that they remain unaffected by a pressure level that could wipe out the vision of another eye less ruggedly designed. Measurements determine how much of the visual field—the all-around broadness of one's gaze—has or has not been narrowed.

A procedure called *gonioscopy* is an examination with a special contact lens that enables the doctor to see the angle between the iris and cornea, the trouble spot where fluid normally filters out of the eye. This area cannot normally be seen by the examiner because light is reflected from the inner surface of the cornea, away from his eye. The special contact lens brings the angle into view and helps to determine the type of glaucoma.

Treatment. The initial treatment of chronic simple glaucoma is medical, in the form of drops put into the eye, or tablets that reduce the rate of secretion of fluid into the eye. Surgery is reserved for patients who cannot be controlled on maximal medical therapy.

Drops must be used faithfully as the doctor directs and may have to be continued indefinitely. There are several classes of drugs. Pilocarpine drops constrict the pupil and draw the iris away from the angle. This facilitates the exit of fluid from the eye, but the constriction of the pupil means that less light enters the eye. If cataracts are present, vision may be blurred.

Other drops such as epinephrine reduce the rate of fluid formation. They tend to dilate the pupil and cannot be used in eyes with narrow angles that have not yet had an iridectomy. Tablets lower pressure by reducing the rate of fluid formation.

Card-carrying patients. Every glaucoma patient should carry in his or her wallet an identification card stating that he or she suffers from glaucoma, and what medications are being used.

Certain drugs can cause dilation of the pupils, which is hazardous in patients with angles so narrow that they can close in an acute attack. Such medications should be avoided unless the patient has had an iridectomy. Medicines with this proclivity usually carry cautionary notices on the labels. Always read the label! When prescribing medication, the family doctor should know what medicines a patient with potential angle-closure glaucoma is taking—including non-prescription drugs.

Glaucoma patients should not drink large quantities of liquids in social situations. There is no need to go thirsty, but robust imbibing should be shunned. Drinking a pint or two of beer or tea can cause a large rise in intraocular pressure.

The most important thing to remember about glaucoma is that the patient cannot tell whether the condition is under control by how well he sees or feels. The eyes must be monitored by an ophthalmologist. Self-management of glaucoma is an invitation to blindness. Vision that has been lost from glaucoma cannot be restored. Treatment can only be aimed at preserving the vision that remains.

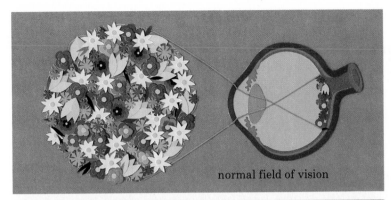

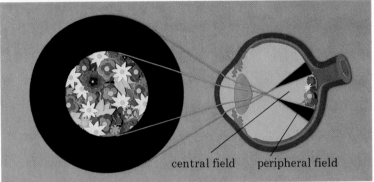

normal field of vision

central field   peripheral field

TUNNEL VISION

At top, the full field of vision is reproduced on the retina of a normal eye. A classic sign of glaucoma is a narrowing of the field of vision so that objects are seen as if looking through a tunnel or gun barrel (below left). Tests of the visual field may disclose a narrowing that the patient is not aware of.

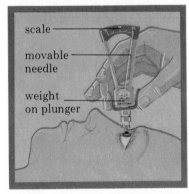

scale

movable needle

weight on plunger

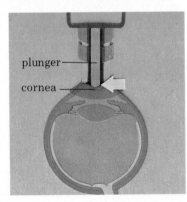

plunger

cornea

THE SCHIUTZ TONOMETER

The Schiutz tonometer is a simple device for measuring internal pressures of the eye. It is placed on the eyeball, as shown, after the cornea is anesthetized. The action is somewhat like that of a tire gauge. A weighted plunger indents the anesthetized cornea against resistance of pressure within the eye. The amount of indentation is shown on a scale.

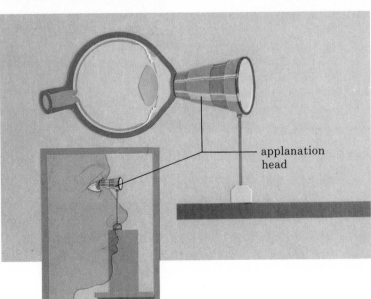

applanation head

OTHER TECHNIQUES

Sophisticated applanation techniques, including electronic measuring devices and some that make no contact with the cornea, give precise measurements of internal eye pressure. The drawing shows a contact applanation tonometer depressing the anesthetized cornea. A microscope head (not shown) permits visualization of measurement.

WHAT CAN I DO TO PRESERVE MY SIGHT?

There is no simple answer, nor are there magic drops to protect one against blindness. However, here are some pointers:

Guard Your Eyes Against Accidents

- Wear safety glasses when striking objects with a hammer, especially metal against metal (a wooden mallet is often advisable). Tiny chips of metal flying at high speed can penetrate the eyeball. Also wear safety glasses whenever using power tools of any kind.
- Use extreme caution when dealing with a weak auto battery. Auto batteries contain hydrogen and oxygen, a deadly explosive. Never inspect a battery for fluid level with a lit match; use a flashlight. If you must use jumper cables, remove the vent caps from both batteries to allow gases to escape. Follow your car owner's manual instructions exactly to avoid striking a spark, and shield your eyes.
- Use lap and shoulder safety belts when driving or riding as a passenger. Auto accidents can cause blindness.
- If you are playing tennis, wear safety glasses or safety rims. When you are at the net and turn to see if your partner is about to serve, cover your face with the tennis racket.
- Exercise extreme caution in the presence of firearms, including air rifles and shotguns loaded with bird shot. These frequently cause accidents leading to blindness.
- Avoid fights. Blows to the eye frequently cause blindness.

Take Care of Your General Health

- Don't neglect diabetes, high blood pressure, and blood diseases, all of which can cause blindness.
- Eat a well-balanced diet.
- Avoid excessive exposure to strong sunlight. Wear dark sunglasses on the beach or over the water, and a cap or hat with a large brim.

Have Your Eyes Examined Periodically

- You cannot tell whether you have glaucoma by how you feel. Your ophthalmologist can advise you how often to be checked, depending on your age and condition.

Seek an Eye Examination in the Presence of New Symptoms

- If your vision is blurred, if your eyes become red or painful, or if you see halos or a cut in your visual field, make an appointment to have your eyes thoroughly examined without delay. Your symptoms may amount to nothing, but rapid diagnosis and treatment can save your eyes if a disease is present.
- Improperly fitted glasses will not do physical damage to your eyes but they can be very disturbing to comfortable seeing. Remember that vision changes with time and that glasses that served well in the past may need updating of the prescription for efficient vision.

CATARACTS

Often a patient with failing vision will say with dread, "Doctor, I hope it's not a cataract." The fear is not justified. Of the common causes of failing vision, it is cataract that affords the best chance for dramatic improvement.

Cataract is a loss of transparency of the lens of the eye. Parts of the lens become opaque and shut out light. Ultimately, the entire lens may become opaque, but this is rarely permitted to happen today. Cataracts vary a great deal in their rate of progression and their imperceptible, moderate, or severe impairment of vision.

Who gets cataracts? Everybody who lives long enough. It takes 90 or more years for some people to develop significant cataracts, but only 40 years for others. Causes are mysterious. There are congenital forms of cataract, and other forms hastened by injuries and internal inflammations of the eye. Diabetics are especially prone to cataracts. But by far the most common variety is *senile cataract,* which does not at all imply an infirm mind, but an association with aging. Some researchers suspect that excessive exposure to bright sunlight helps predispose to cataract.

The Aging Lens

We have already incriminated the lens of the human eye as the villain that forces us into bifocals or reading glasses. The same lens is the culprit in cataracts. One can think of cataracts as extensions of changes in the lens that begin to make small print hard to read around age 40.

The lens continues to grow throughout life, becoming larger, more rounded, and heavier. Onion-like layers in a confined space compress the nucleus or center of the lens, making it denser and harder. Cataracts are a normal part of the aging process, although stresses and other factors undoubtedly play some part. Nearly all persons over 65 have some detectable opacities in their lenses, though many are not in the least troubled. The 300,000-odd patients a year who have cataract surgery are mostly over 60.

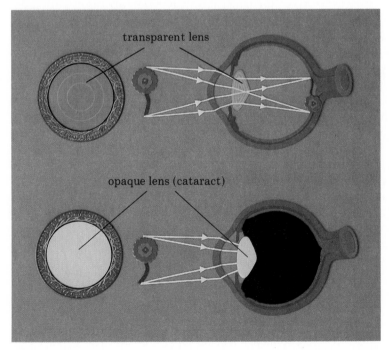

transparent lens

opaque lens (cataract)

CATARACT

The normal crystalline lens of the eye (top drawing) is perfectly transparent, permitting light to reach the retina without impediment to give a clear image, as of a flower. Below, opacities in a lens shut out light like a dirty windowpane. Light waves from a flower reach the lens normally but are partially or completely stopped there so that a fuzzy image or no image at all is received by the retina. Effects on vision vary with the extent and location of cataracts. Opacities at the edge of the lens may not impair vision at all, but those near the center interfere with direct vision. Close vision may be blurred, while distant vision is good, or vice versa.

Symptoms

Some cataracts have no effect on vision. They may be discovered by the doctor who, after dilating the pupils to get a good view, observes opacities in the outer edge of the lens, too far from the center to impair eyesight. With luck, the opacities may remain there for years. A considerate practitioner would probably not alarm the patient unnecessarily by mentioning them.

The extent and location of cataracts in the lens have different effects on vision. Opacities in or near the center of the lens blur direct vision. A patient may be greatly dazzled by bright lights. Vision may be better in subdued light than bright because dilated pupils allow more light to enter. Distance vision may be good but the near image is blurred, or vice versa.

"Second sight." Quite often, someone who has had to wear glasses to read newsprint is able to throw them away and read with his bare eyes. This "second sight" may be construed to be a return of youthful powers. Actually it is a sign of cataracts. Nuclear sclerosis increases the focusing power of the lens and makes the eye more nearsighted.

Examinations for Cataract

Lens opacities cannot be dissolved away. The only "cure" for cataracts is surgical removal of the lens. Prior to decisions about surgery, a complete eye examination is necessary. Abnormalities of the eye—uncontrolled glaucoma, retinal detachment, corneal disease, and other conditions—may make surgery inadvisable. Will cataract surgery improve the patient's vision? In judging the probable outcome, the quality of the patient's vision before cataracts developed is considered as well as the general health of the eye. Intact color vision is a good sign. It indicates that the macula is in good shape and that this important area of the retina should continue to function well after surgery.

The doctor will want to know something about the general health of the patient. Does he or she suffer from diabetes, high blood pressure, or debilitating illness? These should be treated and controlled before the operation is performed.

Infection of the conjunctiva, tear sac, or eyelids must be eliminated, or the eye could be damaged from infection. Sometimes the doctor will order an antiseptic soap to be used on the face several times a day for a week before operation. And often he will prescribe antibiotic or sulfa drugs for a few days to a week before.

Decisions About Surgery

Diagnosis of cataract does not necessarily lead to immediate surgery. The health of the eye, the patient's personal wishes, occupation, age, and intolerance or acceptance of handicap are pertinent factors. There is little possibility that cataracts can cause other diseases of the eye. In rare instances, an overripe or hypermature cataract can cause ocular inflammation or glaucoma.

A retired farmer or housewife or gardener to whom reading has never been very important may be quite comfortable with impaired vision that still permits him or her to walk safely and get around socially. On the other hand, a seamstress, accountant, or writer who must read a lot and see things close up will not long tolerate a visual handicap that threatens his or her job and life-style. Generally, cataracts are extracted when vision is reduced to a level that the patient cannot accept.

The patient should have some understanding of what to expect after cataract surgery so he will not expect vision to be exactly the same as in youth. The eye after surgery has no lens of its own; learning to see with artificial substitutes is described elsewhere (see page 358).

Must cataracts "ripen?" In the past, cataracts were usually extracted by the extracapsular method (the capsule is a membranous structure that envelops the lens, something like plastic wrap). The capsule was opened and the firm substance of the lens pressed out of it. This technique depended on opacification of most of the lens, which was then considered to be "ripe" or mature. Otherwise there was no firm nucleus of the lens to express and too much lens substance would remain if an attempt were made. Ripening took a long time and patients often waited for years, while their vision was seriously impaired, until the cataract was mature enough for surgery.

Today, the intracapsular technique is used. The entire cataract is removed in the capsule, leaving no lens material behind. It is no longer necessary to delay surgery because a cataract is not mature. Patients can be operated on as soon as their vision is sufficiently blurred.

Can cataract surgery be postponed? If one eye retains reasonably good vision, patients frequently elect to defer surgery on the poorer eye. While this gives a respite, it may lead to one of two undesirable situations:

1. Fusion of the two eyes may be lost. The poorer eye may drift in or out, but usually out. Later, if operation plus a contact lens restores vision, the eyes will still not be straight and the patient may complain of double vision.

2. The cataract may overripen, becoming swollen with mushy contents that may leak through the capsule, causing internal inflammation, glaucoma, or both. If this occurs, removal of the cataract becomes an emergency, made technically difficult by the inflammation and the fragile swollen cataract.

On the other hand, a nuclear cataract may blur distance vision without impairing closeup reading. An elderly patient who no longer drives a car or goes out to work may enjoy television and reading for years before needing surgery.

Cataract Operations

If you are scheduled for cataract surgery, you will be admitted to the hospital a day before the operation. Laboratory tests are often done before admission, since any abnormality that may be found could be managed better than if it were discovered a day before surgery. A thorough physical examination also is done. Some doctors prefer to have the eyelashes trimmed so they will not get in the way or touch the instruments, while others feel that this is unnecessary.

Classical or "standard" operation. The patient's face is "prepped" with soap and antiseptic solutions, then wiped clean. The face and body are covered with sterile drapes, leaving only the eye exposed. Heart beat, blood pressure, and respiration are monitored during the operation. While a glucose solution is running into the patient's vein, an anesthetist stands by to administer additional sedatives or needed medications into the vein during the operation. Oxygen is usually piped to the nostrils through plastic tubes.

Anesthetic drops are started in the operating room and then two injections of a local anesthetic are given. One is given on the side of the face to block the facial nerve. This temporarily paralyzes the muscles used to squeeze or close the eye. The other is given into the socket of the eye, entering below on the side away from the nose. Not only does this numb the eye, but it renders the patient unable to rotate or see with it for an hour or two.

The patient can hear what is going on and may even exchange words with the surgeon. More often he drowses through the operation because he has been sedated; there is no discomfort beyond the pinprick of the anesthetic injection. Knowing what to expect can make a patient much more relaxed and cooperative.

Some patients, however, are so fearful that no amount of explanation will relax them. For such patients, general anesthesia may be preferable. In the past, there was some hesitation to operate for cataract under general anesthesia because patients were often restless and vomited after the operation. Today, newer general anesthetics allow the patient to awake quickly and comfortably, and many of the old objections are no longer valid. In some hospitals, most cataracts are operated on under general anesthetics, while in others the local anesthetic is still preferred.

Extracting the cataract. The classical intracapsular cataract operation requires an incision of about 150 degrees in the upper part of the eye, just at the border of the cornea where it meets the white sclera. Through this opening the lens will be removed.

A small part of the iris also is removed to assure proper circulation of fluid within the eye after surgery. Afterward, the pupil will be perfectly round, but on close scrutiny a tiny black V-shaped hole can be seen at the top of the iris. In some cases it is necessary to make a larger vertical hole through the iris *(sector iridectomy)* and the shape of the pupil then resembles a keyhole. Sutures are placed ready for tying later.

An instrument called a *cryoprobe* is generally used to pull the lens out of the eye. The cryoprobe is a pencil-shaped device with an extremely cold tip that is touched to the cataract. The effect is somewhat like touching the tongue to cold metal on a subzero day. The parts freeze together. The surgeon gently teases the adherent lens out of the eye, endeavoring not to break the delicate capsule. Delivery of the lens may take several minutes during which it is especially important that the patient not move his head.

Pre-placed sutures are pulled up and tied, and additional sutures are placed. In the old days only two or three sutures were used, in contrast to the five to seven or even more used today.

The entire operation takes about half an hour. If both eyes are to be operated on, a recovery interval of a few days is allowed between operations.

Phacoemulsification. This impressive word describes a newer technique for cataract extraction that many patients have heard or read about. Its appeal is that only a very small incision requiring a single stitch is necessary, allowing complete activity in a very short time, even immediate return home from the hospital.

Through a three- or four-millimeter incision, the lens nucleus is dislocated into the front chamber of the eye through an incision of the capsule. Then a probe that oscillates 40,000 times a second is inserted to chew up and suck out the fragments. Most of the cataract is removed, but a small amount and some of the capsule usually remain. It is often necessary to make an opening in the capsule, either at the end of the operation or at a second admission to the hospital.

This technique requires expensive instruments and special training. The operation itself is technically more difficult than the conventional operation and the number of surgeons who get consistently good results is not great. Also, it is not suitable for all cases of cataract. If the cataract is very dense and hard, if the chamber of the eye is shallow, or if the pupil cannot be fully dilated, the operation is contraindicated because of the risk of complications.

Like conventional cataract surgery, phacoemulsification has its risks and limitations. It is not a cure-all, and judgment as to the best procedure for a particular patient is best left to the surgeon.

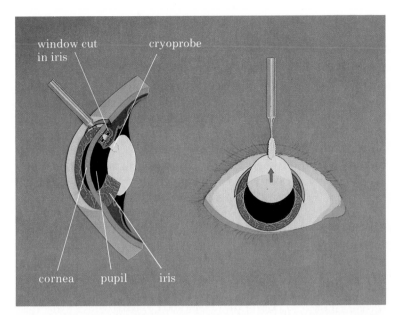

window cut in iris   cryoprobe

cornea   pupil   iris

THE CATARACT OPERATION

In the classical operation for cataract, an incision at the upper border of the cornea provides an opening through which the lens will be extracted. A small part of the iris is removed. Usually the lens is pulled gently out of the eye with a cryoprobe, a pencil-like device with an extremely cold tip that "freezes" firmly to the lens.

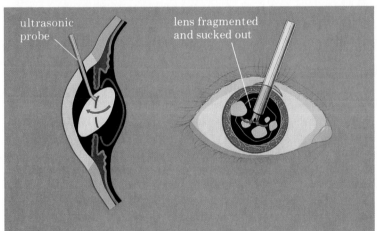

ultrasonic probe

lens fragmented and sucked out

PHACOEMULSIFICATION

Through a small scleral incision, the lens capsule is cut and the lens nucleus is delivered into the front chamber of the eye. An ultrasonic probe with irrigating and suction connections is then inserted to break the lens substance into fragments and suck out the emulsion.

Can my cataract grow back? When a cataract has been removed by conventional surgery, it does not grow back. If some capsule is left behind, either deliberately or otherwise, it may sometimes thicken and have to be needled. Fortunately, this is a relatively minor procedure that takes only a few minutes to perform, and requires a short hospital stay.

What if only one eye has cataract? The operation is the same, but the patient will have to wear a contact lens instead of glasses, or have a plastic lens implanted in the space occupied by the removed crystalline lens. This is necessary to equalize the different magnifying powers of the untouched eye and the one operated on.

After the Operation

After surgery, usually only the operated eye is patched and covered with a hard shield. However, the patient will feel more comfortable after the operation if he keeps both eyes gently closed. With the eye securely sutured, the patient may be allowed out of bed later the same day or early the next morning. If absorbable sutures are used, they will not need to be removed as they fall out by themselves or are absorbed. Silk or nylon sutures can be left in as long as they remain buried, but as they work their way to the surface, the surgeon will probably remove them in the office under local drop anesthesia.

If no lens has been implanted, vision without a cataract glass is very poor in the operated eye, about sufficient for the patient to count fingers. Light will seem brighter and more bluish because the light-filtering lens is gone. "Loaner" cataract glasses for temporary use can be worn a day or so after the operation if the other eye has very poor vision. It is important that the patient learn to get around with glasses before the second eye is operated on for cataract.

Hospital stay. Length of stay in the hospital after surgery varies with the surgeon and local practice. Most patients go home in four days. However, some fine doctors let their patients out of the hospital in two or three days. In some communities, cataract surgery is done on an outpatient basis.

The trend to shorter stays comes from the high cost of hospitalization and an effort to compete with the short stays allowed by newer cataract operations such as phacoemulsification. But while it is gratifying to get home soon, in the long run the patient's improved vision makes the length of hospital stay fade from memory.

It is advisable to wear a hard shield over the operated eye during sleep for the first six to eight weeks. During the day the patient wears his own glasses with a black tape or occluder over the lens for the operated eye. This protects the eye against bright light, which can be disturbing because the pupil is kept dilated by drops for the first few weeks. The drops keep the eye at rest, much as a splint keeps a sprained limb at rest. Sometimes steroid drops are also given to quiet some of the postoperative inflammatory reaction.

Back to work. While the patient is waiting for the eye to heal, there is no reason why he cannot watch television; it will not harm the eyes. Reading involves prolonged jerky movements of the eyes and may cause discomfort, but scanning of mail and light material can be done to the limit of comfort.

With multiple sutures of the eye, there is no reason why a patient in a sedentary occupation cannot spend a few hours a day at work almost immediately after coming home. Most patients feel better if they ease into work in a month or so. And if the activity requires heavy lifting, stooping, and straining, it is best not resumed until two months after operation.

How the World Looks After Cataract Extraction

Removal of a cataract does not restore vision completely to normal. It substitutes a minor handicap for a truly major one. Removing a cataract makes the eye very farsighted, so that it needs a strong convex lens to help focus light rays on the retina. This may be a spectacle lens, a contact lens, or a plastic lens implant.

Permanent cataract glasses can be fitted two months or more after surgery. The lens will be thicker and heavier than an ordinary lens, and objects seen through it will look magnified—about one-third larger than in normal vision. This makes things look closer than they are. The new glasses will cause you to bump into things, knock over glasses of water, reach short of objects, and step too high for stairs.

Also, there will be a ring-shaped blind zone surrounding the objects viewed. In a living room, another person may disappear, then reappear like a jack-in-the-box. Misjudgment of distance requires one to learn to walk and use a knife and fork all over again. Most people learn to manage—and how much better that is than not seeing at all!

Today most cataract lenses are molded in plastic on a corrected curve known as "aspheric." Aspheric curves reduce the blur and distortion when the eye looks off-center. Lightweight aspheric plastic lenses are greatly superior to the heavy glass lenses of the past.

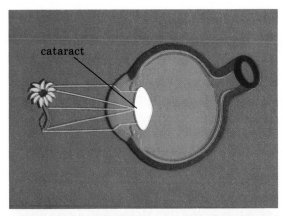

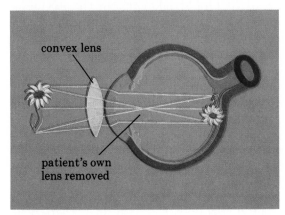

AFTER CATARACT SURGERY

Before cataract extraction, opacities of the lens obstruct, to varying degrees, the transmission of light to the retina. The lower drawing shows the eye after its lens has been removed. The light-bending (refractive) power of the missing lens is lacking, so the image falls behind the retina and the eye is very farsighted.

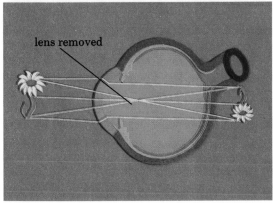

CATARACT GLASSES

Farsightedness after cataract surgery is corrected by a strong convex lens (contact lens or glasses) that brings the image into sharp focus. Persons who were previously nearsighted may not need strong correction and their glasses may be relatively thin.

The trick in wearing cataract glasses is always to look through the center of the lens. When looking up, down, or to the side one should turn the head and not the eye. Thus one always looks through the clear center of the lens.

Once a person learns to wear cataract glasses, he or she may drive a car, sew, read, and watch television as much as desired. Persons who were very nearsighted before cataract surgery may be pleasantly surprised to find that they now take a weak, thin lens. The farsightedness created by removal of the cataract neutralizes the nearsightedness. The retinal image is larger so the patient may enjoy better vision than he has ever had.

Persons who were very farsighted will become even more so. Their new glasses will be very strong, thick, and difficult to learn to use, and these patients will do better with contact lenses.

Frames. Because of its great strength, the effective power of a cataract glass varies with its distance from the eye. A little closer to or a little farther from the eye, vision is less sharp. Therefore the prescription specifies the distance from the eye when the trial lens was fitted. If this distance is not exact in the finished glasses, vision will be less satisfactory than it should be. Either an adjustment of the frame or a change in the power of the lens will be necessary. Some optical companies will make a lens change at a small charge if done within six months. And the stronger the cataract glass, the more likely such an adjustment will be necessary.

Cataract Contact Lenses

Contact lenses (see page 342) have special advantages after cataract surgery. Contact lenses magnify the retinal image only 5 to 8 percent, which is negligible compared to the 25 to 35 percent magnification of cataract glasses.

If one eye is normal and the other has had cataract extraction, a contact lens is almost imperative. Images from the normal and the operated eye fitted with a contact lens are close enough in size so that the brain can blend them for stereoscopic vision. The much larger image from cataract glasses, however, gives such a disparity in size, with double vision, that the brain cannot successfully fuse or tolerate the competing images.

Side vision with a contact lens also is much better than with a spectacle lens. In fact, the field of vision is almost normal, and there is no doughnut-shaped blind area. And a contact lens is not conspicuous. For reading, a thin spectacle lens with bifocal correction can be worn over the contact lens, rather than the thick cataract lens.

There are possible disadvantages, however. One is that it takes time and patience to adapt to contact lenses, which at first feel like foreign bodies in the eye, and their care is more fussy. Another disadvantage is that some elderly patients may be too unsteady, uncoordinated, or unmotivated to go through the daily ritual of inserting and removing contact lenses. A steady hand is necessary, and someone in the wearer's family may provide it, after a bit of instruction. But if a person is perfectly satisfied with cataract glasses, there is no reason to push contacts.

Although contact lenses often excite initial apprehension in cataract patients, their success rate is actually the highest of all contact lens wearers. Persons who go to work or actively pursue a hobby adapt most successfully.

Intraocular Lenses

A small but increasing number of surgeons are implanting an artificial plastic lens or "pseudophacos" before closing the incision. This has the advantage of creating a normal-sized retinal image without the use of a contact lens. There may be a residual refractive error, which can be corrected by a spectacle lens.

Many different models of artificial lenses have been tried over the past 25 years, only to be discarded because of complications resulting from their use. Recently the success rate has improved tremendously, but the procedure remains more difficult and tricky than the conventional operation. The long-term effects of introducing a plastic lens within the eye are uncertain, so many surgeons will not implant one into a young patient, or into more than one eye in an older patient.

Such lenses could be especially helpful to persons too uncoordinated or feeble to fumble with glasses or contact lenses, or to those who wish to appear not to need any help with their vision.

RETINA AND VITREOUS

Cataracts and glaucoma involve fairly accessible structures at the front part of the eye. The "back half" of the eyeball—more than half, really—has different structures subject to different disorders that can affect vision.

The many-layered, exquisitely thin retina is supported at its back side by the choroid; its front side is kept flat by gentle pressure from the *vitreous* humor. The vitreous, which is a transparent jellylike substance very much like the gelatin we have for dessert, fills the posterior chamber. You may have noticed that when gelatin stands in a mold for a few weeks, it shrinks. So does the vitreous degenerate, shrink, and become more fluid with age.

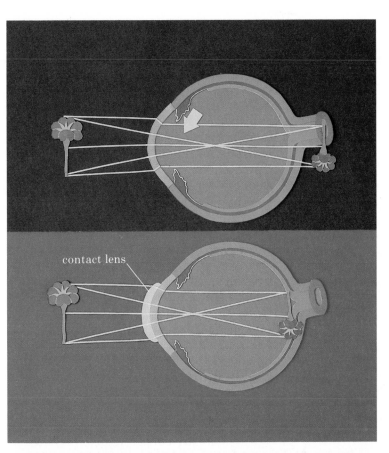

CONTACT LENS

The yellow area shows where a cataractous lens was removed, resulting in farsightedness. An external lens will be needed to bring objects into sharp focus. In contrast to cataract glasses, which greatly enlarge the image and restrict side vision, a contact lens gives an almost normally wide field of vision with negligible magnification.

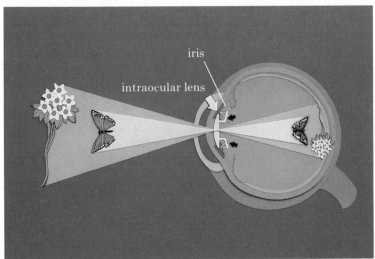

INTRAOCULAR LENS

The drawing shows an intraocular lens (white arrow), which is an artificial plastic lens implanted in the space formerly occupied by the natural lens. The intraocular lens is sutured permanently to the iris. Distant objects (flowers) can be seen clearly, but close objects (butterfly) fall short of the retina and are blurred. The intraocular lens cannot change focus for distant and near vision; close seeing will require glasses.

Flashes and floaters. "Floaters" are seen as floating spots or threads, most annoying when looking at a bright background such as the sky or a sheet of white paper. Cells and strands of tissue in the vitreous cast shadows on the retina and move with eye movements. Floaters are quite common, especially in very nearsighted eyes, and may persist for years. Sometimes they fall out of the line of sight and become less annoying, or one learns to live with them.

Patients over 40 may notice momentary lightning flashes in one eye. Typically, they see a flash of light in a dark place when they move the eye or head. This happens when the shrinking vitreous tugs at the retina wherever it is attached to it. The retina has no pain sense, and a tug on it is perceived as a flash of light.

If the tugging pulls a particle away from the retina, the fragment floats in the vitreous and is seen as a dark shadow against a bright background. Sometimes a shower of floaters occurs. Occasionally, tugging by the vitreous will tear a small hole in the retina, leading sometimes, but not always, to retinal detachment. Patients with light flashes should be examined at intervals for retinal tears and detachment.

Detached Retina

If you think of the eye as a room, the retina can be thought of as wallpaper. If the paper starts to peel away from the wall, it is analogous to retinal detachment. The peeled-loose sheet of the retina cannot "see" anything.

Early symptoms of retinal detachment are flashes of light and floating spots, followed by blurring in one area of the field of vision. If you notice when you look at a person's face with one eye that part of the face is blurred or missing, hasten at once to an ophthalmologist. An untreated retinal detachment will usually progress to total detachment and blindness.

If the detachment is diagnosed and treated before the macula has peeled off, it is often possible to save central detailed vision. Once the macula has peeled off, even if the retina is reattached, vision may not be fully restored.

In the past ten years, new techniques for treating retinal detachment have revolutionized the field, and have dramatically improved the results. Laser beams and other advanced techniques are used to seal tears and get retinal tissue back in place. Hospital stays are relatively short, very different from the old days when patients with retinal detachment often had to lie for weeks with the head kept immovable between sandbags.

New techniques are so sophisticated that a subspecialty of retinal surgery has developed. Many ophthalmologists feel that a patient is best off in the hands of someone with special training in exacting retinal surgery.

Diabetic Retinopathy

Diabetes can cause sudden blurring of vision in several ways. Any sudden large change in blood sugar will cause blurring. If the blood sugar suddenly rises several hundred points, the eyes will become nearsighted. On the other hand, a diabetic who has been running a very high blood sugar and starts vigorous treatment that drops the blood sugar several hundred points will suddenly become very farsighted and unable to read.

In patients who have had diabetes for ten years or more, changes called *diabetic retinopathy* may begin in the retina. Little coils of blood vessels called microaneurysms may develop. There may be retinal hemorrhages, inflammatory deposits called soft exudates, or waxy deposits called hard exudates.

If the hemorrhages damage the macula, vision may fail suddenly. Occasionally the hemorrhage may break into the vitreous, filling the cavity of the eye. This is gradually absorbed, but new vessels grow into the vitreous and bleed again. Scar tissue that forms in the vitreous may cause it to shrink, pulling the retina into the vitreous and detaching it.

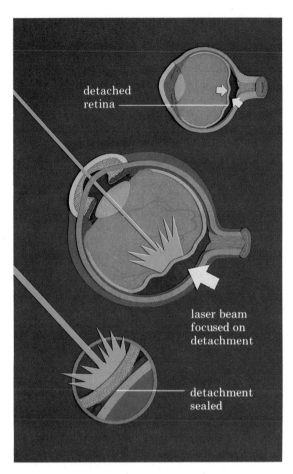

DETACHED RETINA

The most frequent cause of a detached retina is a hole or tear in the exquisitely thin tissue that permits vitreous humor to seep through and separate the retina (yellow arrow) from its underlying choroid layer (white arrow). Dramatic advances in surgical and other techniques have made it possible to reattach the retina successfully in most cases, if treatment is prompt. One technique, shown schematically in the drawings, employs a precisely focused laser beam to seal the detached retina to the choroid (large white arrow), something like a welding operation.

In its early stages, diabetic retinopathy can sometimes be treated by photocoagulating blood vessels that tend to leak. Encouraging results have been obtained from the use of an argon laser beam, which is used to burn and destroy weak new blood vessels in the eye before they have a chance to hemorrhage.

Massive hemorrhage into the vitreous may occur from rupture of new blood vessels that have grown along fibrous bands which are the end stage of a previous hemorrhage. This can become a vicious cycle.

In the past, the management of massive vitreous hemorrhage was expectant. One had to wait patiently for the hemorrhage to undergo spontaneous absorption. This might take six to twelve months, or forever. And meanwhile, more new vessel formation might be expected.

Recently, a new operation called vitrectomy has made it possible to remove most of the vitreous, and with it the blood, replacing it with clear saline. This might improve the vision dramatically. The vitreous is removed through an instrument that cuts it off in small chunks, sucks it out, and replaces it simultaneously with saline. Surprisingly, it has been found that the eye can get along quite nicely without vitreous.

Vitrectomy has made it possible to salvage eyes formerly considered hopeless, such as an eye filled with blood after penetration by birdshot. Now the bloody vitreous can be removed, and an attempt can be made to remove the birdshot under direct visualization using special tiny forceps to grasp the pellets.

Fluorescein Angiography

A newer tool for study of disorders of the retina, such as diabetic retinopathy and many others, is fluorescein angiography. A fluorescent dye is rapidly injected into an arm vein. As this dye reaches the retinal blood vessels, a series of pictures taken with blue light documents the passage of the dye through the retinal arteries, and then the veins and capillaries. Leaking capillaries, very fine newly growing vessels, tumors, and a number of other conditions can be demonstrated by these studies, which are done on an outpatient basis.

Ultrasound

Another recently developed diagnostic tool is the study of the eye and the orbit, or socket, by very high frequency sound waves, which can take a picture similar to, but often more informative than X rays. Thus, even if the view of the interior of the eye is obstructed by a cataract or hemorrhage, foreign bodies or tumors within the eye can be demonstrated and localized. If the eye is abnormally prominent and bulging, ultrasound studies can show whether the bulge is caused by a tumor, by swollen extraocular muscles from thyroid disease, or by a diffuse swelling of the soft tissues of the orbit.

Computerized Axial Tomography

A new technique, rather formidably called computerized axial tomography, uses computer technology to intensify many times the minuscule difference in resistance to passage of X rays by different soft tissues, so they can be demonstrated on film. Thus while conventional X rays show all soft tissues of the eye to be the same, a computerized scan outlines the crystalline lens from its surrounding aqueous humor, which has almost the same specific gravity. It can show a tumor of the choroid, normally invisible to X rays.

The scan can outline a slice only eight millimeters thick through the eye, orbit, and brain, and more recent models can outline a slice just three millimeters thick. The device has made it less necessary to use expensive, more risky, and time-consuming techniques requiring hospitalization for injection of contrast media such as air or radiopaque dyes. These used to be necessary to provide sufficient contrast to demonstrate structures of the eye, socket, and brain by conventional X rays. Now the necessary contrast is delineated and intensified by the computer.

Macular Degeneration

The macula, the tiny area of the retina responsible for sharp detailed vision, may be damaged gradually or suddenly. This impairs the ability to read small print but does not affect ability to get around. Most patients with macular degeneration can be assured that even though they cannot see fine details, they will not go blind, and will be able to move about and attend to their personal needs. Often they can be helped to read with magnifiers.

BIG & LITTLE EYE TROUBLES

Numerous symptoms can be manifested in the eyes. Some are mere nuisances; others are of more serious portent. It is important not to delay reporting any symptoms to your doctor. Often he can give peace of mind by explaining that some frightening manifestation—for instance, flickering, expanding, zigzag flashes that occasionally appear in the field of vision—is not a sign of eye disease and very rarely of any serious trouble.

Watery Eyes

Watery eyes can result from loss of tissue tone in aging. Another cause is obstruction of the duct from the eye into the nose. One of the first things an eye doctor may do is to irrigate the passages with salt water to see if tears will pass through into the nose.

Tears are secreted by the lachrymal gland in the upper outside corner of the eye socket. They collect in two fine ducts at the inner corner of the eye and empty into a sac that drains through a long duct into the nose. Normally, every time we blink we activate a pump that sucks tears into the sac. As we age, the eyelids relax and the tear-pump becomes less efficient. Tears accumulate in the eyes, especially in a cold wind. This is annoying but not serious.

If tear drainage is persistently blocked, pus can form in the tear sacs and bathe the surface of the eye. This is potentially dangerous because any injury to or operation on the eyeball could lead to serious infection and even loss of an eye. An operation connecting the tear sac with the nose will usually restore tear drainage, and with it the infection disappears. The constant flushing of the passages by fresh tears washes away the infection.

Eyelids. Occasionally, in older persons, the lower eyelid may turn in on itself *(entropion),* allowing the lashes to rub against and irritate the eye. If the condition persists it may require surgical correction. The opposite condition occurs if the lower lid loses its tone and sags away from the eye *(ectropion).* Persons with ectropion often have watery eyes because the opening of the lower tear duct no longer communicates with the overflowing pool of tears at the inner corner of the eye. This too can be corrected surgically by a relatively minor operation.

Dry eyes. Tears are important. They keep sensitive surfaces from drying out. Sometimes the protective film of tears is defective and does not cling to the eye as it should. It may run off too quickly and leave dry spots that feel sandy, gritty, and most uncomfortable. In such cases, artificial tears are helpful. These are eye drops formulated so they cling to the eye. Numerous preparations are on the market and may be bought over the counter, as they are quite bland.

Zigzag Scintillations

One's first experience with *scintillating scotoma* is likely to be strange and alarming. A sort of visual fireworks begins in a spot so tiny that it is hardly noticed until it grows larger and larger as it expands toward the outside of the field of vision. One sees a zigzag, lightning-like pattern of flickering brilliance that typically has a circumference of about a quarter circle. The display moves outward from the nose until it disappears in 15 to 30 minutes. Often it is colored—red, yellow, blue.

The shimmering pattern can be seen with both eyes open, with both eyes closed, or with one eye open and the other closed. The eyes have nothing to do with it; the "seeing" takes place in the part of the brain concerned with vision. The cause is a spasm of blood vessels that produces temporary anemia in that part of the brain. Later, the spastic vessels relax and may stretch enough to cause nausea and migraine headache. But often there is no headache—in fact, the condition is sometimes called "migraine without a headache." Rarely is there any serious portent, and certainly the eyes are not involved. The blood pressure should also be checked, as often it is high.

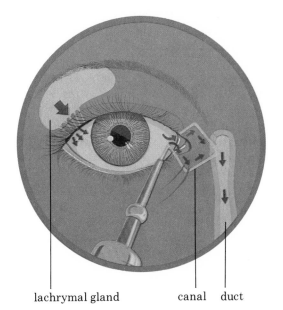

lachrymal gland   canal duct

WATERY EYES

Distressing wateriness of the eyes may come from dammed-up drainage of tears or lax tissues that allow a pool of tears to overflow the eyelid. Tears normally flow from the lachrymal gland, across the eye (black arrows), and through the lachrymal canal and duct to drain through the nose. The drawing shows the technique of flushing clogged lachrymal canals. A syringe placed in the conjunctival sac flushes antibacterial medication into the lachrymal canal and duct.

Xanthelasma

Yellowish fatty plaques may develop in the skin of the eyelids. They can be removed if desired, but may recur. In any case, they do not harm the eyes, but suggest an impaired ability of the body to handle fats and cholesterol (a trait that sometimes runs in families). Presence of such plaques, called *xanthelasma,* should prompt one to have blood studies for fat and cholesterol. If levels are abnormally high, medical treatment may lessen the risk of heart attack.

The Red Eye

Some causes for a red eye are trivial and unimportant. Others are serious and threaten vision. It is hard for a layman to tell which is which, and a red eye is usually good reason to seek a professional examination. It is sometimes impossible to know why an eye is red until it is examined under the slit lamp and corneal microscope.

Subconjunctival hemorrhage. A frequent cause for a red eye is a small hemorrhage under the membrane covering the white part of the eye. This is seen as a sudden red blotch that appears overnight on the white of the eye. There may be a slight sticking sensation, but usually there is no pain. The blotch is caused by the leaking of a brittle blood vessel that tends to spread and get larger until it is absorbed in three or four weeks. The condition is harmless and often occurs in persons who are in good health.

Foreign body; corneal abrasion. A foreign body embedded in the cornea or stuck to the conjunctival membrane will cause redness, watering, and sensitivity to light. A cinder embedded in the cornea will feel as if it is under the upper eyelid—a trick played on us by the nervous system.

If you suspect that a particle is stuck to the surface of the eye and you cannot see a doctor right away, someone can inspect your eye for a foreign body. A pocket flashlight helps. If nothing is seen on the eyeball, the particle may be on the undersurface of the upper lid.

To evert the lid, the patient must look down at his feet but must *not* squeeze the eye. The examiner grasps the lashes of the upper lid and with an applicator stick, or even his forefinger, he presses against the middle of the eyelid while pulling down on it. When the lid is turned inside out, any small cinder that is present may be seen stuck to the eyelid's inner surface. If so, a cotton-tipped applicator wet with water can be used to remove it.

A *corneal abrasion* may cause the same symptoms as a foreign body. If no foreign body can be seen, a doctor should examine the patient promptly. But if you know for sure that something has scratched the surface of the cornea, you should seek help quickly even if you have little discomfort. Corneal abrasions are more painful and harder to treat if they become infected. You may then have a corneal ulcer.

Corneal ulcer. The symptoms of corneal ulcer are the same as those for a corneal foreign body or abrasion, but more severe. Any injury of the cornea is dangerous and not suited to do-it-yourself care. This is especially true for a corneal ulcer.

Don't use some antibiotic drops you find in the medicine cabinet to treat your red eye. Your diagnosis may be wrong, and in certain conditions the wrong drops could cost you the sight of the eye. For example, the most common corneal ulcer is caused by the cold sore virus, herpes simplex. If you should happen to use cortisone drops on such an ulcer, it might seem to improve but in fact would be seriously worsening.

Conjunctivitis. Probably the most common cause for a red eye is an infection of the thin conjunctival membrane that lines the lids and covers the white of the eye. Many different organisms can be responsible, as well as allergies to dusts and pollens. Often there is a discharge of mucus or pus, and here again, self-treatment can be hazardous.

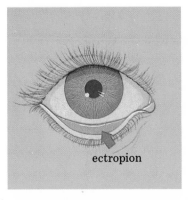

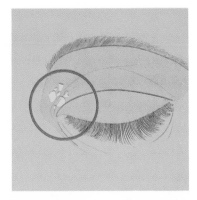

ectropion

ECTROPION

Ectropion is a condition in which the lower eyelid droops away from the eye, collects tears, and prevents them from draining through normal channels.

XANTHELASMA

Xanthelasma is not a disease of the eyes, but yellowish raised patches on the eyelids, associated with disturbed metabolism of fats and cholesterol.

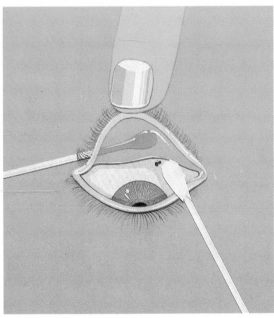

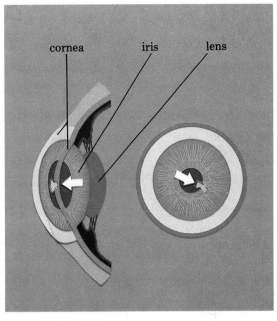

cornea   iris   lens

SPECK IN THE EYE

To remove a cinder from the eye, fold the upper lid inside out over an applicator stick. If a particle is seen, remove it with a cotton-tipped applicator moistened with water.

CORNEAL ULCER

A corneal ulcer may result from infection by the herpes simplex (cold-sore) virus. The drawing shows side and front views of such an ulcer, which can cause serious scarring. Medical care is urgent.

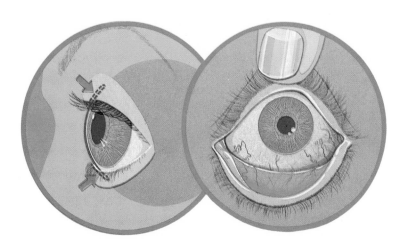

CONJUNCTIVITIS

The conjunctiva is a thin membrane that covers the inside of the eyelids, the cornea, and the white of the eye (green arrows). Allergies, infections, irritants, and many other things can inflame the conjunctiva, giving the eye a bloodshot appearance. The cause should be determined.

Iritis. As the name suggests, iritis is an inflammation of the colored part of the eye. It causes severe pain in or above the eye, brow ache, sensitivity to bright light, and a red watery eye. Usually it is impossible to recognize an early case of iritis without examining the eye under the slit lamp and corneal microscope.

In iritis, the eye is soft and internal fluid pressure is low. The condition is treated with drops such as atropine that dilate the pupil and put the eye at rest. If the red eye were caused by glaucoma, pupil-dilating drops could make matters much worse instead of better, hence the importance of diagnosis in treating a red painful eye.

Glaucoma. This serious threat to vision has been discussed at length (see page 346). Here let us say only that a sudden rise of pressure within the eye can cause a red, painful eye that has to be distinguished from other causes. Improper treatment may not only be ineffective, but may make the condition worse.

Optic Neuritis

Inflammation of the optic nerve can cause sudden blurring of vision. Optic neuritis calls for a complete neurological examination to determine whether it is an isolated phenomenon, related to disease elsewhere in the nervous system, or related to a toxin.

The older we get, the less likely it is that optic neuritis will be caused by inflammation, and the more likely that it is related to an impairment of blood supply.

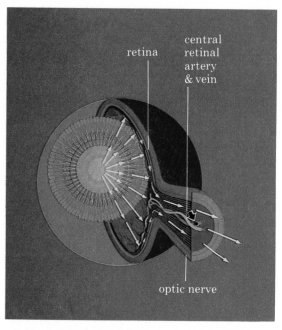

NERVES AND VESSELS

This drawing of the eye shows the optic nerve and blood vessels that supply the retina. Blockage of the central retinal artery (black arrow) stops circulation, so light waves (white arrows) cannot excite nerve cells. Inflammation of the optic nerve can cause sudden blurring of vision.

Blockage of Retinal Vessels

If the central artery supplying the retina is blocked, loss of vision will occur in an instant. This is usually caused by hardening of the arteries, but can result from a particle lodging in the central artery. If treated within hours, circulation can sometimes be restored.

If the central vein or one of its branches is blocked, sudden blurring will occur, but treatment does not usually restore lost vision. Eyes that have suffered this condition are subject to secondary glaucoma and should be watched. Several medications are available that may reduce the agglutinability of the blood platelets and so lessen the tendency for the blood clot to spread. One of these is ordinary aspirin. These may be helpful in an impending vein occlusion that has not yet become total.

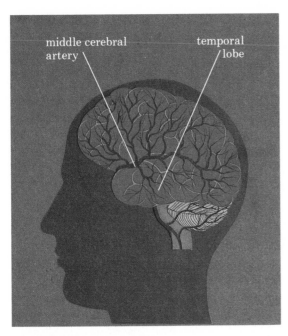

TEMPORAL ARTERITIS

Temporal arteritis seldom occurs before age 60. Inflammation of arteries in the region of the temple can cause boring, intractable headaches lasting for weeks or months and, infrequently, sudden blindness that early diagnosis and treatment can prevent.

Temporal Arteritis

Inflammation of arteries of the brain also can cause blurring of vision. Diagnosis is made by a blood test (sedimentation rate) and by microscopic examination of a biopsy sample of a superficial artery. The condition can be treated by oral cortisone-like drugs.

Blackout Spells

Spells of blurred vision lasting several minutes to several hours deserve investigation. Often they are caused by impaired circulation to the brain.

This is not a hopeless condition and much can be done to help such patients and reduce the likelihood of a stroke. If studies show an obstruction of a carotid artery in the neck, newer surgical techniques can ream out the clogged vessel and improve blood supply to the brain.

Not all spells of blurred vision require such drastic treatment. Some are merely spasm symptoms of arteries supplying the brain.

In the past, the only way such a block of the carotid artery could be demonstrated was to inject radiopaque dye into the artery and take X rays. This is a delicate procedure involving hospitalization, discomfort, and some risk of precipitating a stroke.

Recently, a perfectly safe and painless "non-invasive" test has been under development. Known as "Doppler Studies," these tests determine the speed of moving red blood cells within arteries by bouncing sound waves off them and measuring the wavelength of the returning sounds. It is based on the classic Doppler phenomenon, which makes the pitch of a locomotive horn sound higher as it approaches and lower as it recedes.

Haloes or Rings Around Lights

The normal cornea and crystalline lens of the eye are miraculously constructed to transmit light rays without scattering the light. It does not take much disturbance of either organ to scatter light rays a bit and affect vision.

If fluid pressure within the eye is too great, the cornea swells so that its fibers are not arranged in orderly distortion-free fashion. Swelling of the cornea can also follow injury or chemical irritation such as can be caused by over-chlorinated water in a swimming pool. When the patient looks at a light he sees a halo surrounding it. Similar haloes can be seen if the lens has some imperfections—traces of very early cataract. Haloes around lights do not always mean glaucoma, but they should serve as a signal to visit an eye doctor.

VISION:
TESTS & PROCEDURES

Visual acuity. The familiar eye chart has letters in diminishing sizes. A person with 20/20 vision is able to read at 20 feet what a normal eye should see at 20 feet. A reading of 20/20 does not prove that the eye is free of disease. Near vision is evaluated by reading from a test card with diminishing sizes of type. The lens of the eye in young people is sufficiently flexible to accommodate for near and distant vision without the need for correction with bifocals.

Color vision is tested with special color plates. Defects in color vision that may develop in middle age and beyond may be caused by degenerative changes in the retina, particularly in the macula, which is rich in color receptors. Even in the presence of mature cataract, the eye will usually be able to tell colors and the direction from which a light is shining. If the eye does not have this minimum of vision, some disease of the retina that would make the results of cataract extraction unsatisfactory is suspected. Congenital color blindness is not a disease of the eyes nor does it in any way affect visual acuity.

Visual field. Measurements of ability to see above, below, and to one side of the field of central vision are made with a perimeter or a large black screen called a tangent screen. Among the conditions that restrict the visual field are glaucoma, retinal detachment, stroke, inflammation of the optic nerve, retinal degenerations, and brain tumor. Cataract glasses also restrict peripheral vision, a normal effect that is reduced if contact lenses are worn.

Tonometry. Fluid pressures within the eye can be measured by several methods. A tonometer is an instrument with a weighted plunger that is placed on the eye after it has been numbed by drops. The degree of indentation of the eye measures its softness or hardness. Applanation tonometers measure the force necessary to flatten a small area of the cornea. A computerized electronic tonometer measures the pressure by blowing a puff of air at the cornea and monitoring its flattening. Other electronic tonometers measure pressure by evaluating the reaction of the eye to a quick thrust by a sensor.

Tonography is a specialized technique that measures the resistance of the eye to the outflow of fluid, a reading helpful in eyes suspected of glaucoma. An electronic tonometer rests on the eye for several minutes, while the decrease in ocular pressure caused by the weight of the instrument is recorded on a graph.

Laser coagulation is a technique of welding a torn retina back in place and of obliterating tiny blood vessels by directing an extremely intense and brief burst of parallel light waves at the target.

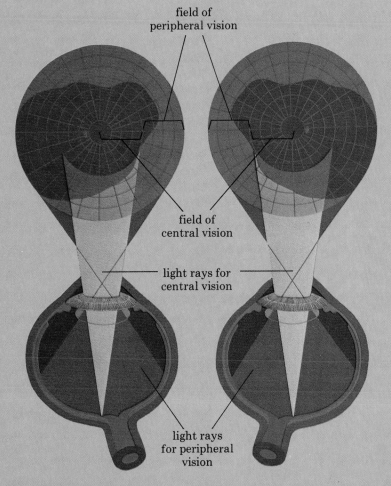

field of
peripheral vision

field of
central vision

light rays for
central vision

light rays
for peripheral
vision

VISUAL FIELD

The visual field of the right eye is shown at far left. The field covers the space seen when the eye is fixed on an object in its direct line of vision. The visual field of the left eye is shown at near left. Both the central fields of detailed vision and the peripheral ("corner-of-the-eye") fields are shown. Blindness in half of each eye can result from obstruction of an artery serving one side of the visual centers in the brain.

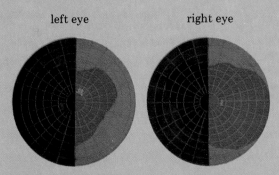

left eye   right eye

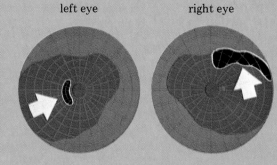

left eye   right eye

IMPAIRED VISUAL FIELDS

The drawing shows the visual fields of a patient who has suffered a stroke from an obstruction (thrombus) of an artery to the visual center on one side of the brain, causing blindness in one half of each eye.

SIGNS OF TROUBLE

Indications of various abnormalities may be discovered from examination of visual fields. Early signs of glaucoma (arrow) appear in the visual field of a left eye. Early signs of a pituitary tumor (arrow) appear in the field of a right eye.

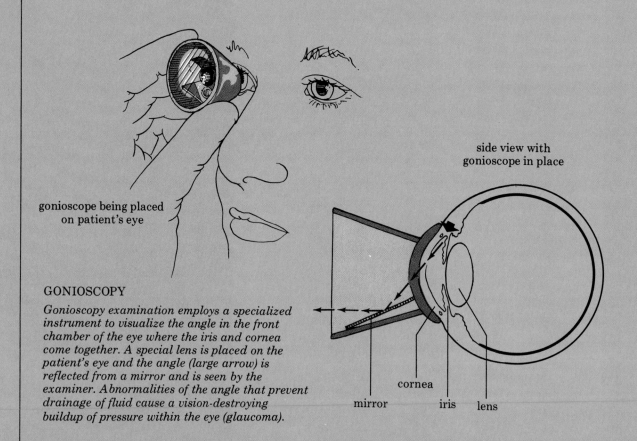

gonioscope being placed
on patient's eye

side view with
gonioscope in place

mirror cornea iris lens

GONIOSCOPY

Gonioscopy examination employs a specialized instrument to visualize the angle in the front chamber of the eye where the iris and cornea come together. A special lens is placed on the patient's eye and the angle (large arrow) is reflected from a mirror and is seen by the examiner. Abnormalities of the angle that prevent drainage of fluid cause a vision-destroying buildup of pressure within the eye (glaucoma).

Gonioscopy. Using a special type of contact lens, often with built-in mirrors, the doctor can look into the hidden angle between the iris and cornea, where fluid drains from the eye, and examine it for adhesions or other abnormalities. The angle is graded for its width, from I to IV. Very narrow angles are capable of closure, which, if it occurred, would then cause an attack of acute glaucoma.

Slit lamp and corneal microscope. This instrument focuses a bright slit of light into the eye where it is viewed with a microscope that magnifies 16 to 32 times. In darkness, this gives the effect of examining a magnified slice through the eye.

Ophthalmoscope. The ophthalmoscope is an instrument for examining the back of the eye (fundus). The doctor holds a *direct* ophthalmoscope in his hand and shines a light into the patient's eye. The light is

reflected from a tiny mirror through an aperture just above it through which the doctor looks (otherwise his head would get in the way of the light). The *binocular indirect* ophthalmoscope is worn on the doctor's head, and resembles a miner's lamp. With it the doctor can see inside the patient's eye with both of his own eyes, thereby getting depth perception. Also, he can see farther out in the peripheral retina than with a direct ophthalmoscope.

Eye drops. The main reason for using pupil-dilating eye drops, even in older people, is to create a larger opening so that internal parts of the eye can be seen as through an open door instead of a keyhole. Drops may also be used as a provocative glaucoma test in the doctor's office, where an acute attack, if elicited, can be controlled. The dilated pupil is quite sensitive to bright light, but this sensitivity wears off in a short while.

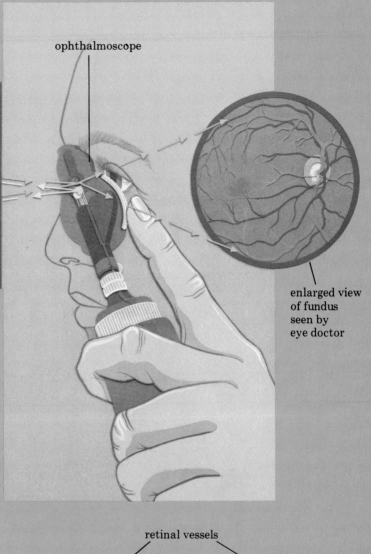

ophthalmoscope

enlarged view
of fundus
seen by
eye doctor

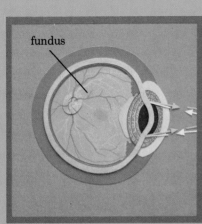

fundus

OPHTHALMOSCOPE

*An ophthalmoscope gives a view
of the deep interior of the eye.
The instrument has a light and a
mirror with a hole in it, through
which the examiner looks. Light
reflected from the mirror (yellow
arrows) illuminates the inside of
the eye and is reflected back
through the hole in the mirror
(green arrows). Lenses of
different power enlarge and
sharpen the observer's view of
the back of the eye (fundus).*

YELLOW SPOT

*The macula lutea, the yellow
spot of the retina, is the point of
clearest vision. Normal macular
and retinal vessels are shown at
right. At far right, degeneration
of the macula blocks out fine
central vision and perception of
colors, but does not impair side
vision. Degeneration results from
deprivation of the blood supply
to the central part of the retina.*

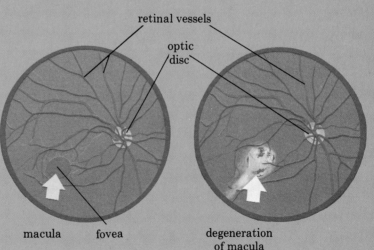

retinal vessels

optic
disc

macula   fovea

degeneration
of macula

CHAPTER **11**   DAVID A. CULP, M.D.
BERNARD FALLON, M.D.

THE OLDER URINARY TRACT

Unlike the heart that throbs, the digestive system that rumbles, and joints that can creak, the genitourinary (GU) tract works in utter silence. Periodically it reminds us, with some urgency, of its excretory function, but in health, that's about all we're aware of.

We are dealing with a system that forms and excretes urine and rids the body of harmful wastes produced in the course of everyday living. The system includes the external genital organs, which give sexual identity and function. The specialist who treats diseases of the tract is a urologist. He differs from some specialists in that he sees a broad range of patients of all ages, from infancy to old age.

The average patient, however, is likely to be middle-aged or older. Particularly, an older man has a high chance of developing some urological disorder. As we grow older, so does the GU tract. Associations with high blood pressure and heart disease may appear; stubborn infections may do damage; growths and obstructions may arise; and genital impediments may occur.

Genitourinary-system ramifications are far-flung, and are a component of the leading causes of death, cardiovascular-renal diseases, the "renal" standing for "kidneys." GU disorders are more common than most people suppose; about 10 percent of admissions to general hospitals are primarily for some urological problem. None is trivial.

Diseases of the tract affect different structures, some of which are as exquisitely delicate and chemically complex as can be found anywhere in the body. These will be identified as various disorders are discussed; however the drawing on page 376 gives a general idea of structures and their principal functions.

THE KIDNEYS

It is our kidneys that enable us to live on dry land. A current belief is that life originated in primeval seas where the external environment provided an abundance of essentials—dissolved salts, minerals, and elements. The transition of life from sea to land required that higher organisms have a working substitute for the abandoned ocean. We have such an environment today—an internal sea of fluids quite similar in composition to ancient oceans—and it is primarily the kidneys that sustain this critical internal environment. The kidneys not only filter wastes out of the blood, but selectively screen and return essential materials to the body.

Anatomy of the kidney. We have two kidneys but could get along very nicely with only one, or indeed with only half a kidney. Some people are born with only one kidney, some have had one removed, and some have one so defective that it cannot function. As long as one good kidney remains, the quality of life and its duration are perfectly normal, and no protective precautions are necessary. The kidney will tend to enlarge and may attain the same functional capacity as the usual set of two.

The kidneys are bean-shaped organs located behind the abdominal cavity just underneath the rib cage. Every day they process about 1,700 quarts of blood (an adult has from 5 to 6 quarts total), which enter through the renal artery and return through the renal vein. The drawing of a cross section of a kidney on page 376 shows its gross structure—a thick mass of maroon-colored tissue curved around a cavity, the *kidney pelvis,* into which urine is funneled via *calyces.*

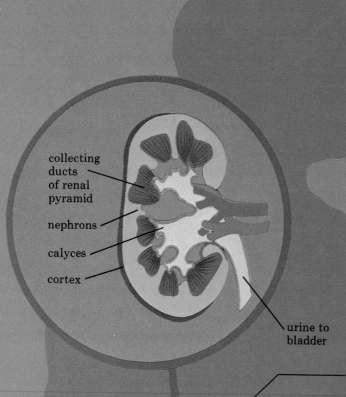

collecting
ducts
of renal
pyramid

nephrons

calyces

cortex

urine to
bladder

KIDNEY STRUCTURE

In the circle, the cross section of a kidney shows its major structures. Nephrons (see opposite page) filter wastes from the blood and return useful materials to it. Wastes are concentrated in urine, which is funneled from collecting ducts to cuplike chambers (calyces) and thence to the ureter, which in turn carries urine to the bladder. The direction of urine flow is shown by arrows. The cortex is the outer layer of the kidney. The kidneys process about 1,700 quarts of blood a day, and produce a quart and a half of urine.

purified blood returns through renal veins

blood input through renal arteries

THE GU TRACT

The genitourinary tract includes the kidneys, bladder and accessory structures, as well as the external genital organs. Blood circulating to the kidneys via the renal arteries is purified and returned via the renal veins. Urine flows to the bladder through slender muscular tubes, the ureters. The urethra is the exit channel from the bladder to the outside. The hormone-producing adrenal glands rest on top of the kidneys but are not part of the GU system.

kidney

ureter

bladder

urethra

The filtration plant. In each kidney, we have upward of a million microscopic filtering units, called *nephrons*. These tightly packed units purify the blood, remove wastes, form urine, deliver it to collecting chambers, and return needed substances to the body.

Under a microscope, an individual nephron is seen to be an intricately convoluted structure with specialized parts. A cup-shaped capsule with double walls partially encircles a ball-shaped network of interlaced capillaries that contain blood to be purified. This tufted network of vessels is called a *glomerulus* ("little ball"). Blood constituents are "pushed" from the capillaries into the space between the double walls of the capsule. The fluid within the walls is called a filtrate. It is very dilute, comprised mostly of water. The kidneys produce about 180 quarts of filtrate a day, out of which about a quart and a half of urine is concentrated.

The capsule is continuous with a kidney *tubule*, which descends, makes a hairpin bend, and meanders in twists and turns until it opens into a collecting chamber or *calyx*. In its course through the tubule, most of the filtrate is reabsorbed and returned to the body along with essential substances. Urine is gradually formed and concentrated from the filtrate and is delivered from the end of the tubule into collecting chambers, thence into the kidney pelvis and down a ureter into the bladder.

Normal urine is a faintly acid, sterile liquid, pale straw to amber in color. *Urinalysis* is one of the most useful and frequent laboratory tests of kidney function and disease lower in the tract, as well as of diseases such as diabetes that are not primarily genitourinary. Study of urinary sediments may reveal particles that shouldn't be there—blood cells, casts, proteins—and help to determine whether trouble lies in the tubules, glomeruli, or elsewhere. Chemical tests can evaluate hormones in the urine, breakdown products of drugs, and other substances that may be significant. Along with the liver, the kidney is a principal excretor of drugs.

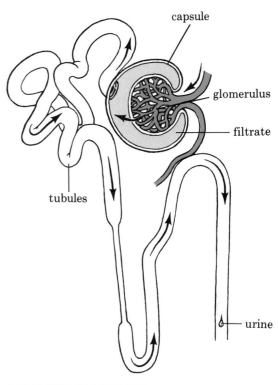

A MARVELOUS FILTER

The working parts of a nephron, the filtration unit of the kidney, are shown above. Constituents of blood from capillaries in the ball-shaped glomerulus are absorbed into the space between the double walls of a surrounding capsule. The content of the capsule, a dilute watery fluid, is called filtrate. Arrows show the flow of filtrate on its long journey through the tubules, which are much longer and more convoluted than shown. As the filtrate moves along, most of it, together with important substances, is reabsorbed, and waste-containing urine is gradually concentrated. Nephrons are densely packed in the curved, maroon-colored mass around the kidney cavity (pelvis). Our paired kidneys contain about two million nephrons. One healthy kidney can easily do the work of two if its companion ceases to function or has to be removed.

Renal Failure

If kidney function declines, there is a steady accumulation of wastes that the body can tolerate up to a certain point. But eventually coma and death may result unless something is done to relieve the pileup of toxic materials that can do serious damage. This state is called renal failure. ("Renal" is a word of Latin origin; words with the prefix "nephr-" derive from the Greek. Both refer to the kidneys.)

The illness accompanying renal failure is *uremia,* a condition in which toxic products accumulate sufficiently to poison the system. There are different degrees of uremia, mild to severe to life-threatening, and acute or chronic. Underlying renal disease may cause no symptoms for a long time, other than vague feelings of tiredness and lack of energy. Progressive uremia evinces such symptoms as headache, lassitude, poor appetite, itchiness, nausea, vomiting, and even convulsive seizures and eventual coma.

There are various causes of kidney failure; probably the most frequent is renal infection. Second to this is *glomerulonephritis,* an allergy-like reaction to infection that causes inflammatory changes in the glomeruli as well as in capillaries elsewhere in the body. Other causes are circulatory diseases, severe diabetes, polycystic disease, and prolonged obstruction of the drainage system.

Diagnosis with good medical care can do much to prevent insidious kidney damage by correcting repairable conditions, controlling infections, and removing any obstructions.

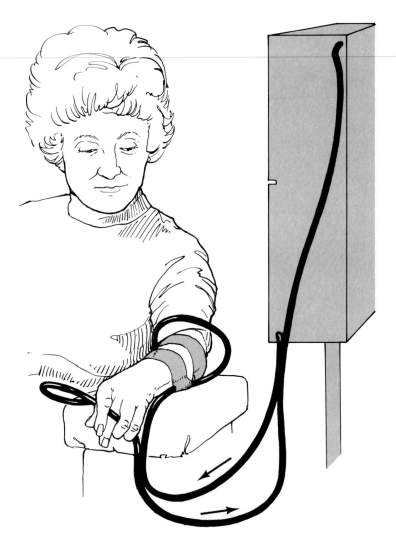

ARTIFICIAL KIDNEYS

Dialysis is a way of purifying blood by circulating it through a machine that exposes blood to fluids that absorb toxic substances and then returns purified blood to the body. Dialysis can be carried out comfortably at home or in dialysis centers. Connections (arteriovenous shunt) are made inside the wrist for easy plugging-in of tubes. Arrows show the flow of blood from an artery to the machine and its return to a vein.

Dialysis. The initial phase of treatment of renal failure is usually dialysis. This is an artificial way of purifying the blood by exposing it to large volumes of fluid that will slowly extract toxic products.

Renal failure is frequently a temporary condition. There is every expectation that the kidneys will return to normal if the patient can be tided over an emergency. In such cases, temporary dialysis is eminently suitable. This is accomplished by infusing fluid into the abdomen through a catheter and removing the fluid several hours later. This procedure, repeated several times, transfers much of the waste across the abdominal lining, which acts as a substitute for kidney membranes.

Artificial kidney. Permanent loss of kidney function generally takes a long time to develop. When the kidneys are hopelessly damaged, or nearly so, preparations for continued dialysis with an artificial kidney can be made in advance. The artificial kidney is a device through which the patient's blood is circulated, cleaned, and returned to the body.

The patient will have to be "hooked up" to the machine quite frequently. This connection is facilitated by a minor surgical procedure that creates what is called an arteriovenous shunt at the inside of the wrist. In effect, the shunt provides a surface connection so that tubes can be plugged in quickly when dialysis is necessary. Interconnection of an artery and a vein at the wrist does not interfere with the function of arm or leg. It allows blood to be withdrawn easily from the artery, run through the artificial kidney for purification, and returned to the vein.

If kidney function is totally destroyed, dialysis for about six hours, two or three times a week, is necessary. In the intervening time, the patient can continue normal work and activities. There are dialysis centers in hospitals around the country. The treatment is expensive, but regardless of the patient's age, most of the costs are covered under special provisions of Medicare, which also covers the costs of kidney transplantation.

It is also possible for the patient to perform the procedure at home with a compact home dialysis unit. The patient needs some training and the assistance of a family member, but home dialysis is less costly and considerably more convenient, inasmuch as the blood can be cleansed in the evening or at other times that do not interfere with work or social schedules. However, at present the expense is borne by the patient, so that home dialysis competes with Medicare-assisted hospital treatment.

Kidney Transplants

Dialysis has some disadvantages and limitations. Life depends upon a machine. One cannot be long away from it. Regular treatments are remindful of this dependency and restraint on freedoms. An alternative is kidney transplantation, a procedure that has advanced quite remarkably in the past 20 years. A good kidney is transplanted into a patient with poor renal function. Of all organ transplantations, those of the kidney are most numerous and most successful.

Someone, living or dead, must donate a good kidney, and the donated organ must have blood group and other factors compatible with the recipient's. Because the chance of a good match is better, a living related member of the family is usually the preferred donor (after making sure that he or she has two good kidneys).

Another source is a cadaver donor—a person who has died suddenly as from a gunshot wound or automobile accident—from whom a kidney can be retrieved quickly before it is damaged from lack of blood flow.

The operation. The transplanted kidney does not occupy the position of a normal kidney. The operation is done through the lower abdomen. The kidney is positioned beside the bladder, since this is the easiest place to hook it to a new blood supply and connect the drainage channel to the bladder.

Technically, the operation is not extraordinarily complex, and its details have been well mastered. The main problem is the chance that the body will recognize the new kidney as an intruder or foreign body and take steps to reject it, through the same immune system that rejects measles viruses in persons with an acquired immunity to measles.

This threat of rejection can be lessened by preoperative irradiation and the use of immuno-suppressive drugs that, as their name indicates, depress the body's immunizing system. Temporary suppression is intended to persuade the body to accept the new kidney as if it were its own, but it also reduces the patient's natural resistance to infections.

The new kidney should begin to form urine quite promptly after it is connected. In the recovery phase, renal function is closely checked, infections guarded against, and omens of rejection watched for. Occasionally, rejection may occur quickly after the operation and require removal of the donated kidney, or rejection may occur after quite a long time has passed.

Nevertheless, a great many kidneys work competently after transplantation and promise many years of survival with good quality of life and relatively little medical supervision. The earliest operations were generally done on relatively young persons, preferably identical twins—one a donor, the other a recipient—but survival of a transplanted kidney in persons in their 50s and 60s now compares favorably with the record of recipients of all ages.

Kidney Tumors

The word "tumor" implies "cancer" to many persons. A tumor may be a cancer. More often than not, it is a mass, growth, or swelling quite unrelated to cancer.

Cysts. The most frequent kidney tumor is a cyst, which is a sac that may contain gas, fluid, or a semi-solid substance. A kidney cyst is usually benign and rarely causes any symptoms unless it should become so large as to block the drainage pathways of the kidney.

A cyst is often found in older persons, incidental to routine examinations or tests for urinary tract problems. Initial X rays may somewhat resemble cancer and arouse apprehension. However, with modern X-ray techniques, judgment as to whether a mass is a benign cyst or cancer can be made with certainty in more than 90 percent of cases. If it is a cyst, no treatment is necessary. In the few uncertain cases, exploratory surgery may be needed to determine the diagnosis.

Some persons have numerous bubble-like cysts in both kidneys, a congenital condition known as *polycystic kidneys*. In middle age, the growth of large numbers of these cysts may compress and destroy normal kidney tissue, with slow development of chronic renal failure. No treatment to prevent progression of this illness is known, except for dietary and medical measures that may help to slow the accumulation of toxic substances in the blood. Dialysis or transplant may ultimately be necessary.

If one member of a family has polycystic kidneys, close relatives also should be screened for the condition.

Kidney Cancers

The most frequent type of kidney cancer in adults is *hypernephroma,* which primarily affects persons over age 40. This form of cancer may sometimes be confused with a cyst.

Symptoms. Occasionally, hypernephroma may be found incidentally at an early stage. More often the patient complains of blood in the urine, pain or ache in the back or side, weakness, loss of appetite, or awareness of a lump in the abdomen.

Blood in the urine is always a symptom that demands immediate urological investigation. It does not necessarily indicate kidney cancer, or disease of the kidney itself, since the source may be anywhere in the GU tract. Obvious blood in the urine is startling to the patient and should be an instant command to get medical attention.

Tests for hypernephroma most often performed are the intravenous pyelogram, tomogram, ultrasound examination, and arteriogram (see page 400). Possible spread of cancer cells to other organs (metastasis) is investigated with the aid of chest X rays, a bone scan, and perhaps a liver scan.

Treatment. If there is no evident spread to other organs, treatment is surgical: removal of the kidney and surrounding fat and lymph glands.

The operation, under general anesthesia, is performed through an incision in the abdomen or flank. Time in the hospital is about ten days, and in absence of complications, the patient can return to work in approximately four weeks. A kidney also may be removed for other reasons than cancer, such as chronic infection or stones.

If cancer cells have spread, surgery may nevertheless be helpful; for instance, if there is excessive bleeding or pain from the affected kidney. More often, in cases where there is spread, radiation or drug therapy is used in attempts to control the tumor. Treatment for cancer that has spread beyond the kidney is rarely curative, but may prolong survival and make the patient more comfortable.

Transitional-cell cancer. A less frequent but major type of kidney malignancy in adults is transitional-cell cancer, so-called from the kinds of cells affected. It originates in the urine-collecting system—the cuplike calyces and bowl-shaped pelvis of the kidney.

This type of cancer occurs most frequently in the 60- to 70-year age group, and is three to four times more common in men than in women. Smoking may be a causative factor, as the tumor is about three times more common in smokers than in nonsmokers.

In most cases, this cancer shows itself by causing blood in the urine, often accompanied by pain from obstructing blood clots. Thus it may reveal itself fairly early, with good chance for cure by surgical removal. However, the operation is more extensive than kidney removal. It is also necessary to remove the ureter—the vessel that carries urine from kidney to bladder—because the ureter is lined by the same type of transitional cells and there is a relatively high chance that cancer will occur later in this structure. Occasionally, a less radical operation—removal of only the involved portion of the collecting system—may suffice if the tumor is small, low-grade, and conveniently located.

Follow-up of patients with this type of cancer is very important, as they tend to develop similar cancers in the other kidney or in the bladder. When the initial cancer is discovered, the bladder should be examined by cystoscopy at intervals of three to six months thereafter, for five years or more.

Other kinds of kidney cancer in older people are relatively rare and are basically treated by removal of the kidney.

Kidney Stones

More people than one might suspect have kidney stones *(calculi)*. Some of us have stones but don't know it and perhaps never will. Some have a huge stone that does serious damage to the kidney but causes no symptoms for a long time. And some have excruciating pain and frightful body twitching when a stone tries to get out through a ureter.

Symptoms vary according to the size and location of stones. Treatment may require only mild and watchful measures, or if stones are causing serious trouble, surgery may be required.

Who gets stones? The peak occurrence of urinary calculi is probably in the 30- to 40-year-old age group, and more frequently in men than in women. Stones form from condensation around microscopic nuclei in urine—a saturated solution of many salts and substances.

Why are some persons—chronic stone-formers—repeatedly troubled by stones, while thousands of others live a long calculus-free life? Nobody really knows. Curiously, there are "stone belts" in the United States—mainly in the southeast, with a secondary belt in the northwest—where the incidence of kidney stones is much higher than in the general population. This peculiar susceptibility may be related to diet, fluid intake, type of soil, climate, or something else, but no specific factor has been identified as yet, despite much research.

Some probable factors that may expedite stone formation are obstructions that cause a backup of stagnant urine, infections, insufficient fluid intake resulting in highly concentrated urine, and certain abnormalities of metabolism or of the urinary tract.

What kinds of stones? Kidney stones are composed of different materials, but most form in the uppermost part of the urine-collecting system (calyces). A small, smooth stone may become dislodged, pass quickly down the ureter to the bladder, and be voided with the urine. "Gravel," which is very fine crystals of stone material, is usually sluiced easily from the tract.

If a stone gets caught in the ureter, which is a narrow muscular tube, it will partially or totally obstruct the kidney, causing severe pain. The urine may contain visible blood, or occult blood detected by analysis. Often the stone will pass through the tube unassisted.

Should a stone become intractably lodged, or the kidney infected with continued pain, the obstruction may be approached from below, via the bladder, employing cystoscopy (see page 386). A catheter may be passed up the ureter to a point above the obstruction. This allows the kidney to drain, like a culvert that bypasses a dam. Or the urologist may insert a stone basket, a cystoscopic device with several wires at its end, which, when opened in the ureter, can grasp the stone so it can be pulled out. If these conservative measures fail, an open operation to remove the stone will be necessary.

Another kind of stone is too large to enter the ureter and cannot be passed spontaneously. It begins as a smaller stone that stays in the kidney and gradually gets larger and larger, especially in the presence of infection, as layers of calcium are deposited. Such a large stone may block the kidney directly at the point where urine enters the ureter (ureteropelvic junction) and will frequently need to be removed surgically.

The stone may cause blood in the urine and severe pain, like a smaller stone. It may also cause intense intermittent pain as it rolls around inside the kidney, occasionally lodging at the outlet and obstructing the kidney temporarily.

The largest stone is the "staghorn" type, so-called from its antler-like projections that are an almost-perfect likeness of the entire collecting system of the kidney, or most of it. A staghorn stone may cause pain, blood in the urine, or fever, or it may present no noticeable symptoms at all. The main danger of such a stone is gradual destruction of the kidney. Therefore, many urologists feel that such stones in younger persons should always be removed. But in an older and perhaps less robust person who has adequate kidney function, a better procedure may be to do serial X rays every six months or so and to intervene only in the event of a crisis.

Surgery for stones. Some details of urological surgery are described elsewhere (see page 399). As for stones, it may be desirable to remove an entire kidney if it is badly damaged and stone-infested. At times, only a part of the kidney, usually the lower part, is removed through an abdominal incision. This involves a two-week stay in the hospital and about five weeks before return to work. A stone in the kidney pelvis is removed through a flank incision.

A stone that is stubbornly stuck in a ureter, unresponsive to conservative measures, is exposed through abdominal or flank incision. Possible complications of removal are leakage of urine and obstructive narrowing of the ureter.

As a temporary measure, obstruction may be relieved by inserting a drainage tube into the kidney. Further treatment is often needed.

In general, one should expect to spend from ten days to two weeks in a hospital for kidney surgery, with another month of recovery before resuming activity. Complications, not usual but possible, include such things as excessive bleeding, prolonged urine drainage, infection of the wound or urinary tract, and difficulties or unexpected circumstances that require more extensive surgery than was originally anticipated.

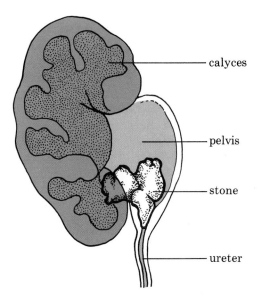

calyces

pelvis

stone

ureter

A STONY DAM

A kidney stone lodged at the junction of the ureter and pelvis may completely block the outflow of urine. Dammed-up urine distends and damages tissues of the kidney. Obstruction and pain may be intermittent if the stone rolls around inside the kidney. Tiny kidney stones (gravel) usually pass without great difficulty.

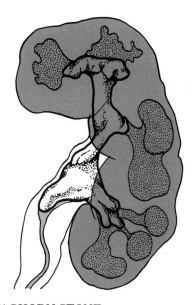

A STAGHORN STONE

A staghorn calculus fills all or most of the kidney pelvis and forms a nearly perfect cast of the cavity. Irregular projections of the stone somewhat resemble antlers, hence the name. The huge stone may cause pain, fever, and blood in the urine, but sometimes there are no noticeable symptoms at all.

Can kidney stones be dissolved?
Through the years, innumerable attempts have been made to find medications that could harmlessly dissolve kidney stones, but they've met with little success except for stones of uncommon composition.

The great majority of stones, at least 90 percent, contain calcium and materials such as oxalate, phosphate, and magnesium ammonium phosphate, precipitated from urinary salts. These common stones can usually be seen in a plain X-ray film of the abdomen, unless they happen to overlie a bone. They cannot be dissolved.

A small proportion of stones are formed from cystine. This is an amino acid, furnished by common food proteins, which is excreted in abnormally large amounts by persons who have a hereditary disease called *cystinuria*. Stones formed by precipitation of great amounts of cystine crystals in the kidneys may be large or small and often need surgery. But sometimes these stones can be dissolved by medication that binds the cystine and, by making the urine less acid, increases the solubility of the crystals. Such medications need to be taken indefinitely and can prevent the formation of further stones if the treatment is faithfully followed.

About 5 percent of stones are condensed from uric acid, a normal constituent of urine. They tend to occur in people with high blood levels of uric acid, as in gout (see page 254). Urate stones are translucent and generally not visible on a plain X-ray film, but can be brought to view by an intravenous pyelogram. The stones may be large or small and may require surgery.

Further formation of urate stones can be prevented, and stones that are in the kidneys but not causing symptoms may be dissolved. This is accomplished by indefinite treatment with the drug, allopurinol, which inhibits the body's production of uric acid.

Sometimes, following surgery, a tube may be left temporarily in the kidney, through which any remaining stone fragments may be washed directly with acid solution and dissolved.

Prevention of stones. Persons who form cystine or urate stones can prevent further formation by proper therapy. Those who form the much more common calcium-containing stones can take comfort from the fact that many patients form only one or two stones during a lifetime. Extensive testing is not often done on patients who have had a single stone, but if stones recur, investigation may disclose overgrowth of the parathyroid glands in the neck.

These tiny glands influence the body's handling of calcium, and if enlarged, can cause excessive excretion of stone-forming calcium in the urine. Removal of the enlarged gland should cure the problem.

People who have excessive amounts of calcium in the urine, for unknown reasons, may be helped by taking a diuretic drug that decreases the urinary concentration of the mineral. Increasing the intake of fluids may also help. But cutting down on calcium-rich foods, such as cheese and milk, makes little difference unless the person is an enormous consumer of these dairy products.

Stones can be prevented with proper urological care, as in the control of urinary-tract infections (see page 395) which tend to accelerate stone formation. Sometimes, if the composition of a stone is known, the urine may be made more acid or more alkaline to make the environment less favorable for precipitation.

THE BLADDER

Technically, the urinary bladder is a cyst; hence its varied inflammations come under the general term *cystitis*. The bladder is an expandable sac lined with transitional cells surrounded by a thick layer of muscle. Ureters opening into the bladder on either side deliver urine, not by gravity, but by muscular spurts.

The bladder is a temporary storage area for urine. As it fills, it reaches a pressure point that triggers the urge to void. Contraction of the bladder muscle empties the contents through the urethra to the outside. Apparently there is no absolute physiological need for such a reservoir, but its social value is immense.

The ureters. The narrow muscular tubes that conduct urine from the kidney to the bladder are not often the seats of primary disease. The tubes are lined by the same kind of cells (transitional) as the bladder and kidney pelvis, in which cancer may originate. Cancer of the ureter requires removal of the ureter and kidney.

Somewhat like an innocent bystander, a ureter may be requisitioned by a trouble-making kidney to pass stones that may scar or constrict the tube, or it may have to be opened surgically to remove a stone, as previously mentioned. In tuberculosis, the ureter may become infected, resulting in stricture and backup of urine, however, this is much less frequent with present-day tuberculosis treatment.

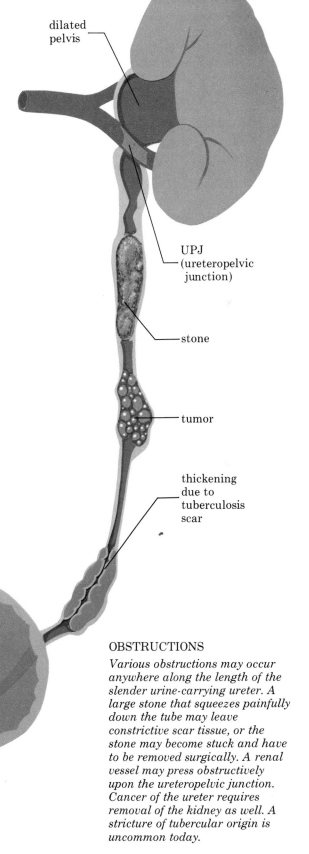

dilated pelvis

UPJ (ureteropelvic junction)

stone

tumor

thickening due to tuberculosis scar

bladder

OBSTRUCTIONS

Various obstructions may occur anywhere along the length of the slender urine-carrying ureter. A large stone that squeezes painfully down the tube may leave constrictive scar tissue, or the stone may become stuck and have to be removed surgically. A renal vessel may press obstructively upon the ureteropelvic junction. Cancer of the ureter requires removal of the kidney as well. A stricture of tubercular origin is uncommon today.

The Cystoscope

The cystoscope is one of the most sophisticated and important urological instruments, and one that many patients are introduced to unexpectedly. Loosely, the word means "a look into the bladder," and the cystoscope itself is a long metal instrument with a light at the end and a magnifying lens. When introduced into the bladder through the urethra, the interior of the bladder and the prostate gland can be viewed.

The point of entry of the ureter into the bladder can also be seen. Small catheters can be passed into the ureters to take X rays of one or both kidneys, or to collect urine separately from each kidney for diagnostic study. Many refinements, such as cutting units or attachments that grasp or crush stones, enable the cystoscope to be used for surgery as well as diagnosis.

Cystoscopy—examination of the bladder and prostate—may be done in the urologist's office or in a hospital, with local or general anesthesia. With local anesthesia, the procedure is not exactly pleasant—especially for a man, since the instrument must traverse the penis—but examination is usually brief and the information gained may be invaluable.

Trouble With Dribble and Spurt

Control of urination after infancy is an acquired skill that we give no thought to unless it gets embarrassingly out of order. Urinary incontinence in its various forms —dribbling, wet undergarments, uncontrollable sudden urge to void, inability to hold back, and leakage after laughter— is a truly great and secret problem of afflicted adults.

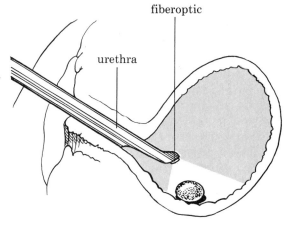

CYSTOSCOPY

A cystoscope inserted through the urethra enables the operator to inspect the interior of the bladder and related structures, and, with accessories, to do surgical procedures. In the drawing, a cystoscope passed through the short female urethra makes a bladder stone visible at the viewing end of the instrument.

Incontinence is relatively infrequent in men, but there is some risk of it after certain types of prostate surgery. If the prostate is totally removed for cancer, the anatomy of controlling sphincter muscles of the bladder is inevitably changed to some extent. *Stress incontinence*, which is provoked by lifting, straining, or laughing, may result. This often improves greatly within a few months of surgery, but occasionally, loss of control may be severe and irreversible. In such case, the patient may require that a catheter be placed in the bladder continuously.

Incontinence is a fairly common problem in older women, particularly if they are obese and have borne several children. Pelvic-floor muscles may be weakened, causing a descent of the bladder with shortening of the urethra. Increased pressure in the abdomen from coughing, laughing, or lifting a heavy object may cause urine to leak in small or even fairly large amounts. In mild cases, relief may be affected by losing weight or avoiding tobacco, which aggravates coughing and bronchitis. In more severe cases, there is good success from surgical treatment or wearing a pessary (see page 399).

Neurogenic bladder. If nerves that control bladder function are damaged by injuries, strokes, or disease, muscular contractions that empty the bladder on command will be disordered. One of two problems will result: the bladder muscle will become overactive or underactive.

If the bladder becomes overactive (spastic), urine may be expelled sporadically with no voluntary control. This incontinence, associated with small bladder capacity, may result in severe infections of the urinary tract or impeded drainage of the kidneys.

Underactivity of the bladder muscle (flaccid bladder) will have similar consequences. The bladder, which is constantly full, will have overflow dribbling, perhaps infection due to a stagnant pool of urine, or possible partial obstruction of ureters and kidneys.

Common causes of neurological malfunction (neurogenic bladder) are spinal injuries, slipped discs, strokes, syphilis, and diabetes. Treatment depends on the nature and severity of problems. Medications may suffice in milder cases, but in more severe cases, a catheter may be used to drain the urine. The catheter may be permanent (indwelling), or it may be inserted into the bladder to empty it every few hours.

Sometimes the bladder will have to be surgically bypassed by stitching the ureters to a piece of bowel that is brought onto the abdominal wall. This acts as a conducting tube on which a bag is placed to collect the urine.

Bladder Stones

Bladder stones are not nearly as frequent in the United States as in some other countries, such as Japan. They are less common than they were a half century ago, perhaps because of improved nutrition, hygiene, and general medical care. "Cutting for stone" is an ancient operation, and a drastic one, performed without anesthesia by operators who got in and out of the bladder as fast as they could and hoped for the best.

Stones are usually associated with some obstruction to the outlet of the bladder. Surgery does not impose the agonies that famous persons such as Samuel Johnson, Benjamin Franklin, and Samuel Pepys suffered at the hands of stone-cutters. Most often, bladder stones are removed without making an incision, with cystoscopic instruments that crush and extract the stones. But sometimes stones are removed through an abdominal operation.

Bladder Cancer

Cancer of the bladder occurs at a rate of 20,000 new cases a year in the United States. It is not a rare disease; about one person in a hundred will develop bladder cancer in his or her lifetime. It may occur at any age, but most patients are between 60 and 75 when symptoms of cancer are first recognized.

Men are affected about three times as often as women. Exposure to certain industrial dyes has been linked to bladder cancer. Tobacco also may have an influence; smokers are affected about three times as often as nonsmokers. The bladder is host to innumerable chemicals excreted by the kidneys.

Bladder cancer may occur as a relatively benign lesion that progresses very slowly, or as a highly malignant type that spreads rapidly to other parts of the body. Most cancers arise in the lining cells of the bladder, and rarely in the muscle wall.

Symptoms. The predominant initial symptom of bladder cancer is blood in the urine. Other symptoms may be frequent urination, difficult urination, or a urinary infection. Or there may be pain in the back from obstruction of a kidney. The diagnosis is confirmed by cystoscopy and removal of a piece of the tumor for study by a pathologist. If it is small, the entire tumor may be resected and no other surgery may be required.

Treatment. We have only one bladder and it is not replaceable. Therefore, treatment of smaller lesions, particularly if they are of low-grade malignancy, is generally conservative. The tumor can often be fully removed by an electrical cutting unit through the cystoscope. But watchful follow-up cystoscopy will be necessary for a lifetime because of the tendency of tumors to recur in other areas of the bladder. Radiation is sometimes used as a primary treatment, but more often as an adjunct to surgery.

Removal of the entire bladder *(total cystectomy)* is a major operation with a mortality rate of about 10 percent. Urinary drainage must be diverted to the outside into a collecting bag. A disturbing side effect is impotence, and the patient has major physical and psychological handicaps. Thus, total cystectomy is reserved for cancers that are large, show evidence of progressing through the bladder wall, or have a high grade of malignancy. For widespread cancer, drugs offer hope of prolonging life, but not of cure.

Bladder Operations

Total removal of the bladder and adjacent organs, with diversion of the urinary stream to the outside, is a lengthy operation performed through an abdominal incision. The hospital stay is about a month, with return to work after three months. Removal of a portion of the bladder is a less drastic operation, requiring about ten days in the hospital; later recurrence of cancer is possible.

Sometimes a tumor is scraped off the bladder wall *(transurethral resection)* with cystoscopic instruments inserted through the penis. The hospital stay is only a week, with return to work in two weeks. Again, possible recurrence of cancer will be watched for.

A drainage tube may be inserted into the bladder for temporary relief of obstruction, or permanent drainage in incontinence. Hospital stay is only a week, but further treatment will often be necessary.

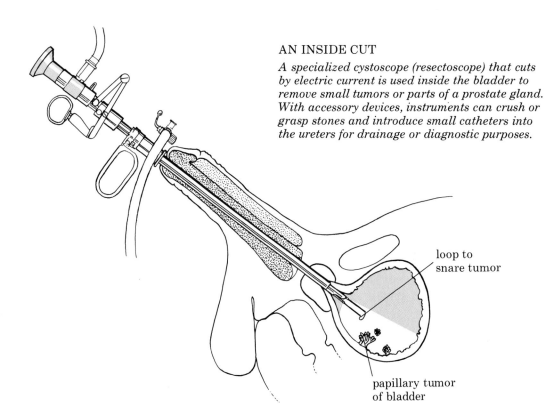

AN INSIDE CUT

A specialized cystoscope (resectoscope) that cuts by electric current is used inside the bladder to remove small tumors or parts of a prostate gland. With accessory devices, instruments can crush or grasp stones and introduce small catheters into the ureters for drainage or diagnostic purposes.

loop to
snare tumor

papillary tumor
of bladder

THE PROSTATE

The prostate gland is linked to male sexual function and its disorders are of no concern to women, except as consorts. The gland is an accessory sex organ that is generally trouble-free until around middle age. Increasingly with the years, it becomes an important and common site of urological disease in men.

The main function of the prostate is to secrete a fluid that is a constituent of semen, the sperm-carrying ejaculate that effects fertilization. Prostatic fluid provides volume and substances that preserve and sustain activities of the male germ cells, spermatozoa.

Anatomy. The prostate gland completely encircles the urethra, which discharges urine through the penis, at the outlet of the bladder (posterior urethra). Another part of the urethra (anterior) is largely in the shaft of the penis. The part surrounded by the prostate contains muscles that hold back urine until it is ready for expulsion. The gland has three main lobes and ducts that open into the urethra.

Its encircling position enables the prostate, if enlarged, to squeeze the urinary channel that passes through it, causing partial or complete obstructions of bladder emptying that are common in older men.

Examination. Before discussing specific conditions of the prostate, we should emphasize the special importance of regular physical examinations for men after 40 with respect to prostatic disease. Rectal examination takes only a minute or so. The doctor inserts a lubricated gloved finger into the rectum and feels the size, firmness, or softness of the gland. Stony hard areas may suggest cancer and require further examination. Gentle massage of the gland produces a few drops of fluid that can be studied in a laboratory if necessary.

Rectal examination will often detect prostate cancer that has given no symptoms and is in an early stage when it can be cured completely. Unfortunately, only 5 to 10 percent of prostate cancers are discovered at the earliest stage when total cure is most likely.

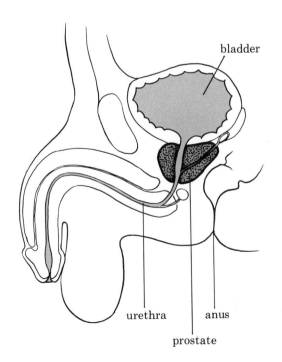

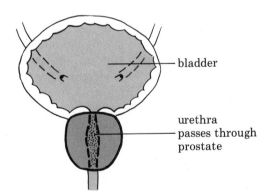

THE MALE GLAND

At left is shown the size and location of the prostate gland in relation to the bladder, penis, urethra, and anus. Above, the prostate completely encircles the portion of the urethra (posterior) at the bladder outlet, which contains muscles that control urination. The prostate empties into the urethra and, when ejaculation occurs, the gland contracts. Its secretions combine with sperm-carrying fluids, which also enter the posterior urethra, to form semen.

Benign Prostatic Hypertrophy (BPH)

In most men, the prostate begins to enlarge at about age 40. Its growth is generally benign (that is, not cancerous) and rather slow. The cause is not known, but is probably based on hormone relationships. It is estimated that two-thirds of men over 60 have some degree of prostatic enlargement. "Benign" does not necessarily mean "kindly" or "harmless."

Sufficient enlargement of the gland produces prostatism: obstruction of the bladder outlet by the prostate. The prostate may protrude into the bladder cavity, causing a dam-up of stagnant urine from failure to empty the bladder completely. Bladder stones or infections may result. Urine under pressure in the bladder may back up into the kidneys (*hydronephrosis)* with severe damage to kidney function. In many cases, urinary retention will ultimately result: the patient cannot urinate despite having a full bladder and a strong urge to empty it. This distress can usually be relieved by passing a catheter into the bladder.

Symptoms. There are different degrees of urinary obstruction. The stream may be slow to start, feeble, and intermittent, or the urge may be more frequent, especially at night. It may take a long time to complete the act or much straining to start it. Hernias and hemorrhoids frequently result from straining with high pressures in the abdomen. The stream may be narrow and end in dribbling. Insidious enlargement of the prostate over the years may erase a man's memory of what a full free-flowing stream used to feel like.

Treatment. Palliative measures may help to relieve congestion if the kidneys are not endangered and there are no stones or other complications.

It may be helpful to avoid prolonged sitting on soft, cushiony seats and exposure to cold and dampness. The urge to urinate should be obeyed immediately; indeed, intentional urination every couple of hours may avert overdistention of the bladder.

Moderate amounts of alcohol do not seem to be specifically irritating, but heavy beer drinking, perhaps because of sheer volume and delay in urinating, seems unwise. Hot spices appear to irritate the prostatic urethra; a man may experimentally forgo chili and pepperoni. A drink of water several times through the day produces dilute urine that helps to flush the bladder outlet. Such temporizing measures are not curative and should be discussed with one's doctor, who will give counsel appropriate to the individual patient.

More drastic treatment may not be necessary for a long time if symptoms are tolerable and health of the urinary tract is not threatened. When and if symptoms become severe enough, surgery is indicated.

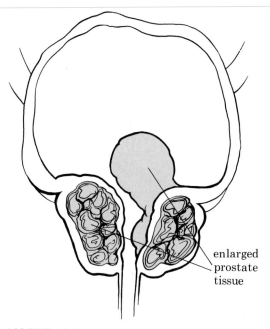

enlarged
prostate
tissue

AN ENLARGED PROSTATE

Some degree of enlargement of the prostate gland is common in men after 40. The slowly increasing size of the gland (hypertrophy) may in time cause it to protrude into the bladder cavity as shown, partially or even completely impeding the outflow of urine. Moderate difficulties of urination may be tolerated for some time if obstruction is not severe enough to threaten the health of the urinary tract. Surgery for this condition is almost never urgent enough to constitute an emergency.

Operations for BPH. There are two types of surgery for benign enlargement of the prostate (BPH). The choice depends mostly on the size of the gland and the experience of the surgeon.

If the gland is small or of moderate size, a *transurethral resection* (TUR) will usually be done. No incision is made. An instrument similar to a cystoscope, but with a wire loop at its end through which an electric current runs, is introduced into the bladder through the penis. The wire loop is used to cut away chips of the inner portion of the prostate until all overgrown tissue is removed. Any bleeding from the gland can be controlled by the current.

A catheter is usually left in the bladder for several days after the operation, to drain the urine until the prostate has begun to heal. The patient is usually out of the hospital in a week and back to work in three weeks.

If the prostate is very large, a different approach *(suprapubic prostatectomy)* may have to be taken. The prostate is exposed through an incision in the lower abdomen. Overgrown tissue is removed, but the outer rim of the gland, the capsule, is left intact. Two catheters may be left in place, one to be removed after a few days and the second after a week.

Hospital stay (12 days) and convalescence (four weeks) are somewhat longer after this operation than after TUR. Impotence or difficulties of urination rarely result from either of these operations.

If prostatic overgrowth is extreme and urinary-tract complications have occurred or are threatened, it may be necessary to place a catheter into the bladder and leave it there for several weeks before doing surgery. The hope is that kidney function will be improved by better drainage, which the catheter provides.

Cancer of the Prostate

The longer a man lives, the more likely that he will develop prostate cancer. This cancer is very common in older men. At age 90, one would expect three out of four men to have prostate cancer, discoverable by microscopic examination of prostate tissue. These oldsters may never know that they have prostate cancer and will probably die of something else.

But what of younger men? In many men, it appears that a small focus of cancer in the prostate may not progress extensively, either by local spread or to distant parts of the body. However, some 20,000 men die each year from prostate cancer.

Detection of a small area of cancer gives the best chance that prompt surgery can eliminate a potentially life-threatening condition. Many prostate cancers are discovered incidentally on rectal examination, or in follow-up of symptoms of difficult urination, similar to those of benign hypertrophy. The latter is not related to cancer but can occur along with it.

If a hard nodule is discovered in the prostate, a piece of tissue should be taken from it (biopsy). Examination by a pathologist may confirm that the nodule is indeed cancerous. If so, further tests will be done to determine whether the cancer has spread. X rays may reveal evidence of spread to bones or lymph nodes. Blood tests may indicate distant invasion, and rectal examination is important to evaluate local spread. Cancerous tissue may have grown large enough to cause bladder obstruction, or coexistent benign overgrowth may lead to frequent voiding day and night with possible infection or urinary retention.

Treatment may vary according to the age of the patient, his life expectancy, and severity of symptoms. In a 50- or 60-year-old man, prostate cancer would be treated much more aggressively than in one of 80.

Total prostatectomy. If cancer is confined to the prostate, the entire gland is removed, as well as surrounding tissues. Surgery is performed either through an incision in the lower abdomen, or through a perineal incision between the scrotum and anus. The hospital stay for total prostatectomy is about three weeks, with another two months of recuperation before resuming usual activities.

Impotence almost always results from this operation, because of the necessarily extensive removal of tissues and the disturbance of nerve pathways. There may be complications of infection and leakage of urine while control is being reestablished. But if the area of cancer is small and total removal is successful, no more treatment is necessary, other than periodic checks for possible recurrence.

Other therapies. If prostate cancer has spread, total excision may not be feasible, and adjunctive therapy may be necessary. External radiation treatments may be given, or radioactive material—commonly, radioactive gold or iodine—may be implanted directly into the cancerous tissue to destroy it.

Destruction of prostate tissue by contact with extremely cold probes *(cryosurgery)* has been increasingly used in recent years. This treatment controls localized tumors and relieves obstruction by shrinking the gland.

If the cancer is widespread and bladder obstruction is present, the previously described transurethral resection can give relief, but it does not cure the cancer. Prostate cancer is said to be "hormone dependent" (as is breast cancer)—aggravated by male hormones and depressed by female hormones. Appropriate hormone therapy is valuable in controlling disseminated prostate cancer.

The testicles may be removed to interrupt the patient's production of male hormone, or female hormones may be given, or both. This may stabilize or arrest the progression of prostate cancer for long periods of time, even several years. Like total prostatectomy, hormone treatment frequently results in impotence, and may produce some signs of feminization. These should not deter a man who is enabled to enjoy other good things of life for a good many years.

With current methods of treatment, there is good hope of cure of early cases of prostate cancer, and of extended control in later cases that have spread widely before diagnosis. Even in far advanced and seemingly hopeless cases, new drugs that are being evaluated give hope for the future and even the possibility that someday medical therapy for prostate cancer will replace surgery.

Like other forms of cancer, early discovery and prompt treatment of prostate cancer give an excellent chance of permanent cure. Unfortunately, prostate cancer usually originates in outer parts of the gland where it can grow silently for a long time before causing symptoms, such as bladder obstruction, that would lead a man to consult a doctor. We again emphasize the importance of periodic rectal examinations for men over 40.

THE TESTIS

The testis is not often the site of primary disease in men over 40; the most serious problem is cancer, which occurs mostly in men under 30 years of age. A middle-aged man has generally outgrown the risk, but testicular cancer occasionally occurs in older men and warrants a technique of self-examination comparable to self-examination of the breasts by women. The predominant sign is the presence of swelling or a hard mass, usually painless.

There are several types of testicular malignancies. The most common may be treated surgically by removal of the testes, followed by X-ray therapy to lymph nodes of the abdomen. With other types, surgical removal of abdominal lymph nodes is necessary, along with radiation to the area.

Other Scrotal Masses

Not every mass in the scrotum is a cancer. *Hernia* is the most common reason for scrotal swelling. The soft mass gives an impulse when the patient coughs. Treatment is surgical.

Hydrocele is a swelling around the testis containing clear fluid. The fluid accumulates in the sac of the membrane that covers the testis. The swelling varies in size, can be painful, and does not give an impulse when the patient coughs. Congenital hydroceles in children tend to disappear. In adults, hydroceles usually occur spontaneously but may be secondary to inflammation. A *spermatocele* is a similar structure near the testis containing fluid in which sperm are present.

If a flashlight is placed over a hydrocele or spermatocele, the clear fluid inside will transmit the light, helping to make a diagnosis. Treatment may not be necessary, although surgical removal is relatively easy if discomfort is severe.

Epididymitis is inflammation and enlargement of the epididymis, a structure lying beside the testis. It may be associated with urinary infection, fever, extreme pain, and inflammation of the scrotal skin. This is the most difficult scrotal swelling to differentiate from a tumor. If diagnosis of epididymitis is positive, treatment by bed rest, support of the scrotum, and appropriate antibiotics usually gives rapid improvement. If diagnosis is uncertain, surgical exploration of the scrotum may be necessary to determine the condition.

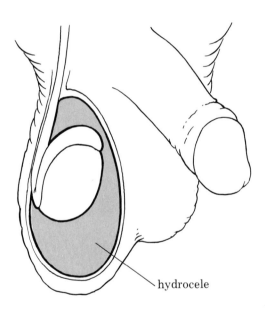

hydrocele

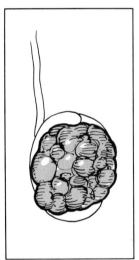

tumor   epididymitis

SCROTAL MASSES

A hydrocele is a swelling of the scrotum, usually painful, produced by accumulation of clear fluid in the sac that surrounds the testis. The swelling may subside spontaneously but relief by tapping or surgery is relatively easy. Spermatocele is essentially the same condition, except that the fluid contains sperm. Hernia is a frequent cause of scrotal swelling. At right above, cancer of the testis is rare in men over 40. Epididymitis is an inflammation of part of the seminal duct beside the testis; surgery is used to effect a more rapid recovery and relieve pain.

The Urethra

The urethra is the channel through which urine is propelled from the bladder to the outside. The female urethra is short, less than two inches, and is the source of many problems referred to later. The longer male urethra, about nine inches, runs through the penis and has obligations in addition to urine transport—as a receiver and carrier of prostatic fluid, sperm, and semen, and an extensible participant in their emission.

Life-threatening illness rarely originates in the urethra, but it may be a seat of chronic disease.

Stricture. Gonorrhea frequently affects the urethra in men, and if not properly treated, may result in chronic inflammation and scar tissue that narrows the channel—a stricture. This may be a 20-years-after surprise, sometimes taking that long to develop after a gonorrheal infection.

Obstruction by stricture may cause difficulties in voiding, similar to those of bladder-outlet obstruction by an overgrown prostate, as well as infections of stagnant urine and even back pressure extending to the kidneys.

Stricture may be managed over a long period by gradual dilation of the narrowed urethra with sterilized rubber or metal instruments that stretch the area. In severe cases, surgery may be necessary to restore the channel to normal caliber.

Nonspecific urethritis. Although gonorrhea is one common cause of urethral inflammation, it's not the only one. Sometimes, especially in men, culture of the urethral discharge shows no growth of bacteria at all, or only of the kinds that are normal inhabitants of the area. Except for frequency and burning when voiding, the patient generally feels fine. Thus the label "nonspecific."

Treatment of the acute condition with an antibiotic may clear up the symptoms, pending culture studies that turn out to be negative. The patient's medical history and factors that might contribute to his complaint or require treatment are, of course, considered.

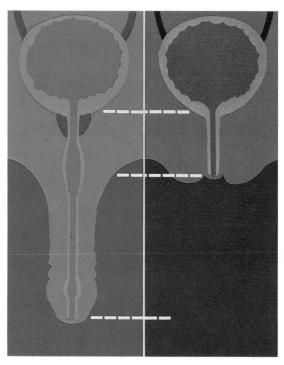

MALE AND FEMALE URETHRAS

The male urethra, with its posterior section where prostate secretions and sperm enter the duct, is longer and functionally more complex than that of the female. The short female urethra is not subject to prostate troubles, but is somewhat more susceptible to ascending infections.

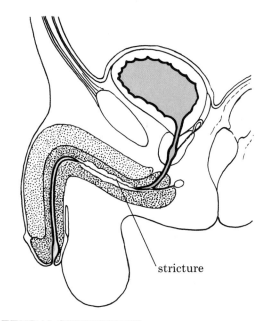

stricture

URETHRAL STRICTURES

A stricture of the urethra is a narrowing and tightening of the channel, resulting from injury or inflammatory changes, as from an old gonorrheal or other infection that leaves constricting scar tissue. Difficulties of urination are similar to those caused by prostatic obstruction.

URINARY-TRACT INFECTIONS

Probably the most frequent and potentially most serious problem seen by urologists is infection. This may occur at any point in the urinary tract, as an isolated illness, or at several locations at once.

Symptoms. Frequent symptoms of severe urinary-tract infection may be fever, chills, back pain, frequency of voiding with burning or stinging, lethargy, and a general feeling of illness. There may be tenderness in the affected area.

Infections are often associated with conditions such as stones or other obstructions. The pool of stagnant urine thus produced is ideal for bacterial growth.

Antibiotics are the treatment of choice for acute infections. But surgery may be necessary for conditions that, if uncorrected, could lead to complications and eventual kidney failure. Prevention of future trouble is one of the main reasons for removal of kidney stones, correction of obstructions at the ureteropelvic junction, removal of overgrown prostate tissue, and correction of urethral stricture.

Pyelonephritis. The location and severity of infection are significant. Acute infection of the kidney and its pelvis *(pyelonephritis)* can be life-threatening unless antibiotic treatment is given promptly. Drainage of dammed-up urine through a catheter in the bladder or around an obstruction may be necessary. Chronic pyelonephritis is a slowly progressing infection that may run on for years, with occasional acute episodes of fever or back pain. The patient may not be aware of any problem until late in the illness, which can progress to cause severe kidney damage and is probably the most common cause of kidney failure. As with acute infection, search should be made for complicating abnormalities of the tract that can be corrected to prevent serious trouble.

Bladder infections are rarely life-threatening, although inflammations that come under the general term *cystitis* can be highly distressing and quite dramatic in their acute stage: grossly bloody urine, pain in the bladder area, and very frequent and painful voiding. Usually antibiotic treatment is quickly successful. The same cannot be said about chronic bladder infections, which produce nagging symptoms of frequency, burning, and discomfort that can be very difficult to eliminate, even with antibiotics. What the patient calls "cystitis" may be partly or mainly an inflammation of the urethra (see below).

"Urethral Syndrome" in Women

Women do not have a prostate gland to encircle and squeeze the bladder outlet and cause obstructive symptoms; they have a short urethra near the vagina and anus. Bacteria of the rectal and contiguous skin have but a short distance to reach the urethra and spread upward toward the bladder. Local hygiene may not be the best. Decreased production of female hormones in postmenopausal women tends to result in thin, tender, painful vaginal tissues. These conjunctions, plus unknown factors, contribute to a quite prevalent condition that has achieved the title "urethral syndrome."

Typical symptoms are frequency, burning, and urgent need to void. There are recurrent attacks of cystitis. The bladder may indeed be involved, but often it is an inflamed urethra that is the site of the most distressing symptoms.

Acute infections usually respond well to antibiotics, but chronic infection is a more difficult problem and hard to eradicate. Some correctable condition may be found, but often there are no obstructions or abnormalities. Some women with chronic symptoms have no detectable infection.

Every urologist has several patients with this syndrome whose complaints are exceedingly difficult to manage. Long-term medication with antibiotic drugs may be tried to prevent recurrent attacks. And recurrences may be instances of reinfection. A simple practice, worth trying and assuredly harmless, is to take showers instead of tub baths, and perhaps even to forgo swimming. Bath water washes the rectal area and can carry bacteria into contact with vaginal and urethral tissues.

Prostatitis

Urinary tract infections are rather infrequent in men until the prostatic age is reached, which is any time after middle age. Then, obstruction to bladder flow by an enlarged prostate frequently predisposes to infections.

Infection of the prostate itself is not uncommon. The gland may be the site of severe, acute infection that can make the patient dangerously ill, or possibly of a chronic recurrent infection that is difficult to eradicate and may cause severe discomfort and pain.

Antibiotics do not penetrate into prostatic tissue very well. Because of this, one of the mainstays of treatment is prostatic massage, designed to drain infected fluid from the gland. Newer drugs of the sulfonamide and tetracycline groups are more effective, and greater relief from medical treatment can now be hoped for.

URINARY-TRACT OBSTRUCTIONS

Throughout this chapter, it has been noted that obstructions of the urinary tract occur with some frequency. They are exceedingly important as causes of kidney damage and eventual renal failure if not treated properly and in time.

The kidneys continue stubbornly to produce urine as long as they can, even though there are obstacles in spillways farther down the tract. The obstruction may be anatomical, such as a stone or enlarged prostate, or physiological, such as a neurogenic bladder. In either case, the results are similar. A little urine may trickle around a partial obstruction, or the blockage may be complete.

Urine accumulates above the obstruction while the kidneys keep on producing. Urine overfills structures too small to contain it, and the stagnant pool is prone to infection. Back pressure dilates the tract and is transmitted to the kidneys where it does damage. At worst, if blockage is prolonged, kidney tissue is squeezed to death by hydraulic pressure.

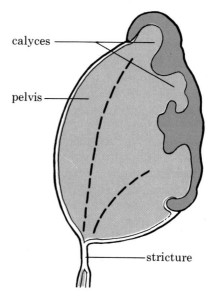

calyces

pelvis

stricture

PELVIC DILATION

A backup of urine above a stricture high in the ureter distends the kidney pelvis beyond its normal boundaries (dotted lines) and, unless relieved, inflicts serious damage on the kidney.

A complete obstruction is a urological emergency. It may occur anywhere from the pelvis of the kidney down to the urethra, and usually the patient is in extreme pain. Urinary infection may have spread to the bloodstream.

It is imperative that the obstruction be relieved quickly. If appropriate, this may be done by inserting a catheter to drain distended structures. Or the obstruction, such as a stone in the ureter, may be removed surgically.

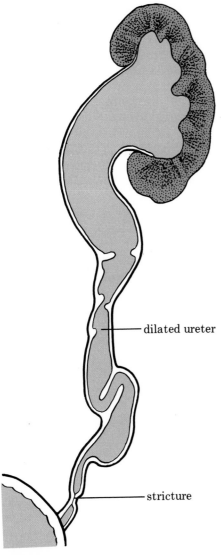

URETHRAL OBSTRUCTION

Obstructions may occur anywhere in the genitourinary tract. Obstruction of the lower ureter, as from a stricture near the bladder, dilates the ureter with dammed-up urine, which the kidney continues to produce but cannot expel. A partial obstruction may permit some urine to trickle around it.

In some emergency instances, it may be advisable to provide immediate drainage and do surgery later. This is commonly done in cases of urinary retention secondary to benign overgrowth of the prostate.

If an obstruction is partial, pain may demand immediate relief, but it is also possible for damage to progress quietly, silently, and without a sign. In such cases, the functioning ability of the kidneys must be evaluated before doing surgery. Prolonged medical and fluid therapy is sometimes needed to restore such a patient to a condition where he or she can tolerate an anesthetic.

Relief of an obstruction is usually followed by improvement of kidney function, but sometimes damage is permanent.

SEXUALITY

Notions that people should decrease or forgo sexual activity as they get older, that there is some vague inappropriateness of ardor in older age groups, that impotence is inevitable, or that post-menopausal intercourse is dangerous, are, of course, false. While sexual drive tends to diminish with age, particularly if unexercised, it often remains quite strong and there is no reason why it should not be satisfied.

Psychological and social factors commonly underlie sexual complaints and are discussed elsewhere. But sometimes there are primary or associated physical impediments or disease that fall within the urologist's specialty, and he may be able to assure a worried patient that his or her GU tract is quite normal.

Vaginal Problems

Many women are disturbed about sexual intercourse after the menopause because of discomfort associated with vaginal dryness and irritability, resulting from decreased production of female hormones and lubricating secretions. If this is a problem, it can be corrected (see page 445).

Impotence

Impotence—inability to carry out the sexual act because of a penis too flaccid for penetration—is quite frequent in older men and happens in young men, too. Often the main factors are psychological and quite complex: feelings of inadequacy, rejection, lack of self-confidence, or fear of trying again if one attempt at intercourse has failed.

Men don't have a menopause, but they may develop vague nervous and emotional symptoms attributed to the "change of life" or *male climacteric*. Some call it "middle-age crisis"—a time when a man may be depressed by a dead-end job, domestic boredom, obstreperous offspring, money worries, competition of younger men, feelings of being over the hill, waning allure, and impotence.

Diminished output of male hormone is rarely great enough to justify supplements. If tests show significant deficiency, testosterone therapy may be tried cautiously. More often, the best help comes from reassurances of a physician or from psychological counsel that may bring apprehensions to light so the patient can take action and end them.

Alcohol. It is popularly believed that alcohol is an incitement to sexual prowess. But it is neither popularly nor widely realized that alcohol in amounts sufficient to affect the liver tends in an opposite direction—toward impotence.

There are non-alcoholic causes of liver disease, but advanced liver disease and cirrhosis of the liver are commonly related to alcoholism (see page 210). Male and female hormones (sex steroids) are metabolized in the liver. Changes seen in male alcoholics with cirrhosis of the liver, as well as less-advanced liver disease, are feminizing: breast enlargement, diminished chest and body hair, and atrophy of the testicles. The extent of alcoholic impotence is not precisely known, but it would seem to be frequent enough to warrant investigation in male complaints of sexual disability. Treatment other than abstinence would be the same as for liver disease (see page 208).

Organic causes. A number of organic conditions can be associated with impotence. If possible, these should be recognized and corrected before attributing impotence to purely psychic reasons. Some of these conditions are: diabetic impotence; circulatory disease; neurological disease, such as stroke or spinal-cord injury; trauma of pelvic structures; and aftereffects of surgery (prostatectomy).

An uncommon but sexually handicapping, not to mention embarrassing, male ailment is called *Peyronie's disease*. It occurs most often in men between ages 40 and 60. Scar tissue in the penis causes severe pain on erection and a curvature of the organ that makes sexual intercourse impossible. The cause is not known, but it may be of genetic or vascular origin.

Medical treatment offers little help, although sometimes the condition improves spontaneously and no treatment is necessary. Reconstructive surgery is indicated for severe cases, where the scarred area is removed and replaced by a skin graft from the abdomen.

However, treatment should be postponed for at least six months after diagnosis to see what course the disease will take in an individual patient, as there may be spontaneous resolution with satisfactory sexual performance.

Prostheses. If impotence is associated with organic disease and sex drive is still present, surgical help is available. Plastic devices can be inserted in the penis to maintain stiffness for intercourse. This procedure is relatively free of complications, and if the device proves uncomfortable, it can be removed.

Vasectomy

Many men of 70 or older are capable of impregnating a woman of childbearing age. Consequently, older as well as younger males may consider the desirability of *vasectomy,* a permanent and trustworthy method of male sterilization.

The surgical procedure is quite simple. Many urologists perform it in their offices or in the outpatient department of hospitals. Through a small incision in the scrotum, the sperm-carrying ducts are severed and the ends sealed, so that fertilizing cells are barred from the seminal emission. Follow-up a short time after the operation is necessary to be sure that sperm are no longer transported.

Vasectomy does not affect the hormone-secreting parts of the testis or interfere with sex drive and potency in any way. What if a man later changes his mind and wants to become unsterilized? Very rarely, the cut ends of the ducts have been rejoined and fertility restored, but anyone considering vasectomy should think of it as permanent and irreversible.

UROLOGICAL SURGERY

Aspects of hospitalization and surgery have been mentioned in discussions of particular conditions. In addition, there are some general aspects of urological surgery that a patient should understand. Knowledge that the procedures of doctors and nurses are not really mysterious, but are vital to your safety and comfort, can be a great aid to peace of mind.

Urological operations of significance are mostly on the kidney, prostate, or bladder. Some very major procedures—total removal of the bladder is the most dangerous—have a relatively high mortality rate. Most procedures now are quite safe and mortality from surgery has diminished as anesthesia, antibiotics, supportive and monitoring equipment, and surgical techniques have improved. The mortality rate for the most frequently performed operations is now less than 1 percent.

Preparation. Preoperatively, the patient will usually have a chest X ray, electrocardiogram, and routine blood tests to determine how well the kidneys, heart, and liver are functioning, and to check for possible anemia or bleeding problems. On the evening before surgery, the site of incision is shaved and carefully washed with antibacterial soaps. No fluid intake is allowed after midnight on the day of surgery.

After surgery. With most procedures, the immediate postoperative period is not very comfortable, but within a few days the patient usually feels well. Complications are relatively infrequent, and the patient is usually home within a week or two of surgery.

Immediately after the operation, no food is allowed for one or several days, depending on the extent of surgery and the condition of the patient. The patient is likely to be a host for various tubes, and often will need drainage from a temporary catheter for from several days to two weeks or more.

Frequently there is some blood in the urine after bladder or prostate operations, and the catheter allows blood to drain freely rather than to form clots inside the bladder. The catheter also prevents urine from leaking through recent incisions in the bladder and thus promotes more rapid healing.

After open surgery, rubber drains are left protruding from the incision down to the site of surgery. If there is any leakage from the urinary tract, the fluid can escape through the drain to the outside, rather than accumulate in a deep area where an abscess could form. The drains are usually removed in a few days when healing is progressing well.

Recovery at home. After discharge from the hospital, the patient needs a period of rest and convalescence. Recuperation time varies with the age of the patient, general health, and the kind of operation performed, and is very important for the full healing of incisions and the return of a normal sense of well-being.

If full activity is resumed too soon, it may take a long time for tiredness and incisional pain to disappear. Incisional hernias may occur, requiring further surgery. The advice of one's doctor on how long to "take it easy" at home should be followed.

THE URINARY TRACT: TESTS & PROCEDURES

Intravenous pyelogram. This primary means of urological investigation is an X-ray study performed by injection of an X-ray dye into a vein, with serial X rays taken at intervals. These X rays outline the kidney, particularly its collecting system, and also reveal the ureter and give an outline of the bladder. This procedure is very valuable in the diagnosis of stones and tumors in the tract. Because chronic kidney failure and obstructive disease tend to produce changes in the X rays, they are helpful in diagnosis.

Lymphangiogram. This X-ray test is used to visualize the lymph nodes, particularly in the pelvis and the abdomen, which may be involved in prostate or bladder cancer. The X-ray contrast medium is injected into each foot and then is transported through the lymphatic system to the nodes in the pelvis and abdomen.

Cystoscopy is the procedure of examining the interior of the bladder and prostate gland with a cystoscope, a long metal instrument with a magnifying lens and a light at its end, which is introduced into the bladder through the urethra. This may be done under local or general anesthesia, and no incision is made. Cystoscopy enables the interior of the bladder to be viewed and diagnosis made of prostate or bladder disease. Accessory devices used in conjunction with a cystoscope make it possible to cut tissues, grasp stones, and do other procedures.

Resectoscope. This instrument is used in the cystoscope to remove bladder tumors or an overgrown prostate via the urethra (transurethral resection).

Rectal examination is performed by insertion of the physician's finger into the patient's rectum. The entire circumference of the lower bowel can be felt, allowing possible detection of cancer of the rectum. In the front portion of the rectum, the prostate gland can be palpated and any suspicious hard areas that may indicate cancer can be felt.

Scan. In this test, a radioactive isotope is injected into a vein. The isotope will settle selectively in the kidneys or other desired organs, and the density of its emanations, registered on film, helps to detect any abnormalities that may be present.

Ultrasound is a procedure by which sound waves are passed through the body and their echoes are picked up on an electronic receiver. The echoes can outline a mass or tumor in the body, and can help to distinguish between solid tumors and those filled with fluid, such as cysts.

Urinalysis is a chemical and microscopic study of the urine. Particular constituents seen or looked for are white blood cells, red blood cells, proteins, and concentration of the urine, all of which may reflect changes in function of the kidneys, bladder, or other parts of the urinary tract.

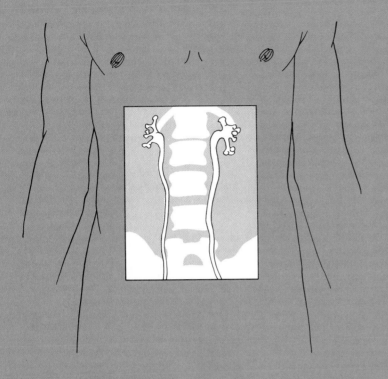

PYELOGRAM

X rays of the urinary tract, made with injection of a radiopaque dye into a vein, delineate structures and abnormalities such as stones and are of great value in diagnosis. X rays of local areas can be taken by introducing radiopaque substances into particular regions through cystoscopes and catheters. It also is possible to take X-ray motion pictures of the urinary tract, and of other organ systems, in action (cinefluorography).

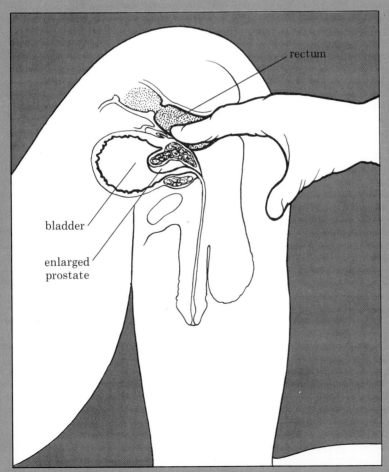

rectum

bladder

enlarged prostate

PALPATION

A rectal examination is a brief and painless procedure, especially important for men over 40, that gives important information about the prostate gland and lower bowel. The patient bends over and the physician inserts a lubricated gloved finger into the rectum to feel (palpate) the prostate and surrounding structures. The examiner's trained sense of touch tells him much about the gland—its size, firmness, and bogginess—and may detect the presence of stony hard areas that require further examination to rule out the possibility of cancer.

DIABETES IN THE MATURE PERSON

Diabetes is one of the more prevalent diseases in the world. Although it can affect young people, even the very young, the most common form is often called "maturity-onset" diabetes because it shows up in middle life. There are overlapping similarities between so-called juvenile- and maturity-onset diabetes, as we shall see. But we will assume that juvenile diabetics are already under treatment (since, in most cases, the onset of their condition is so obvious that it is rarely missed) and that readers of this book are in the after-40 age group, for whom a diagnosis of diabetes may come as an unwelcome surprise.

Incidence. The National Commission on Diabetes reported in December, 1975 that "diabetes mellitus is a major health problem directly affecting as many as ten million Americans. The prevalence of the disease is increasing rapidly. Between 1967 and 1973 its prevalence increased by more than 50 percent in the United States. It now affects five percent of the population. Its incidence appears to be increasing by six percent each year."

The Commission estimated that the number of persons with diabetes will double every 15 years and that an American baby born today has better than a one-in-five chance of developing the disease unless a means of prevention is found. They also pointed out that diabetics are 25 times more prone to blindness than non-diabetics, 17 times more prone to kidney disease, and their life expectancy is about one-third less than that of the general population.

Something has happened to diabetes in the 50 years since insulin became available for treatment. Before insulin, the vast majority of diabetics did not live long enough to develop long-term complications. Even in those days, however, those diabetics who could still produce some of their own insulin could indeed survive for varying periods of time, but at a price: semi-starvation. If the person reduced food intake to the level of his own meager insulin production, he might survive, but it would be an emaciated survival, like a starved prisoner of war.

If diabetics developed an infection (this was before the days of antibiotics), they were often doomed, as infection inflates the need for insulin. When this demand could not be met, the result was often diabetic coma and death. In addition to diabetic coma, the usual causes of death of diabetics in the era before insulin were infection, gangrene of the extremities, and other acute catastrophes. Today, they are heart disease, stroke, kidney complications, and cancer. These are also the causes of death in the general population, except that they tend to occur somewhat earlier in the diabetic. In other words, diabetics now most often succumb to the same terminal illnesses as non-diabetics.

This is progress!

The much longer and satisfying lives of today's diabetics are indeed a tremendous tribute to present methods of treatment and control. But there are also some sobering facts. In a sense, the long-term complications of diabetes are the price of successful treatment. Diabetics now live long enough to be susceptible to the complications that did not befall diabetics of the past who died at a much younger age. Complications may affect the blood vessels, heart, eyes, nerves, kidneys, and indeed most parts of the body, and diabetes in combination with other diseases causes difficulties in treatment.

Untreated, uncontrolled diabetes strikes as devastatingly as it has for at least 3,000 years. But when the first drops of insulin were isolated a half-century ago, treatment took a dramatic new turn and the mysteries of the disease began slowly to be unraveled.

WHAT IS DIABETES?

It is often said that the fundamental causes of diabetes are unknown. The same can be said of the weather. Scientists do not know all the basic and complex causes of changes in climate and weather, but what they do know is of considerable value in everyday living. A great deal *is* known about diabetes, and intricate pieces of the puzzle are constantly being found and fitted together. Moreover, diabetes is almost always readily identifiable, and something can be done about it.

Insulin Fifty Years After

In very general, oversimplified terms, diabetes at present is defined as insufficient, ineffective, or unavailable insulin, whatever the cause.

The basic theory is simple, but its workings are complex. Specialized cells in the tail of the pancreas gland *(beta cells)* produce the hormone known as insulin, store it, and release it upon demand. The beta cells are localized in the areas of the pancreas known as *islets of Langerhans,* whence the term "insulin." This hormone is necessary for the assimilation of basic food elements—carbohydrates, fats, proteins— and the storage of surpluses. Insulin also acts as a chemical messenger that directs various organs to store or release *glucose,* the simplest form of sugar readily used by the body. In the absence or ineffectiveness of insulin production, deleterious changes occur in innumerable tissues and organs due to the resulting glucose imbalance.

A beautifully orchestrated system turns the insulin supply on and off in a non-diabetic person. The first swallow of food (even the thought of it) prepares the ever-ready insulin system to start manufacturing the hormone, the release of which is actually just triggered by the release of a gastrointestinal hormone. As food is absorbed into the bloodstream, the rising blood-sugar level stimulates further insulin release. A normal person can produce 40 to 50 insulin units daily and has about 200 more units available in the pancreas for emergencies. The blood-sugar level of a non-diabetic is almost always tightly confined within a normal range that is nearly impossible to elevate, and this is true in every species.

The insulin factor. Dr. Frederick Banting and Dr. Charles Best, working in a grubby Toronto laboratory, produced the first usable preparation of insulin in 1921, and showed that lack of insulin is the main factor in the onset of diabetes.

Their experiments involving removal of the pancreas from dogs left the animals with no insulin whatsoever. The dogs became diabetic, their blood-sugar levels were grossly elevated, and they urinated constantly as their bodies attempted to remove the excessive blood sugar. The huge loss of fluid, unreplaced even by drinking large amounts of water, led to dehydration. Inability to assimilate food without insulin led to the inefficient, "smoky" burning of body fats. These acidic "ashes" resulted in *acidosis,* vast accumulations of ketones (acids), which is an abnormal state. The dogs died—as did human diabetics—from dehydration and acidosis, until the discovery of insulin. When prepared insulin was injected, blood sugars became normal and the experimental dogs survived.

Insulin was briefly hailed as the solution to all diabetic problems, but it soon became obvious that the hormone insulin by itself did not cure the disease. What it did, and does, is to prolong life and sustain functional health for many years, and indeed for some, nearly a full lifetime. That is essentially its role today, although some forms and refinements of insulin have been developed since the Banting-Best breakthrough.

pituitary gland

thyroid gland

one islet of
Langerhans

alpha cell

beta cell

delta cell

CHEMISTRY OF DIABETES

Hormone interactions in diabetes are subtle and complex. The pituitary gland releases growth hormone, which antagonizes insulin function, and somatostatin, which is an insulin helper. The thyroid gland speeds metabolism and creates a demand for more insulin. Emergencies trigger the adrenal glands to put out a burst of adrenaline, which raises blood-sugar levels.

ISLET CELLS

A single islet of Langerhans, one of a million or so in the pancreas, is shown diagrammatically in the circle. Specialized cells within the minute area of an islet produce an ebb and flow of hormones that maintain delicate balances in response to demands of the body. Beta cells produce insulin, store it, and release it as needed. Alpha cells produce glucagon, a hormone that raises blood-sugar levels, the opposite effect of insulin. Still other cells (delta cells) produce somatostatin, which assists insulin. In maturity-onset diabetes, the beta cells often produce enough insulin, or more than enough, but the diabetic cannot use it effectively.

adrenal glands

pancreas

Symptoms

Three "polys" are cardinal symptoms of diabetes. *Polyuria* is a great increase in the volume and frequency of urination, from the body's unceasing effort to wash excessive sugar and wasted food materials from the blood. In an uncontrolled diabetic, urination can become almost a full-time occupation. Loss of so much food material in the urine causes *polyphagia,* almost insatiable hunger. The third poly is *polydipsia,* constant thirst and incessant drinking. Accompanying signs are weight loss, dehydration, and extreme tiredness. Weakness is also quite understandable, since the untreated diabetic literally starves in the presence of plenty of food that cannot be assimilated without sufficient insulin.

Usually the most definite sign of diabetes is *hyperglycemia,* high levels of sugar in the blood. This by itself may not cause any symptoms, but if sugar levels continue high, the kidney glucose-filtering-retrieval system is overwhelmed and much sugar is spilled into the urine. *Glycosuria* (sugar in the urine) is characteristic of diabetes, and was historically a means of diagnosis. Ancient physicians noticed that flies gathered around discarded urine, which proved to be sweet to the taste.

Sugar in the blood. Everybody has sugar in the blood, in the form of glucose. Without it we would starve. The bloodstream is actually an intricate series of canals that deliver food elements to cells, and this cannot be done without insulin. The bloodstream also delivers wastes to the filtering systems of the liver and kidneys, which excrete the wastes in the urine and then reabsorb and return essential materials to the blood (see page 375). Glucose, being valuable to the body, is normally reabsorbed, but if the load becomes overwhelming, as in diabetes, the overtaxed recovery system cannot function effectively and sugar spills into the urine.

Diagnosis. Ordinarily, diabetes is readily identifiable. Suspicion is aroused if there is sugar in the urine, and confirmed if a blood test shows abnormal glucose levels. The laboratory tests are simple and should be a part of routine physical examinations. All routine physical exams should include diabetes screening. A more accurate diagnosis may require that tests be repeated or be given at timely intervals after test meals.

Mild symptoms of diabetes or "preclinical" diabetes (see page 407) may make diagnosis elusive. In borderline cases, a *glucose tolerance test* may be needed. This consists of measuring the blood-sugar level in the fasting state, having the patient drink a measured amount of liquid containing glucose, then monitoring the blood-glucose level at hourly intervals. If the level is abnormally high and remains elevated for a prolonged period, the patient presumably has diabetes.

WHICH DIABETES?

Diabetes, as we have used the word, is the common everyday term for *diabetes mellitus* or classical diabetes. The technical term can be loosely translated as "running through of sugar." A quite different disease, called *diabetes insipidus,* has nothing to do with usual diabetes but shares one of the cardinal symptoms: constant thirst, excessive water drinking, and the excretion of a great volume of pale urine, but without an increase in blood sugar or the appearance of urine sugar.

Diabetes insipidus results from a lesion affecting the production of one of the hormones of the pituitary gland. Persons with this condition may lose as much as 15 to 25 quarts of urine daily. There is no relationship to insulin production, and the condition can be readily treated with pituitary-hormone preparations.

Varieties of diabetes. Modern classifications of diabetes mellitus are rather confusing, not only to physicians, but also to patients who encounter baffling terms in the literature. Different names often represent the same thing, or describe various stages of diabetes. Sometimes the classifications derive from confusion concerning the onset, duration, or other problems of diabetes. We shall attempt to clarify terms.

"Juvenile diabetes," or juvenile-onset diabetes, mostly affects persons younger than 17, although this age may vary with individuals. The insulin-producing cells of such persons are damaged or even destroyed so that no insulin is produced and replacement injections are essential. Juvenile-onset diabetes is also called "labile" or "insulin dependent," and the objectionable term "brittle" is sometimes applied. Some adults have this juvenile-type diabetes, meaning simply that their diabetes is very difficult to regulate.

Maturity-onset diabetes or adult-onset diabetes generally afflicts people over 40 years of age; the peak age of diagnosis is during the fifth decade of life or later. The onset is often insidious, as contrasted to the juvenile type, which may occur quite rapidly. These older patients often produce enough of their own insulin, but for complex reasons that are the subject of much research, they cannot utilize it effectively.

The inference is that most adult-onset diabetics can be treated easily by diet alone or by oral tablets that lower the blood sugar. However, distinctions between juvenile and adult forms of diabetes are not ironclad. Some patients whose diabetes started at an early age may have a serene adult-like course with no difficulty in management, while others whose diabetes started in middle or later life have difficulty in maintaining a stable course. Hence, the term "juvenile diabetes" (really a misnomer) is sometimes used for any unstable, difficult-to-regulate diabetes.

Time-Spans of Diabetes

Diabetes can also be classified by its relationship to time.

Pre-diabetes. Essentially, pre-diabetes is a research term that has little real meaning since persons so labeled will not inevitably become diabetic. The term is used to label persons who appear susceptible to diabetes in the future (susceptibility to diabetes is discussed below). However, even highly suspect persons do not invariably become diabetic. At this stage, no abnormalities can be found in usual blood or urine tests. One "pre-diabetic" group, for example, would be those with parents who are both diabetic.

"Pre-clinical," "covert," "asymptomatic," or "chemical" diabetes. These terms designate persons ranging from those whose blood sugar is occasionally elevated after the stress of a large meal, to those whose blood glucose is nearly always elevated at such a time. These people ordinarily have no obvious symptoms and can be detected only if elevated blood glucose is found after a large meal or after drinking glucose. Sometimes glucose may be found in the urine. These findings are not always consistent and may be missed entirely, since there is little to raise the suspicion of either doctor or patient. This stage of the disease (also called "latent") often progresses to typical adult-onset diabetes.

Clinical diabetes, overt diabetes, or diabetes mellitus. Clinical diabetes is discovered by blood and urine testing, often because of symptoms. Untreated patients in this group nearly always have the symptoms previously detailed, and most diabetes is diagnosed at this stage. When classical symptoms are present, the diagnosis is almost impossible to miss.

WHO GETS DIABETES?

The spectrum of diabetes is so broad that one is tempted to state that almost anyone can get it. This is not quite true, however, as millions of people do not become diabetic. But a number of factors are known to predispose to diabetes.

Heredity

Heredity is a major factor in the onset of diabetes, but while the influence of heredity is unquestioned, it is not a simple and clear-cut influence. While most authorities believe that diabetes occurs only in persons with a hereditary predisposition to it, not all such persons will succumb to it, regardless of how long they live. Other factors are apparently necessary to provoke symptoms in the predisposed. The inherited predisposition could be a "pre-diabetic" state that may or may not erupt into overt disease. Exactly what is inherited is not known; possibly it is an incapacity of the pancreas to secrete enough insulin at appropriate times, which is not manifested until environmental factors augment the genetic predisposition and then precipitate the disorder.

There is a heavy predominance of diabetes in the family histories of diabetics. In the simplest genetic pattern, diabetes is thought to be an incomplete recessive disease. Theoretically, if the father and mother both have diabetes, all their children should develop the disease eventually. If only one parent has diabetes, half their children should develop the disease and the others should be carriers. But it does not quite work out that way. In fact, not more than one in eight or ten will become diabetic, and that may be at an older age.

One problem is that a hereditary diabetic background is not always known. Who knows for sure that a great uncle or cousin had diabetes, and how long ago? Few accurate medical records were kept several generations back. Many persons with newly found diabetes know of no one in their families who had this condition in the past, but ten or twenty years later, relatives *are* found with diabetes. More diabetes within families appears as people live longer, although not everyone tells relatives of his "infirmities." In an Oxford, Massachusetts diabetic study in 1946, about 20 percent of patients with newly found diabetes knew of diabetic relatives, but 12 years later, 70 percent or more knew of such relatives.

Heredity is undoubtedly an important factor in diabetes and certainly one to be aware of, but its influence cannot be specified in hard-and-fast ways. It might be thought of as an influence that lies dormant, even for an entire lifetime, unless other factors awaken it.

Stress

Various stresses are significant influences in inducing diabetes to "break out" in a predisposed person. Aging itself is a stress since many body functions are somewhat less efficient after age 40 than before. Blood-sugar levels may gradually become a bit elevated in the decades after 50, not necessarily achieving diabetic levels, but at least indicating decreased insulin output.

Severe infections are a common form of stress. Women who have given birth to large babies (over nine pounds) or to many children are more likely to develop diabetes than the average woman.

Obesity, which creates a demand for more insulin than the body can provide, is the most common and greatest stress factor in our society, and it is known also that the overweight use insulin much less effectively. There are many other possible stress situations, of course, but if a person inherits a potentially imperfect insulin-producing system, the effects of aging, obesity, multiple childbirth, multiple infections, and other forms of stress may bring the diabetes potential to an active phase.

Viruses

The possibility that viruses may be linked to the onset of diabetes has long been considered. Mumps has been indicated as an occasional cause of diabetes in some. English scientists noted that diabetic children had antibodies to certain viruses, indicating past infection, more frequently than their non-diabetic peers. It was also observed that diabetes in the young was more frequent when viral infections were rampant, and that the prevalence was much greater at ages five to seven and twelve to fourteen, periods when children enroll in primary and secondary schools.

The virus connection is not proved but is tempting to speculate on, for if a virus could be implicated, a vaccine might be effective against it. Unfortunately, a large number of viruses are now thought to have this capability. This would make it more difficult to produce an effective vaccine against multiple offending viral agents.

It is probably true that diabetes is more common in certain ethnic groups, but not because of racial or ethnic origins. Populations in which people have intermarried over long periods of time apparently have greater susceptibility, which, coupled with overweight, insufficient exercise, rich diet, and other such factors, makes it easier for diabetes to surface from the latent or "prediabetes" area.

TREATMENT OF DIABETES

If diabetes is considered to be a problem related to lack of enough useful, active, effective insulin at proper times, then the treatment is quite simple: restoration of insulin in amounts to do the job that it alone can do. There are, however, very complex hormonal and other influences that confuse the issue (see page 425) and that may lead to new or modified treatments as researchers delve into them. But all of today's treatment methods replace insulin in one way or another, albeit sometimes in less obvious ways.

Juvenile-onset diabetics do not produce any insulin, or virtually none, and almost always must have insulin replaced by injection. So must many long-term adult diabetics. Insulin must be injected because, if swallowed, it is digested like any protein food and does not enter the blood as insulin.

In milder forms of diabetes, where the problem is only a *relative* lack of insulin, diet may be the only treatment necessary. For instance, if an obese diabetic does not produce enough insulin to be effective in the face of excess weight, reduction of excess weight may provide sufficient insulin. When diet is effective, the person can use his own insulin, which is at least as good as that from outside sources.

For some diabetics who do not produce enough insulin, and in whom weight reduction and diet are not effective, certain oral *blood-sugar-lowering tablets* are available. These are also called *oral hypoglycemic agents*. Compounds called *sulfonylureas* stimulate the pancreas to either make or release more insulin. These compounds are not effective in all patients, but when they are they may aid in keeping blood-sugar levels normal. Other substances, called *biguanides,* have been used to lower the blood-sugar levels. They do not increase insulin production, but work by augmenting any available insulin.

Determining treatment. If a middle-aged person who hasn't been feeling well goes to a doctor who diagnoses diabetes, the patient is often quite understandably surprised and upset. What lies ahead? Treatment of mild diabetes of the adult-onset type in an obese patient usually begins with diet alone, since diet and weight loss are the keystones of treatment.

Tests and evaluations will be done to fit the treatment to the patient, as the spectrum of diabetes, from mild to severe, is very broad. Sometimes the patient may be hospitalized for a week or so while blood and urine tests are done, the need for insulin injections is assessed, forms and dosages are determined, a history of allergies and reactions is taken, and even one's life-style is scrutinized. Life-style is important, however, because if a diabetic exercises vigorously or does hard physical work, he will need less insulin than if he were sedentary. Increasingly, these tests are being done on an outpatient basis.

In almost no other chronic disease is the faithful, dedicated following of a prescribed program by the patient more rewarding than with diabetes. The physician can direct and oversee, but the diabetic lives with his condition day by day, and what he does daily is vital to his welfare. Instruction and information are important—self-testing of urine by dipping "test sticks" into it, knowing when and what to eat, and spacing insulin injections—and all are learned with the aid of a doctor. The reward? One is reminded of the advice of Dr. Oliver Wendell Holmes on how to live a long life: "Acquire a chronic disease early in life and take care of it."

Exercise

Exercise, too, has an important role in diabetes. The disorder does not foreclose one from hard work, a smashing tennis game, or a good jog. On the contrary, there are famous professional athletes who are diabetic. It has long been known that vigorously active persons require much less insulin than those who are sedentary. During exercise, there is much greater uptake of the basic fuel, glucose, by the muscles. Exercise burns sugar, like insulin, and lowers blood-glucose levels, even more so in diabetics than in non-diabetics. Patients who need insulin injections learn, with a doctor's help, how to adjust to exercise by taking less insulin before strenuous activity, or perhaps by eating more.

Diet

"Diet" is a word that turns people off, implying rigid, even inhumane restriction. Yet diet is merely what we eat, and innumerable persons follow special diets for many sound medical reasons. It is more gracious and encouraging to call a diet a "meal plan" or "eating plan."

The great majority of adult-onset diabetics are obese when the disease is discovered. Many, if not most of them, make enough of their own insulin to avert or suppress symptoms of diabetes if their body weight were normal. For them, a basic well-balanced reducing diet (see page 150) to bring their weight down to normal, thus equalizing their insulin output with their needs, may be the only treatment needed. Those adult-onset diabetics who are lean to begin with usually need insulin injections along with meal plans to maintain their normal weight and activity. It is important for both the fat and the lean to have the goal of keeping their weight normal.

Suitable meal plans for individual diabetics are furnished by physicians and clinics to patients under treatment (an *untreated* diabetic is at considerable risk), and we will not give a long list of specifics. The principles of diet, however, are quite simple:

- It must contain enough calories to fuel the body's activities, but not so many as to pile on body fat.
- It should have a proper balance of carbohydrate, protein, and fat.

All foods contain one or all of these. A pizza, for example, is made up of carbohydrate, fat, and protein.

Of the three components, *carbohydrate* (sugars and starches) may be most misunderstood. It is the main fuel for body energy use the world over. Sugars are quickly assimilated; marathon runners can be seen sucking an orange or eating a candy bar for a rapid spurt of energy. Starchy components—grains, vegetables, breads, "staffs of life"—are not overwhelmingly sweet and some people do not think of them as carbohydrate at all. Starchy carbohydrates, in forms of wheat, rice, potatoes, corn, and vegetables, supply major energy needs of world populations. *Protein* builds and repairs tissues and can be drawn on, somewhat wastefully and more slowly, for energy. Fat, including oils, is usually visible in foods and is the form in which excess energy, from overeating, is stored in often unflattering deposits in the body.

Carbohydrate, protein, and fat are required in every healthful meal plan. So are vitamins and minerals, which are normally provided by a well-balanced diet but which may need supplementation in those rare cases where there is loss or depletion.

Timing of eating is extremely important for diabetics. If a normal person eats nothing all day, very small amounts of insulin are released as he slowly digests himself. Since the diabetic cannot make insulin as needed, the amount of insulin injected in the morning is planned to last exactly 24 hours, until the next insulin injection is due. If it does, meals must be spaced to maintain an adequate level of blood sugar. One way of proportioning the food is to allow one-fifth of the calories for breakfast, two-fifths for lunch, and two-fifths for dinner. In addition, many insulin users need mid-morning and mid-afternoon snacks to avoid low-blood-sugar reactions.

Although this balancing of food intake to match the available insulin is an artificial way of living, it's necessary to balance insulin and diet. There is a similar need for such timing of food intake when oral tablets are used. The insulin level provided by injection in diabetics will not accommodate large sudden masses of food intake. As a result, mostly-carbohydrate meals are often largely spilled into the urine.

SELF-DISPENSED INSULIN

Normally, insulin is dispensed from the pancreas gland as fluctuations of food intake, fasting, and exercise demand it. An average adult has some 200 units of insulin in reserve and produces about 40 units a day. Breakfast triggers the release of perhaps 5 units of insulin, and other meals "turn on" insulin in automatic response to food intake and activities of the day.

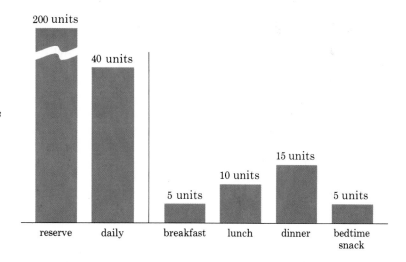

200 units · 40 units · reserve · daily · 5 units · breakfast · 10 units · lunch · 15 units · dinner · 5 units · bedtime snack

INJECTED INSULIN

A diabetic who needs one injection of insulin a day (some need more) has a pool of insulin that lasts 24 hours. He cannot fine-tune it to changing balances. Thus, meals must be spaced to prevent low-blood-sugar reactions, which can occur if the insulin has little or no food to act upon. The graph shows one way of proportioning food intake to keep diet and insulin in balance.

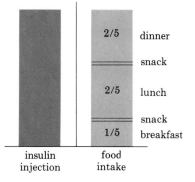

insulin injection · food intake · 2/5 dinner · snack · 2/5 lunch · snack · 1/5 breakfast

Types of food are also important. The fastest to be absorbed is a glucose solution such as orange juice, which is utilized almost immediately. Massive sweet, sugary concentrations are difficult to contain in an effective diet, but more complicated carbohydrate, as found in vegetables and grains, can be used since it is broken down and absorbed more gradually. A good diet does not require peculiar, fad-like foods. In fact, except for those foods that contain massive amounts of sweets, the diabetic can eat most foods that others eat.

Amount and variety. A first consideration in planning a diabetic meal plan is what the person's ideal weight should be, related to activity. Nine times out of ten, the newly discovered adult-onset diabetic is obese, and the object is to reduce weight while providing sufficient food for energy. Others will need to gain weight or remain at normal weight.

The fact is that diabetes treatment must be "tailor-made" for the individual patient. Persons who are active and make some or much of their own insulin can use fairly generous diets. But those who are completely insulin-dependent will have great difficulty in maintaining any type of control if their diet is too liberal or irregular.

A doctor considers calories and proportions of carbohydrate, fat, and protein in fitting a diet to the needs of a particular patient. A good deal of caloric adjustment for weight control can be done with fats, which have more than twice as many calories per gram (9) as carbohydrate and protein (4 each). The present tendency is to use less fat, more protein, and relatively more generous portions of carbohydrate than were used previously.

There is some disagreement as to the ideal amount of carbohydrate. A fairly liberal amount of carbohydrate may work out satisfactorily for patients who are active or take sufficient insulin.

How much food is enough? If a person loses nutrients in the urine through poor diabetes control, hunger will be insatiable and weight will still be lost. Smaller amounts of food may be satisfying and adequate if this loss of nutrients is diminished by diet or insulin.

Meal planning. A typical diet for a moderately active person might contain 200 grams of carbohydrate, 90 grams of protein, and 80 grams of fat for a total of 1,800 calories. Since gram measurements are difficult for most Americans to understand, ordinary household measures will do as well. Better yet is the Exchange System, originally encouraged for the convenience of diabetics by the American Diabetic Association.

In this system, foods are classified according to their carbohydrate, protein, fat, and calorie values. Equivalent foods are grouped into a common category, let us say a Meat Exchange or a Bread Exchange, for which values are pre-counted in grams and calories. Figuring daily intake accurately is a matter of simple addition. For instance, a Meat Exchange furnishes 7 grams of protein, 5 grams of fat, negligible carbohydrate, and 73 calories. It isn't necessarily meat, either—instead of an ounce of chicken, substitute one egg, which has the same nutrient value. The Exchange System allows one to substitute equivalent foods that are preferred or happen to be in the refrigerator. And the gram- and calorie-counting is automatic. For details, see page 143.

Realistically, the meal plan must contain foods that the person likes and is used to eating. It does not require strange or peculiar foods—just foods that are properly balanced and distributed to prevent waste of calories through the urine, or undesirable weight gain. With time and enough effort, it is even possible to have a diabetic diet of gourmet quality, although simpler foods are obviously much easier to prepare on a routine basis.

Insulin

Millions of units of insulin have been self-injected by diabetic patients over the years. Many thousands of diabetics have now lived longer than 30 years, which, if they take two injections daily, as many do, would mean something like 25,000 injections — far from pleasurable, but a reasonable price for life and health. The number of 50-year-duration diabetics is also increasing.

There are still some problems with insulin. Several forms, variable in onset and duration of effect, have been developed. The purest type of insulin is *regular,* clear, or crystalline insulin, very much like the natural product of the pancreas gland. It is absorbed rapidly and is effective almost immediately, but duration of effect is usually not more than six hours. The life of insulin produced by the body is very much shorter, but it is constantly released as needed. If regular insulin were the only one in use for injection by diabetics, it would have to be injected three or four times daily. It is most useful in diabetic emergencies.

Changes have been made to make insulin effective for longer periods. One of the most common intermediate forms is *Lente insulin* (meaning slowly). The other most commonly used insulin is *NPH,* which is regular insulin premixed with protamine zinc in order to prolong its action. Both of these are usually effective within an hour and are planned to last 24 hours.

A problem is that, in many patients, the intermediate insulins don't start their activity soon enough, while in other patients, they are too short in duration. By mixing short- and longer-acting insulins, and/or by taking intermediate-acting insulin twice a day, fuller coverage may be provided. Many patients require two daily injections for stable control. Other insulins *(Ultra-Lente* and *Protamine Zinc)* are quite long-acting with a duration of longer than a day. There is also a *Semi-Lente,* which acts a bit longer than regular insulin, but for a lesser period of time than the intermediate insulins.

While most diabetics on insulin therapy use NPH or Lente, many, and nearly all juvenile-onset patients, require mixtures of various types of insulin, usually injected as one dose in the same syringe. Many factors are involved in the insulin requirements of an individual patient, and at times the requirements may increase, as from stresses, infections, and illnesses that increase the need for insulin. A diabetic also needs special schedules of insulin when undergoing surgery, and regulation must obviously be left in the hands of a physician during these stress periods.

Self-tests of urine. Patients are instructed how to make rather simple tests of urine to measure the effectiveness of blood-sugar control. Tests before meals and at bedtime, continued for a period of time, may be desirable when diabetes is just diagnosed in order to adjust treatment to the patient's customary range of activities and possible wide fluctuations in blood-sugar levels. Later, this may be accomplished with fewer tests.

The urine-test materials are tablets or "test strips" of chemically treated paper or tape, which are dropped or dipped into urine as directed on the package. A change in color of the testing material indicates the amount of sugar in the urine.

"Diabetes Pills"

Properly called *oral hypoglycemic agents,* "diabetes pills" are tablets or capsules that, in many patients, reduce blood-sugar levels—a benchmark of control of the disease. A group of blood-sugar-lowering compounds called *sulfonylureas* came into use about 20 years ago. They have the property of stimulating release of insulin from the beta cells of the pancreas, and are effective only if the patient's pancreas can produce some insulin. This limitation ruled out their usefulness for many long-term diabetics who often require large amounts of insulin, and certainly ruled out younger juvenile-onset diabetics who produce no insulin of their own.

The sulfonylureas proved to be most effective in treatment of diabetics whose onset was after age 40, who had diabetes for less than ten years, and who required less than about 30 units of insulin daily. While there were some exceptions to these criteria, in general the tablets were most effective for the milder diabetics.

Another group of oral agents called *biguanides* later became available. These tablets do not stimulate the pancreas to release more insulin, but work in different ways, which might be summarized as amplification of what little natural insulin is available.

The tablets have been used by millions of diabetics throughout the world. Since the two types of pills work differently, combinations were sometimes used. The good news about the tablets was that they freed suitable patients from the distress of injecting themselves with insulin, and if effective, they used the person's own insulin, which presumably is at least as good as that from an animal source. They also had a public health benefit by encouraging persons who feared diagnosis, because of apprehension about insulin injection, to "come out of the woods" for a checkup.

A negative effect of the pills was that patients who had been using them were very difficult to change over to insulin injections, if and when the tablets became ineffective. Significant numbers of patients had a secondary failure—that is, while treatment with oral agents was successful for a time, they later needed insulin because the tablets became less effective. Most often the reason for such failures is the fact that diabetes may become less readily treatable without insulin after a period of years, or after failure to observe diet.

The simple convenience of the oral agents led to a certain amount of mediocre treatment. Many patients neglected diet, itself an effective treatment in most overweight adult-onset diabetics, and an important factor in successful treatment with oral agents. There were some annoying side effects from the pills, but at one time about 40 percent of diabetics in the United States were treated with oral compounds, possibly another 40 percent with insulin, and 20 percent with diet alone.

All seemed serene until a study labeled UGDP (University Group Diabetes Program) was publicized several years ago. The study was organized by twelve university-affiliated clinics for the laudable purpose of determining whether treatment with oral compounds prevented long-term diabetic complications. Some 800-odd patients, supposedly of the same diabetic status, were divided into four groups among twelve large diabetes clinics. One group received a fixed dose of a sulfonylurea pill (tolbutamide), while another received placebos—pills with no active ingredients. A third group was treated with a fixed daily dose of insulin, and the fourth received variable doses of insulin as needed.

The study concluded that there was an excess of deaths from cardiovascular disease in patients treated with oral drugs, and that the death rate was 2½ times greater in this group than in those treated with a placebo. Publication of findings, initially in the lay press, roused a great pro-and-con furor, with a polarization of physicians and non-physicians, informed and uninformed, into two camps. One group believed the use of oral hypoglycemic agents to be potentially dangerous; the other felt that they were a boon in treatment of diabetes and should be used as needed.

Although no other project of comparable magnitude has been attempted, studies by other groups around the world, while admittedly not strictly comparable, generally do not substantiate the UGDP data. Opponents have questioned the choice of patients for the UGDP groups, the validity of statistical analysis, the fact that an unchanging dose of medication was used regardless of patients' needs, and the extrapolation of data from 800 patients to the millions of diabetics under treatment. The Committee for the Care of the Diabetic, a large group of diabetes specialists, strongly opposed the Food and Drug Administration's plan to make oral treatment difficult by requiring stringent package inserts.

Meanwhile, the debate has raged in and out of courts, in scientific circles and elsewhere, and some years later the controversy has not been resolved. The two polarized camps of physicians are now augmented by a third group that feels the oral agents could be used with relative safety but should be prescribed prudently, that there are many patients who cannot or will not take insulin (which is also not without some hazard), and that the oral agents, if used intelligently and carefully, have a definite place in the treatment of diabetes.

If nothing other than a sense of caution and careful evaluation of the goals of individual treatment evolves from the controversial UGDP study, it will have been worthwhile. Other studies, possibly yielding more definitive answers, are being done. But to date, the study findings have not been generally accepted throughout the rest of the world where use of the tablets continues, apparently without reservations.

SHORT-TERM PROBLEMS

Sooner or later, many persons with diabetes are likely to experience some acute or short-term problems. Most of these give warnings that should be recognizable by the patient and, just as important, by informed members of the family.

Insulin Reaction

(Low Blood Sugar)

This is the most common complication in diabetics who use insulin or oral tablets. The condition has also been called "insulin shock"—in effect, too much insulin, causing rapid or gradual lowering of blood sugar below the normal levels.

What causes this relative excess of insulin? It can be too much insulin, not enough food, unusual amounts of exercise, or any combination of these.

Symptoms. A lowered blood-sugar level causes typical reaction symptoms such as sweating, nervousness, extreme hunger, anxiety, headache, confusion, weakness, and, if prolonged and untreated, even unconsciousness. Most insulin reactions are minimal and mostly annoying, are nearly always preventable, and are completely harmless if treated early. On the other hand, if severe and prolonged, the reaction can be dangerous. Another danger is the possibility of a reaction occurring while driving a car or during any activity requiring coordination and clear judgment. Another area of potential danger is the incapacitation of a reaction during swimming or skiing. Persons treated with insulin should not participate in these sports alone. Family and friends should understand the nature of insulin reactions, which can cause great alarm and the unnecessary treatment of a condition that is easily corrected in its early stages.

Treatment. An immediate treatment is the ingestion of quickly assimilable sugars, preferably sweet liquids such as orange juice, ginger ale, or anything else containing sugar. Diabetics should carry candy or sugar cubes that are quickly available. Even crackers or similar forms of less quickly assimilated carbohydrate will serve in a pinch. Filling stations with machines that dispense sugary soft drinks (not the diet kind) are oases for diabetics who feel an insulin reaction coming on.

Severe reactions when a patient cannot respond (never try to force liquids into an unconscious person) will require at least an injection of *glucagon,* a secretion of the pancreas gland that raises blood sugar. In still more severe cases, intravenous glucose may be necessary. Frequently, the "education" of a diabetic's family includes instruction as to when and how to give a glucagon injection with an insulin syringe.

Ketoacidosis

This is a more serious problem, terminating, if untreated, in *diabetic coma,* the most frequent cause of death of diabetics in the days before insulin. Diabetic coma is quite rare today because of prompt effective treatment, but it is a threat to untreated diabetics who may not be aware of the dangers of their disease and to persons whose control of the disease is poor. It is the opposite of an insulin reaction. Diabetic acidosis occurs when, because of insufficient insulin, blood-sugar levels increase greatly and acids such as acetone become increased in the blood. This sets up the chain reaction of events outlined below.

Symptoms. Fortunately, ketoacidosis does not usually occur suddenly, but takes place over a period of hours or even a day or more. There is increased urination, dehydration, loss of body fluids, and the appearance of large amounts of glucose and acetone in the urine. The patient becomes drowsy, tired, and thirsty, and vomiting or diarrhea often occur. As symptoms progress toward coma, breathing becomes labored and the breath takes on a sweetish odor (acetone). Unconsciousness may appear on short notice or after a period of hours. All of this, however, is reversible if treatment is begun early enough.

Ketoacidosis frequently occurs when a diabetic becomes ill from some common infection, does not eat, and skips the insulin dose at a time when even more insulin is needed. True diabetics need insulin even when not eating, and massive loss of body fluids from urination, vomiting, or diarrhea can bring on acidosis.

Treatment of ketoacidosis is of an emergency nature, usually requiring hospitalization. A doctor should be called at once; home measures cannot help and can only delay treatment and recovery. Insulin is given as needed, sometimes in large amounts, and intravenous fluids are needed to replace salts and vital electrolytes depleted by the tremendous loss through the massive urination.

There are other types of acidosis as well. A threat to older patients is *hyperosmolar acidosis,* which is related to dehydration and concentration of body fluids rather than to an insulin deficit alone. Although it is treated with insulin, the basic correction is of fluid imbalance.

There is also a *lactic acidosis* caused by excessive lactic acid in the blood. Lactates, which are salts of lactic acid, are usable as fuel, but if excessive amounts are present or cannot be used, severe acidosis will result. This condition also is treatable when recognized early.

One of the problems clouding the treatment picture is the recent publicity concerning the oral compound DBI and its implication as the alleged cause of lactic acidosis. Actually these biguanide preparations have been in use by millions of patients for 15 or more years. Apparently lactic acidosis takes place especially when these compounds are used to treat persons who have defective kidney or other organic function. In these situations, the lactic acid can be increased to dangerous levels.

The use of phenformins (biguanide drugs) has been restricted to patients with special needs certified by an attending physician.

Infection

One of the threats to diabetics is the increased susceptibility to infection. One reason is that body defense mechanisms do not function optimally in the presence of high levels of blood glucose. However, a diabetic whose condition is well controlled generally has no exceptional difficulty with infections, nor should he, providing there is adequate circulation of blood. Antibiotics have helped to reduce this threat so that the numerous boils and carbuncles formerly seen in diabetics are now rarely seen.

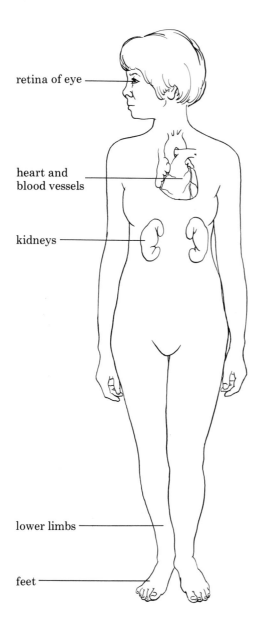

retina of eye

heart and
blood vessels

kidneys

lower limbs

feet

LONG-TERM COMPLICATIONS

The association of diabetes with many "degenerative" diseases is repeatedly mentioned in other chapters of this book by specialists who discuss disorders of the heart, circulation, eyes, kidneys, and other organ systems. A belief that all diabetics will surely develop these complications in a crippling manner is widespread but ill-founded. While many with diabetes do develop complications after a period of years, and should be aware of and informed about them, many escape them or are not incapacitated by them. Fear of complications can impose a great burden of unnecessary worry.

Uncontrolled diabetes unquestionably increases the risk of early and serious complications. Whether good control can avert late complications is not proved, but the consensus of authorities is that the patient who conscientiously follows a program designed for him has much greater likelihood of avoiding or postponing them.

VULNERABLE ORGANS

Parts of the body especially susceptible to diabetic complications are shown in the drawing. Deterioration of blood vessels may ultimately impair circulation to any tissue or organ, particularly the retina of the eyes, the heart, and the kidneys. The feet and lower limbs are vulnerable to poor circulation; good foot hygiene is important. Tingling sensations or pain may be caused by effects on the nervous system. Excessive fear is unwarranted if the diabetic has good medical supervision and is informed about the importance of self-care.

The Eyes

Diabetes is one of the leading causes of blindness originating in adults, yet relatively few diabetics become legally blind. The statements do not conflict. There are many who have markedly impaired vision or whose retinopathy has destroyed their sight, but these are a small percentage compared to eight or ten million probable diabetics in the United States. The chance of a diabetic's becoming blind if he or she lives long enough is real, but quite small, percentage-wise. Moreover, newer types of treatment give hope that the threat of blindness can be further reduced.

Hemorrhage. The eye is essentially like a hollow table tennis ball with a membranous covering, filled with fluid that keeps the eyeball distended. Increases in fluid pressure cause a condition called glaucoma, another leading cause of blindness that is not especially related to diabetes.

One danger is that after many years of diabetes (at least ten or more), changes may take place in blood vessels of the eyes. At first the changes appear to be little red dots (microaneurysms). These may or may not progress and are reversible. More threatening is the formation of brittle new vessels (called neovascularization) that may rupture and leak blood into the eye fluid. Small, early hemorrhages may be absorbed and improve, but if enough blood leaks into the eyeball, vision is obviously obstructed.

Can good control of diabetes lessen the possibility of hemorrhage or reduce the amount of visual loss? There is some evidence that it may, but it is very difficult to relate the quality of care directly, since relatively few diabetics have had really good care over a period of many years. The eyes sometimes deteriorate to a point, then remain on a stable plateau for many years, and sometimes improve spontaneously.

Diabetic retinopathy. Disease of the retina, the image-receiving, light-sensitive tissue at the back of the eyeball, is termed *retinopathy.* The retina is a vulnerable area in diabetics. Rupture-prone, extraneous blood vessels may grow on its surface, bleeding points may appear, and scars can occur, sometimes detaching the retina.

Symptoms and treatment of detached retina are discussed elsewhere, as are the uses of *lasers* for treatment (see page 362). Of the latter, the type known as *xenon arc* produces a true photo-coagulation that can actually destroy tissue but, skillfully used, can prevent further bleeding in selected cases. *Ruby* and *green* lasers act differently to improve circulation through the eye and indirectly decrease the number of threatening extraneous blood vessels.

A recent study conducted in a number of clinics by the National Eye Institute reported that proper use of lasers showed promise in treatment of retinopathies and could be helpful in preventing blindness. The techniques are too recent for full evaluation, but the outlook is indeed hopeful.

What of the person whose vision is already impaired or destroyed by massive hemorrhage into the eye? A dramatic new type of surgery called *vitrectomy* has recently come into prominence (see page 363). It employs a combined probe and drill-and-suction instrument to suck out hemorrhagic material and replace it with normal saline solution.

This procedure is generally reserved for patients who have completely lost their vision in at least one eye for a prolonged period. Sometimes this surgery may restore some degree of vision, or at least give a clear field through which the ophthalmologist can see if lasers or other treatment might be effective. Vitrectomy demands great skill and, as techniques are perfected, could advance the treatment of visual complications of diabetes.

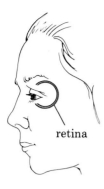

retina

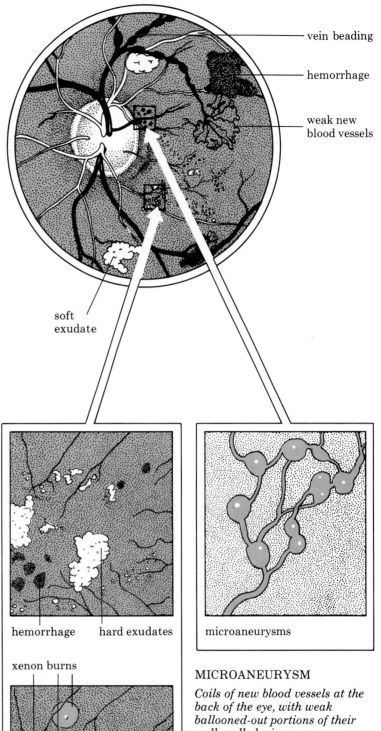

vein beading

hemorrhage

weak new
blood vessels

soft
exudate

hemorrhage   hard exudates

microaneurysms

xenon burns

RETINOPATHY

*Diabetic retinopathy affects the
retina and blood vessels at the
back of the eye. The drawing in
the circle shows various manifestations. An early change is the
appearance of tiny red "blood
blisters" (microaneurysms).
Weak new blood vessels may
form, rupture, and leak blood
into the eye. Hard and soft
materials (exudates) may pass
through the walls of vessels. The
eye reflects all of the degenerative ills of diabetes.*

HEMORRHAGE

*Leakage of blood into the eye ob-
structs vision partially or
completely. Small hemorrhages
may be absorbed and improve,
but a massive hemorrhage is like
a blinding curtain of blood.
Vitrectomy is a last-hope procedure for sucking blood and clots
out of the eye through an instrument and replacing sucked-out
material with saline solution.*

PHOTOCOAGULATION

*The drawing at right shows
bleeding points in the retina that
have been sealed off (photo-
coagulated) by rays from a type
of laser (xenon arc) to prevent
further bleeding. The treatment
is most successful when done
early while the patient still has
good vision. Tears in the retina
also can be sealed by laser
techniques.*

MICROANEURYSM

*Coils of new blood vessels at the
back of the eye, with weak
ballooned-out portions of their
walls called microaneurysms,
may develop in persons who
have had diabetes for ten years
or more. The tiny blood-filled
blisters are rupture-prone and
may leak blood into the eye. An
eye examination can reveal the
condition in early stages before
vision is impaired.*

Blood Vessels

The circulatory system ages in diabetics and non-diabetics alike. The main difference is that blood-vessel deteriorations occur earlier in diabetics than in non-diabetics, and underlie complications that may occur in the eyes, heart, kidneys, and in the blood supply to any tissue or organ.

Many diabetics have cardiovascular disease at an earlier age than their non-diabetic peers, consistent with the observation that diabetics often age earlier than non-diabetics. This is thought to be especially true if diabetes is poorly regulated, although it has not yet been shown that good control of blood-sugar levels, a keystone of treatment, can prevent premature aging of vessels. Perhaps this is because, with treatments now available, it is very difficult to fine-tune the responses to the continually fluctuating need for insulin, which a healthy pancreas does with ease.

Suffice it to say that a person with diabetes should have an evaluation of heart and blood-vessel status as part of a proper medical examination for early treatment. Diabetics often have increased blood levels of *lipids* (cholesterol, triglycerides, and other fatty substances) that frequently improve with good diabetic care. Treatment of high blood pressure and other conditions associated with cardiovascular disease is discussed on page 65.

While it is true that cardiovascular disease is a major problem in diabetes, excessive fear and apprehension are hardly warranted, assuming that the "whole patient" has good medical care. Increasing numbers of diabetics have lived 50 or more years since the onset of their diabetes without exhibiting evidence of serious degenerative disease.

The Kidneys

Another frequent complication resulting from diabetes is kidney disease (nephropathy). Initial damage occurs in the basement membrane and small vessels of the kidney, and later involves the entire kidney structure. The ultimate outcome is uremia, which is probably the leading cause of death of juvenile-onset diabetics.

Management of serious kidney disease has advanced greatly in recent years through the increasing use of dialysis and successful transplantations, giving improved quality and duration of life to many who had no such hope before (see page 379). The function of the kidney is to purify the blood, removing many of the waste products.

Disease of the Nervous System

(Neuropathy)

One of the most annoying and, in fact, unsolved problems of diabetes is damage to the nervous system (neuropathy). Symptoms may occur early or late in the course of the disease. Often the manifestations are minor nuisances—sensations of numbness, tingling, or the feeling that a limb has "gone to sleep." But sometimes the condition can cause severe pain, as well as loss of strength and muscle tone.

The condition is exasperating, particularly since there is no specific treatment. The cause is unknown, but recent research has shown that when blood-sugar levels are continually elevated—which is to say, poorly controlled—an undesirable end-product called *sorbitol,* which is a form of carbohydrate degeneration, is stored in nerves and other tissues as well. This *may* be a factor in diabetic neuropathy.

Current treatment consists of relieving pain, attending to diabetes control, and encouraging the patient. In most cases, the pain eventually disappears. Neuropathy, while an annoying condition, is not the destructive process that kidney or eye complications can be.

Diabetic impotence. Not always publicly discussed but rather frequent in middle-aged diabetic males is the problem of sexual impotence. It differs from impotence of psychogenic origin in that it has a definite organic basis. Failure to recognize the fact of a probable organic basis for premature impotence in some diabetics can lead to marital stress. A wife suffering from flagging attentions may believe this is proof of infidelity. A husband can be humiliated by waning virility and inability to maintain an erection although his sex drive is as strong as ever.

Impotence is not usually a problem until diabetes has existed for a long period, although it sometimes may be a symptom of undiagnosed diabetes in a middle-aged man who has previously been normally potent. The man is fully responsive to erotic stimuli, but insidiously and progressively loses his ability to have erections.

The underlying cause is a form of neuropathy. Erection usually results when blood collects in and distends the penis, and dilation of arteries is under nervous control. Inability of nerve impulses to dilate arteries of the penis and maintain the engorgement of the organ with blood may cause this condition, highly suggestive that impotence is of diabetic origin. Other indications of neuropathy in addition to numbness, tingling, and pain are absence of nocturnal emissions and morning erections.

Can diabetic impotence be avoided or postponed? There is no specific treatment. The impotence is usually permanent if it is truly of diabetic origin, but it may not be. Other causes of impotence affect diabetics and non-diabetics alike. Diabetes that is untreated, leaving the patient badly out of control with resulting weakness and debilitation may result in a type of impotence that is reversible, but this is not the typical impotence of neuropathy.

What can be done about the loss of sex life due to neuropathy? Unfortunately, nothing specific. The other causes of this condition should be ruled out. Ordinarily there is no diminution of male hormone. Proper psychic support and understanding are vital. The problem should be discussed jointly with husband and wife, since many times this loss of ability is accepted when both parties realize it is not the fault of any one of them but rather an inevitable state caused by a physical situation beyond their control, or as the ancient Greeks put it, "the Gods didn't smile on us." Understanding and acceptance brings other compensations. Moreover, urologists now have access to certain prosthetic devices that might be helpful in some circumstances.

Feet and Limbs

Most of us have heard harrowing stories about diabetics who had their toes amputated, or a foot, or even a leg, because of gangrene (death of tissues). Blood-vessel narrowing does make the possibility of gangrene more of a threat to diabetics than to others. However, in recent years there have been dramatic improvements in surgical techniques so that the threat has been greatly minimized.

There are many reasons for this improved outlook—better medical care by physicians, the effectiveness of antibiotics, and tremendous advances in surgical techniques such as blood-vessel grafts and bypass operations. Indeed, innumerable feet have been saved. Fewer amputations are needed, and when they are, they may be only partial. Not the least important treatment is education of the patient to make him aware of potential difficulties and of good hygiene and foot care.

The foot, the farthest extremity from the heart, is a natural target for poor circulation and infection. As we grow older, blood vessels become more hardened, narrowed, and atherosclerotic (see page 77). This narrowing of arteries with decreased circulation is worsened by many years of diabetes, particularly where vessels become smaller near the end of the leg and foot. If infection occurs in the foot, there is insufficient blood at a time when more blood is needed to assist the healing process. A neglected small scratch or blister may worsen and eventually become gangrenous if excellent care is not instituted. Furthermore, many diabetics have decreased sensation due to neuropathy and may not readily feel pain, which warns of impending problems.

Diabetics need to watch their feet very carefully, and preventive measures are obvious. Shoes should not be tight, ill-fitting, or productive of corns or blisters, which must be treated early and well. Toenails should be trimmed with care, and people with poor vision should not try to trim their toenails with sharp objects. If a sore is present on the foot, even though painless, wash it with soap and water—never apply iodine or strong medications—put on a dry dressing, and check with your physician. Common garden-variety athlete's foot can also be a hazard, since it is a focus for more serious infection.

Chronic ulcers most commonly arise on the sole or "ball" of the foot. The earliest change is a callus that may recur despite regular foot care. Thickened skin may be removed by rubbing with a coarse towel after bathing, but ulcers sometimes lurk underneath calluses. An ulcerated foot needs a doctor's attention and antibiotics, as well as bed rest to relieve pressure areas or deformities that tend to make an ulcer chronic.

Problems that begin in the toes or feet may involve the leg if nothing is done about them. A doctor should be seen if there is any discoloration of the skin. Skills of a podiatrist or an orthopedist may be needed to correct ingrown toenails, bunions, claw toes, pressure points, and other sites of potential trouble.

Goals of Treatment

The goal of treatment is to keep the patient in a normal state of body chemistry and physiology, although this ideal is often difficult to achieve with the treatment available today. As good as insulin is, it is difficult to keep blood- and urine-sugar levels and other measurements always normal. Compromises sometimes have to be made to lessen the likelihood of annoying or disabling low-blood-sugar reactions ("insulin shock").

Many informed and determined diabetics have learned to live with their condition and maintain a reasonably controlled state along with an active life. Some physicians feel that the physiology of the diabetic would more nearly approximate that of the non-diabetic if injections of regular, short-duration insulin were used several times daily, thereby stimulating the body's normal "on demand" release of insulin. Many diabetics need injections twice daily even with the use of intermediate insulin.

The Diabetic Life

Unquestionably, the person with diabetes lives longer and better than ever before. At one time, the life-span was measured in days, weeks, or months; today it is measured in many years. Although the average life-span of diabetics is less than that of non-diabetics, an amazing number of persons with diabetes now live long, productive, satisfying lives, often with few complications. To mention a few of many, they include Bobby Clarke, star hockey player; Ron Santos, baseball infielder; and Mary Tyler Moore, actress. Billy Talbert, the tennis player, has had diabetes for nearly 50 years.

The diabetic life, useful and rewarding though it can be, is not quite a normal life. It is not wholly normal when one has to think continually of diet and daily insulin injections and to otherwise be nearly always aware of diabetes. But diabetes need not be the severe handicap that it often was in the past.

THE FUTURE OF DIABETES

Insulin came into medical use almost overnight when discovered in 1921, and a similar revolution in management of diabetes may emerge from many of the exciting aspects of current research. Some promising advances are technological, with the possible employment of mini-computers and sensors to supply minute amounts of insulin in automatic response to changing blood-sugar levels, much as the body normally does. Newer knowledge of hormone and insulin interactions gives better understanding of the complex fundamental nature of diabetes. Developments mentioned briefly below are not yet available, and some may never be practical. However, the progress is encouraging since in medical history, the dreams of researchers have frequently turned into therapeutic facts.

Pancreas transplants. Whole pancreas glands have been transplanted into a very few persons, a score or so, but none of the patients survived long. The pancreas deteriorates readily, and the operation is difficult and risky, with the donated gland ultimately rejected as a foreign body. If large doses of immunosuppressive agents are used to deter rejection, then the danger is that of massive infection. And there is an insurmountable practical problem as well: if five million or more diabetics need a new pancreas, where would the organs come from, even if the rejection problem were overcome? Whole pancreas transplantation is not a realistic possibility for the future, except as research models.

Beta-cell transplants. Why not, then, transplant only the insulin-producing beta cells of the pancreas? There has been some limited success in culturing beta cells taken from rats and transplanting them into other genetically compatible rats. The transplanted cells survived in the liver and produced insulin on demand when blood-sugar levels became elevated. But rejection of the cells is still a major obstacle here, too, and the procedure is certainly not feasible for human beings in the near future. Tremendous numbers of cells would have to be grown and transplanted from one species to another—until now, not possible. However, great strides have been made in this field and beta-cell transplants might someday be practical.

Glucose sensor. This is a device about the size of a quarter, designed to be implanted in the abdominal area of the patient, not unlike a cardiac pacemaker, that attempts to measure blood-sugar levels much like a beta cell does. The disk-shaped unit generates small electric currents in reaction to changing blood-sugar levels. A miniature computer can relate this to blood-glucose levels. Eventually, it is hoped that it will be possible to broadcast these data to a receiving unit small enough to be worn on a belt or carried in a pocket. On demand, it would be possible to determine the approximate blood-sugar level. The patient could then inject insulin or take nourishment as needed without the delay and nuisance of testing the blood for sugar. Such implantable glucose sensors are undergoing laboratory tests, and hopefully if and when perfected, may give diabetics an effective means of continually monitoring fluctuating blood-sugar levels. This is indeed hopeful for the future.

Artificial pancreas. A more sophisticated unit, called an *artificial beta cell,* would combine a glucose sensor with an insulin dispenser. "Mechanical pancreases" built on this principle are in fact now used in some hospitals to cope with dire emergencies, such as during surgery. These devices are much too large and cumbersome to be used outside a hospital, but progress is being made in designing smaller units. Researchers are working with as-yet unperfected models that combine a glucose sensor and a minicomputer. To this someday will be added a power supply, pump, and insulin reservoir. The sensor would monitor the blood-sugar levels, the computer would compute how much insulin is needed, and the pump should then release a precise amount of insulin from the reservoir into the body—pretty much what a normal pancreas gland does. To refill the reservoir, insulin would be injected into the reservoir as needed. A reservoir of glucose would be incorporated to counteract low blood sugar.

Such is the ideal artificial pancreas. Problems of miniaturization, power, ruggedness, reliability, and stability are being attacked with hope and considerable ingenuity. If perfected, an implanted mechanism might prevent or minimize progressive damage to blood vessels if, as many specialists think, such damage may occur because of imperfect insulin replacement.

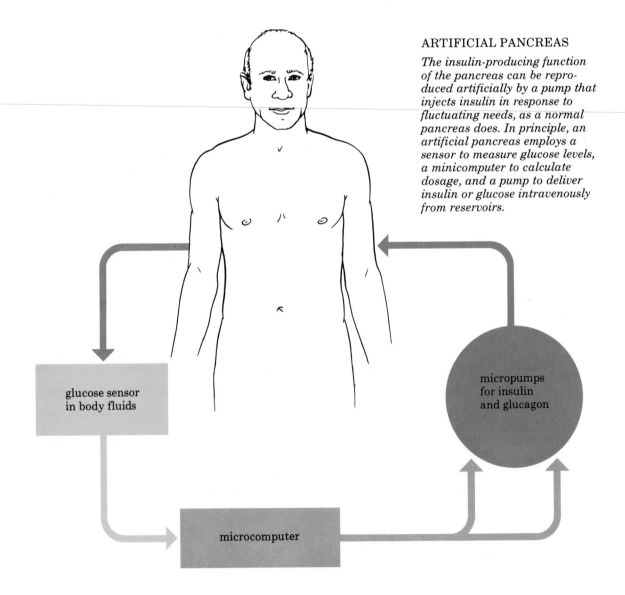

ARTIFICIAL PANCREAS

The insulin-producing function of the pancreas can be reproduced artificially by a pump that injects insulin in response to fluctuating needs, as a normal pancreas does. In principle, an artificial pancreas employs a sensor to measure glucose levels, a minicomputer to calculate dosage, and a pump to deliver insulin or glucose intravenously from reservoirs.

glucose sensor in body fluids

micropumps for insulin and glucagon

microcomputer

The hidden chemistry of diabetes. The pancreas, a complex member of the endocrine orchestra, does other things than produce insulin. Its *alpha cells* produce *glucagon,* a hormone that opposes the effects of insulin by breaking down the storage form of sugar *(glycogen)* into usable glucose. In effect, it raises the blood sugar, and glucagon injection is one way of treating overdoses of insulin. Some investigators think that diabetes may be a condition in which too much glucagon is present.

Many obese adult diabetics produce normal amounts of insulin or even more, but cannot use it effectively. Various "anti-insulin" processes may be involved: the diabetic may have fewer receptor cells for insulin, or too much glucagon, or his insulin may somehow be defective in quality.

But there are other hormonal influences too. The thyroid hormone speeds up metabolism and creates a demand for more insulin. Acute stress releases adrenaline from the adrenal glands, preparing a person for "fight or flee" emergencies by increasing the heart rate and raising the blood sugar. Longer stress releases cortisone-like hormones that also raise blood sugar. And the pituitary gland releases *growth hormone,* which is antagonistic to insulin function. Since this hormone is vital to the growth of young people, it is a possible factor in the rapid onset of juvenile diabetes during years of peak growth.

On the other hand, the pituitary also produces a "friend of insulin," a hormone called *somatostatin* (growth-stop). It helps insulin by blocking the effects of growth hormone, glucagon, and some other hormones. Recent research has uncovered the fact that delta cells in the pancreas probably also make somatostatin. In a very few patients in whom it has been used, somatostatin enabled the insulin dose to be decreased. At present, the short-lived hormone is primarily a research tool, but it and other substances may someday help overcome the various insulin antagonists.

Chemical trails in diabetes are devious and take unexpected turns. The scope of research is so broad and intensively pursued that no one can foretell what the nature of the next major breakthroughs will be. Perhaps they will involve a way to make sluggish insulin receptors of cells use insulin effectively, which many diabetics cannot do. Or, more fancifully, they may explore the genetic manipulation of immature cells or non-pathogenic bacteria to train them to produce insulin inside or outside of the body.

The background of research is lengthy, tedious, often frustrating, and sometimes seems dead-ended, but its fruits can sometimes emerge with dramatic suddenness. One day in 1922, a 17-year-old diabetic named Leonard Thompson was gravely ill. He weighed just 75 pounds and early death was inevitable. The next day when he became the first person to be treated with the newly discovered insulin, he began to regain weight and strength and the downhill course was suddenly reversed.

It is safe to say that not only are the lives of diabetics better than ever before, but they and their families have every reason to hope for even better prospects in the future.

CHAPTER **13**   GEORGE E. SHAMBAUGH, JR., M.D.

THE DEVELOPED SENSES: HEARING

Of all physical handicaps, impaired hearing is by far the most frequent. Yet it is a hidden handicap, without the white cane of the blind or the crutches of the lame to betray its presence. When a deafened but normal-appearing person does not answer a question, or gives an inappropriate reply, the reaction is one of impatience rather than compassion. The hard-of-hearing person feels excluded and easily becomes suspicious that people are laughing and talking about him behind his back.

Helen Keller, who became totally blind and totally deaf in early childhood, had this to say: "The problems of deafness are deeper and more complex, if not more important, than those of blindness. Deafness is a much worse misfortune, for it means loss of the most vital stimulus—the sound of the voice—that brings language, sets thoughts astir, and keeps us in the intellectual company of man."

There are many causes of hearing loss: congenital deafness, infections, tumors, drugs, and even simple wax in the ears. And man's hearing impairments become more common as the ears grow older. One form of progressive loss of hearing sensitivity, called *presbycusis,* is practically "normal" in that it occurs sooner or later in all of us, just as the skin wrinkles and the hair thins with aging. The degree of impairment varies greatly in different persons. But the most frequent cause of hearing loss in both young and old adults is a condition commonly called *otosclerosis,* in which an abnormality of bony parts of the ear muffles the transmission of sound. The condition is quite common in middle years and later, though the disease process may have begun some time before a hearing handicap is recognized.

How We Hear

Our hearing mechanism has three distinct interlinked parts: an outer ear, a middle ear, and an inner ear. The inch-long canal of the outer ear, through which sound waves enter, terminates at the eardrum or *tympanic membrane.* The membrane is translucent like waxed paper, and kept taut by muscles. Beyond it is the small air-filled chamber of the middle ear, in which a chain of three very small bones is suspended. These bones *(ossicles)* conduct sound across the middle ear and magnify its force some twenty times.

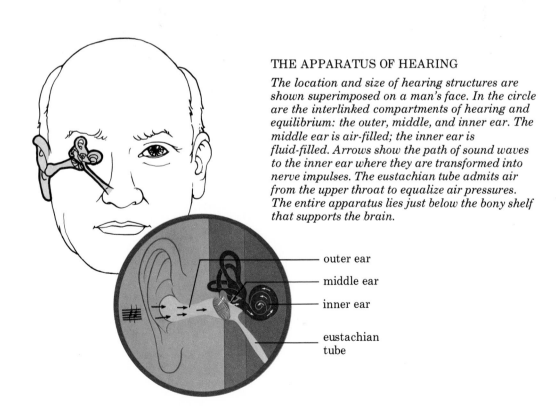

THE APPARATUS OF HEARING

The location and size of hearing structures are shown superimposed on a man's face. In the circle are the interlinked compartments of hearing and equilibrium: the outer, middle, and inner ear. The middle ear is air-filled; the inner ear is fluid-filled. Arrows show the path of sound waves to the inner ear where they are transformed into nerve impulses. The eustachian tube admits air from the upper throat to equalize air pressures. The entire apparatus lies just below the bony shelf that supports the brain.

outer ear

middle ear

inner ear

eustachian tube

HOW WE HEAR AND KEEP OUR BALANCE

The center drawing shows the anatomical structures of hearing and equilibrium; smaller drawings show enlarged details. Incoming sound waves make the taut eardrum vibrate (front view, A). A chain of three tiny bones in the middle ear (B) amplifies the *vibrations and transmits them via the stapes bone to the oval window of the fluid-filled cochlea. Vibrations, which now are fluid-transmitted, stimulate the minute hair cells in the organ of Corti (F) where they are then converted into nerve* *impulses that travel over the cochlear nerve to the hearing centers of the brain. Fluid in the semicircular canals (C) is responsible for transmitting sensations of bodily balance. The inner ear is imbedded in extremely hard bone.*

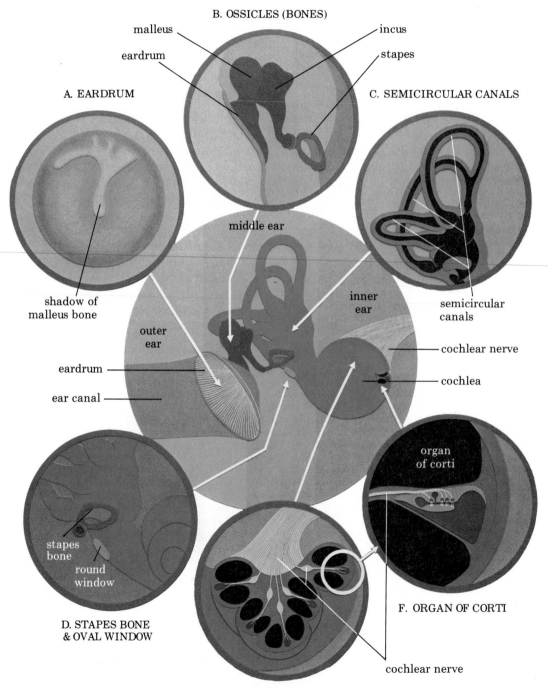

B. OSSICLES (BONES)

malleus

incus

eardrum

stapes

A. EARDRUM

C. SEMICIRCULAR CANALS

middle ear

shadow of
malleus bone

inner
ear

semicircular
canals

outer
ear

cochlear nerve

eardrum

ear canal

cochlea

organ
of corti

stapes
bone

round
window

F. ORGAN OF CORTI

D. STAPES BONE
& OVAL WINDOW

cochlear nerve

E. COCHLEA

Attached to the inner side of the eardrum is the hammer bone *(malleus).* When sound waves strike the eardrum, it vibrates and moves the hammer, which taps on the anvil bone *(incus).* The anvil vibrates the stirrup-shaped bone *(stapes)* that moves in and out of the oval window, the entrance to the fluid-filled inner ear. You can imagine the tininess of the bones from the fact that the middle ear is about the size of an aspirin tablet.

Thus sound is conducted to the inner ear, or *labyrinth,* which consists of a complicated series of fluid-filled passageways embedded in rock-hard bone. It includes three semicircular canals, one for each plane in space, that modulate our sense of balance.

The part concerned with hearing is a snail-shaped structure called the *cochlea.* Inside it is the *organ of Corti,* which, for simplicity, can be thought of as a complex of cells lying upon a thin membrane, with another membrane overhanging. In between are rows of fantastically delicate hair cells, some 17,000 of them, connected to fibers of the hearing nerve. The hair ends of the cells are embedded in the overhanging membrane. The organ lies within a spiral passageway of the cochlea.

Incoming sound impulses, now fluid-transmitted, exert unimaginably minute pulls upon hair ends. At this point, the energy of sound, which has been mechanical, is transformed into electrical impulses that stimulate the hearing nerve and propagate nerve impulses to the brain. And so we hear.

Conditions that diminish or prevent the transmission of sound to the inner ear cause the type of hearing loss known as *conduction deafness.* There is a transmission gap. Conditions that damage or destroy the hearing nerve cause hearing loss commonly called *nerve deafness.* Both types of impairment can coexist.

The nerve of balance with endings in the semicircular canals arose earlier in evolution and is much more durable than the fragile hearing nerve. Thus many conditions that cause nerve deafness spare the nerve of balance. An exception in which both hearing and balance are affected is Ménière's disease (see page 437).

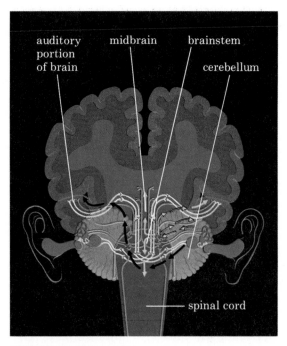

NERVE PATHWAYS

Nerve impulses from the inner ear (white lines and black arrows) travel to the switching centers of the brainstem and cross to the auditory centers of the brain on the opposite side, where sound is perceived. Impulses from the balance mechanisms of the inner ear (green lines and yellow arrows) travel up to parts of the brain, to the brainstem, down the spinal cord, and to the cerebellum, where muscle movements are controlled.

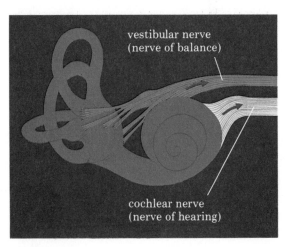

DIZZINESS

Attacks of dizziness may result from involvement of both the nerves of balance and hearing, shown in the drawing above emerging from their respective points of origin. The two nerves merge into the acoustic nerve and travel together to the brainstem.

Am I Losing My Hearing?

Often a hearing loss comes on so slowly that it is hardly recognized. One's family may be first to notice and suggest that something be done. Unfortunately, too many people do not get professional help. The first recourse should not be a hearing aid dealer but a physician. Medical examination is important because conditions not arising primarily in the ear may be involved. Or a simple hidden cause may be discovered. For instance, a suspected loss of hearing may in fact prove to be simple inattention, or "husband deafness." And what a relief if one's deafness is simply the result of excess wax in the ears!

Evaluating hearing. If hearing loss is real and diagnosis uncertain, the physician will probably refer his patient to an ear specialist (otologist). The otologist will take a detailed medical history, which may be related to ear problems, and examine the ears, mouth, and throat.

The actual hearing tests range from simple to complex. For instance, tuning forks placed upon the forehead and the mastoid bones behind the ears can give useful information: the relative hearing ability of the two ears, and the nature of the impairment (conductive, nerve type, or mixed). Other tests help to determine the exact site along the hearing pathway where trouble lies. The ear specialist can then advise about treatment, surgery, or a hearing aid, with respect to a patient's particular needs.

The patient will probably be referred to an *audiologist,* who is a university-trained specialist with skills and equipment for evaluating hearing problems and prescribing rehabilitative measures. One such piece of equipment is an audiometer, an instrument that gives a graphic record *(audiogram)* of hearing sensitivity from the lowest to the highest sound frequencies. With it, the audiologist can give impartial advice as to whether or not a hearing aid will help and what type of aid should serve best. He also can refer patients to an appropriate dealer and follow up on results. Such an evaluation can avert the purchase of an expensive but unsatisfactory hearing aid that ends up in a bureau drawer.

CONDUCTION DEAFNESS

As previously mentioned, conditions that impede the transmission of sound to the inner ear cause varying degrees of hearing impairment classed as conduction deafness. The simplest example is blockage of the outer ear canal by ear wax or other material that muffles sound. Impacted ear wax is quite common in older people and is "cured" almost instantly in a doctor's office by flushing out the wax.

The middle ear is also a common site of conduction difficulties. Since it is air-filled, like the outer ear canal, air pressures must be kept equal if the intervening eardrum is not to be pulled inward, impairing its movement. This is normally accomplished by the *eustachian tube*, which connects the middle ear with the upper part of the throat. Each time we yawn or swallow, the tube opens momentarily and lets a little air in or out to equalize internal and external pressures on the eardrum.

Failure of the tube to open causes an uncomfortable full or blocked feeling in the ears, with severe pain if it occurs suddenly. At first, hearing is only slightly impaired. But if the tube remains closed, air in the middle ear is gradually absorbed and replaced with fluid, with even greater impairment of hearing. By removing fluid through a small incision in the eardrum membrane, sometimes with the insertion of a tiny ventilating tube, hearing can be successfully restored.

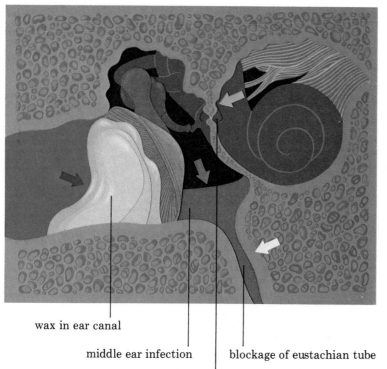

wax in ear canal

middle ear infection   blockage of eustachian tube

stapes fixed to overgrown bone

CONDUCTION DEAFNESS

Conduction deafness results from conditions that muffle vibrations and prevent the adequate transmission of sound to the inner ear. These conditions include wax in the ear canal pressing on the eardrum (blue arrow); infection in the middle ear (orange arrow); blockage of the eustachian tube (white arrow); or stapes fixation by bony overgrowth (yellow arrow).

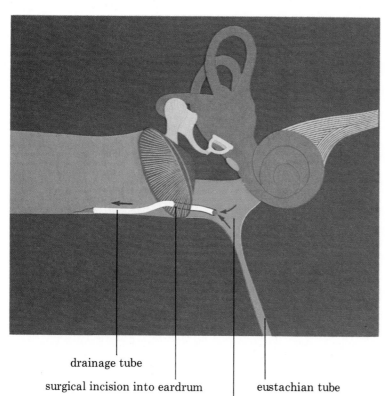

drainage tube

surgical incision into eardrum   eustachian tube

fluid in middle ear chamber

DROWNED SOUND

One form of conduction deafness is caused by persistent blockage of the eustachian tube that permits fluid to accumulate in the normally air-filled middle ear. Hearing can be restored by drainage through an incision made in the eardrum, sometimes aided by inserting a tiny tube.

INFECTION

Infections can travel from the lungs, mouth, and nasal passages to the middle ear cavity (black arrows) via the eustachian tube. Acute infections usually are controlled quickly by antibiotics, and once-dreaded mastoid complications are rare. However, chronic infections with persistent discharge may lead to cyst formation and require surgery to correct.

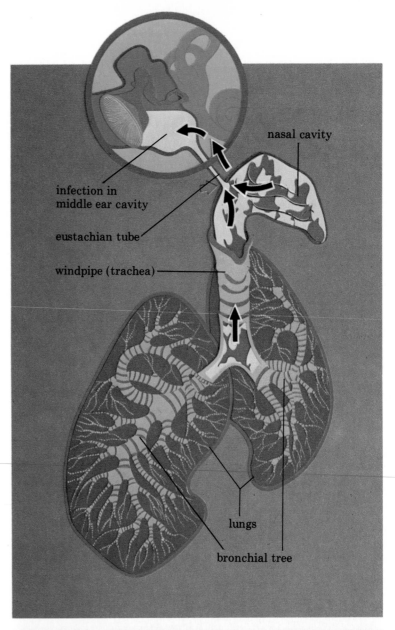

nasal cavity

infection in middle ear cavity

eustachian tube

windpipe (trachea)

lungs

bronchial tree

A PERFORATED EARDRUM

A perforated eardrum (U-shaped tear) is shown in relation to middle ear bones, which also may be damaged so that sound is not carried to the inner ear. The perforation may be covered by a skin graft over the eardrum (yellow arrow) and the chain of bones may be reconstructed surgically (tympanoplasty) to restore hearing.

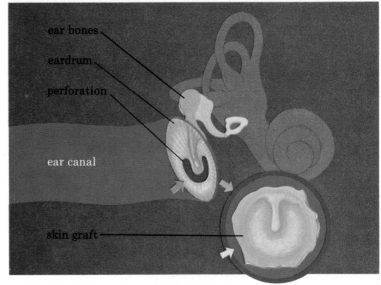

ear bones

eardrum

perforation

ear canal

skin graft

Infections of the middle ear cavity, often called "abscessed ear," occur more often in children than in older adults. Prompt antibiotic treatment quickly controls the infection and hearing returns to normal. Rarely nowadays does a middle ear infection lead to the dreaded mastoid complications of years ago.

Chronic infections of the middle ear are another story, however. Affected ears continue to drain because of invasion of the bone by a cyst called *cholesteatoma.* Antibiotics are of no value, and surgery is required to remove the disease, stop the malodorous discharge, and eliminate the risk of extension to the brain.

Tympanoplasty. Old middle ear infections no longer active may have left a large hole or perforation in the eardrum membrane, or may have destroyed part of the chain of tiny bones that carries sound to the inner ear. In either case, conduction of sound is severely impaired. Usually hearing can be restored by surgical reconstruction of the damaged areas—a procedure known as tympanoplasty.

Otosclerosis

Contrary to what its common name implies, this is not a hardening but rather a localized softening in the hard shell of bone that encloses the inner ear. The formal scientific name is *otospongiosis.*

Actually, the condition is quite common. By middle age, approximately one in five women and one in ten men have developed a small nodule of otospongiosis in the wall of the cochlea. In most cases, fortunately, the nodule rehardens and remains small and harmless. But in about 12 percent of cases it continues to expand very slowly until it reaches and presses upon the stirrup bone (stapes)—the last, smallest, and most important in the chain of tiny sound-conducting bones. The slowly expanding nodule gradually dampens the vibratory movements of the stapes, and progressive impairment of hearing finally becomes quite severe.

Symptoms. An early indication of this type of hearing loss is inability to hear a whisper or voices at a distance. Bone conduction of sound is usually good, so the person's own voice seems quite loud to him and he tends to speak softly, being at times hard to understand. Usually he can hear fairly well on the telephone, sometimes with the help of a booster to amplify soft voices.

Persons with this type of hearing difficulty are well suited for a proper hearing aid, as the clarity of sound is not impaired, just its loudness. It is necessary only to amplify speech to make it understandable.

Stapedectomy. The condition of stapes fixation by otospongiosis was considered hopeless and incurable not too long ago. But today in most cases, hearing can be restored rather dramatically by surgery, provided that the hearing nerve is functioning normally.

The operation, known as *stapedectomy,* is performed through an operating microscope—the middle ear chamber, as has been mentioned, is aspirin-sized. Under local anesthesia, the surgeon removes the nonfunctioning stirrup bone and replaces it with a tiny synthetic rod or stainless steel wire, bridging the conduction gap. Once again, vibrations can be transmitted freely to the inner ear. Restoration of hearing by successful stapedectomy is quite prompt; at times, the patient begins to hear well on the operating table.

After the operation, the patient may feel a little transient giddiness. He or she is advised to lie on the unaffected side of the head for 24 hours and then, when out of bed, to avoid sudden movements. The hospital stay is three to five days, followed by a quiet week or ten days at home.

Although loss of hearing due to otospongiotic fixation of the stapes usually begins before age 40, impairment can progress long beyond that age, and in some cases it may not begin to be noticed until after the menopause. But if the hearing nerve is in good condition, older people are just as suitable for surgical restoration of hearing as younger persons.

One should know, however, that neither stapedectomy nor tympanoplasty is always successful. Depending upon the severity of the disease and the condition of the hearing nerve as determined by special tests, chances of success in a particular patient can range all the way from one or two chances in ten to as many as nine chances in ten. With this knowledge, the informed patient can make a wiser decision with respect to surgery and/or a hearing aid.

NERVE DEAFNESS

The other major type of hearing loss is *nerve deafness* (sensorineural or inner ear deafness). In its unmixed form, sound is conducted perfectly well across the middle ear. The trouble is in the "receivers" of the inner ear: membranes, hair cells, nerve fibers, and other delicate structures.

Some slight hearing loss for high-pitched sounds is common in the 40s and 50s. A good young ear can hear sounds of high frequency, up to 20,000 or more hertz, that an older ear can't. It is unlikely, for instance, that a middle-aged man or woman can perceive the finest nuances of a piccolo. Fortunately, sounds of the very highest pitch are less important in human affairs than lower sounds of speech.

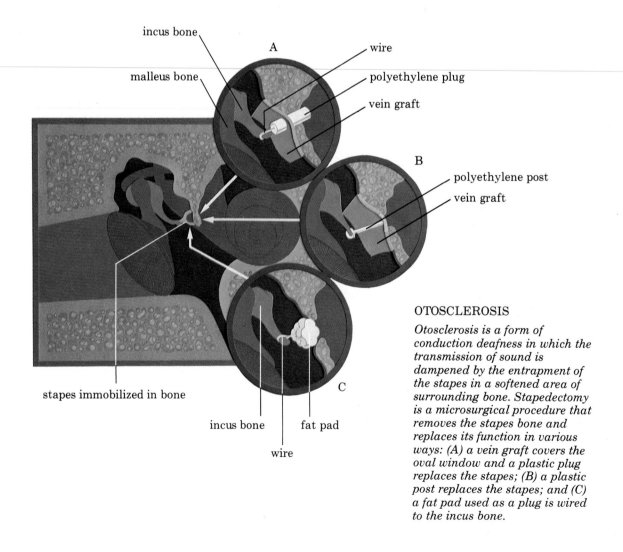

incus bone
malleus bone
A
wire
polyethylene plug
vein graft
B
polyethylene post
vein graft
stapes immobilized in bone
incus bone
fat pad
C
wire

OTOSCLEROSIS

Otosclerosis is a form of conduction deafness in which the transmission of sound is dampened by the entrapment of the stapes in a softened area of surrounding bone. Stapedectomy is a microsurgical procedure that removes the stapes bone and replaces its function in various ways: (A) a vein graft covers the oval window and a plastic plug replaces the stapes; (B) a plastic post replaces the stapes; and (C) a fat pad used as a plug is wired to the incus bone.

At any age, structures of the inner ear can be damaged or destroyed by severe infections, by certain lifesaving antibiotics, or by a virus. The mumps virus can destroy hearing in one ear, but nearly always spares the other. People with monaural or one-ear hearing cannot locate the direction of sound and have difficulty in concentrating on the speaker in a noisy background—or indeed, in hearing him at all if he's on the side of the "bad" ear. Otherwise, hearing is quite satisfactory.

Conditions other than viral and drug causes of nerve deafness are rare in young people but more frequent after age 40. These age-related causes include natural deterioration of nerve sensitivity, prolonged exposure to loud noises which can permanently harm delicate ear structures, and a variant form of otospongiosis.

Cochlear Otospongiosis

Many cases of progressive hearing loss of the nerve type are caused by a somewhat different form of otospongiosis than previously described (see page 433). The nodule of softened bone grows inward into the cochlea rather than, or in addition to, immobilizing the stirrup bone. The condition is not easily recognized and is probably more common than is thought. An ear specialist must make the diagnosis.

Diagnosis requires inspection of the eardrum membranes for a pinkish glow from the spongy nodule, administering various hearing tests, obtaining a family history of the patient's relatives who have had a stapes operation, and the use of a recently developed method for X-raying the inner ear known as *polytomography*.

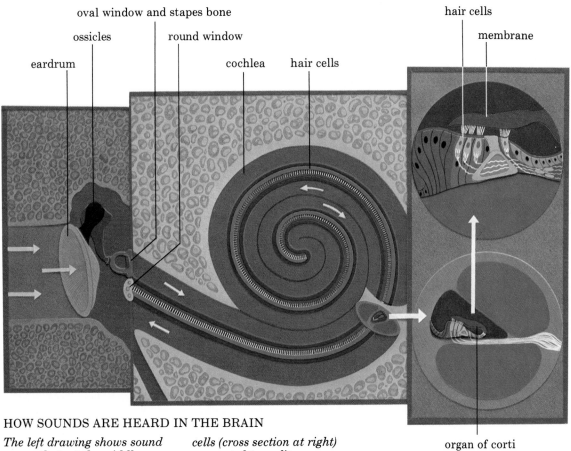

HOW SOUNDS ARE HEARD IN THE BRAIN

The left drawing shows sound waves that set the middle ear bones to vibrating. The terminal stapes bone "shakes" the oval window and fluids beyond it in the chochlea (center). Between the two partitions of flowing fluid are rows of minute hair cells (cross section at right) connected to auditory nerve fibers. Vibrations of a membrane in contact with hair cells are converted into nerve impulses that travel to the brain. Nerve deafness results from impairments along neural pathways.

Treatment. Fortunately, there is a new and promising method to promote rehardening of the softened nodule of bone, which then becomes inactive, with arrest of further nerve deterioration. The treatment utilizes fluoride, a trace element necessary for strong bones and teeth. Larger doses of fluoride than provided by fluoridated water are necessary, but they're still well within the range of safety. The beneficial action is greater when a soluble calcium preparation made from oyster shells is also prescribed. It has been found that this same combination is effective in strengthening the bones of older persons with osteoporosis (see page 458).

The fluoride treatment is still undergoing research, and it does not bring back hearing. But in four out of five cases, it is successful in arresting further deterioration of the hearing nerve. Early diagnosis is of course important, as it is for other types of hearing loss.

Presbycusis

This type of nerve deafness comes with advancing years. One might think of it as "wear and tear" of the inner ear resulting from years of faithful service.

Symptoms. Usually the earliest loss of sensitivity is for sounds of highest pitch, and progressive loss gradually includes sounds of lower pitch. As a rule, presbycusis is not a significant handicap until after age 60, but there is individual variation in either direction.

The affected person can usually hear voices but has difficulty in understanding speech. He or she hears certain tones of the scale reasonably well, but others poorly or not at all, tending to distort the incoming sound load. Spoken consonants such as *s* and *f* may be indistinguishable. There is loss of clarity, background noises can be confusing, and loud sounds may be distressing or actually painful.

Treatment. There is no treatment to restore lost hearing in presbycusis, and as yet no known way to arrest or retard this type of hearing loss, other than good nutrition and avoidance of excessive noise.

However, a diagnosis of presbycusis, for which nothing can be done medically or surgically, should not be accepted without a thorough examination. In a recent analysis of 100 consecutive over-65 patients examined for impaired hearing, half were indeed found to have presbycusis. But the other half proved to have a remediable defect, such as impacted ear wax, fluid in the middle ear, or cochlear otospongiosis where hearing loss could be arrested.

A properly fitted hearing aid (see page 438) may be of some help to persons with presbycusis, but too much should not be expected of a hearing aid alone. Of equal or greater importance is speech reading, where the movements and expression of the whole face, not just the lips, supplement the limited help from a hearing aid. Since presbycusis usually impairs hearing of high-pitched tones more than tones of low register, substitution of a buzzer for a telephone bell or door chime can be of help.

Noise Deafness

Noise deafness is a form of nerve deafness that is preventable. It is caused by prolonged exposure to noise levels greater than the inner ear can tolerate without damage. The ears can recover from brief exposure to noise, but chronic exposure wears down the delicate hearing nerve endings and causes hearing impairment, at first temporary, but later permanent.

The unit of loudness measured by audiologists is the *decibel*. A whisper is about 20 decibels, and ordinary conversation, 50 to 60. The limit of loudness that can be tolerated indefinitely without damage is commonly put at 85 decibels. Most of us are at least briefly exposed to sounds louder than that without being aware of it. Noise of a subway or heavy truck rumbling by registers about 100 decibels, and a riveting machine, 110. A snowmobile, emitting 115 decibels, is very hard on the ears. And some rock bands and stereo sets playing at maximum loudness give off an ear-splitting 140 decibels.

Some hearing loss is quite frequent in persons exposed to excessive noise over long periods of time: workers in noisy factories (prone to "boilermaker's deafness"), riveters, or jackhammer operators. It occurs in carpenters using electric saws and in some dentists using high-speed drills. And it is especially common among trapshooters, hunters, and military personnel.

Symptoms. The earliest sign of noise-induced hearing loss is a sharp drop in the audiogram for tones of high pitch. Ringing in the ears is another early symptom. If noise exposure continues, the dip in the audiogram deepens and broadens to include the tones needed to understand speech.

Prevention. There is no treatment—only prevention, by changing one's occupation or using ear protection when bombarded by noise. The ear protectors worn by airport personnel are very efficient protection, but tightly fitting ear plugs also are effective. Ordinary cotton is not too helpful, but a specially prepared sound-absorbing cotton known as Swedish wool, obtainable in drugstores, is quite helpful as well as convenient and comfortable to wear when around noise.

Ménière's Disease

Dizziness does not necessarily originate from disease of the inner ear, but it is one symptom of a disorder known as Ménière's disease, which is particularly frequent in persons of middle age or older. Confirmatory symptoms are roaring noises in the ear *(tinnitus)* and distortion and impairment of hearing. Both the nerves of hearing and of balance are involved.

The underlying condition is an excess of inner ear fluid *(endolymph)*. The fluid, produced chiefly in the cochlea, flows through narrow channels to fill the semicircular canals and ends up in a small pouch called the endolymphatic sac, where it is resorbed. If the sac is defective—probably from a long-ago childhood virus infection—the resorption of fluid is sluggish and it tends to back up under pressure.

Symptoms. The first symptom is fullness or pressure in the ear and side of the head, often mistaken for eustachian tube obstruction. But attempts to relieve the pressure by holding the nose and blowing air into the middle ear are of no avail. Attacks of dizziness or vertigo, coming on with little or no warning, can be frightening and incapacitating. The room seems to be spinning; usually there is pallor, sweating, or nausea. Head noises are often described as rumbling, surf-like sounds, and the hearing loss tends to increase with successive attacks.

Treatment. An acute attack of vertigo is tided over by bed rest, sedation, and assurance that the attack will run its course. But another unpredictable attack is likely sooner or later. Most persons with Ménière's disease respond well to medical treatment. General measures that reduce the retention of body fluids may relieve some of the pressure in the inner ear. These include strict limitation of salt intake, moderate limitation of fluid intake, correction of any hormonal imbalance, and management of allergic reactions to inhalants or foods. Also recommended is complete cessation of cigarette smoking, which causes constriction of small blood vessels of the endolymphatic sac, further impairing its function. A physician may prescribe a diuretic to hasten fluid elimination from the inner ear.

Surgery. If attacks of vertigo continue despite medical treatment, surgical opening of the endolymphatic sac may be necessary. If this fails, and if attacks of vertigo are profoundly handicapping and the affected ear has already lost most of its hearing, an operation known as *labyrinthectomy* gives permanent relief. The function of the inner ear is surgically destroyed. This cures the vertigo but leaves the ear totally deaf, virtually as it was before surgery. In the great majority of cases of Ménière's disease, only one ear is affected; the other ear retains its hearing.

The sooner the correct diagnosis of Ménière's disease can be made and medical treatment begun, the better the outlook for control of symptoms and recovery of useful hearing without surgery.

Head noises. Ringing in the ears, known as *tinnitus,* is a very common complaint, especially in the elderly. It usually occurs along with a hearing impairment. If hearing can be improved by stapes or tympanoplasty surgery, or by medical means, the tinnitus will likely diminish and sometimes stop altogether. In other cases there is no effective remedy for ringing in the ears and the person must learn to accustom himself to his head noises that are always worse in quiet surroundings. However, tinnitus is rarely so constant and unbearable that it is necessary to cut the hearing nerve.

Hearing Aids

The situation for the hard of hearing is infinitely better today than it was a half century ago. Hearing aids then were bulky contraptions with wires leading to a heavy battery worn under the clothing. Now they are amazingly small and efficient.

An electrical hearing aid is, essentially, a miniature microphone and loudspeaker powered by batteries. It amplifies sound. There are many makes and designs available with technical differences to accommodate a broad range of hearing problems.

Professional help in selecting a comfortable and efficient hearing aid is obviously desirable, as a poorly fitted aid is too often consigned to a bureau drawer in frustration and disappointment. An ear specialist, diagnosing the condition of a particular patient, can advise about hearing aids, and may even discover a condition that is correctable. Sometimes a hearing aid is quite unnecessary, or cannot be expected to be of benefit. Again, an audiologist can advise about a proper hearing aid to fit a patient's needs, and check the performance of a chosen aid.

We have already mentioned that persons with conduction deafness usually find a proper hearing aid to be quite satisfactory. The situation is somewhat different in cases of nerve deafness, where a frequent difficulty is a "skipping" of perception of sounds of different frequencies along the tonal scale. Sounds of certain pitch are heard better than others, tending to distort and muffle the overall clarity of what is heard. A hearing aid that makes sounds louder may only increase the distortion and make matters worse instead of better. However, it may be possible for an audiologist, on the basis of a patient's audiogram, to recommend a hearing aid that compensates to some extent for distortions. Another circumstance that may affect the choice of a hearing aid is the presence in varying degree of both the conduction and nerve types of hearing impairment.

A practical bit of advice is to rent—and use—a hearing aid for a month's trial before committing one's self to an investment of several hundred dollars.

The outlook is bright for people with the types of partial deafness that become more common with age. Improvements in hearing aids are only one aspect. All of the delicate operations performed through the operating microscope for conductive type losses have been perfected during the past 25 years. Further progress is certain to be made in the years ahead to overcome these most frequent of all physical handicaps.

DIZZINESS AND MOTION SICKNESS

Receptors of the balance system lie in ridges at the dilated ends of the semicircular canals (A, B), and tiny sacs (utricle and saccule) contain terminations of the auditory nerve. Moving fluid in these structures sends information to muscles. Shifting position excites disorderly nerve messages, felt as dizziness.

fluid

A. AMPULLA

fluid

nerve fibers

B. CRISTA OF AMPULLA

endolymphatic sac

semicircular canals

utricle

saccule

nerve of balance

hair cells

E. ORGAN OF CORTI

hearing nerve

fluid

C. MACULA OF
UTRICLE & SACCULE

fluid

nerve fibers

D. DETAIL OF MACULA

MÉNIÈRE'S DISEASE

Vertical and sidewise accelerations of body movements are modulated in small areas of the utricle and saccule (C). Vertical acceleration presses fluids that stimulate tiny beads, which then move down on hair cells (D). Sidewise acceleration causes the beads to move across hair cells, stimulating nerve impulses (E). Ménière's disease involves both the nerves of hearing and balance. Classic symptoms are vertigo, impaired hearing, and roaring noises.

CHAPTER **14** ROBERT P. HEANEY, M.D.
ROBERT LUBY, M.D.

FOR WOMEN ONLY

Some 27 million women in the United States are 50 years old or older. On the average, a woman of 50 has a good three decades of life ahead of her. The years to come should and can be enjoyable and fulfilling. They are ushered in by a biological event of middle age—the menopause or "change of life"—that is a normal benchmark of maturation denied to the male.

No doubt some myths and apprehensions about the menopause still persist, but far less so among today's enlightened women than among physicians of the past century who listed 135 conditions allegedly caused by the menopause, including "hysterical flatulence, blind piles, boils in the seat, pseudo-narcotism, and temporary deafness." The fearsome array of menopausal disorders dwindled remarkably when it was realized that, if two events occur at the same time, one does not necessarily cause the other.

How a woman reacts to the onset or anticipation of menopause depends as much upon her temperament and life patterns as upon physical changes. There is extreme variability in emotional reaction and hence in symptoms complained of. In part, this is related to the age at which menopause occurs—mid-40s to early 50s—and the emotional significance of the change to the person. Major changes in a woman's lifestyle often occur at the precise time when the menses cease. She thus is confronted with unmistakable physiologic evidence of advancing age at a time when her social and family roles, and the meaning those roles have had for her, are undergoing subtle alterations.

A few women react to the menopause—quite mistakenly—as a physical and emotional disaster, particularly if they view it as a harbinger of imminent senescence, of lessened femininity, or of waning sexuality. The great majority of women have no menopausal difficulties of any importance and not a few rejoice in a newfound feeling of freedom and independence.

And the change of life does bring its advantages: a transition from child*bearing* to child *rearing*. Pregnancy, contraception, menstrual cycles, and obstetrical exams are in the past, and so are most afflictions common to the young. In fact, by attaining middle age, an ordinarily healthy woman demonstrates great vital capacity. For many women, freedom from the nuisances and rigors of the reproductive phase of life gives freedom for work and services that bring fresh satisfactions. Frequently there is a reawakening of sexuality.

Of course some capacities diminish as we get older, but hardly ever at breakneck speed. Certain physical ailments have a peak incidence around the middle years and it is well to know something about them. We will discuss the management and prevention of major conditions that may concern women at middle life and after.

THE MENOPAUSE AND AFTER

Technically, the menopause is the time when menstrual periods stop for good.

Perhaps one-third of women "bump into" the menopause abruptly. Menstruation is here one month, gone the next. More commonly, the menses become irregular for a few months or years before ceasing altogether. But even though menopause may occur suddenly, the probability is that it has been creeping up unbeknownst for some time. Most likely there have been ups and downs of hormone production, and as a result, menstruation is irregular. Thus some menopausal symptoms begin before the concluding event.

FEMALE CYCLES

Woman's reproductive system is a finely tuned orchestra of organs and hormones. Ovaries produce female hormones and contain follicles of primitive egg cells, one of which normally swells and bursts to release a mature egg (ovum) each month during childbearing years. Pituitary gland hormones stimulate an immature egg follicle to grow during the first half of the menstrual cycle and initiate complex interactions (see opposite page). The mature egg is carried through the fallopian tubes (where fertilization normally occurs) into the uterus. If fertilized, the egg is implanted in the lining of the uterus and the placenta forms; if not, the egg is shed with products of menstruation. The cervix or neck of the uterus projects into the upper vagina. Adrenal glands produce steroid hormones, which can be converted into small amounts of estrogens after the menopause.

pituitary gland

adrenal glands

fallopian tubes (oviducts)

ovary

uterus

vagina

What Triggers the Menopause?

The immediate reason the menstrual periods stop is that the ovaries cease to produce hormones at their previous high levels. It is perfectly normal for ovaries to "wear out" at this time of life and to stop functioning. Their major functions are two: the production of ova or egg cells, and the production of female hormones, estrogen and progesterone. The egg, if fertilized, becomes another human being. The female hormones prepare the lining of the uterus to receive and nurture a fertilized egg. Both of these functions cease at menopause; it is the end of fertility. The ovaries were not designed to function throughout a long lifetime.

A young ovary contains several thousand primitive egg cells. Each month, after puberty, an egg cell begins to enlarge, swell, and "ripen" into readiness for fertilization. How one cell is chosen from thousands is a mystery. If the egg is not fertilized, the monthly effort fails and menstruation signals the failure. During her reproductive lifetime, an average woman matures about 400 egg cells; after the menopause, none.

Normally, estrogen levels in the menopausal woman do not fall to absolute zero. They simply drop below the levels needed to stimulate growth of the lining of the uterus. Some estrogens are apparently needed for vital cell functions throughout the body, in both men and women. At menopause, a woman's estrogen output dwindles to about the level of a normal man of the same age. This does not mean that she becomes any less a woman, however, for the sexual characteristics that have shaped her are already formed.

Where do estrogens come from after menopause? We used to think the source was the tired old ovaries, continuing some desultory work. Now we believe that the source is basically the same as in men—that is, the estrogens are derived from other hormones that are chemically similar but have quite different functions (for instance, hormones of the adrenal glands related to cortisone). These other hormones can be reshaped by body chemistry into small amounts of estrogens. Women differ greatly in how much estrogen they produce in this way, which probably accounts for variations in symptoms as they go through menopause.

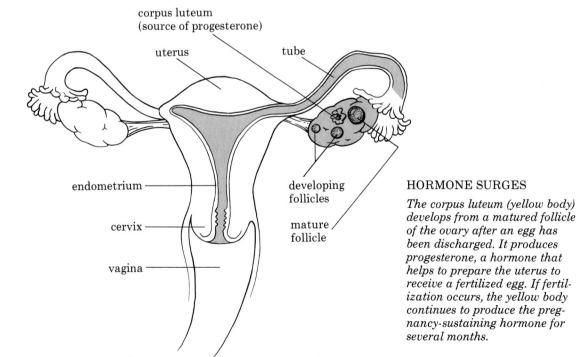

HORMONE SURGES

The corpus luteum (yellow body) develops from a matured follicle of the ovary after an egg has been discharged. It produces progesterone, a hormone that helps to prepare the uterus to receive a fertilized egg. If fertilization occurs, the yellow body continues to produce the pregnancy-sustaining hormone for several months.

Symptoms

Two major symptoms are associated with the menopause. They are *"hot flashes"* (a more dignified term is *vasomotor instability*) and *genital atrophy*. Many other subjective symptoms may just happen to be concurrent with the menopause, rather than a direct physical consequence.

Hot flashes are the most typical symptom, mildly annoying to some women but very disturbing to others. "Flash" is a good descriptive word for this sensation of heat, something like a super-blush, that generally courses through the blush areas of the body: face, neck, and upper chest. Often accompanied by sweating and followed by a chill, flashes may occur sporadically or recur several times a day, possibly provoked at times by hot surroundings, hot drinks, alcohol, or mental stress.

What causes hot flashes? Here we turn to another family of hormones called *gonadotrophins,* produced by the pituitary gland. An active ovary is normally stimulated by gonadotrophins to produce estrogens, which signal the pituitary to reduce its gonadotrophin output, thus keeping interacting hormones in balance. At menopause, when ovarian hormone production falters, pituitary hormones rise to high levels, trying to turn on an ovary that is too tired to care. This is the specific factor that appears to excite hot flashes, felt as a rush of blood through dilated vessels. The mechanism is not well understood, but in instances where gonadotrophin levels are normal, hot flashes are usually not encountered, regardless of estrogen levels.

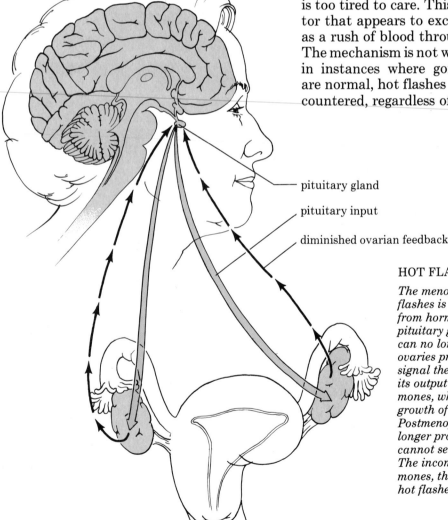

pituitary gland

pituitary input

diminished ovarian feedback

HOT FLASHES

The menopausal nuisance of hot flashes is thought to originate from hormonal commands of the pituitary gland that the ovaries can no longer respond to. Active ovaries produce estrogens, which signal the pituitary to reduce its output of gonadotrophic hormones, which in turn stimulate growth of an ovarian follicle. Postmenopausal ovaries that no longer produce much estrogen cannot send a feedback message. The incoming pituitary hormones, then, appear to excite hot flashes.

Genital atrophy. This is a slow process, occurring much later than hot flashes, if it is recognized at all. In this condition, "atrophy" implies a wasting and shrinking of tissues and mucous membranes deprived of adequate hormonal support. There is a drying effect—a decline in secretion of lubricating fluids, a counterpart of erection in the male—and pelvic tissues lose tone (tension present in resting muscles). This lack of soft tissue support and the gradual thinning of vaginal and vulvar linings may give rise to burning sensations, increased susceptibility to local infection, and pain or discomfort with sexual intercourse.

Genital bleeding. Unexplained bleeding from the genitals after menopause is definitely an abnormal symptom, calling for immediate investigation. The assumption is that some malignant (cancerous) process is responsible, until it is disproved, as it usually is. A common diagnostic procedure is D & C (dilation and curettage), a relatively minor operation often performed under general anesthesia that ordinarily requires no more than a day or two in a hospital. The opening into the womb is dilated and a spoon-shaped instrument (curette) is used to scrape the lining of the uterus, giving tissue for analysis.

Treatment

Estrogenic hormones, which suppress the gonadotrophic activity described above, give significant if not complete control of bothersome symptoms.

Inexpensive and effective forms of estrogens that can be taken by mouth are available. There is no advantage in receiving estrogens by injection, unless for whatever dubious psychological benefit might ensue from the extra inconvenience, added cost, and discomfort.

A number of estrogen-containing creams are available for local application to the vulva and vagina in cases in which the major symptom is genital atrophy. These may be used as the sole treatment or as a supplement to low oral doses of estrogen. Recent developments suggest that administration of long-acting progesterone products by intramuscular injection may also control hot flashes.

Many physicians, while taking Pap smears to detect abnormal cells on the cervix, also take another specimen from the wall of the vagina itself. Certain of these cells (superficial) are produced as a result of estrogen stimulation and their numbers give a crude indication of estrogen levels. However, the procedure is not always reliable and may be affected by unrelated factors such as infection and intercourse.

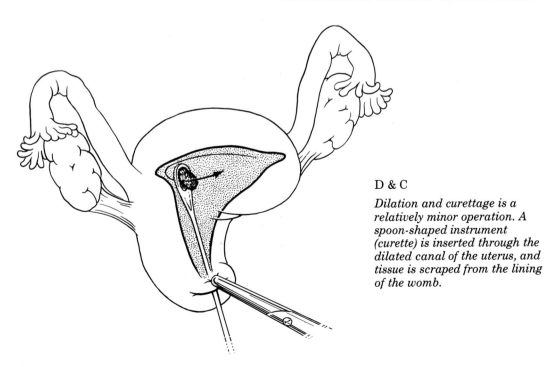

D & C

Dilation and curettage is a relatively minor operation. A spoon-shaped instrument (curette) is inserted through the dilated canal of the uterus, and tissue is scraped from the lining of the womb.

A Word About Estrogens

Attitudes of physicians regarding the management of menopausal and post-menopausal patients vary enormously. At one extreme is the philosophy that "the change" should be interfered with completely—estrogens for everyone, even into advanced years, creating a hormonal facsimile of perpetual youth. At the other extreme is absolute refusal to give any type of hormones or medications under any circumstance to any woman at this transitional period of life. A middle course in which the expected benefits of estrogens are made available to a woman who needs them, with due respect for their potencies, is more usual.

What is the risk of estrogen treatment? Considerable, sometimes sensationalized concern has been expressed in popular literature. Compounds such as diethylstilbestrol, a synthetic estrogen-like agent, have been called a cause of cancer. More recently, natural estrogenic products have been statistically associated with increased incidence of cancer of the endometrium (the uterine lining) in postmenopausal women. There have even been charges that overexuberant prescribing of estrogens is an example of rampant male chauvinism.

What is a woman to believe? How can she participate intelligently with her physician in reaching decisions about these matters?

Substrate of cancer. To begin with, cancer is not a single disease and does not have a simple cause, in the sense that an infection is caused by a specific microbe. Nor is an infection all that simple. Besides the causative germ, other factors, such as tissue resistance, debility, route of entry into the body, and so on, are important. In the various forms of cancer, these "other" factors have an overwhelming role.

One such factor is especially relevant to the question of estrogen and cancer. This is the process of cell multiplication that normally occurs in any actively working lining tissue of the body. By "lining tissue," we mean the sheet of cells that covers internal or external surfaces, such as the skin, the gastrointestinal tract, the ducts of glands (for example, in the breasts), or the reproductive tract. Certain of these lining tissues, when they are actively working, continuously shed their surface cells. These must be replaced by cell multiplication from a deeper layer. The most striking examples of this activity are afforded by the linings of the intestine and uterus.

Medical science has long recognized that even potent cancer-producing chemicals would not affect such lining tissues unless they are actively working—that is, undergoing active cell multiplication. If we were to remove the ovaries from girls before puberty and never gave them estrogens, their uterine and breast duct lining cells would never become active, and we could virtually wipe out breast and uterine cancer (and incidentally, the human race) in a single generation. This is not because estrogens *cause* cancer, but because estrogens are nature's stimulant of lining tissues of the breast and uterus. Without this entirely normal stimulation, those tissues are quite resistant to the known or unknown cancer-causing agents a woman may be exposed to.

We believe that decisions about postmenopausal estrogen therapy should be made in this context. Prolonging estrogen exposure of the susceptible lining tissue past the menopause simply prolongs the exposure that has been a natural risk during premenopausal years. It is, naturally, a cumulative affair, just as the longer one drives an automobile, the greater the risk of accident.

If, for the sake of illustration, cancer of the uterus is caused by something like a virus that is dormant in the tissues and needs years of estrogen stimulation to have a chance to produce an actual cancer, then a woman who harbors that virus may well increase her risk somewhat by estrogen treatment. But a woman who does not have the virus incurs no risk at all by taking estrogen. Medical science now suspects such strange virus-like agents in many forms of cancer. But even if proved to be a cause, there is as yet no way of telling who harbors such viruses and who does not.

Despite recent reports of an increase in endometrial cancer, vital statistics data do not yet indicate an increase of such cancers identified at the time of death. Statistics of human biology are such a potpourri of innumerable known and unknown factors that it is hardly possible to evaluate recent endometrial cancer reports with any certainty. Among the factors that make evaluation difficult are the increasing age of the population, changing criteria of diagnosis, and the retrospective or backward-looking type of case study on which existing reports have been based.

Method of administration. Does the form of estrogen treatment make a difference? Probably. Continuous, uninterrupted estrogen administration seems clearly to be associated with some increase of breast and endometrial cancer. It may be that the unrelenting stimulation of *continuous* treatment is more responsible for cancer risk than the stimulation itself.

Thus, estrogens should be given in *cyclic* fashion—that is, interrupted and resumed as medical judgment indicates. It is probable that a progesterone compound (another ovarian hormone) should be administered several times a year to assist the uterine lining through its growth phase and to shed its products more completely. It is clear that hormonal medication should be monitored closely by both patient and physician.

The principal benefits of hormone administration are the control of hot flashes and the thinning of the lining of the genital tract. Good medicine demands that the lowest effective doses to accomplish these goals be used. With precautions of low doses, cyclic administration, and progesterone-induced shedding, the possibility of serious side effects is greatly minimized.

PROTECTIVE EXAMINATIONS

The art of medicine is such that we cannot cure all diseases or prevent all diseases even if we knew they were about to develop. But we can prevent some, and the chances of curing others are better if they are recognized early. This is the reason for periodic medical examinations.

Nevertheless, we sometimes think that the need for checkups has been oversold. Many women we don't reach at all, but campaigns for checkups have been so urgent as to produce in some part of the public a kind of cancer phobia, or at least a state of unmitigated apprehension, which is quite out of proportion to medical realities. Cancer is unquestionably a serious disease, but it is often controllable, and in any event, some cancers are far from the worst disorders seen by physicians.

Thus, routine periodic checkups should be directed at the total woman. Advice about such problems as blood pressure, weight, exercise, nutrition, and other factors less dramatic than cancer may be far more important to an average woman than the tests that check her for cancer. Very often she doesn't understand that.

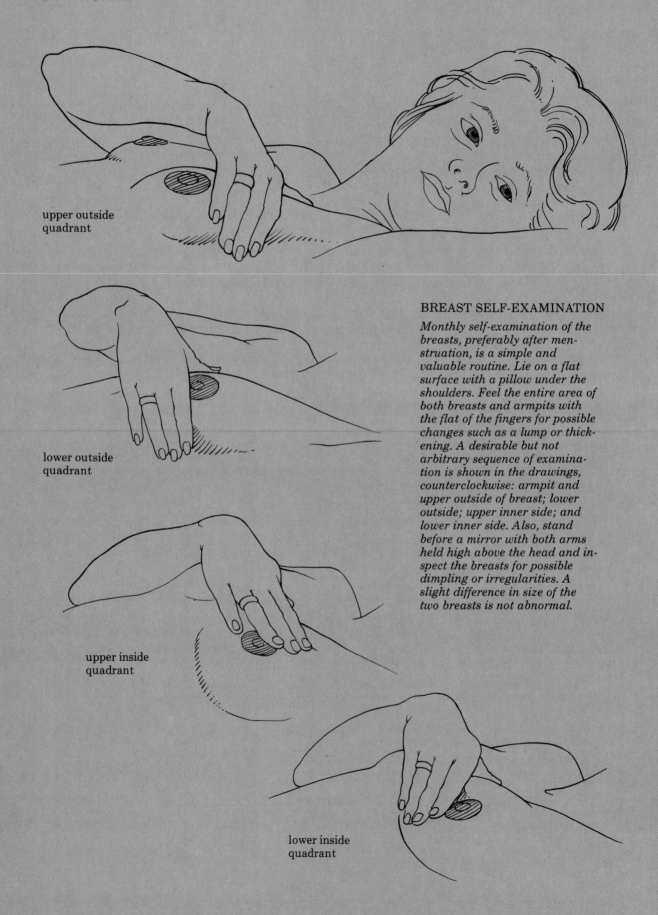

upper outside
quadrant

lower outside
quadrant

upper inside
quadrant

lower inside
quadrant

BREAST SELF-EXAMINATION

Monthly self-examination of the breasts, preferably after menstruation, is a simple and valuable routine. Lie on a flat surface with a pillow under the shoulders. Feel the entire area of both breasts and armpits with the flat of the fingers for possible changes such as a lump or thickening. A desirable but not arbitrary sequence of examination is shown in the drawings, counterclockwise: armpit and upper outside of breast; lower outside; upper inner side; and lower inner side. Also, stand before a mirror with both arms held high above the head and inspect the breasts for possible dimpling or irregularities. A slight difference in size of the two breasts is not abnormal.

What should be checked? In addition to such routine items as heart, lungs, blood pressure, nervous system functions, blood and urine tests, and many others, the physician will examine a woman's breasts for lumps, the genital area for evidences of estrogen deficiency, and the cervix, uterus, and ovaries for possible abnormalities. Prior to menopause, a woman who has no particular complaints need be checked only once every two to five years, or if she is receiving oral contraceptives, once every 12 months. After menopause, a complete checkup is recommended every year or every two years.

Although cancer danger signals may have been overplayed, it is indeed true that a woman should seek medical help for such unexplained findings as a lump in the breast or abnormal bleeding, particularly if the latter occurs after menopause. Breast self-examination is an excellent routine to learn. (In fact, the woman has a significant advantage over the examining physician, inasmuch as she can feel both with her fingers *and* her breast, whereas the physician can use only his fingers).

Other diagnostic tests such as *mammography,* a technique for X-raying breast tissues, may help to detect very early cancers in the breast. Mammography is ordinarily not recommended for symptomless women under age 35, in whom breast cancer is relatively rare, or for frequent routine use in older women. The reason is that some amount of radiation is added to amounts already accumulated in the body. No test is without risk, and the actual risk of cancer of the breast is low enough so that too-frequent exposure may impose a greater risk of damage from the test than the risk of the hunted-for disease. However, recent improvements of X-ray film for mammography reduce the amount of radiation to one-ninth of that previously necessary, and significantly reduce the risk of a valuable diagnostic technique, employed with discrimination.

Who should be examined? How often? And what should be done? There are no generally agreed-upon answers, but we can offer a few commonsense suggestions:

- Women with a history of cancer in the family, particularly in close female relatives and particularly if these cancers involve the breast or uterus, should be examined earlier and more often.
- Women who have never borne children tend to have a higher incidence of breast cancer than those who have given birth, and might profitably be examined more frequently and be diligent about breast self-examination.
- Cancer of the cervix is less frequent in women who have never had sexual intercourse and in women who have had only a single sexual partner, whereas it is more common in women with multiple partners. It would make good sense for the latter group to have vaginal examinations and Pap smears earlier and more often than virginal or single-partner women.
- Any woman who has abnormal bleeding, especially after menopause, or discovers a lump in the breast or bleeding from the nipple, should seek medical advice without delay.

GENITAL REPAIRS

Inconvenient or very distressing problems that occur after menopause are broadly categorized as "relaxation"—not recreational or restful, but a sagging, laxness, "letdown," and loss of firmness of structures that make up the floor of the pelvis, the great bowl that supports abdominal organs. In popular language, various conditions are often referred to as "fallen womb."

Contributing causes are lessened muscle tone with age, old tears and lacerations of childbirth, decreased estrogen levels, and the fact that standing, straining, and lifting put all the weight and pressure of abdominal organs upon the pelvic floor.

Symptoms

The different pelvic structures affected and the extent of relaxation produce a variety of symptoms and differences of mildness or severity. Sometimes we see a woman with marked relaxation who is essentially free of discomfort and unconcerned about doing anything about it. More often, symptoms gradually become sufficiently distressing or embarrassing that help is sought for what our grandmothers called "female troubles."

What are some of these troubles?

The uterus itself may sag or "drop" into the upper part of the vaginal canal or even protrude from it *(prolapse)*.

Relaxation of structures at the neck of the bladder may permit involuntary escape of urine. This is likely to occur when standing, or when coughing or sneezing. Urine out of control may cause only a slight moistening or a real soaking.

Relaxation of the pelvic floor around the vaginal or rectal openings may allow the rectum to bulge through the rear wall of the vagina, a partial hernia called a *rectocele*. If mild, the condition may not be very bothersome, but when severe, it may result in soiling or difficulties in defecation.

Weakened support of the bladder may permit its base to sag into the vaginal canal and bulge through its opening. This is called a *cystocele*.

Predominant symptoms are disturbances of urination or bowel movements.

Treatment

Whether or not a woman chooses to have active treatment for the conditions mentioned depends very much upon her own attitudes and the extent to which she feels that her life-style and feelings of well-being are unnecessarily clouded. In themselves, the conditions are not threatening to life—only to the style of life.

Temporizing measures may be quite satisfactory to some women. These consist of devices called *pessaries,* which give mechanical support to the uterus or walls of the vagina, or both. The rubber or plastic devices require careful fitting to individual needs and removal at frequent intervals, and, of course, the underlying condition is not corrected.

Surgery gives a permanent correction. The operations, though not minor, are well tolerated even by elderly women, and age itself is no deterrent unless there are other medical problems. Several types of surgical procedures are equally satisfactory.

A sagging bladder or rectum (cystocele or rectocele) may be corrected by shortening or tightening the supporting muscles. This can be done independently, but the usual preference is to combine it with removal of the nonfunctioning uterus by vaginal *hysterectomy*. The bladder is temporarily separated from the vaginal tissues and supporting tissues around the bladder and its neck, in much the same way that surgeons repair an abdominal hernia. Repair of a rectocele is similarly accomplished by temporarily separating the vaginal tissue from the rectum and reducing the bulk of the tissue. The operations require a hospital stay of a week to ten days, followed by rest at home.

Entirely adequate sexual function occurs following these procedures, which could be called "genital rehabilitation." Patients generally feel much better after the abolishment of distresses, which at best were bothersome, and at worst disabling.

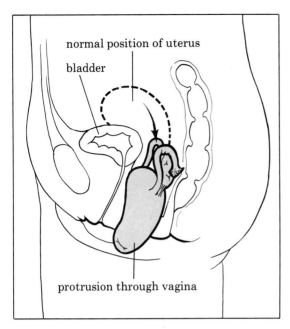

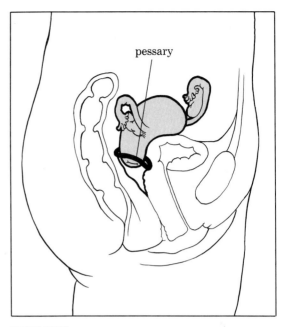

PROLAPSE

"Fallen womb" is a common term for prolapse of the uterus. Weakening or relaxation of structures that support the uterus, often aggravated by stresses such as lifting and gravity, permit the womb to sag into the vault of the vagina. In extreme cases, the neck of the uterus may protrude from the vagina.

PESSARY

A prolapsing or a retroverted uterus (one that is tipped backward from its normal position) may be given mechanical support by a pessary placed in the vagina. Variously shaped pessaries of rubber or plastic do not correct the underlying condition but may serve satisfactorily. Surgical repair is usually permanent.

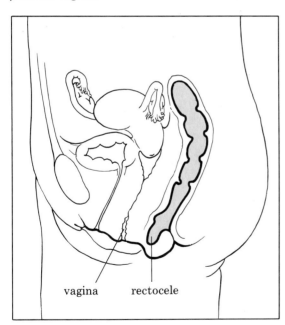

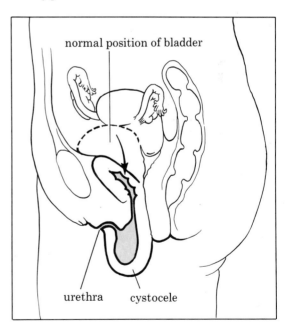

RECTOCELE

If supporting tissues of the lower bowel become weakened, the rectum may bulge (partially herniate) through the rear wall of the vagina. This is called a rectocele. Slight herniation may not be very troublesome, but if it is severe enough, the predominant symptoms are soiling and difficulties in bowel movements.

CYSTOCELE

The base of the bladder may sag into the vaginal canal and bulge into its opening if supporting tissues become weakened. This is called a cystocele. As the condition progresses, there may be frequency of urination and involuntary passage of urine. There is some increased risk of bladder infection (cystitis).

HYSTERECTOMY

Hysterectomy—surgical removal of the uterus—is an emotion-laden topic among the public and within the medical profession. On the one hand, many women believe, and perpetuate through bridge-table conversation, the idea that hysterectomy is a very risky operation with many irreversible consequences and prolonged side effects (not true, especially after the menopause). On the other hand, hysterectomy is charged with being the most frequent of "unnecessary" operations, profitably foisted upon women by surgeons who love to sacrifice female organs.

Perhaps some light can be shed by trying to define some terms. A great many elective operations, done at a convenient time, do not involve life-threatening emergencies; they are performed in expectation of easing pain or discomfort, minimizing handicaps, correcting deformities, improving appearance, and establishing functional efficiency with a bit of reinvigoration of joy in life. Such operations are unnecessary in the sense that patients could get along in some fashion without them. Many persons refuse surgery for varicose veins, hemorrhoids, a sagging uterus, a deviated septum, a trussed-up hernia, or other chronic nuisances. They endure with fortitude and come to no bad end, barring complications. All that is forgone is the relief that "unnecessary" surgery might well provide.

So with hysterectomy. Removal of a cancerous uterus is unquestionably necessary, and accounts for about 15 percent of hysterectomies. But let's examine other situations in which a physician might recommend or discuss the pros and cons of hysterectomy.

Indications

Hysterectomy is a major operation. The risk in modern surgery is small, but all surgery entails some risk.

Fibroid tumors are a frequent indication for hysterectomy. These are growths of muscle and connective tissue in the muscular wall of the uterus. A middle-aged woman has at least a 50 percent chance of having "fibroids," which quite possibly have caused no symptoms and are discovered on routine physical examination. The tumors may be as small as a pea or unbelievably large, although huge sizes are very rare today because of timely intervention.

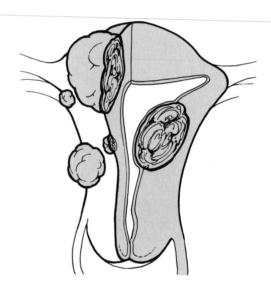

FIBROIDS

Fibroid tumors are noncancerous growths of muscle and connective tissue in the wall of the uterus, characteristic of middle life. Fibroids may be present for years without causing distress but may cause various symptoms if they become large enough to press on nearby structures. Symptomless fibroids in women near the menopause may be left alone and watched since the tumors tend to regress after the change of life. In postmenopausal women, if surgery is indicated, the entire fibroid-containing uterus usually is removed.

Fibroid tumors are rarely cancerous, but they exist in a susceptible environment. In a young woman, fibroids can be removed without removing the uterus if she wishes to preserve the childbearing function. If the tumors were present before menopause, they tend to get smaller afterward. Fibroids may be large enough to cause sensations of pain or pressure in the abdomen, or be associated with abnormal bleeding. If the tumors enlarge after menopause and if bleeding occurs, the uterus will be gently scraped (D & C) to obtain tissues for analysis. With such information, hysterectomy may be recommended.

Relaxation. We have previously discussed pelvic relaxations: slippage of the uterus, cystocele, rectocele, escape of urine, and abnormal bleeding. The desirability of hysterectomy depends on the severity of discomfort or on the severity and frequency of abnormal bleeding. If the only justification for removing an organ is that it is a real and present threat, many hysterectomies are unnecessary in the strictest sense. What the operation offers, when appropriate, is improvement of the quality of life.

In considering hysterectomy, one should ask what the alternatives are and consider that symptoms will never get better by themselves.

Backache is not an indication for hysterectomy. An operation solely for that purpose is unlikely to give expected benefits and is hardly necessary.

The Operation

In the past, hysterectomy was often done by removing the top part of the uterus and leaving its neck or cervix in place, still susceptible to cervical problems. Today, hysterectomy is almost always "total" or "complete"—that is, the body of the uterus and its attached cervix are removed together. Very rarely, the cervix may be allowed to remain if it has suffered disorders, such as endometriosis with dense adhesions, or infections.

What about the ovaries? Unless there is something the matter with them, the ovaries are not removed in women under 40. Their ovaries are still producing hormones and contribute to general well-being. Also, if the ovaries are removed, it is more difficult to get satisfactory effects from hormone replacements than in older women.

If the patient is approaching or past the menopause, ovary removal is usually advised. The ovaries have virtually ceased to function, or soon will, and will not really be missed. There may or may not be a need for temporary hormone replacements, depending on age and other factors. A woman should discuss such matters with her physician and, with full understanding, agree to procedures before surgery.

Cancer of the ovary is difficult to diagnose, and too often is well advanced at the time of discovery. Removal of the ovaries eliminates the possibility of this form of cancer, just as hysterectomy eliminates the possibility of future cancer of the uterus. After hysterectomy, there will be no more menstrual periods or further need for routine Pap smears. All of these are plus benefits of surgery undertaken for more urgent reasons.

The actual operation is performed through one of the two routes, the abdomen or the vagina.

Abdominal hysterectomy is performed by cutting through the abdominal wall and removing the uterus. This route is usually taken if the uterus is very large or distorted by tumors, or in exploration for cancer.

The incision may be vertical if wide exposure is necessary for the surgeon to see what he is doing. Otherwise, and more commonly, the incision is made crosswise along the top of the pubic hair line. Its scar is generally invisible beneath the Plimsoll line of a reasonably discreet bikini.

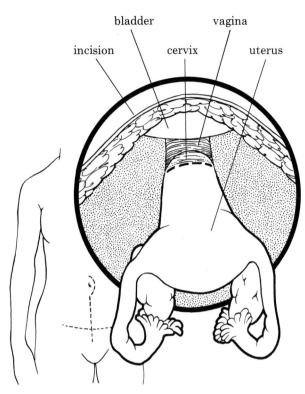

bladder   vagina

incision   cervix   uterus

ABDOMINAL HYSTERECTOMY

If the uterus is quite large, adheres to other organs, is distorted by fibroids, or indicates suspicion of cancer, removal through incisions in the abdomen, as shown, is usually preferred. This method allows the surgeon ample room to work in. In older women, the tubes and ovaries usually are removed along with the uterus.

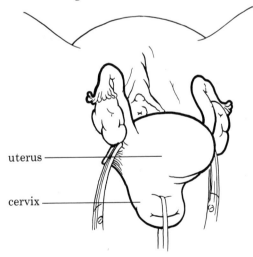

uterus ——

cervix ——

VAGINAL HYSTERECTOMY

The incision for vaginal hysterectomy is made deep in the vagina and does not leave a scar visible on the outside. There is minimal handling of other organs, and postsurgical gas pains are not so annoying. Stretched and sagging tissues that support the vagina, rectum, and bladder are accessible to direct repair.

Vaginal hysterectomy is performed through an incision deep in the vagina. It leaves no external scar. The vaginal route is well suited to conditions frequent in women past childbearing age: hysterectomy because of excessive bleeding not due to cancer, and hysterectomy with repair of sagging supports of bladder, rectum, and vagina. The vaginal technique allows somewhat less manipulation of organs that have to be moved out of the way, and the postoperative days are likely to go more smoothly.

Hysterectomy by either route is normally done under general anesthesia. The hospital stay is around ten days, toward the end of which the external clips or sutures are removed.

After the operation. Hysterectomy *per se* should not cause any serious side effects. It does not cause superfluous hair to grow or change a woman as a person. If weight is subsequently gained, it has a caloric rather than a missing-organ origin. Sexual intercourse can be resumed in a month to six weeks, and is probably beneficial to suppleness of vaginal tissues. Indeed, sexual pleasure is often enhanced by restoration of youthful tone to vaginal structures.

Whether or not a woman will feel seriously depressed after hysterectomy is unpredictable, unless on a premise that emotional stability before hysterectomy augurs for emotional stability afterward. A normal reaction to removal of a gallbladder, appendix, or other organ that has behaved unkindly is "good riddance!"

Justified hysterectomy in a postmenopausal woman involves an organ that has gone out of business, serves no function—one hesitates to say "useless," but the word is apt—and contributes not a whit to femininity. Happily, most patients understand that after full recovery, if not before.

CANCER

To come to middle life is to arrive at an age when cancer is an increasing statistical threat. Cancer is the leading cause of death of women between the ages of 30 and 54, and the second most common cause from ages 55 to 74. The most common site, however, is not sex-biased but is shared with men. It is the gastrointestinal tract, which accounts for about 30 percent of cancer deaths in this age group.

We have previously noted that lining cells of the gastrointestinal tract continuously and rapidly replace themselves throughout life. This is also true of lining cells of the breast and uterus. It is the "female cancers" of the latter organs that this chapter will discuss.

Uterus

Cancer of the endometrium (the lining tissue of the uterus) is diagnosed with increasing frequency today. In all probability, this increase reflects general aging of the population—more women live to susceptible age—as well as earlier application of diagnostic tests to patients who have suspicious symptoms.

The most significant symptom is abnormal bleeding. If vaginal bleeding occurs a year or more after cessation of menstruation, a malignant cause should be presumed until excluded. The pattern of normal bleeding before menopause is important; frequency, duration, and amount should all diminish. If there is an increase in frequency or if bleeding lasts longer or is heavier, evaluation of the uterine lining by curettage (D & C) is essential. Ordinarily this is done in a hospital, but a technique of curettage in the physician's office is gaining favor and appears to be satisfactory in the hands of experienced physicians.

The Pap smear is of little value in detecting cancer of the endometrium. *Endometrial biopsy,* an office procedure by which a sample of tissue is taken directly from the lining of the uterus, is the most effective screening technique in a patient without symptoms. This can usually be done at the time of routine examination without appreciable discomfort. In the hands of many physicians, it is a very effective and accurate diagnostic technique.

Cancer of the cervix, the neck of the uterus, is declining as a cause of death. Much of the credit can be given to routine Pap smear tests, which detect early symptomless cancer of the cervix with great reliability. Unknown numbers of women have not died from carcinoma of the cervix because malignancy was discovered in early stages when it is readily curable.

Availability of tests unfortunately does not mean that all women avail themselves of them. The years around menopause are a time when many disorders, not only cancer, become statistically more likely to affect women. But the need for medical attention and alertness to symptoms is not so urgent as in younger years when matters of conception, pregnancy, childbirth, and supervision of family health required regular visits to a physician. Some older women tend to avoid checkups as postponable nuisances, at the very time when early discovery of some correctable condition could give them comfort and peace of mind.

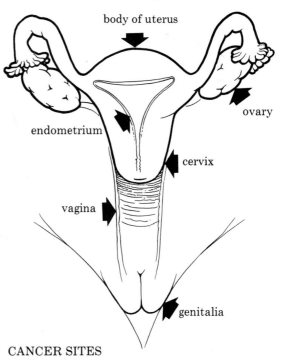

CANCER SITES

Of the sites of malignant tumors of the female genital tract, shown in the drawing, cancers of the body and lining of the uterus and its cervix are most frequent. Checkups are important as one grows older.

Breast

Breast cancer is almost nonexistent in women under 35 years of age—only two cases per 100,000 population. The odds are much worse in the 40s and 50s, the perimenopausal years. No woman is immune, but some seem more liable to breast cancer than others. Factors that appear to increase the risk are: not giving birth before age 25, family history of breast cancer (sister, mother, grandmother, or maternal aunt), and presence of a disorder called cystic fibrosis, which consists of cyst-like dilations of duct tissue in a dense fibrous surrounding. Women in the high-risk category probably should be screened annually from age 35 on. The desirability of mammography (see page 449) for younger women is questioned because of some irradiation risk, but a fair consensus is that the technique, which sometimes detects very small and highly curable cancers before they are discoverable by touch, is justified and useful after age 50.

Self-examination of the breasts (see page 448) is a first line of defense. Most lumps in the breast are discovered by women themselves, though some can only be detected by a physician. Most lumps in the breast are harmless, but some are not. If a suspicious lump is found to be cancerous by a pathologist, surgery is recommended.

There is considerable controversy, some of it among surgeons but a great deal among laymen, about "simple" vs. "radical" mastectomy. In simple mastectomy, the breast alone is removed. In radical mastectomy, muscles of the chest and adjacent lymph nodes are removed as well. The heart of the matter is not the degree of disfigurement but cure of the disease.

In the most grave situation—advanced disease with lymph node involvement—radical mastectomy apparently does not achieve a better rate of cure than simple mastectomy with radiation therapy. Of course, the more advanced the disease, the less the prospects of permanent cure. In very early breast cancer, small and apparently localized, simple mastectomy may be all that is required. Complex factors are involved—speed of invasion, degree of malignancy, and others—however, objective answers to "simple-radical" controversies may come from ongoing evaluations of alternative methods of breast cancer treatment.

Breast cancer surgery. If your physician detects a mass in the breast and determines that it should be excised, as most would do, you are admitted to the hospital for this procedure. In most instances, the mass is removed through a small incision; while you are under anesthesia, the tissue is examined by the pathologist, using a technique of freezing and studying microscopic sections. If the lesion is benign, no additional surgery is performed. If it is malignant, the surgeon usually will proceed with the appropriate operative procedure, which may be radical or modified radical mastectomy.

In these operations, the entire breast and varying amounts of the underlying and adjacent supporting structures and the lymph nodes associated with the breast will be removed. The usual duration of this surgery is between one and two hours, and the convalesence is generally quite prompt. It is important that the patient maintain ability to move her arms, and physical therapy to keep the shoulder joint supple and the arm strong is often of value. Soon after healing, a suitable garment providing a breast prosthesis is used, and the individual resumes an active life. Most women who have this type of surgery leave the hospital somewhere between the fourth and seventh postoperative day.

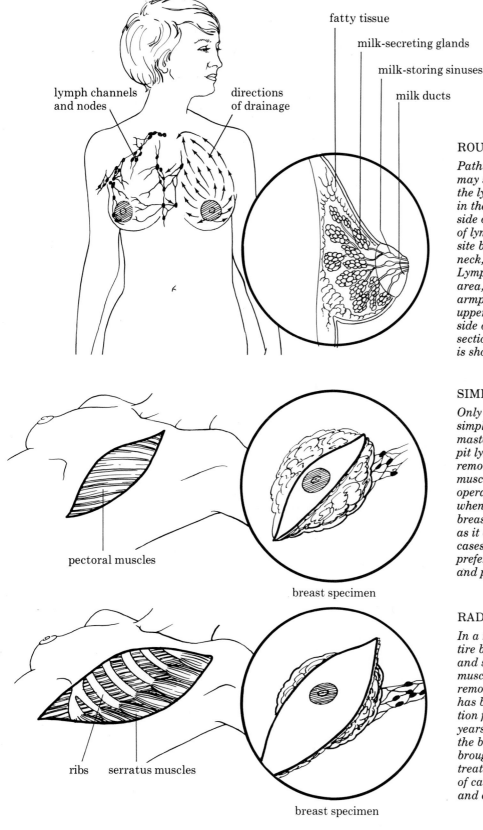

fatty tissue

milk-secreting glands

milk-storing sinuses

milk ducts

lymph channels
and nodes

directions
of drainage

pectoral muscles

breast specimen

ribs   serratus muscles

breast specimen

ROUTES OF SPREAD

Pathways by which cancer cells may spread from the breast in the lymph (and blood) are shown in the drawing. Arrows (right side of drawing) show directions of lymph drainage to the opposite breast, chest, lungs, armpit, neck, and general circulation. Lymph channels of the breast area, with lymph nodes in the armpit, neck, and inner and upper chest, are shown in the left side of the drawing. A cross section of a normal adult breast is shown in the circle.

SIMPLE MASTECTOMY

Only the breast is removed in a simple mastectomy. In a total mastectomy, the breast and armpit lymph nodes also are removed but underlying chest muscles are preserved. The latter operation is increasingly used when tumors are small and breast cancer is discovered early, as it often is nowadays. In such cases, total mastectomy may be preferred by both surgeon and patient.

RADICAL MASTECTOMY

In a radical mastectomy, the entire breast, armpit lymph nodes, and sections of arm and chest muscles beneath the breast are removed. Radical mastectomy has been the "standard" operation for breast cancer for many years, but new knowledge about the biology of the disease has brought reconsiderations of treatment according to the type of cancer, its size and location, and evidence of spread.

OSTEOPOROSIS

Osteoporosis is an affliction that unfairly attacks older women; men are not entirely immune, but are not very prone to it. The condition is so common in women after middle life that it is often called "postmenopausal osteoporosis." One out of four white women in the United States will develop osteoporosis and suffer bone fractures between the menopause and age 70. By far the most common form of osteoporosis occurs in postmenopausal women as a primary disorder, apparently not associated with any other disease.

Osteoporosis is to the skeleton what anemia is to the blood—incapacity to sustain normal functions. Bones become thinner, weaker, and more fragile, and while perfectly normal in quality, they just aren't substantial enough to resist stresses that normal bones take in stride. So they break very easily.

Symptoms

There are no symptoms—until a fracture occurs. Then the symptoms are due solely to the fracture and the disability it causes.

Sometimes the fractures may be so minor, and the damage they produce may accumulate so slowly, that the woman may be unaware of actual fracture. Such cumulative small fractures are responsible for the "dowager's hump" and the loss of height that often occurs. An osteoporotic woman can easily shrink two or three inches in stature as she ages, and shrinkage of as much as eight inches is not unknown. The changes mentioned are primarily due to collapses of the spine, which osteoporosis principally involves, although all the bones of the body are affected.

Fractures occur without warning, on exertion of moderate physical effort or none at all. Bones may break from little more stress than rolling over in bed or picking an object off the floor in advanced cases.

Who is susceptible? Large, heavy, obese women are relatively free from serious osteoporosis. Those most at risk seem to be women who, in their prime, were small-boned, fine-featured, highly feminine, light-skinned, often of Celtic or North European background, and women whose mothers, maternal aunts, or grandmothers developed osteoporotic fractures.

Women with dark skin or of Southern European extraction seem to be somewhat protected. The disorder is quite rare in American black women. Heavy physical work throughout life also seems to confer protection, probably because the skeleton is "exercised" and becomes heavier in persons who do hard work. Nutrition also may be a factor, but specifics are elusive.

Causes

The cause of postmenopausal osteoporosis is unknown. It is not even certain that it is a disease. It may be a normal part of the aging process, since some bone loss does occur with aging. However, it is hardly normal for bones to break from ordinary daily activities.

Bones are perpetually remodeling themselves and moving structural materials in and out. After growth is complete in the late teens, there is a great deal of remodeling to be done, both to keep the bony substance fresh and strong and to modify its shape and adapt it to changing uses of our limbs as we age.

The amount of bony material in our skeletons actually increases in both men and women until about age 35 to 40. Thereafter it begins to decrease in both sexes because, as bone is remodeled, more old bone substance is removed than is replaced by new material. In postmenopausal women, this imbalance becomes exaggerated and the amount of bone substance decreases much more rapidly than in men. Why this difference? There are many speculations but precious little hard evidence. A plausible suspicion is that decreased estrogen production has something to do with it.

Where Fractures Occur

Although all the bones of the body are affected by osteoporosis, there are certain favored locations of breaks. Often the first manifestation of bone loss is fracture of the wrist-end of one of the forearm bones. There is a sharp increase of such fractures in women after the menopause. The breaks are usually sustained in a fall, as in slipping on an icy sidewalk. Usually these fractures heal well and leave no disability.

Spine. Another major site of fractures is the spine. These are more serious, possibly causing permanent disability, and begin to appear in women in their late 50s and early 60s. A fracture may result from a jolt in a car on a rough road, or from stepping off a high curb. Most often the precipitating incident is physical effort exerted with the body bent forward, as in tugging to open a stuck window, lifting a heavy pan out of an oven, or hoisting a corner of a mattress in making a bed.

What happens is that, as the body is bent forward, the front edge of a vertebra (or more than one) is squeezed beyond its strength and partially collapses. Hence these are called "compression fractures." The fractured bone pieces do not separate. On the contrary, the bone is squashed together and telescopes into itself. For this reason, casts are not used in treatment.

The instant symptom of compression fracture is excruciating pain and severe backache. Acute pain gradually eases as healing occurs, but the shape of the spine has been somewhat altered and change in the shape of affected vertebrae is permanent. As repeated fractures occur in several vertebrae, the spine becomes permanently bent forward and a prominent hump may appear in the middle or upper back. An accumulation of many such fractures is the main reason for the stooped, shortened stature of many older persons.

Compression fractures tend to nag at a woman by way of persistent *chronic backache.* This can be a significant disability in an otherwise vigorous and healthy 60-year-old woman.

Hip. The most serious osteoporotic fracture is that of the hip, but fortunately, it is less common than spinal fractures. What usually breaks is the rounded upper end of the thigh bone where it angles in to fit into the hip socket.

Broken hips most frequently occur fairly late in life, commonly after age 70, and almost always in women who have previously sustained other osteoporotic fractures. Hip fracture usually occurs as a result of a minor fall and indicates quite severe bone loss.

BONE LOSS

Frequently, an early sign of bone loss (osteoporosis) in older women is fracture of a forearm bone at the wrist, shown in the drawing. The break usually occurs when the hand is outthrust to cushion a fall. Limb fractures treated in conventional ways usually heal normally. The ongoing process of osteoporosis is painless and causes no symptoms until a break occurs.

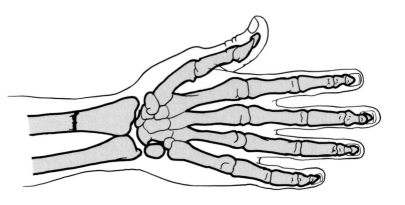

DOWAGER'S HUMP

A major site of osteoporotic fracture is the spine. A slight jolt or lifting effort in a bent-forward position may cause the front edge of a weakened vertebra to collapse into itself, as shown in the drawing. This changes the shape of the spine. A major fracture causes excruciating pain, but repeated small fractures of vertebrae may be so minor that the woman is not aware of them. Ultimately, the spine is bent forward permanently and a prominent hump ("dowager's hump") may appear in the upper or middle back. Shrinkage in height of an inch or two or even more occurs as the front of the spine is squeezed into itself by numerous compression fractures.

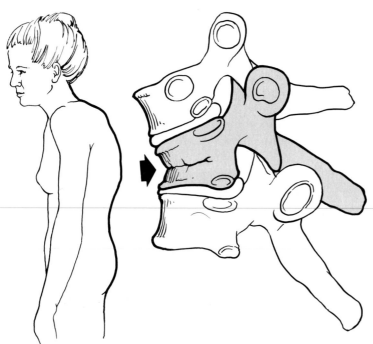

BROKEN HIP

The most disabling osteoporotic fracture involves the hip. Usually what breaks is the upper part of the thigh bone where it fits into the socket, as shown in the drawing. Broken hips commonly occur late in life in women who have suffered previous osteoporotic fractures. Most broken hips require surgery, which may employ nails to secure parts. Or, an artificial hip joint may be held in place by a special bone cement.

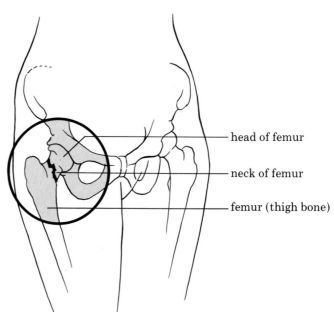

head of femur

neck of femur

femur (thigh bone)

Treatment

No known treatment will put more bony material back into the skeleton after it has become osteoporotic. Nor can compressed vertebrae of the spine be expanded back to normal shape once they have collapsed.

However, various forms of treatment are commonly tried after osteoporotic fractures have occurred. These include estrogens, calcium supplements, anabolic ("upbuilding") steroid hormones, and even male hormones, alone or in combinations. They may well help the patient to feel better, and may possibly prevent further bone loss, but they almost certainly do not restore the quantity of bone to normal. A number of experimental treatments are being evaluated, such as fluorides alone or in combination with high calcium intake, but it is too early to tell whether they can actually reverse the disorder.

Limb fractures are treated in conventional ways with casts and slings, and usually heal quite normally.

Spine fractures usually require bed rest and pain relievers for several days. After severe initial pain has subsided, the patient should receive physical therapy and a bit of retraining in activities of daily living.

Physical therapy is directed toward alleviating the painful muscle spasm and strengthening the muscles of the back, which straighten the spine. Most osteoporotic women have let these muscles become weak and flabby (if they ever developed them at all). When they can learn to build up these muscles, they improve their posture and lessen the chronic back pain, which is a major disability. Sometimes a firm foundation garment helps to provide support for a painful back.

Retraining in daily living activities is directed toward avoiding situations that may further compress the vertebrae. Specifically, the woman must learn *not to bend forward at the waist*. When she must pick something off the floor or from a low shelf, she should bend at the knees, keeping the back straight. Numerous simple devices that make bending unnecessary are available. There are long-handled shoe horns and long-handled scissorlike tongs that allow one to stand upright and pick up an item from the floor.

It is also important to avoid sudden jolts to the spine, such as occur when sitting down suddenly on a hard bench or riding in a car on a bumpy road.

Hip fractures usually require surgery, though some may heal simply with bed rest. Usually a special nail is inserted to fix the head of the thigh bone to the shaft where the two broke apart. In certain cases, an artificial hip joint may be inserted (see page 248). This route would likely be chosen if damage to the head and neck of the thigh bone is so serious, or the bone so weak, that satisfactory healing with a nail is improbable.

While recognizing that there is no guaranteed or certain form of protection against osteoporosis, it nevertheless seems reasonable that women at risk be given the benefit of estrogen treatment or high calcium intake or both. Calcium intake should be at least 1.5 grams a day. This amount is provided by ordinary good diet plus a full quart of whole or skim milk daily, or its equivalent in other dairy products except cottage cheese, which is low in calcium.

Estrogen treatment would appear to be most indicated in women who show signs of severe estrogen deficiency, such as genital atrophy. The dose required for osteoporotic protection is not established, but since it's not entirely certain that estrogen can really prevent bone loss, small doses seem best. Estrogen therapy must of course be prescribed and managed by a physician, but a woman can adjust her diet herself.

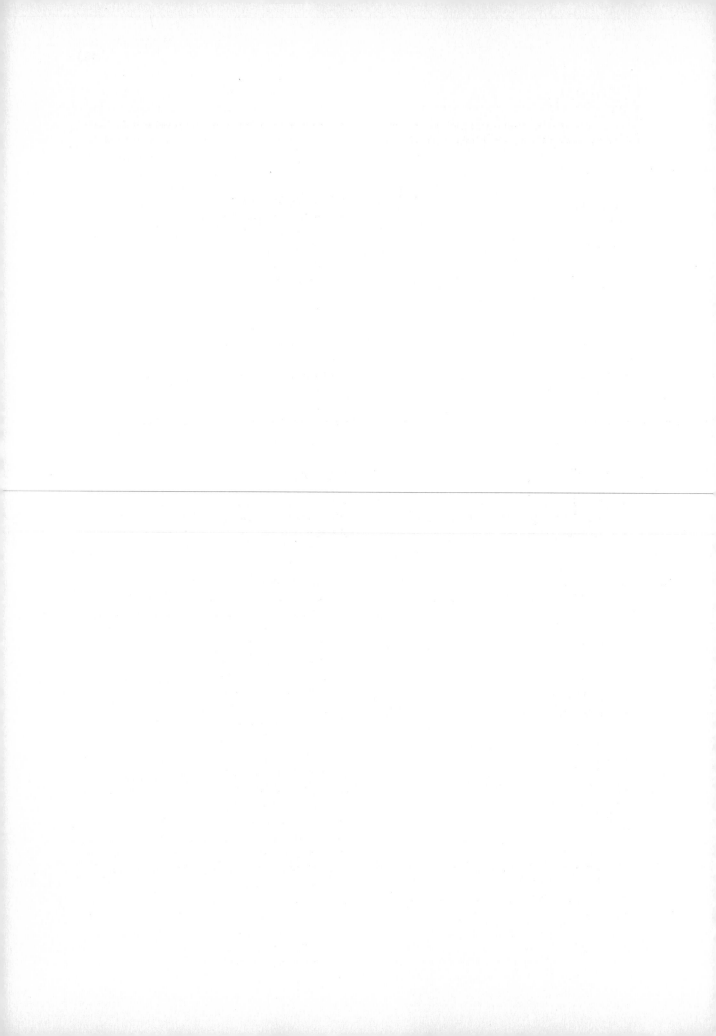

INDEX

Boldface references indicate illustrated text.

I

J

K